Advancements in the Diagnostics and Therapeutics for Non-Small Cell Lung Carcinoma (NSCLC)

Pallavi Singh
https://orcid.org/0000-0003-4537-4607
Graphic Era University, India

Shiva Prasad Kollur
https://orcid.org/0000-0003-3914-3933
Amrita Vishwa Vidyapeetham, India

Raghavendra G. Amachawadi
https://orcid.org/0000-0001-9689-1124
Kansas State University, USA

IGI Global
Scientific Publishing
Publishing Tomorrow's Research Today

Vice President of Editorial	Melissa Wagner
Director of Acquisitions	Mikaela Felty
Director of Book Development	Jocelynn Hessler
Production Manager	Mike Brehm
Cover Design	Jose Rosado

Published in the United States of America by
IGI Global Scientific Publishing
701 East Chocolate Avenue
Hershey, PA, 17033, USA
Tel: 717-533-8845 | Fax: 717-533-7115
Website: https://www.igi-global.com E-mail: cust@igi-global.com

Library of Congress Cataloging-in-Publication Data

Names: Singh, Pallavi, 1983- editor | Prasad Kollur, Shiva editor | Amachawadi, Raghavendra editor
Title: Advancements in the diagnostics and therapeutics for non-small cell lung carcinoma (NSCLC) / edited by Pallavi Singh, Shiva Prasad Kollur, Raghavendra G Amachawadi.
Description: Hershey, PA : IGI Global Scientific Publishing, [2026] | Includes bibliographical references and index. | Summary: "This book aims to provide crucial insights on future Directions in NSCLC Treatment and Research and a forward-looking perspective on ongoing clinical trials, new drug development, and emerging treatment paradigms"-- Provided by publisher.
Identifiers: LCCN 2025021032 (print) | LCCN 2025021033 (ebook) | ISBN 9798337320960 hardcover | ISBN 9798337320977 paperback | ISBN 9798337320984 ebook
Subjects: LCSH: Lungs--Cancer--Diagnosis | Lungs--Cancer--Diagnosis--Technological innovations | Lungs--Cancer--Treatment | Lungs--Cancer--Treatment--Technological innovations
Classification: LCC RC280.L8 A36 2026 (print) | LCC RC280.L8 (ebook)
LC record available at https://lccn.loc.gov/2025021032
LC ebook record available at https://lccn.loc.gov/2025021033

British Cataloguing in Publication Data
A Cataloguing in Publication record for this book is available from the British Library.

Table of Contents

Detailed Table of Contents

Amongst various cancers, lung cancer is the most aggressive cancer type indiscriminative of the gender. According to the International Agency for Research on Cancer (IARC) in GLOBOCAN 2022, around 2.5 million new lung cancer cases were detected and 1.8 million deaths occurred. Lung cancer is classified into two types: small-cell carcinomas, and non-small cell carcinomas. NSCLC is the most common type contributing to up to 85% of lung cancers. Lung cancer cells have alterations in the mechanisms governing proliferation of normal cells and commonly observed genetic alterations in NSCLC include KRAS, EGFR, HER2, MEK, BRAF, and PI3K. Smoking is the main risk factor for lung cancer and is more common in men than in women. Chemotherapy, radiation therapy, and surgical resection are commonly used therapies for NSCLC but due to their few limitations, discovery of newer targets and anticancer drugs with improved bioavailability and lower systemic toxicity is required for NSCLC treatment.

Non-small cell lung cancer (NSCLC) represents the greatest prevalent sort of lung cancer. NSCLC constitutes nearly eighty percent of the overall incidence of lung cancer. Squamous cell carcinoma (SCC), adenocarcinoma (ADC), and large-cell carcinoma (LCC) are among the three predominant classifications of NSCLC. NSCLC is primarily triggered by anomalies in the epithelial growth factor receptors

(EGFR). The genes that encourage malignancy and are affiliated with several kinds of pathways include EGFR, BRAF, KRAS, MET, ALK, and ROS. The primary risk factor of NSCLC is mutations in these genes. The most effective therapy for NSCLC is based on histological outcomes; nevertheless, its progress, predisposition to metastases, and possible treatment are not well recognized. Recently, there has been a considerable increase in the use of targeted medications with low toxicity and high potency for cancer treatment due to mutations in receptor tyrosine kinases such as the EGFR, ALK, MET, and BRAF genes. This chapter explore the several gene mutations, associated pathways and targeted therapies via epigenetic modification, miRNA mutation, copy number alterations in molecular subtypes of NSCLC.

Non-small cell lung cancer makes up approximately 85% of all lung cancer diagnoses, around the globe. Despite advancements in therapeutic interventions, accurate prognosis for advanced-stage NSCLC is unsatisfactory and consequently, the 5-year survival rate in cases of metastasis is worrisome, amounting to less than 10%. This book chapter, aimed at providing a detailed review of the tumour microenvironment in NSCLC, highlights the contributions of stromal cells, immune infiltrates, metabolic reprogramming, and extracellular matrix remodelling. The authors explore the possible immunosuppressive mechanisms exploited by the tumors, including immune checkpoint activation, regulatory T-cell expansion, myeloid-derived suppressor cells, and dysfunctional antigen presentation. Furthermore, current trends in immunotherapeutic strategies have been examined and challenges including resistance and the pressing need to develop effective combination regimens has also been addressed.

Non-small cell lung cancer (NSCLC) remains a significant health challenge despite therapy advances. The lung and gut microbiome are crucial in NSCLC development and treatment response. This chapter reviews microbe integration in NSCLC management, focusing on: (1) identifying lung and gut microbes linked to NSCLC; (2) developing microbiome-based diagnostics using liquid biopsy and AI; (3) exploring microbiome-targeted therapies like fecal transplants to improve treatment; and (4) addressing clinical challenges of implementation. Microbial imbalances contribute to NSCLC through inflammation and immune changes via the gut-lung axis. Unique microbial profiles could serve as biomarkers for detecting and predicting NSCLC outcomes. AI helps link microbial data with clinical information for predictive models. Microbiome-targeted strategies aim to improve therapy outcomes but face challenges in proving causality, standardization, and regulation. Research collaboration is needed to utilize the microbiome for personalized NSCLC care.

K. Gayathri, Department of Microbiology, Sacred Heart College, Tirupattur, India
Pallavi Singh, Graphic Era University, India
M. Manigandan, Department of Microbiology, Sacred Heart College, Tirupattur, India
B. Lokeshwari, Department of Microbiology, Sacred Heart College, Tirupattur, India
P. Saranraj, Department of Microbiology, Sacred Heart College, Tirupattur, India

Non-small cell lung cancer (NSCLC) is the most common type of lung cancer and accounts for about 85% of all lung cancers, and it is still a significant cause of cancer death globally. It is intimately related to environmental, genetic, and chemical exposures as well as smoking. While recent development in liquid biopsy allows for classification utilising biological fluids like blood and saliva, TNM (Tumour, Node, Metastasis) staging system plays a crucial part in prognosis and treatment. Each with unique pathological traits, the disorder consists in adenocarcinoma, squamous cell carcinoma, and big cell carcinoma. Non-invasive, quick, highly specific detection is provided by methods like biosensor technology and biomarker analysis. Imaging techniques including early discovery utilising Computed Tomography (CT), Histological validation with Biopsy, Bronchoscopy to visualise and Cytology to examine the cells define diagnostic approaches for NSCLC. Recent developments in liquid biopsy let one classify utilising biological fluids such as saliva and blood. Early detection and focused treatment may be made easier by Biomarkers including Proteins linked with NSCLC and circulating tumour DNA (ctDNA). Using Nanotechnology and Electrochemical sensing, biosensors let one detect cancer-associated molecules in real time with great accuracy. Artificial intelligence (AI) will be included into future NSCLC detection to provide better image analysis of multi-analyte biomarkers as well as diagnoses. Discovery of genes and proteins is probably going to keep improving therapeutic targeting and diagnostic accuracy. Combining new technology has great power to improve early detection, patient survival in NSCLC. Along with new detection strategies, the present chapter covers epidemiology, categorisation, and diagnosis of NSCLC.

There is rising interest in CAR-T therapy as a potential treatment of non-small cell lung cancer (NSCLC) that comprises about 85% of all lung cancer and has a high mortality rate. This is a new technology whereby T cells are engineered to attack certain tumor-specific antigens. However, it tends to be undermined by other factors (i.e., the immunosuppressive tumor microenvironment and antigen heterogeneity). More recent data have found epidermal growth factor receptor (EGFR) and mesothelin as future targets of CAR-T therapy. The development of cars such as dual-targeting CAR improves the efficiency of treatment. However, there also exist some challenges such as safety concerns such as cytokine release syndrome (CRS). To overcome immunosuppressive barriers, CAR-T/immune checkpoint combination therapy can be used as an added advantage. Further research on new CAR-T regimens and trials is needed to improve patient treatment outcomes and survival in patients with NSCLC, a complex and advanced disease.

Lung cancer is a life threatening disease, particularly when it comes to non-small-cell lung cancer (NSCLC), and tends to have an unfortunate outlook for patients who are diagnosed with it. With surgeries and therapies such as chemotherapy, radiotherapy, targeted therapy, and immunotherapy, coupled with an enhanced grasp of genetic and molecular markers, treatment approaches can now be tailored to individuals. This chapter highlights case studies with illustrations and clinical scenarios in non-small cell lung cancer, including instances of long-term survival, disease modification, and treatment response, in an attempt to underscore the challenges in managing non-small cell lung cancer (NSCLC) and to point to areas that may be addressed in the future to improve patient outcomes. Regardless of these advances, issues remain, such as financial limitations and the ethical issues of cost-effectiveness. The future of NSCLC treatments aims to deliver more effective and personalized care, thereby improving patient outcomes and quality of life.

K. Kesavardhini, Department of Microbiology, Sacred Heart College, Tirupattur, India
K. Gayathri, Department of Microbiology, Sacred Heart College, Tirupattur, India
E. Tharani, Department of Microbiology, Sacred Heart College, Tirupattur, India
P. Saranraj, Department of Microbiology, Sacred Heart College, Tirupattur, India

Approximately 85% of lung cancer incidences are classified as non-small-cell lung cancers associated with elevated death and morbidity rates. Over the past decade, significant advancements have been made in the treatment with non-small cells lung tumours, resulting in improved early detection and therapy of pre-invasive and early-stage cancers. Surgery is the primary therapeutic modality in the initial phases of non-small cells lung cancer. Thoracoscopic lobectomy as an optimal option for early-stage non-small cell lung carcinoma patients, as it minimises the likelihood of complications, discomfort, and haemorrhage postoperatively. However, problems with thoracoscopic lobectomy, like sputum retention and decreased respiratory muscle function, ranged from 19 to 59%. The significant function of pneumonectomy in managing early-stage Non-Small Cells Lung Cancer (NSCLC) is its effectiveness as a surgical therapy. Stages III and IV lung cancer are often the ones that are identified as incurable. A complicated disease, stage III lung cancer can affect some people with technically resectable Non-Small Cell Tumours in the Lungs (NSCLC), multimodal options for treatment, including chemoradiotherapy post-surgery, constitute the most efficacious strategy. Salvage therapy is the principal surgical method for unresectable stages III/IV NSCLC, entailing the removal of residual or recurring lesions following non-surgical intervention. Surgical intervention may be utilised for the treatment of oligometastatic stage IV Non-Small Cell Lung Cancer (NSCLC). The management of NSCLC frequently presents difficulties for postoperative pulmonary rehabilitation. Recent advancements in surgical lung rehabilitation for those with NSCLC were disclosed, aimed at assisting researchers in identifying more efficacious therapies.

Cancer deaths globally are most common from lung cancer. Up to 57% of patients are diagnosed late; the 5-year survival rate is 10%-16%. ML has been extensively studied to provide patient data-based solutions to improve results. ML and AI have improved non-small cell lung cancer (NSCLC) diagnosis, therapy, and prognosis. Treatment resistance has made advanced-stage NSCLC nearly incurable, despite the development of signal transduction system blockers that target driver mutations. Understanding the common molecular patterns that support targeted therapy resistance in NSCLC subtypes is essential to developing successful treatments and overcoming tumor heterogeneity. We must understand these qualities to optimize treatment and overcome therapeutic challenges for squamous NSCLC patients to improve outcomes. Lung cancer imaging and early diagnosis have improved because of AI approaches like Natural language processing (NLP) and convolutional neural networks (CNNs). CNN distinguishes benign and malignant nodules to aid early detection and reduce biopsies. NLP extracts clinical information from unstructured medical texts and EHRs to improve patient histories and treatment planning. AI algorithms have shown great predictive accuracy in personalized treatment strategies. AI algorithms can help clinicians screen at-risk asymptomatic patients, investigate and triage symptomatic patients, and diagnose cancer recurrence. Possible limits and hazards include ethics, resource requirements, data security, and reporting criteria.

Vivek Pazhamalai, Department of Bio Engineering, School of Engineering, Vels Institute of Science, Technology, and Advanced Studies, India
Manideepa Govindarajan, Department of Bio Engineering, School of Engineering, Vels Institute of Science, Technology, and Advanced Studies, India
Meenupriya Venkatesan, Department of Bio Engineering, School of Engineering, Vels Institute of Science, Technology, and Advanced Studies, India
Jayasri Rajkumar, Department of Bio Engineering, School of Engineering, Vels Institute of Science, Technology, and Advanced Studies, India
Mathumida Rajendran, Department of Bio Engineering, School of Engineering, Vels Institute of Science, Technology, and Advanced Studies, India
S. Ivo Romauld, Department of Bio Engineering, School of Engineering, Vels Institute of Science, Technology, and Advanced Studies, India
S. S. Meenambiga, Department of Bio Engineering, School of Engineering, Vels Institute of Science, Technology, and Advanced Studies, India

Non-small-cell lung cancer (NSCLC) stands as a predominant and complex malignancy, constituting approximately 85% of all lung cancer diagnoses. The etiology of NSCLC is multifactorial, with tobacco use emerging as the primary risk factor, while air pollution and radon exposure also significantly contribute to its development. The therapeutic landscape for NSCLC has undergone a paradigm shift with the advent of targeted therapies, facilitated by advancements in genetic and biomarker testing. These innovations have enabled the identification of specific mutations, thereby informing personalized treatment strategies tailored to individual patient profiles. This chapter aims to elucidate the current state of NSCLC management, with a particular focus on multimodal treatment approaches for locally advanced disease. It will also explore the role of innovative surgical techniques and contemporary pharmacological interventions in the context of early-stage NSCLC. This chapter aims to provide a nuanced understanding of the current therapeutic options and future directions in NSCLC management.

The majority of non-small cell lung cancer (NSCLC) patients are diagnosed at advanced stages, where curative treatments may no longer result in optimal outcomes, and the quality of life is limited by disease- or treatment-related adverse events. This chapter explores the principles and practices of palliative and supportive care in NSCLC, emphasizing the importance of early integration into standard oncology care. Core discussed topics include clinical symptom management (including pain, dyspnea, fatigue, cough, nausea/vomiting, anorexia, and cachexia), psychological and psychosocial support (including psychological distress, caregiver burden, financial toxicity, cultural considerations, and spiritual suffering), management of disease- and treatment-related complications (including coagulopathy, malignant pleural effusion, superior vena cava syndrome, spinal cord compression, hypercalcemia, and hematologic, neurological, and dermatologic complications), ethical decision-making, and the role of a multidisciplinary palliative care team.

Lung cancer, particularly non-small cell lung carcinoma (NSCLC), poses significant challenges in oncology. Accounting for approximately 85% of lung cancer-related deaths, NSCLC's aggressive nature demands comprehensive management strategies. Environmental factors like smoking and air pollution, alongside genetic mutations in genes such as EGFR, KRAS, and ALK, contribute to its development. Recent advancements in diagnostic modalities, including low-dose CT scans and molecular profiling, facilitate early detection. Treatment paradigms have evolved to incorporate multimodal approaches, encompassing surgery, radiotherapy, chemotherapy, targeted therapies, and immunotherapy. Collaboration among healthcare professionals is crucial for effective patient care. As research continues to unfold, novel therapeutic strategies and personalized medicine approaches hold promise for improving outcomes in NSCLC patients.

Several treatment methods have been proposed for lung cancer, each exhibiting different success rates. Efforts in this field aim to enhance the effectiveness of these treatments while reducing their side effects. New technologies are being utilized to improve treatment methods and facilitate early diagnosis, ultimately increasing

Preface

Non-Small Cell Lung Carcinoma (NSCLC) is the most common form of lung cancer, accounting for approximately 85% of all lung cancer cases. Despite advances in detection and treatment, NSCLC remains one of the leading causes of cancer-related deaths worldwide. This book aims to provide a comprehensive, multidisciplinary perspective on NSCLC, integrating current research and clinical practices in diagnostics, therapeutics, and patient care management. This book will provide a Detailed Understanding of NSCLC, Examine the pathophysiology, molecular biology, and epidemiology of NSCLC, including risk factors such as smoking, environmental toxins, and genetic mutations. It will explore Cutting-Edge Diagnostic Techniques and Review advancements in imaging, molecular profiling, liquid biopsy, and genomic testing that have revolutionized early detection and personalized treatment planning. It will delve deeper into various treatments like surgery, radiation, and chemotherapy, alongside the newer landscape of targeted therapies, immunotherapy, and combination therapies. Further, the book will address the evolving role of precision medicine and biomarkers in creating individualized treatment regimens. It will focus on Multidisciplinary Care whereby it will emphasize the importance of a collaborative approach involving oncologists, pulmonologists, surgeons, radiologists, and palliative care specialists. This book will provide crucial insights on future Directions in NSCLC Treatment and Research and a forward-looking perspective on ongoing clinical trials, new drug development, and emerging treatment paradigms. It will address challenges such as drug resistance, tumor heterogeneity, and the need for novel therapeutic agents in NSCLC.

This book will fill a significant gap in the current literature by providing an evidence-based yet practical guide for both seasoned oncologists and those newer to the field. Several books on lung cancer exist, but most are either highly focused on specific therapies, outdated in their approach, or written in a highly technical style inaccessible to non-specialists. This book stands apart by providing a balanced, multidisciplinary approach to NSCLC, combining the latest scientific findings with clinical insights and a focus on patient care.

Various Chapters of this book provide the following insights:

CHAPTER OVERVIEW

Chapter 1: Non-Small Cell Lung Carcinoma (NSCLC) and Underlying Causes

This chapter establishes a foundational understanding of NSCLC by exploring its epidemiology, environmental risk factors, and molecular basis. It connects molecular insights into carcinogenesis with their clinical implications, underscoring how causative factors influence disease development and patient prognosis, thereby setting the stage for targeted prevention and personalized treatment approaches.

Chapter 2: Genetic Mutations Associated with NSCLC and Molecular Subtypes

Focusing on pivotal genetic alterations such as EGFR, KRAS, and ALK mutations, this chapter delineates the molecular subtypes of NSCLC that guide precision medicine. It highlights how genetic profiling has transformed diagnosis and therapeutic stratification, enabling clinicians to tailor treatments that improve survival outcomes and reduce toxicity.

Chapter 3: Tumor Microenvironment and Immune Evasion in NSCLC

Exploring the complex interplay between tumor cells and their microenvironment, this chapter reveals mechanisms of immune escape that hinder treatment efficacy. It emphasizes the clinical translation of these insights into immunotherapies, providing a framework for overcoming resistance and improving patient responses to checkpoint inhibitors and other immune-based treatments.

Chapter 4: Integration of Microbial Systems in NSCLC Emerging Paradigms in Diagnosis and Treatment

This chapter presents emerging evidence on the influence of the lung and gut microbiome on NSCLC biology and treatment outcomes. It discusses how microbial profiles can serve as novel biomarkers and therapeutic adjuncts, revolutionizing diagnosis and immunotherapy through microbiome modulation.

Chapter 5: Different Types of Diagnostic Approaches in NSCLC

This chapter analyzes the spectrum of diagnostic tools—from imaging to molecular assays—critical for accurate staging and personalized therapy planning. It underscores the fusion of advanced diagnostic technologies with molecular pathology to optimize early detection and therapeutic decision-making.

Chapter 6: CAR-T Cell Therapy - Effectiveness and Limitations Against NSCLC: Evaluating CAR-T Cell Therapy Outcomes

Focusing on the forefront of immunotherapy, this chapter evaluates CAR-T cell strategies in NSCLC, assessing both pioneering successes and clinical challenges. It bridges cutting-edge molecular engineering with patient-centered outcomes, providing insight into its evolving role and future potential in lung cancer treatment.

Chapter 7: Case Studies and Clinical Scenarios in NSCLC

Through detailed clinical cases, this chapter illustrates the real-world application of molecular diagnostics and therapies in diverse patient contexts. It highlights decision-making complexities and treatment personalization, enhancing understanding of how molecular science informs tailored clinical management.

Chapter 8: Surgical Management of NSCLC and Postoperative Care and Complications

This chapter reviews the pivotal role of surgical intervention in NSCLC management, integrating advancements in minimally invasive techniques with perioperative care. It combines molecular staging insights with clinical protocols to optimize surgical outcomes and address complications, improving long-term survival and quality of life.

Chapter 9: Role of Artificial Intelligence and Machine Learning in the Diagnosis and Treatment of NSCLC

Highlighting transformative technologies, this chapter explores how AI and machine learning enable precision diagnostics and predictive analytics in NSCLC. It discusses applications ranging from image analysis to treatment optimization, demonstrating their impact on enhancing clinical decisions and personalized care.

Chapter 10: Therapeutic Approaches in NSCLC: Navigating Side Effects and Outcomes

This chapter focuses on managing adverse effects associated with contemporary NSCLC therapies, emphasizing multidisciplinary strategies that balance treatment efficacy with quality of life. It integrates molecular insights into toxicity mechanisms with clinical guidelines to guide supportive care and improve patient adherence.

Chapter 11: Palliative and Supportive Care for Advanced Non-Small Cell Lung Cancer

This chapter underscores the importance of comprehensive palliative care in advanced NSCLC, focusing on symptom management, psychosocial support, and integration of emerging therapies. It highlights how molecular and clinical advancements can improve end-of-life care, aiming to enhance patient dignity and comfort.

Chapter 12: Advancements in the Diagnosis and Therapeutics for NSCLC: From Genetic Mutations to Public Health Perspectives

Synthesizing breakthroughs across the spectrum of NSCLC research, this chapter links molecular discoveries to their clinical and public health impacts. It provides an integrative overview of how evolving diagnostics and therapies collectively transform disease management and outcomes.

Chapter 13: Future Trends in NSCLC and Care

This final chapter projects future directions in NSCLC research and treatment, including innovations in molecular targets, personalized therapeutics, AI-driven care models, and global health strategies. It encourages continuous scientific exploration and collaboration to advance precision oncology and improve patient survival worldwide.

The Target Audience for this book includes:

- Oncologists, pulmonologists, and other medical specialists treating patients with NSCLC.
- Medical students and residents with an interest in oncology and respiratory diseases.
- Researchers focused on lung cancer biology, diagnostics, and therapeutic innovations.

- Healthcare providers involved in palliative care, supportive care, and patient advocacy.

Acknowledgement

We, the editors of this volume, wish to express our deepest gratitude to all those who have contributed to the successful completion of this book, ***Advancements in the Diagnostics and Therapeutics for Non-Small Cell Lung Carcinoma (NSCLC).***

First and foremost, we extend our sincere thanks to all the contributing authors for their dedication, expertise, and commitment. Their scholarly contributions form the foundation of this work and have been a comprehensive resource on the subject. We also gratefully acknowledge the efforts of the reviewers, whose valuable feedback and constructive suggestions have helped us maintain the scientific rigor and quality of the chapters.

We take this opportunity to thank our respective institutions — **Graphic Era (Deemed to be University), Dehradun, Uttarakhand, India; Amrita Vishwa Vidyapeetham, Mysuru, Karnataka, India; and Kansas State University, Manhattan, USA** — for their constant encouragement, resources, and support that made this endeavour possible.

We also wish to acknowledge the assistance of our Ph.D. Scholars and B.Tech. Biotechnology students whose sincere efforts in formatting and organizing the documents greatly facilitated the editorial process.

Finally, we are indebted to our families, colleagues, and well-wishers for their encouragement and support throughout this journey. We hope that this book serves as a meaningful contribution to the field and inspires further advancements in the treatment of pancreatic cancer.

Editors

Prof. (Dr.) Pallavi Singh

Dr. Shiva Prasad Kollur

Dr. Raghavendra G. Amachawadi

Chapter 1
Non-Small Cell Lung Carcinoma (NSCLC) and Underlying Causes

Kanika Phutela
https://orcid.org/0009-0006-7447-6281
Postgraduate Institute of Medical Education and Research, Chandigarh, India

Sadhna Sharma
https://orcid.org/0000-0002-6631-1704
Postgraduate Institute of Medical Education and Research, Chandigarh, India

ABSTRACT

Amongst various cancers, lung cancer is the most aggressive cancer type indiscriminative of the gender. According to the International Agency for Research on Cancer (IARC) in GLOBOCAN 2022, around 2.5 million new lung cancer cases were detected and 1.8 million deaths occurred. Lung cancer is classified into two types: small-cell carcinomas, and non-small cell carcinomas. NSCLC is the most common type contributing to up to 85% of lung cancers. Lung cancer cells have alterations in the mechanisms governing proliferation of normal cells and commonly observed genetic alterations in NSCLC include KRAS, EGFR, HER2, MEK, BRAF, and PI3K. Smoking is the main risk factor for lung cancer and is more common in men than in women. Chemotherapy, radiation therapy, and surgical resection are commonly used therapies for NSCLC but due to their few limitations, discovery of newer targets and anticancer drugs with improved bioavailability and lower systemic toxicity is required for NSCLC treatment.

DOI: 10.4018/979-8-3373-2096-0.ch001

1. INTRODUCTION TO LUNG CANCER

Cancer has rapidly become a universal health problem worldwide. The coronavirus disease 2019 (COVID-19) pandemic has majorly contributed in delaying the diagnosis and treatment of cancer because of insufficient health care settings, disruptions in employment and concerns arising due to COVID-19 exposure (Siegel et al., 2023). The prevalence of cancer has increased gradually every year thereby affecting the health of all human societies (Meacham & Morrison, 2013). The prevalence of different cancers varies in males, females, and children. In men, prostate, lung, bronchus, urinary bladder, colon, and rectum are the most prevalent cancers, whereas in women, cancers of lung, breast, uterine corpus, and thyroid constitute a major proportion of cancer (Siegal et al., 2016; Schottenfeld et al., 2006). In children, blood cancer and brain and lymph nodes associated cancers are common (Yoo et al., 2003). The primary cancer is caused by a sequence of subsequent gene mutations that alter cell functions. A variety of chemical compounds have been identified that have a usual role in causing gene mutations and forming cancer cells (Aizawa et al., 2016).

Amongst various cancers, Lung cancer is the most aggressive cancer type that is ranked first in terms of incidence and mortality (18.4%) (IARC, WHO; 2018). According to the latest estimates from the International Agency for Research on Cancer (IARC) in 2022, approximately 2.5 million new cases of lung cancer were diagnosed globally, with over 1.8 million deaths due to this disease (Bray et al., 2024). As with other cancers, lung cancer has the best chance of being cured when it is discovered in early stages of disease. Unfortunately, lung cancer is usually discovered at an incurable stage of the disease, thereby making the treatment challenging (Cersosimo, 2002). The process of cancer development involves uncontrolled cell growth that invades the surrounding tissues and spread to other parts of the body. In proliferating cancer cells, two major mutations observed are those which increase the abundance of proteins they code for, also known as oncogenes or the mutations that hamper function of specific genes, also known as tumor suppressor genes. These events occurring in the cancer cells are critical because they regulate the process of tumorigenesis and many genetic diseases which arises from genes that are originally meant to protect DNA from mutational events (Barr., 2018).

Smoking is the main risk factor for lung cancer and the frequency of smoking determines the progressive increase in risk of lung cancer and once a person quits smoking, the risk declines (Cersosimo, 2002). Lung cancer among never smokers (LCANS) accounts for about 25% lung cancer cases (Parkin et al., 2005), among which 60% to 80% are women. Molecular profiling studies have identified that the tumor genome of non-smokers largely differs from that of lung cancers occurring in smokers. In tobacco smokers with lung cancer, mutations in TP53, KRAS, and

STK11 are commonly seen, whereas among non-smokers mutations in EGFR, HER2 and the ALK-ELM4 fusion events occur frequently (Rudin et al., 2009). Other risk factors associated with lung cancer include chronic inflammation caused by infections and few other medical conditions. Studies have suggested that patients having chronic obstructive pulmonary disease with no past smoking history are more susceptible of developing lung cancer (Von et al., 2006). Also, patients suffering from pulmonary tuberculosis are likely to develop lung cancer in a few years and this risk was correlated with location of tuberculosis lesions (Rudin et al., 2009).

2. NON-SMALL CELL LUNG CANCER

2.1. Epidemiology

The Global Cancer Observatory (GLOBOCAN) estimated an incidence of 19.3 million cancer cases worldwide for the year 2020 (Sung et al., 2021). India has the highest prevalence of cancer followed by China and United States of America (Figure 1 & 2). It was also approximated that from 2020 to 2040, cancer cases in India would increment to 2.08 million accounting for a rise of 57.5 per cent (Ferlay et al., 2020).

In males and females, lung and breast are the most common sites of cancer. It was further proposed that the incidence of cancer cases is likely to rise by 12.8 per cent in 2025 in comparison to 2020 (Kumar et al., 2022). These new estimates can provide support in planning various cancer activities to prevent and confine the spread of cancer by mediating early detection and spreading awareness to restrict progressive increase in cancer cases. Lung cancer is classified into two types: small-cell carcinomas, and non-small cell carcinomas. NSCLC is the most common type contributing to up to 85% of lung cancers. Approximately 350 people die due to lung cancer every day that is much more than the deaths caused because of colorectal cancer, that is another major reason of cancer death overall. According to estimates, in 2023 as many as 103,000 out of the 127,070 lung cancer deaths (81%) occurred due to smoking (Islami et al., 2018).

Figure 1. Estimated proportion of top 10 leading sites of cancer in India by sex – 2022 (Image taken from Kumar et al; 2022)

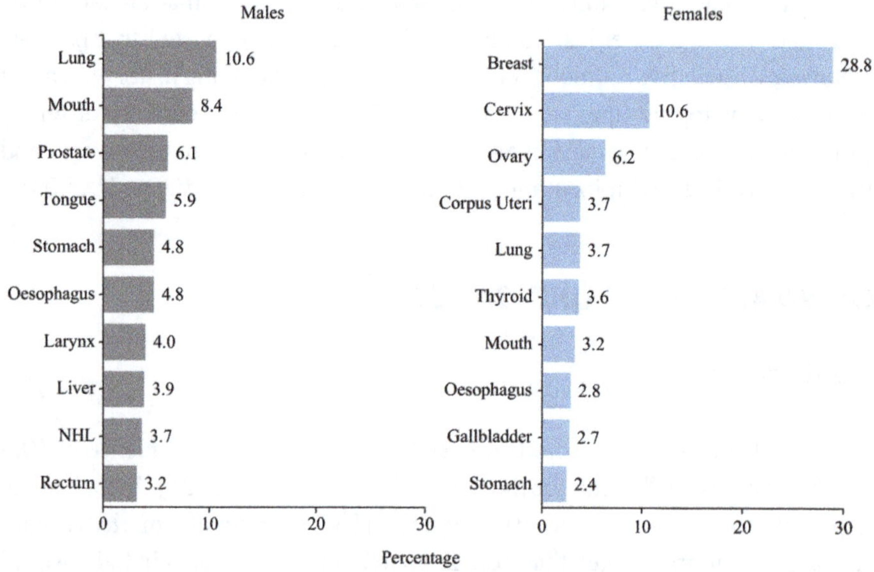

Figure 2. Estimated age-wise number and incidence rate for all sites of cancer by sex – 2022. (Image taken from Kumar et al; 2022)

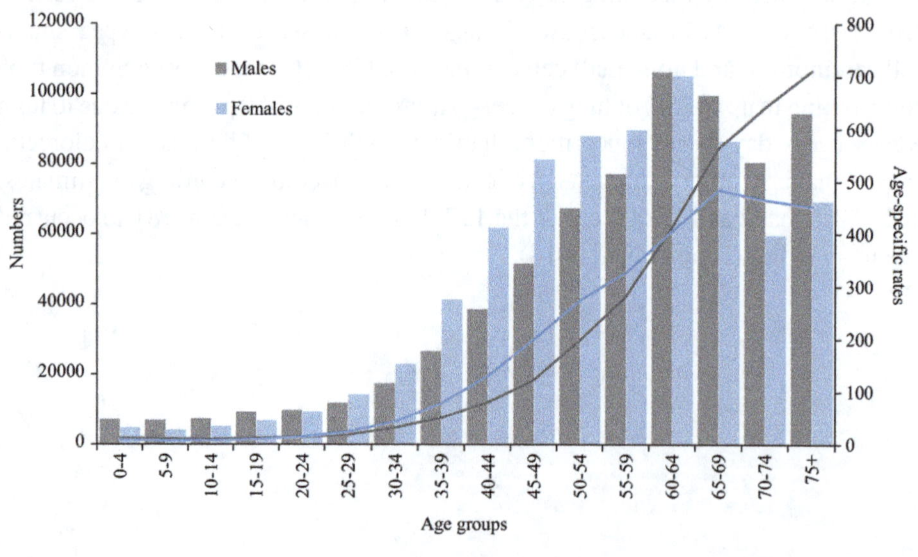

According to the National Cancer Institute's Surveillance, Epidemiology, and End Results (SEER) program, there were an estimated 229,000 new cases of lung cancer in the US in 2020, accounting for 12.7% of all cancer diagnoses. The current incidence of 45.6/100,000 is down from a peak of 69.5/100,000 in 1992, largely due to smoking cessation. Efforts undertaken since 1960s have caused reduction in smoking prevalence among US adults from 42.4% in 1965 to 13.7% in 2018 (Jamal et al., 2018). While many Western nations report a similar trend, developing nations such as China and the nations of the former Soviet Union have not seen similar success with smoking cessation and lung cancer incidence (Howlander et al., 2019).

Developing nations such as China, India, and Russia are estimated to contribute to the burden of lung cancer as 65% of Chinese men currently initiate smoking by their mid-20s, portending a continued increase in lung cancer incidence (Doll, 2010). Moreover, increased industrialization and access to tobacco worldwide, the worldwide incidence of lung cancer is on the rise (Barta et al., 2019).

It has also been observed that cigarette smoking is much more common in individuals with less school education, 32.1%, compared with 9.1% in college graduates (Seigel et al., 2018). Smokers with low educations levels are less likely to even attempt to quit (Torre et al., 2016). The use of tobacco is highest in the Army, 37.3%, and Marine Corps, 35.7% (Smith et al., 2009). The military services have been specifically targeted by tobacco companies (Joseph et al., 2005). Around 27.9% of people below the poverty threshold smoke (Torre et al., 2016). Thus, there is a strong association between lower income and cigarette smoking (Sidorchuk et al., 2009).

2.2. Types of NSCLC

Adenocarcinoma, squamous-cell carcinoma, and large-cell carcinomas are the three subtypes of NSCLC (Figure 3). According to Global cancer statistics, 2020, the most typical type of NSCLC is lung adenocarcinoma which accounts for around 40% of all lung cancers (Zappa et al., 2016).

Figure 3. Incidence of lung cancer subtypes (Image taken from Haggstrom et al; 2014).

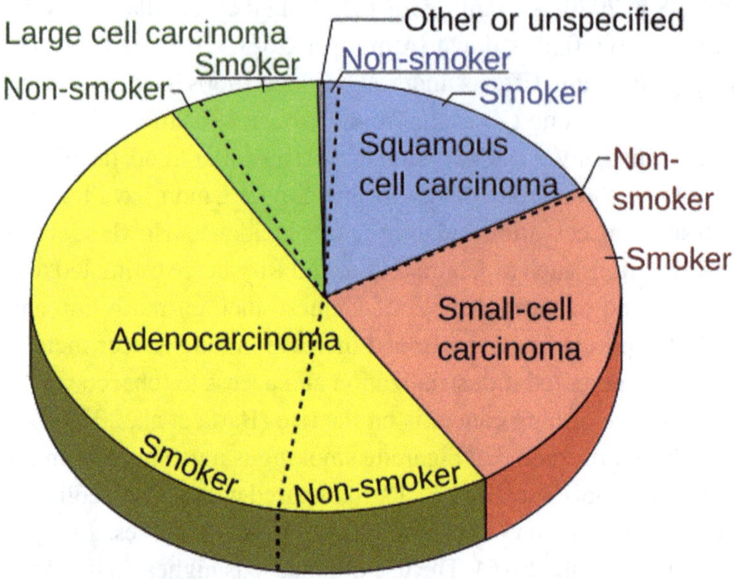

2.2.1. Lung adenocarcinoma

It emerges from epithelial type II alveolar cells in the lung airway that secrete mucus among other substances (Couraud et al., 2012). About 40% of lung cancer cases are lung adenocarcinomas, the most common type of lung carcinoma that affects women and non-smokers. They are confined towards the outer perimeter of the lung and the size gets doubled after 161 days (Gedde et al., 1979). Lung adenocarcinomas have a higher tendency for metastasizing than squamous-cell carcinomas. It tends to express immunohistochemical markers such as TTF-1 and napsin A. According to the WHO classification early stages of lung cancer are recognized as adenocarcinoma in situ (pre-invasive lesion) that is less than 3cm in diameter present in a lepidic pattern, minimally invasive adenocarcinoma that is more than 3 cm in diameter and exclusion factors include presence of lymphovascular invasion and tumor necrosis with size more than 5mm (Travis et al., 2016).

Alterations in several genes are linked to a specific type of NSCLC. In adenocarcinoma common alterations include disarrangement in surfactant-related and small airway-associated genes (SFTPA2, SFTPB, MUC1, and NAPSA) (Bhattacharjee et al., 2001; Garber et al., 2001; McDoniels-Silvers et al., 2002; Beer et al., 2002; Giordano et al., 2001). These functions are mostly linked to the histological characteristics of the cells or origin from where these subtypes originate thus emphasizing the role of histology in carcinogenesis. Like gene expression, miRNA signatures can distinguish across NSCLC histological subtypes with good accuracy (Dacic et al., 2010). miR-155 is observed to be significantly increased only in AC and is associated with wildtype EGFR and KRAS. DNA methylation is also being used as a possible biomarker for diagnosis and prognosis in both malignant and non-malignant tissues, as well as for chemoprevention and therapy (Selamat et al., 2012). It is one of the key epigenetic markers that controls somatically heritable variations in gene expression. Cell cycle control, the epithelial to mesenchymal transition, and the RAS and WNT signalling pathways are among the genes that are enriched in aberrantly methylated AC (Nacht et al., 2001).

2.2.2. Squamous-cell carcinoma

Squamous cell carcinomas (SqCC) represent 25% to 30% of lung cancers and tend to arise from cells located in the airway epithelium. Immunohistochemical markers such as CK5, CK6, p40, and desmoglein-3 are usually present (Nacht et al., 2001). SqCC tumours are frequently characterized by overexpression of cytokeratins and cytokeratin-regulatory genes (GSTT1, CEL, and PRDX6), as well as dysregulation of detoxification genes and antioxidant proteins. Among the miR signatures, miR-205 is found to be highly specific marker for SqCC (Lebanony et al., 2009). As of yet, no long noncoding RNAs (lncRNAs) have shown promise in lung cancer diagnosis or treatment, and the field of studying lncRNAs in this disease is still in its infancy.

Global DNA methylation and expression profiles in SqCC show that HOXA2 and HOXA10 methylation may have predictive value and aberrant DNA methylation has a role in several crucial events such as DNA replication, recombination, and repair processes (Heller et al., 2013; Lockwood et al., 2012).

2.2.3. Large-cell carcinoma

Large cell cancers account for approximately 5% to 10% of all lung cancers, and the incidence is declining due to newer immunophenotyping techniques that allow better classification of undifferentiated squamous cell carcinomas and adenocarcinomas (Kupeli & Koseoglu, 2018; Hou et al., 2017, Rektman et al., 2013; Chan et al., 2019). According to the WHO classification, large cell lung carcinomas are composed of poorly differentiated cells with abundant cytoplasm, big nucleoli and lack typical characteristics observed in lung adenocarcinoma or squamous cell carcinoma (Travis et al., 2015). Six subtypes of LCC are recognized by the current WHO classification: LCC with rhabdoid phenotype (LCC-R), LCC with basaloid carcinoma (BC), lymphoepithelioma-like carcinoma (LELC), large cell neuroendocrine carcinoma (LCNEC), clear cell carcinoma (CCC), and LCC undifferentiated-type (LCC-U) (Copin, 2016). Despite having six distinct morphological features in the 2004 WHO classification, LCC is synonymous with NSCLC, not otherwise specified (NOS). Rather than biopsy and cytological examination, pathological evaluation post-surgery is the primary method used to diagnose LCLC (Bi et al., 2018).

Studies indicate that LCLC is more common in men and smokers, and it typically manifests as a big mass with central necrosis (Weissferdt et al., 2014; Sun et al., 2014). Moreover, majority of LCLC cases are seen in the elderly (>60), involving the upper lobe and its clinical symptoms also correlate with the extent of invasion (Hanagiri et al., 2010; Galffy et al., 2018). These tumors are commonly diagnosed at later stages (III/IV) and the choice of treatment preferred is usually surgery combined with chemotherapy for the prognosis such patients (Cao et al., 2019).

2.3. Lung cancer staging

Cancer staging plays a crucial role in the diagnosis process and helps in designing efficient therapeutic approach. The international TNM-based staging system explains physiological extent of disease. 'T' defines extent and size of main tumor, 'N' defines extent to which regional lymph nodes are involved and 'M' provides information about whether the cancer has metastasized or not (table1). Additional numbers to each of these categories explains about expansion of the cancer. Various combinations of these three categories are utilized to create TNM subsets (Figure 4). NSCLC stages are further categorized from one to four where the lower stage indicates the less spread of the disease (Murray et al., 1993).

Table 1. Definitions for TNM descriptors (Adapted from Detterbeck et al; 2018)

T (primary tumor)			
T0 - No primary tumor	T1 - Tumor _3 cm	T2 – Tumor >3 but _5 cm or tumor involving: visceral pleura, main bronchus	T3 – Tumor >5 but _7 cm or invading chest wall, pericardium, phrenic nerve;
Tis - Carcinoma in situ (squamous or adenocarcinoma)			**T4** – Tumor >7 cm or tumor invading: mediastinum, diaphragm, heart, great vessels, trachea, esophagus, spine
N (regional lymph nodes)			
N0 - No regional node metastasis	**N1** - Metastasis in ipsilateral pulmonary or hilar nodes	**N2** - Metastasis in ipsilateral mediastinal or subcarinal nodes	**N3** - Metastasis in contralateral mediastinal, hilar, or supraclavicular nodes

continued on following page

Table 1. Continued

T (primary tumor)			
M (distant metastasis)			
M0 - No distant metastasis	**M1a** - Malignant pleural or pericardial effusion	**M1b** - Single extrathoracic metastasis	**M1c** - Multiple extrathoracic metastases

Figure 4. Lung cancer stage grouping, 8th edition (Image taken from Detterbeck et al; 2018)

T/M	Subcategory	N0	N1	N2	N3
T1	T1a	IA1	IIB	IIIA	IIIB
	T1b	IA2	IIB	IIIA	IIIB
	T1c	IA3	IIB	IIIA	IIIB
T2	T2a	IB	IIB	IIIA	IIIB
	T2b	IIA	IIB	IIIA	IIIB
T3	T3	IIB	IIIA	IIIB	IIIC
T4	T4	IIIA	IIIA	IIIB	IIIC
M1	M1a	IVA	IVA	IVA	IVA
	M1b	IVA	IVA	IVA	IVA
	M1c	IVB	IVB	IVB	IVB

3. RISK FACTORS AND CAUSES FOR NSCLC

3.1. Tobacco and smoking

Smoking is the main risk factor for lung cancer (Figure 5), accounting for 75–80% of fatalities from the disease and being more common in men (27%) than in women (23%). During the world wars, soldiers were given cigarettes for relieving their anxiety and this trend led to tremendous increase in smoking in the early 90s which was then adopted by women and adolescents. But later in 1950, cigarette smoking was seen to increase the risk of lung cancer (Wynder et al., 1950). Nicotine the main ingredient in tobacco smoke binds to nicotinic acetylcholine receptors present in the brain thereby altering neurotransmitter levels. The carcinogenic compounds present in tobacco are known to cause DNA damage and mutations that enhance the process of tumorigenesis after continuous usage over the years. In addition, second hand smoke, that results from the burning of tobacco products is another major factor for lung cancer. Because of the filters on the user end of cigarettes, some carcinogens in second hand smoke are absorbed in quantities that are higher than those of the smoker; for example, exposure to benzopyrene is four times higher (Hackshaw, 1998). The risk of lung cancer is known to be 20–30% higher for nonsmoking spouses of smokers.

Developmental delays, asthma, and SIDS are among the chronic illnesses linked to exposure by children or pregnant women (Simons et al., 2014; Al-Sayed & Ibrahim, 2014; Oberg et al., 2011). Since they simulate tobacco use without producing hazardous combustion products, electronic cigarettes have become more and more popular in recent years. Nevertheless, research indicates that e-cigarette aerosol particles do include trace metals, nitrosamines, and polycyclic aromatic hydrocarbons in variable amounts, and there is currently no long-term information regarding cancer risk (Dinakar et al., 2016).

Figure 5. Main factors causing lung cancer worldwide

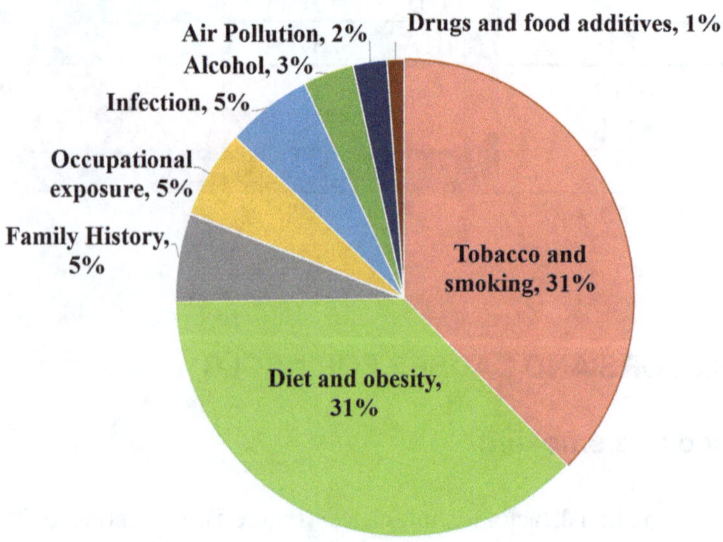

3.2. Diet and obesity

Evidences also suggest that specific components of the diet exert some protective effects against lung cancer for example diet consisting of vegetables and fruits mainly cruciferous vegetables. Chemicals such as isothiocyanates posses' anti-cancer activity that reduces lung cancer risk and this effect is associated with high intake of cruciferous vegetables. Other diet components such as fried or well-done red meat are also linked to elevated risk of developing lung cancer whereas protective effects were found to be related with β-carotene supplementation (Zhang et al., 2023).

3.3. Family History

Many studies have reported that positive lung cancer family history is a crucial risk factor that early-onset lung cancer (Tanoue et al., 2009). A linkage analysis study detected a critical susceptibility locus linked to chromosome 6q23–25 in high-risk pedigrees (Oken et al., 1982). The risk of lung cancer development has been associated with Li–Fraumeni syndrome defined by germline mutation occurring in p53 tumour-suppressor gene (Von et al., 2006).

Tumors acquire intrinsic genetic driver mutations, most of which involve cell signalling pathways including the ErbB protein family (EGFR/HER1-4) and the GTP-ase Kirsten rat sarcoma virus (*K-ras*) gene (Herbst et al., 2008). Other genetic and epigenetic changes can cause inactivation of tumor suppressor genes such as *p53*, *p16* and *PTEN* (Herbst et al., 2008). Mutations rarely occur in the same signalling pathway (Kristeleit et al., 2011). Some mutations are associated with lung tumor histology such as EGFR and EML4-ALK mutations which are associated with adenocarcinomas mainly in nonsmokers (Herbst et al., 2008).

3.4. Occupational exposure

Occupational exposure to carcinogens such as asbestos is another risk factor that contributes for 5% to 10% of lung cancers (Albin et al., 1999). Asbestos, the most common and naturally occurring silicate mineral has been widely used in construction since 19th century. Asbestos exposure is associated with high risk (5-fold) of lung cancer (Alberg et al., 2013). Moreover, exposure of both asbestos and tobacco smoking has a synergistic effect on lung cancer risk (Dela Cruz et al., 2009).

3.5. Infection

Lung carcinogenesis has been associated with cellular damage and inflammation occurring during respiratory infection. Tuberculosis (TB) the dominant cause of deaths worldwide has 1.76 odds ratio of developing lung cancer according to a meta-analysis (Kabbani, 2013). HIV also increases lung cancer risk by 2.5 times and the advent of antiretroviral medications that primarily guard against the infection that causes AIDS, lung cancer has emerged as the primary cause of mortality for HIV patients in the United States (Lee et al; 2011, Alberg et al; 2013 & Broody et al; 2013). Lung cancer rates are increased in patients undergoing immunosuppressive therapy. Moreover, chronic obstructive pulmonary disease (COPD) linked inflammation and scarring is indirectly associated with an elevated risk of lung cancer. The known mechanisms by which COPD can increase lung cancer risk include extended exposure to inflammatory cytokines, DNA repair mechanism suppression, and high cellular proliferation (Volkow et al; 2014). Evidence suggest that COPD increases lung cancer risk by 6- to 13-fold (Berthiller et al; 2008 & Voirin et al; 2006).

3.6. Alcohol

International Agency for Research (2012) on Cancer has categorised alcohol as group I carcinogen. Alcohol drinking is associated with several cancer types including cancers of colon, rectum, breast and the head and neck (Bagnardi et al; 2001 & Corrao et al; 2004). However, it is still unknown if alcohol is a risk factor for lung cancer on its own, and tobacco use may be a significant confounding factor for alcohol exposure. In a study, alcohol consumption was associated with a slight decrease in total lung carcinoma risk when consumed in low quantities (>0–<1 drink/day) and associated with a modest increase in risk when consumed in large quantities (≥7 drinks/day). Few differences were observed in histological subtype (Bagnardi et al; 2015).

3.7. Air Pollution

In early 1920s ambient air quality was proposed to be a critical risk factor for lung cancer (Tylecote et al; 1927). Concerning indoor and outdoor air quality, there are two primary aspects, the combustion of fossil fuels produces several carcinogens such as sulphur dioxide, PAH and trace metals and extended exposure to any of these can elevate lung cancer risk (Alberg et al; 2002). For example, occupational exposures in the trucking industry are linked with approximately 50% increment in relative lung cancer risk (Dela Cruz et al., 2009). In the developing countries, air pollution from burning of soft coal and biomass fuels including wood, plant-based materials and solid waste for purposes like heating and cooking is linked to lung cancer risk (Torok et al; 2011 & Lee et al; 2011). It was also observed that proper ventilation in cooking areas can significantly decrease the risk of developing lung cancer (Alberg et al; 2002).

3.8. Drugs and Food additives

The food additives proven as safe, are authorized after conduction of proper toxicological analyses for consumption in the food sector. The Acceptable Daily Intake (ADI) levels of food additives for human use are calculated from their No-Observed-Adverse-Effects-Level (NOAEL), determined on the basis of toxicological evaluation. Some food additives cause carcinogenicity because of the following reasons including negative synergistic effect (potassium sorbate, ferrous salts and ascorbic acid), changes in chemical structure during enzymatic processing, improper and longer storage (benzoic acid and benzoates) and exceeding the recommended safety limits (Fasihnia et al; 2020). Butylated hydroxytoluene (BHT) commonly used to enhance the shelf life of packed foods was seen to increase the risk of Lung tumors (Fasihnia et al; 2020).

4. GENETIC ALTERATION IN NSCLC

The process of cancer development involves uncontrolled cell growth that invades the surrounding tissues and spread to other parts of the body. Tumors are classified into two types, benign tumors that grow locally and malignant tumors that spread to nearby tissues. While most of the human tumors are benign in nature, some of them can be deadly due to their presence on vital organs such as the brain tumor (Weinberg et al; 2014). Cancer is mostly caused due to mutations that develop spontaneously because of DNA damage leading to altered gene function. These mutations can be of several types (table 2) including, point mutations, mutation in stop codons which disrupt the protein structure, upregulation of a specific gene, loss of gene function mutations and epigenetic modifications to DNA, majorly the methylation of cytosine in CpG islands that causes gene silencing (Bertram, 2000).

Table 2. The promising strategies for overcoming drug resistance to targeted therapies in NSCLC (Xiang et al; 2000)

Resistant to	Resistance Mechanisms	Target	Promising Strategies
Osimertinib	C797S	EGFR L858R	Erlotinib + Afatinib
All EGFR-TKIs	trans-C797S/T790M	EGFR	First generation TKIs + third generation TKIs
Osimertinib	G724S & L718Q	EGFR	Afatinib
Osimertinib	HER2D16	EGFR	Osimertinib + Afatinib

continued on following page

Table 2. Continued

Resistant to	Resistance Mechanisms	Target	Promising Strategies
Osimertinib	MET amplification	EGFR	amivantamab + lazertinib
Gefitinib/ osimertinib.	MET dysregulation	EGFR	Dictamnine (c-Met inhibitor)
Osimertinib/ dacomitinib	AXL overexpressing	EGFR	ONO-7475(AXL Inhibitor) + osimertinib
Osimertinib	FGFR1 overexpressing	EGFR	FGFR inhibitor + AKT inhibitor
Gefitinib	BIM deletion polymorphism	EGFR	Vorinostat (HDAC inhibitor)
EGFR-TKIs	ROS1 rearrangement	EGFR	crizotinib
EGFR-TKIs	HER3 augmentation	EGFR	HER3-DXd
Sotorasib	MET amplification:	KRAS	Crizotinib+ sotorasib
Lorlatinib	the activation of bypass tracks	EGFR, TP53, NRAS-G12D	combination with other inhibitors
Crizotinib	Point mutations, fusion gene amplification	F1174L, L1152R, S1206Y, G1202R, G1269S.	arrangement of the usage of various generations of drugs
Brigatinib	Combined mutation	E1210K+S1206C and E1210K+D1203N	combination with other inhibitors
Crizotinib	Activation of bypass tracks	EGFR, extracellular signal regulated kinase (ERK), Crk-like adaptor protein	combination with other inhibitors
Alectinib	Mutations	G1202R, G1206C, G1206Y, E1210K, and I1171T/N/ S mutations	arrangement of the usage of various generations of drugs
Ceritinib	Mutations	G1123S, F1174C/L/V, and G1202R mutation	arrangement of the usage of various generations of drugs
Brigatinib	Activation of bypass tracks	MTOR T1834-T1837del, and MET amplification	combination with other inhibitors
Ensartinib	Mutations	G1269A, G1202R, and E1210K	arrangement of the usage of various generations of drugs
Alectinib	Activation of bypass tracks	C-MET activation, SRC, YAP 1, ABCC11, Transformation to SCLC, and EMT	combination with other inhibitors
Brigatinib	Mutations and gene tracks	G1202R, I1171T, I1171N, V1180L, G1202R, and ALK amplification	arrangement of the usage of various generations of drugs

continued on following page

Table 2. Continued

Resistant to	Resistance Mechanisms	Target	Promising Strategies
Lorlatinib	ROS1 mutation	ROS1 G2032R, ROS1 S1986F	alternative ROS1 inhibitors (alectinib, brigatinib, or ceritinib, gilteritinib)
Ceritinib	ROS1 mutation	ROS1G2032R	alternative ROS1 inhibitors (Repotrectinib)
Brigatinib	ROS1 mutation	ROS1G2032R	alternative ROS1 inhibitors (Repotrectinib)
Entrectinib	ROS1 mutation	ROS1G2032R, ROS1 L2086F	alternative ROS1 inhibitors (Repotrectinib)
Crizotinib	ROS1 mutation	ROS1 G2032R, ROS1 L2086F	alternative ROS1 inhibitors (Repotrectinib)
Dabrafenib	MEK Continuous activation	BRAF V600E	dabrafenib + trametinib
Trametinib	AKT Signaling pathway up-regulation	BRAF G469A	Trametinib + Vemurafenib
Osimertinib	BRAF V600E mutation	EGFR	dabrafenib + trametinib + osimertinib
BLU-667, LOXO-292	Solvent front mutation KIF5BRET G810R	RET G810S	TPX-0046
Neratinib	YES1 acceleration	HER2	Dasatinib + Neratinib

In proliferating cancer cells, two major mutations observed are those which increase the abundance of proteins they code for, also known as oncogenes or the mutations that hamper function of specific genes, also known as tumor suppressor genes. These events occurring in the cancer cells are critical because they regulate the process of tumorigenesis and many genetic diseases which have a predisposition to cancer which arises from genes that are originally meant to protect DNA from mutational events (Barr, 2018). Cancer is caused due to genetic alterations at the cellular level and involves several genetic and environmental factors. Thus, the understanding of these events has direct clinical relevance. Some of the commonly mutated receptors are discussed below:

4.1. ERBB family

ERBB2 and ERBB1 belong to family of transmembrane receptor tyrosine kinases that are commonly altered in NSCLC. When ligand binds to the ERBB receptors, it leads to their homodimerization thereby initiating intracellular signalling cascades. ERBB2 has been found to be upregulated in approximately 30% of NSCLC cases, mainly adenocarcinoma (Weiner et al; 1990; Rachwal et al; 1995) and its levels were also linked to the development of multiple drug resistance in NSCLC along with other cancers (Kern et al; 1994; Pfeiffer et al; 1996). Another receptor of this family, ERBB1 is involved in regulating epithelial cell proliferation and is observed to be activated in lung cancer but the mechanism is not clear. Moreover, the ERBB1 ligands like epidermal growth factor and transforming growth factor β are produced by the cancer cells indicating autocrine loop system (Rachwal et al; 1995; Rush et al; 1993). In NSCLC, ERBB1 activation was found to be related to the tumor stage and degree of differentiation (Tateishi et al; 1990). Monoclonal antibodies against both ERBB1 (C225) and ERBB2 receptor (Herceptin) are already in clinical trials in combination with standard chemotherapy for both breast and lung cancer treatment (Damstrup et al; 1992).

4.2. RAS

These are proteins (KRAS, HRAS, and NRAS) present in the plasma membrane and are triggered by point mutations resulting in continuous cell proliferation. KRAS is commonly activated in PDAC, colorectal cancer, lung cancer due to mutations in codon 12 and affects 25% of all NSCLC (Richardson & Johnson, 1993). Growth factors, chemokines, and ions such as calcium activate KRAS proteins which lead to activation of various downstream pathways such as RAF-MEK-ERK signalling pathway, and PI3K-PknB-AKT mTOR signalling pathway, revealing KRAS communications with multiple pathways (Hanafusa et al; 2002). It has been observed that KRAS mutations are common in smokers (30%) occurring due to nitrosamines present in tobacco smoke (Chen et al; 2017). In KRAS mutated cancers, PD-L1 expression was found to be upregulated whereas major histocompatibility complex (MHC) expression was downregulated thereby facilitating the immune escape (Chen et al; 2017; Coelho et al; 2017).

4.3. MYC

RAS signalling activates nuclear genes such as MYC, which further drives cell growth. It is the most deregulated oncogene in several types of cancers as its activity is frequently elevated leading to increased MYC protein expression (Ciriello et al; 2013). Its main function is to control the expression of several genes that constitute a regulatory network required for cell growth and expansion (Amanti et al; 1992). It has been observed to be activated in approximately 20% of NSCLCs. In addition, activation of MYC was observed in many cancers including breast cancer (21.6%), ovarian cancer (30.7%), prostate cancer (8%) and pancreatic cancer (14%) (Curtis et al; 2012; Guinney et al; 2015).

4.4. Tumor suppressor genes

4.4.1. p53

The main function of p53 protein is to maintain the genomic integrity and inhibit cancer growth. To suppress the tumor formation, it interacts with specific DNA binding sites and triggers the activation of genes involved in arresting cell cycle, apoptosis, ferroptosis, DNA repair or autophagy (Hafner et al; 2019; Levine, 2019; Janic et al; 2018). Tp53 is inactivated in many human cancers due to presence of mutations in its gene sequence that allows unregulated interaction with downstream proteins like MDM2 (Levine, 2019). Factors such as hypoxia or damaged DNA cause drastic increase in p53 protein levels which further activates downstream genes like p21, BAX, MDM2 that help in regulating the cell cycle transition and apoptosis (Takahashi et al; 1989). P53 is inactivated in nearly 50% of NSCLCs majorly affecting the 17p13 locus and is strongly associated with smoking which cause G-T transversions due to the carcinogen benzopyrene present in tobacco smoke (Denisenko et al; 1996).

4.4.2. Retinoblastoma (RB)

The main function of this gene is suppression of G1-S progression and is found to be mutated in several cancer types. It is observed to be mutated in nearly 30% of NSCLCs majorly affecting the 13ql4 locus (Harbour et al; 1988). Mutations in the RB locus are related to development of retinoblastoma disease and it also increases the tendency of developing lung cancer by 15% thus giving evidence of having genetic tendency to lung cancer (Sander et al; 1989). The mutations altering RB gene function are mostly deletions or nonsense which lead to very little protein expression. Two RB-linked genes also have been implicated in lung cancer such as p107 and pRB2/p130 and downregulation of these proteins is associated with enhanced aggressive behaviour (Minimo et al; 1999).

5. DIAGNOSIS

5.1. Computed tomography

For the diagnosis of lung cancer by chest radiography approach tumors as small as 1 cm can be detected, that have around 109 cells which can disrupt bronchial and vascular epithelia. In comparison to plain radiography or conventional tomography, CT better detects peripheral lung lesions of lung tissue. Spiral CT scans can provide more accurate diagnosis as they are able to collect data continuously in a shorter span of time with less radiation exposure. Nodules that are smaller as 1–5 mm can also be detected with modern spiral CT technology. Due to all these advantages, CT is commonly done for lung cancer screening (Sobue et al; 2002).

5.2. Sputum cytology

Cytological examination of sputa is another diagnostic procedure for lung cancer and helps in detecting central tumors present in the larger bronchi. Also, it was reported that the sputum samples analysis failed to show small adenocarcinomas (approx. diameter 2 cm) that emerged from small bronchi, bronchioles, and alveoli (Toyoda et al; 2008). For early detection of lung cancer, sensitivity of sputum cytology is only 20-30% and factors like number and cell type influence its pre-malignant condition detection capability (Risse et al; 1987). Moreover, the inclusion of sputum cytology by various studies was found to be insufficient in accurately diagnosing suspected cases of lung cancer (Dougall et al; 1992).

5.3. Positron emission tomography

In the recent years, Positron emission tomography (PET) scanning has come up as a new imaging modality which is currently being explored for its role in assessment of lung cancer. But when compared with CT, PET has lower spatial resolution, thereby preventing it from accurately assessing the primary tumour status. It has been observed that false-positive PET findings are commonly observed in tuberculous infection, histoplasmosis, and rheumatoid lung disease (Erasmus et al; 1999).

5.4. Bronchoscopy and Tissue biopsy

Bronchoscopy and lung tissue biopsy are the most utilized diagnostic tools for acquiring a specific histological diagnosis of lung cancer. However, few major limitations are associated with bronchoscopy for pre-malignant lesions which otherwise are difficult to detect because they have thickness of 0.2–1 mm thus identification of these lesions needs a high level of expertise (Nooreldeen & Bach, 2021). This limitation has been addressed by the development of fluorescence bronchoscopy that involves LIFE-lung Fluorescence Endoscopy which is far more superior as compared to the older technique (Kurie et al; 1998).

The best method for cancer confirmation is performing tissue biopsy. The biopsy sample should have enough tissue material to correctly identify the lung cancer subtype by histopathology. Performing the initial biopsy is critical to confirm the early diagnosis and avoiding the complications associated with repeated tests.

Different types of procedural methods used for detecting lung carcinomas include fibre optic bronchoscopy, endobronchial ultrasonography, mediastinoscopy, pleural fluid analysis (thoracentesis), and thoracoscopy. These methods are expensive, associated with high risk of complications, and there is a possible need for more samples (Kennedy et al; 2000).

5.5. Biomarker testing

Biomarker testing makes maximum use of lung tissue biopsies to test various mutations. Some of the molecular testing sequencing platforms that are approved by FDA include Oncomine, MSK IMPACT, and Foundation One CDx (Planchard et al; 2018; Hellmann et al; 2018). However, a critical issue face by the oncologists is the type of biopsy to be used in the clinicals setting. Thus, the barriers in early lung cancer detection can only be overcome by the identification and development of simple, accurate, and inexpensive tools for its early diagnosis.

5.6 Liquid biopsy

Although tissue biopsy is the gold standard for gathering information at the gene level but because of its invasiveness and biasness caused by tumor heterogeneity the focus has been shifted towards the use of liquid biopsy (Kennedy et al; 2000). Blood based liquid biopsies are being used for investigating the genetic profile of tumors, however their use is limited due to less amount of plasma circulating tumor DNA (ctDNA). Therefore, malignant pleural effusion (MPE) is preferred due to tumor cell abundance and it is minimally invasive as compared to tissue biopsy (Guo et al; 2019).

6. CURRENTLY USED TREATMENT STRATEGIES FOR NON-SMALL CELL LUNG CANCER (NSCLC)

Most of the lung cancer patients receive their diagnosis when the disease is already advanced and there is little possibility of recovery. On the other hand, early-stage local treatment is advantageous and improves overall survival chances. The primary treatment option for early-stage disease is surgery (Cunha et al; 2011) which is one of the best strategies for longer survival (Sangha et al; 2010).

- The five-year survival rate in operated cases after the surgery is approximately 80% for stage I and around 50% for stage II NSCLC patients (Tanoue et al; 2009). However, radiotherapy is not given post-surgery for stage II patients.

As of right now, stage II patients have been found to benefit from adjuvant platinum-based chemotherapy, which is also the preferred course of treatment for patients who have undergone complete resection (Oken et al;1982).

- The treatment options for stage III NSCLC include radiotherapy, chemotherapy, and surgical resection (table 3). Radiation therapy and chemotherapy can be administered sequentially or concurrently to patients in stage IIIA who are not able to undergo surgery. For patients who cannot be given combination therapy, the option left is external radiation therapy. The treatment plan for patients at stage IIIB includes external radiation therapy or a combination of chemotherapy administered one after the other.
- Stage IV NSCLC consists for around 40% of the freshly detected NSCLC patients and the treatment recommended considers various factors including, histological type, comorbidity, and genetic features of the cancer (Von et al; 2006).

6.1. Chemotherapy

In NSCLC cases chemotherapy is frequently given in patients with PS 0 and 1, however it is not much effective for patients having PS > 2 so palliative care is preferred in such patients. Chemotherapy has shown to improve the 1-year overall survival rate gradually from 20% to 50% (Cunha et al; 2011). For stage IV NSCLC (PS 0 or 1) combinational therapy is usually recommended as first-line therapy. Another treatment option for stage IV NSCLC is the use of EGFR tyrosine kinase inhibitors (first line). Mutations of EGFRs cause uncontrolled cancer cell growth leading to several types of cancers including NSCLC.

- Studies have depicted that these agents (gefitinib or erlotinib) are more effective than combinational chemotherapy using platinum for stage IIIB or IV lung adenocarcinoma patients as a first-line treatment (Sangha et al; 2010; Tanoue et al; 2009). In cases where the cancer has not spread after administration of first-line therapy, maintenance is continued. The primary goal of this approach is to improve ill-effects related to this disease, and most importantly enhance the survival time (Oken et al; 1982).
- FDA has approved the use of Pemetrexed (Alimta), and Erlotinib (Tarceva) as a maintenance treatment of lung cancer in advanced stages (Socinski et al; 2002; Paz et al; 2012).
- For patients not responding to the first line therapies, second- and third-line therapies are used e.g. gefitinib, pemetrexed, erlotinib, and docetaxel are prescribed as second-line treatment option for advanced stage disease. Pemetrexed was seen to yield similar clinical response in comparison to

docetaxel and provided better results in lung adenocarcinoma patients (Weiss et al; 2006) whereas erlotinib response was frequent in women with adeno-carcinoma or non-smokers, which was linked with often EGFR activating mutations (Shepherd et al; 2005). Erlotinib is widely used for patients as second- or third-line therapy only if they were not earlier treated with erlo-tinib or gefitinib.

Table 3. Treatment options for NSCLC (Alaoui et al; 2015)

Stage	Treatment Options
I, II-resectable	Surgery
I, II-unresectable	Radiotherapy
II-resectable	Surgery followed by chemotherapy (adjuvant)
IIIA-resectable	Surgery followed by chemotherapy
IIIA-resectable	Chemotherapy followed by surgery
IIIA-unresectable	Sequential or combined chemoradiation
IIIB	Chemotherapy or radiation
IV (PS - 0 or 1)	Chemotherapy (combination of two platinum-based cytotoxic drugs)
IV (PS - 0 or 1), with no squamous carcinoma histology and brain metastasis	first line doublet combination chemotherapy with Bevacizumab (VEGF antibody)
IV (PS - 2)	Chemotherapy (single cytotoxic drug)
NSCLC with EGFR mutations	Erlotinib and gefitinib
III, IV (where first-line platinum-based therapy has failed)	Docetaxel, pemetrexed, erlotinib and gefitinib
Recurrent NSCLC	Radiation therapy, Cytotoxic chemotherapy, Surgery, Laser therapy and EGFR inhibitors EML4-ALK inhibitors
Brain Metastases	Whole Brain Radiotherapy (WBRT), Surgery and Systemic Therapy

6.2. Angiogenesis Inhibitors

Mechanisms promoting angiogenesis play a significant role in NSCLC treatment by supporting growth of tumor, thereby causing expansion of newly formed blood vessels. Bevacizumab is the only monoclonal antibody that targets circulating VEGF and is approved for advanced NSCLC treatment (Ellis & Al-Saleh, 2012).

- Sorafenib and sunitinib are one of the several anti-angiogenic agents that are being investigated for their clinical use. They both have shown to be active individually in NSCLC patients but no improvement was seen when either of these was given along with carboplatin and paclitaxel in a phase II trial (Socinski et al; 2010).
- In addition to these various other agents that inhibit VEGFR along with PDGFR are being explored clinically, including cediranib, axitinib, motesanib, and linifinib (Pardoll, 2012). Clinical investigations are being conducted for many agents that have cytotoxic activity against three angiogenic pathways but resistance to anti-VEGF agents develops in all the patients ultimately. This resistance may occur due to increase in some compensatory angiogenic pathways such as PDGF or FGF signalling. Thus, multitargeted combined anti-angiogenesis therapies may present a new treatment option for NSCLC patients.

6.3. Immune checkpoint Inhibitors

Cancer growth is persistent in nature because of its vast repertoire of mutations that lead to the development of resistance mechanisms against commonly used treatment strategies. Lung cancer is among the top five cancers that carry excessive number of somatic mutations (Cersosimo, 2002). Initially overall survival of advanced stage patients of NSCLC was one year but the identification of driver genomic alterations and targeted therapies have caused major improvement in overall survival of a subset of NSCLC patients. The discovery of immune checkpoints led to the development ICIs that were awarded Nobel prize for their remarkable effects in NSCLC treatment (Pardoll, 2012). Many of the immune checkpoints are activated by ligand- receptor interactions (Thomas et al; 2012).

- The best-known immune checkpoints are cytotoxic T lymphocyte antigen-4 (CTLA-4) and programmed cell death protein-1/programmed cell death ligand-1(PD-1/PD-L1) pathways. In NSCLC, ipilimumab and tremelimumab are two monoclonal antibodies that have been used against CTLA-4, an inhibitory T-cell co-receptor present on activated T-cells and regulatory T-cell subsets (Alegre et al; 2001). IC inhibitors that include anti-CTLA-4 and anti-PD-1, are also being investigated in NSCLC (Sundar et al; 2015). Observations from trials of two-phase III studies have proved Nivolumab to be a better option in comparison to docetaxel in both non-squamous and squamous NSCLC (Paz et al; 2015).
- Targeting PD-1 ligands (PD-L1, PD-L2) is another immunotherapeutic option as these are specifically overexpressed in various human cancers such as

lung cancer. Moreover, phase I study depicted the clinical activity of PD-L1 inhibiting compounds in NSCLC (Dong et al; 2002; Topalian et al; 2011). Although PD-1/PD-L1 and CTLA-4 inhibitors are frequently used ICIs in lung cancer, still development of resistance to these agents remains a major challenge (Figure 6). Patients suffering from locally advanced and metastatic NSCLC, ICIs are the most preferred treatment option however due to few limitations' other options such as cellular therapy has gained importance.

Figure 6. Mechanism of action of PD-1 and PD-L1 inhibitors (Image taken from Eno et al; 2017)

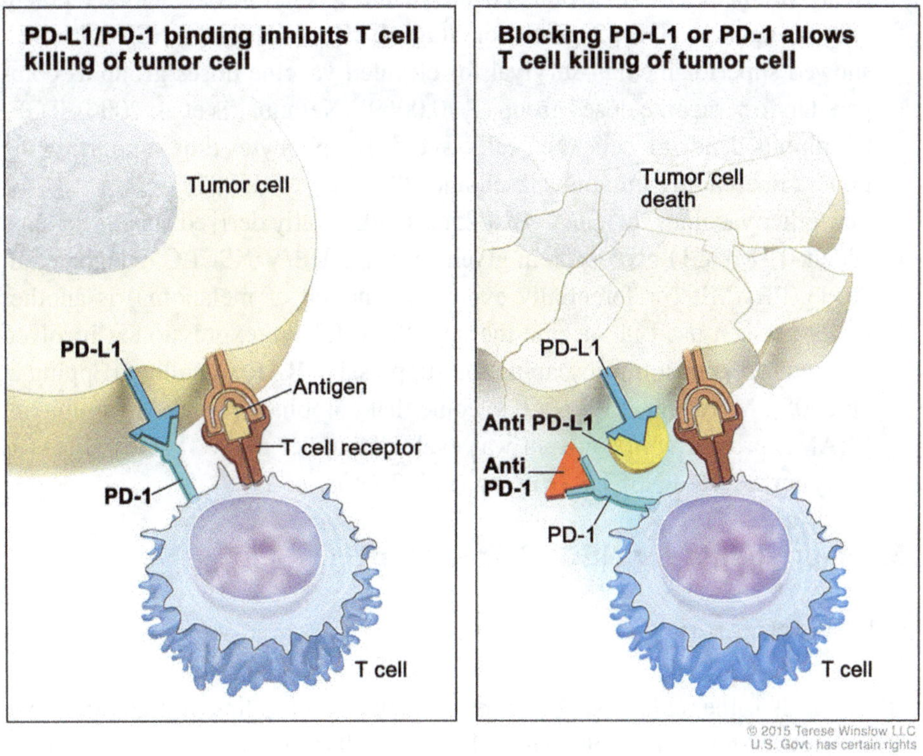

6.4. Available Vaccines for NSCLC Treatment

Vaccines are important developments in present-day medicine which helps in saving millions of lives each year. It consists of an antigen- specific immunotherapy approach in which priming of the immune system leads to generation of antigen-specific antibodies and CD4+/CD8+ T-cells against the relevant tumor antigens (Massarelli E et al; 2014). Several vaccines are under development for NSCLC treatment and have shown potent results in clinical trials. MAGE-A3 and liposomal-BLP25 are two cancer vaccines that are in clinical development for the treatment of potentially curable NSCLC. For vaccine development a variety of immunoadjuvants are used such as phospholipids, viral vectors, liposomes, and dendritic cells. MAGE-A3 (Melanoma-associated antigen A3 vaccine) is expressed on 17-50% of NSCLC tumors and its expression is linked with poor prognosis (Vansteenkiste et al; 2013). This vaccine was initially developed for metastatic melanoma patients but also showed better results after 28 days in early-stage NSCLC (Nemunaitis et al; 2006).

- Belagenpimatucel-L (4 irradiated lung cancer cell lines) is another potent vaccine against TGF-β2 given for Stage II/IIIA/IIIB/IV of NSCLC which showed superior median survival for elevated vaccine doses group as compared to low vaccine doses group (P=0.0069) (Nemunaitis et al; 2006). TGF-b2 inhibits dendritic cells, NK cells, and T_c lymphocytes thus supporting the tumors in escaping immunosurveillance (Thomas et al; 2012).
- Few other vaccines include L-BLP25, a synthetically derived vaccine against Mucin-1 (MUC1) glycoprotein given for stage IIB/V NSCLC (sangha et al; 2011). PRAME (preferentially expressed antigen of melanoma) is another tumor antigen used in vaccine therapy. PRAME overexpression is involved in tumor progression by escaping the suppressive RAR signalling (Epping et al; 2005). Moreover, a PRAME vaccine that combined purified recombinant PRAME protein with adjuvant was evaluated under phase II study (PEARL study) in resected NSCLC (Epping et al; 2005).

6.5. Other agents for NSCLC Treatment

6.5.1. Talactoferrin

Breast milk is the major source of this particular iron-binding protein (Spadro et al; 2008). It was shown to employ naive dendritic cells (DC) into lymphoid follicles present in the gut lymphoid tissue thereby presenting tumor antigens leading to DC maturation (Thomas et al; 2012). The Preclinical studies have depicted suppression of NSCLC tumor growth with talactoferrin (Varadhachary et al; 2004). Talactoferrin showed improved OS in placebo-controlled phase II study, similar results were obtained in advanced stage IIIB/IV NSCLC patients when combined with carboplatin and paclitaxel (Digumarti et al; 2011).

6.5.2. Insulin-like Growth Factor Inhibitors

This system consists of two receptors - Insulin-like growth factor 1 receptor (IGF-IR) and IGF-IIR along with their ligands. These are involved in regulating development of somatic tissues and carbohydrate metabolism (Maki, 2010). It was seen that upregulated IGF-1 levels, and downregulated IGFBP-3/4 levels are associated with increased chances of lung cancer (Capelletto & Novello, 2012). Among the various inhibitors developed against the IGF signalling pathway, Figitumumab, IGF-1R targeting monoclonal antibody depicted enhanced overall response rates in phase II trial when compared to chemotherapy in earlier untreated advanced or metastatic NSCLC cases (Minucci & Pelicci, 2006).

6.5.3. Histone Deacetylase Inhibitors

Histone deacetylases (HDACs) are upregulated in a variety of cancers and are usually involved in repressing gene expression by causing chromatin condensation (Schrump et al; 2009). HDACs have emerged as an interesting target for cancer therapy because epigenetic modifications caused by HDACs are reversible (Owannikoko et al; 2010). Various HDAC inhibitors are involved in modulating the acetylation status of many vital cellular proteins such as p53, STAT3, α-tubulin involve in tumor growth and proliferation (Ramalingam et al; 2010). HDAC inhibitors have shown anticancer activity in animal models of carcinogenesis such as SAHA, Vorinostat and Romidepsin, are FDA approved for cutaneous T-cell lymphoma (CTCL) treatment. Various other inhibitors like entinostat, cI-994, pivanex and romidepsin, are being explored clinically for treatment of NSCLC (Zhang et al; 2009).

7. CONCLUSION

The non-small cell lung cancer incidence is growing with each passing day primarily due to its poor prognosis and delayed detection. Despite the available treatment options that include chemotherapy, radiation therapy, immunotherapy and surgery, the disease rate continues to increase due to factors like systemic toxicity and drug resistance genesis thereby leading to therapy failure. For the management of non-small cell lung cancer, nanoparticle-based systems are being explored for the imaging, screening, and treatment of primary tumors. The global burden of lung cancer is suspected to increase sharply with rising tobacco-smoking rates. While smoking has decreased in the Western world, but it is on the rise globally and in many developing nations such as China. Underprivileged populations are at higher risk of lung cancer, cigarette smoking, infections, due to lower access to healthcare and worsened lung cancer survival rates. Prevention steps taken to control the disease burden should target such risk factors that include smoking, occupational and environmental exposure to carcinogens, and HIV and Tb infection.

8. FUTURE DIRECTIONS

NSCLC is the predominant cancer type and most cases are usually diagnosed at advanced stage of disease making it difficult to treat. Expanding the access to screening, nicotine addiction programs, and experimental lung cancer treatments can help reduce the mortality rates among underprivileged populations. The treatment options of NSCLC have evolved remarkably in the past years. A better understanding of the tumour microenvironment has enabled the development of targeted therapies leading to the rise of personalized medicine. It is important to understand that this benefit from current standard therapies is only observed in few patients, with targeted therapies limited to histological subtypes having actionable driver mutations, and durable responses from immunotherapy occurring uncommonly. Moreover, targeted therapy is also linked to the emergence of secondary clones that are less effectively targeted by the initial treatment directed at the primary clone. Therefore, to improve the treatment outcomes, there is a need to focus on the mechanisms behind acquired resistance to allow their prevention at the early stages.

REFERENCES

Aizawa, K., Liu, C., Tang, S., Veeramachaneni, S., Hu, K. Q., Smith, D. E., & Wang, X. D. (2016). Tobacco carcinogen induces both lung cancer and non-alcoholic steatohepatitis and hepatocellular carcinomas in ferrets which can be attenuated by lycopene supplementation. *International Journal of Cancer, 139*(5), 1171–1181. DOI: 10.1002/ijc.30161 PMID: 27116542

Al-Sayed, E. M., & Ibrahim, K. S. (2014). Second-hand tobacco smoke and children. *Toxicology and Industrial Health, 30*(7), 635–644. DOI: 10.1177/0748233712462473 PMID: 23042595

Alberg, A. J., Brock, M. V., Ford, J. G., Samet, J. M., & Spivack, S. D. (2013). Epidemiology of lung cancer: Diagnosis and management of lung cancer, 3rd ed: American College of Chest Physicians evidence-based clinical practice guidelines. *Chest, 143(5 Suppl)*, e1S–e29S.

Alberg, A. J., Yung, R. C., Strickland, P., & Nelson, J. (2002). Respiratory cancer and exposure to arsenic, chromium, nickel, and polycyclic aromatic hydrocarbons. *Clinics in Occupational and Environmental Medicine, 2*(4), 779–801. DOI: 10.1016/S1526-0046(02)00056-0

Albin, M., Magnani, C., Krstev, S., Rapiti, E., & Shefer, I. (1999). Asbestos and cancer: An overview of current trends in Europe. *Environmental Health Perspectives, 107*(Suppl 2), 289–298. PMID: 10350513

Alegre, M. L., Frauwirth, K. A., & Thompson, C. B. (2001). T-cell regulation by CD28 and CTLA-4. *Nature Reviews. Immunology, 1*(3), 220–228. DOI: 10.1038/35105024 PMID: 11905831

Bagnardi, V., Blangiardo, M., La Vecchia, C., & Corrao, G. (2001). A meta-analysis of alcohol drinking and cancer risk. *British Journal of Cancer, 85*(11), 1700–1705. DOI: 10.1054/bjoc.2001.2140 PMID: 11742491

Bagnardi, V., Rota, M., Botteri, E., Tramacere, I., Islami, F., Fedirko, V., Scotti, L., Jenab, M., Turati, F., Pasquali, E., Pelucchi, C., Galeone, C., Bellocco, R., Negri, E., Corrao, G., Boffetta, P., & La Vecchia, C. (2015). Alcohol consumption and site-specific cancer risk: A comprehensive dose-response meta-analysis. *British Journal of Cancer, 112*(3), 580–593. DOI: 10.1038/bjc.2014.579 PMID: 25422909

Barr, A. J. (2018). The biochemical basis of disease. *Essays in Biochemistry, 62*(5), 619–642. DOI: 10.1042/EBC20170054 PMID: 30509933

Barta, J. A., Powell, C. A., & Wisnivesky, J. P. (2019). Global Epidemiology of Lung Cancer. *Annals of Global Health, 85*(1), 8. DOI: 10.5334/aogh.2419 PMID: 30741509

Beer, D. G., Kardia, S. L., Huang, C. C., Giordano, T. J., Levin, A. M., Misek, D. E., Lin, L., Chen, G., Gharib, T. G., Thomas, D. G., Lizyness, M. L., Kuick, R., Hayasaka, S., Taylor, J. M., Iannettoni, M. D., Orringer, M. B., & Hanash, S. (2002). Gene-expression profiles predict survival of patients with lung adenocarcinoma. *Nature Medicine, 8*(8), 816–824. DOI: 10.1038/nm733 PMID: 12118244

Berthiller, J., Straif, K., Boniol, M., Voirin, N., Benhaïm-Luzon, V., Ayoub, W. B., Dari, I., Laouamri, S., Hamdi-Cherif, M., Bartal, M., Ayed, F. B., & Sasco, A. J. (2008). Cannabis smoking and risk of lung cancer in men: a pooled analysis of three studies in Maghreb. *Journal of thoracic oncology: official publication of the International Association for the Study of Lung Cancer, 3*(12), 1398–1403.

Bertram, J. S. (2000). The molecular biology of cancer. *Molecular Aspects of Medicine, 21*(6), 167–223. DOI: 10.1016/S0098-2997(00)00007-8 PMID: 11173079

Bhattacharjee, A., Richards, W. G., Staunton, J., Li, C., Monti, S., Vasa, P., Ladd, C., Beheshti, J., Bueno, R., Gillette, M., Loda, M., Weber, G., Mark, E. J., Lander, E. S., Wong, W., Johnson, B. E., Golub, T. R., Sugarbaker, D. J., & Meyerson, M. (2001). Classification of human lung carcinomas by mRNA expression profiling reveals distinct adenocarcinoma subclasses. *Proceedings of the National Academy of Sciences of the United States of America, 98*(24), 13790–13795. DOI: 10.1073/pnas.191502998 PMID: 11707567

Bi, Y., Qu, Y., Liang, Z., Liu, Z., Zhang, H., Liang, X., Luo, Y., Cao, J., Zhang, H., & Feng, R. (2018). Clinicopathological analysis of Large Cell Lung Carcinomas definitely diagnosed according to the New World Health Organization Criteria. *Pathology, Research and Practice, 214*(4), 555–559. DOI: 10.1016/j.prp.2018.02.006 PMID: 29525405

Bray, F., Laversanne, M., Sung, H., Ferlay, J., Siegel, R. L., Soerjomataram, I., & Jemal, A. (2024). Global cancer statistics 2022: GLOBOCAN estimates of incidence and mortality worldwide for 36 cancers in 185 countries. *CA: a Cancer Journal for Clinicians, 74*(3), 229–263. DOI: 10.3322/caac.21834 PMID: 38572751

Cao, L., Li, Z. W., Wang, M., Zhang, T. T., Bao, B., & Liu, Y. P. (2019). Clinicopathological characteristics, treatment and survival of pulmonary large cell neuroendocrine carcinoma: A SEER population-based study. *PeerJ, 7*, e6539. DOI: 10.7717/peerj.6539 PMID: 30944773

Capelletto, E., & Novello, S. (2012). Emerging new agents for the management of patients with non-small cell lung cancer. *Drugs*, *72*(Suppl 1), 37–52. DOI: 10.2165/1163028-S0-000000000-00000 PMID: 22712796

Cersosimo R. J. (2002). Lung cancer: a review. *American journal of health-system pharmacy: AJHP: official journal of the American Society of Health-System Pharmacists, 59*(7), 611–642.

Chan, A. W., Chau, S. L., Tong, J. H., Chow, C., Kwan, J. S. H., Chung, L. Y., Lung, R. W., Tong, C. Y., Tin, E. K., Law, P. P., Law, W. T., Ng, C. S. H., Wan, I. Y. P., Mok, T. S. K., & To, K. F. (2019). The Landscape of Actionable Molecular Alterations in Immunomarker-Defined Large-Cell Carcinoma of the Lung. *Journal of thoracic oncology: official publication of the International Association for the Study of Lung Cancer, 14*(7), 1213–1222.

Ciriello, G., Miller, M. L., Aksoy, B. A., Senbabaoglu, Y., Schultz, N., & Sander, C. (2013). Emerging landscape of oncogenic signatures across human cancers. *Nature Genetics*, *45*(10), 1127–1133. DOI: 10.1038/ng.2762 PMID: 24071851

Coelho, M. A., de Carné Trécesson, S., Rana, S., Zecchin, D., Moore, C., Molina-Arcas, M., East, P., Spencer-Dene, B., Nye, E., Barnouin, K., Snijders, A. P., Lai, W. S., Blackshear, P. J., & Downward, J. (2017). Oncogenic RAS Signalling Promotes Tumor Immunoresistance by Stabilizing PD-L1 mRNA. *Immunity*, *47*(6), 1083–1099. e6. DOI: 10.1016/j.immuni.2017.11.016 PMID: 29246442

Copin, M. C. (2016). Carcinome à grandes cellules, carcinome lymphoepithelioma-like, carcinome NUT [Large cell carcinoma, lymphoepithelioma-like carcinoma, NUT carcinoma]. *Annales de Pathologie*, *36*(1), 24–33. DOI: 10.1016/j.annpat.2015.11.006 PMID: 26739900

Corrao, G., Bagnardi, V., Zambon, A., & La Vecchia, C. (2004). A meta-analysis of alcohol consumption and the risk of 15 diseases. *Preventive Medicine*, *38*(5), 613–619. DOI: 10.1016/j.ypmed.2003.11.027 PMID: 15066364

Couraud, S., Zalcman, G., Milleron, B., Morin, F., & Souquet, P. J. (2012). Lung cancer in never smokers--a review. *European journal of cancer (Oxford, England: 1990), 48*(9), 1299–1311.

Curtis, C., Shah, S. P., Chin, S. F., Turashvili, G., Rueda, O. M., Dunning, M. J., Speed, D., Lynch, A. G., Samarajiwa, S., Yuan, Y., Gräf, S., Ha, G., Haffari, G., Bashashati, A., Russell, R., McKinney, S., Langerød, A., Green, A., Provenzano, E., & Aparicio, S.METABRIC Group. (2012). The genomic and transcriptomic architecture of 2,000 breast tumours reveals novel subgroups. *Nature*, *486*(7403), 346–352. DOI: 10.1038/nature10983 PMID: 22522925 da Cunha Santos, G., Shepherd, F. A., & Tsao, M. S. (2011). EGFR mutations and lung cancer. *Annual Review of Pathology, 6*(1), 49–69. DOI: 10.1146/annurev-pathol-011110-130206 PMID: 20887192

Dacic, S., Kelly, L., Shuai, Y., & Nikiforova, M. N. (2010). miRNA expression profiling of lung adenocarcinomas: correlation with mutational status. *Modern pathology: an official journal of the United States and Canadian Academy of Pathology. Inc, 23*(12), 1577–1582.

Damstrup, L., Rygaard, K., Spang-Thomsen, M., & Poulsen, H. S. (1992). Expression of the epidermal growth factor receptor in human small cell lung cancer cell lines. *Cancer Research, 52*(11), 3089–3093. PMID: 1317257

Dela Cruz, C. S., Tanoue, T. L., & Matthany, R. A. (2009). Lung Cancer: Epidemiology and Carcinogenesis. In Shields, T. W. (Ed.), *General Thoracic Surgery* (7th ed., pp. 1281–1298). Wolters Kluwer Health/Lippincott Williams & Wilkins.

Detterbeck, F. C. (2018). The eighth edition TNM stage classification for lung cancer: What does it mean on main street? *The Journal of thoracic and cardiovascular surgery, 155*(1), 356–359.

Digumarti, R., Wang, Y., Raman, G., Doval, D. C., Advani, S. H., Julka, P. K., Parikh, P. M., Patil, S., Nag, S., Madhavan, J., Bapna, A., Ranade, A. A., Varadhachary, A., & Malik, R. (2011). A randomized, double-blind, placebo-controlled, phase II study of oral talactoferrin in combination with carboplatin and paclitaxel in previously untreated locally advanced or metastatic non-small cell lung cancer. *Journal of thoracic oncology: official publication of the International Association for the Study of Lung Cancer, 6*(6), 1098–1103.

Dinakar, C., & O'Connor, G. T. (2016). The Health Effects of Electronic Cigarettes. *The New England Journal of Medicine, 375*(14), 1372–1381. DOI: 10.1056/NEJMra1502466 PMID: 27705269

Doll, R. (2010). Evolution of knowledge of the smoking epidemic. *Tobacco: Science, policy, and public health*, 1-13.

Dong, H., Strome, S. E., Salomao, D. R., Tamura, H., Hirano, F., Flies, D. B., Roche, P. C., Lu, J., Zhu, G., Tamada, K., Lennon, V. A., Celis, E., & Chen, L. (2002). Tumor-associated B7-H1 promotes T-cell apoptosis: A potential mechanism of immune evasion. *Nature Medicine, 8*(8), 793–800. DOI: 10.1038/nm730 PMID: 12091876

Ellis, P. M., & Al-Saleh, K. (2012). Multitargeted anti-angiogenic agents and NSCLC: Clinical update and future directions. *Critical Reviews in Oncology/Hematology, 84*(1), 47–58. DOI: 10.1016/j.critrevonc.2012.02.004 PMID: 22405734

Epping, M. T., Wang, L., Edel, M. J., Carlée, L., Hernandez, M., & Bernards, R. (2005). The human tumor antigen PRAME is a dominant repressor of retinoic acid receptor signaling. *Cell, 122*(6), 835–847. DOI: 10.1016/j.cell.2005.07.003 PMID: 16179254

Erasmus, J. J., McAdams, H. P., & Patz, E. F.Jr. (1999). Non-small cell lung cancer: FDG-PET imaging. *Journal of Thoracic Imaging, 14*(4), 247–256. DOI: 10.1097/00005382-199910000-00004 PMID: 10524805

Fasihnia, S. H., Peighambardoust, S. H., Peighambardoust, S. J., Oromiehie, A., Soltanzadeh, M., Pateiro, M., & Lorenzo, J. M. (2020). Properties and Application of Multifunctional Composite Polypropylene-Based Films Incorporating a Combination of BHT, BHA and Sorbic Acid in Extending Donut Shelf-Life. *Molecules (Basel, Switzerland), 25*(21), 5197. DOI: 10.3390/molecules25215197 PMID: 33171666

Fasihnia, S. H., Peighambardoust, S. H., Peighambardoust, S. J., Oromiehie, A., Soltanzadeh, M., & Peressini, D. (2020). Migration analysis, antioxidant, and mechanical characterization of polypropylene-based active food packaging films loaded with BHA, BHT, and TBHQ. *Journal of Food Science, 85*(8), 2317–2328. DOI: 10.1111/1750-3841.15337 PMID: 32686157

Ferlay, J., Ervik, M., Lam, F., Colombet, M., Mery, L., Pineros, M., Znaor, A., Soerjomataram, I. and Bray, F. (2020). Global Cancer Observatory: Cancer Today. International Agency for Research on Cancer, Lyon.

Garber, M. E., Troyanskaya, O. G., Schluens, K., Petersen, S., Thaesler, Z., Pacyna-Gengelbach, M., van de Rijn, M., Rosen, G. D., Perou, C. M., Whyte, R. I., Altman, R. B., Brown, P. O., Botstein, D., & Petersen, I. (2001). Diversity of gene expression in adenocarcinoma of the lung. *Proceedings of the National Academy of Sciences of the United States of America, 98*(24), 13784–13789. DOI: 10.1073/pnas.241500798 PMID: 11707590

Giordano, T. J., Shedden, K. A., Schwartz, D. R., Kuick, R., Taylor, J. M., Lee, N., Misek, D. E., Greenson, J. K., Kardia, S. L., Beer, D. G., Rennert, G., Cho, K. R., Gruber, S. B., Fearon, E. R., & Hanash, S. (2001). Organ-specific molecular classification of primary lung, colon, and ovarian adenocarcinomas using gene expression profiles. *American Journal of Pathology, 159*(4), 1231–1238. DOI: 10.1016/S0002-9440(10)62509-6 PMID: 11583950

Guinney, J., Dienstmann, R., Wang, X., de Reyniès, A., Schlicker, A., Soneson, C., Marisa, L., Roepman, P., Nyamundanda, G., Angelino, P., Bot, B. M., Morris, J. S., Simon, I. M., Gerster, S., Fessler, E., De Sousa, E., Melo, F., Missiaglia, E., Ramay, H., & Tejpar, S. (2015). The consensus molecular subtypes of colorectal cancer. *Nature Medicine*, *21*(11), 1350–1356. DOI: 10.1038/nm.3967 PMID: 26457759

Guo, Z., Xie, Z., Shi, H., Du, W., Peng, L., Han, W., Duan, F., Zhang, X., Chen, M., Duan, J., Lin, J., Chen, X., Lizaso, A. A., Han-Zhang, H., He, J., & Yin, W. (2019). Malignant pleural effusion supernatant is an alternative liquid biopsy specimen for comprehensive mutational profiling. *Thoracic Cancer*, *10*(4), 823–831. DOI: 10.1111/1759-7714.13006 PMID: 30779318

Hackshaw, A. K. (1998). Lung cancer and passive smoking. *Statistical Methods in Medical Research*, *7*(2), 119–136. DOI: 10.1177/096228029800700203 PMID: 9654638

Hafner, A., Bulyk, M. L., Jambhekar, A., & Lahav, G. (2019). The multiple mechanisms that regulate p53 activity and cell fate. *Nature Reviews. Molecular Cell Biology*, *20*(4), 199–210. DOI: 10.1038/s41580-019-0110-x PMID: 30824861

Hanafusa, H., Torii, S., Yasunaga, T., & Nishida, E. (2002). Sprouty1 and Sprouty2 provide a control mechanism for the Ras/MAPK signalling pathway. *Nature Cell Biology*, *4*(11), 850–858. DOI: 10.1038/ncb867 PMID: 12402043

Hanagiri, T., Oka, S., Takenaka, S., Baba, T., Yasuda, M., Ono, K., So, T., Uramoto, H., Takenoyama, M., & Yasumoto, K. (2010). Results of surgical resection for patients with large cell carcinoma of the lung. *International Journal of Surgery*, *8*(5), 391–394. DOI: 10.1016/j.ijsu.2010.06.003 PMID: 20547250

Harbour, J. W., Lai, S. L., Whang-Peng, J., Gazdar, A. F., Minna, J. D., & Kaye, F. J. (1988). Abnormalities in structure and expression of the human retinoblastoma gene in SCLC. *Science*, *241*(4863), 353–357. DOI: 10.1126/science.2838909 PMID: 2838909

Heller, G., Babinsky, V. N., Ziegler, B., Weinzierl, M., Noll, C., Altenberger, C., Müllauer, L., Dekan, G., Grin, Y., Lang, G., End-Pfützenreuter, A., Steiner, I., Zehetmayer, S., Döme, B., Arns, B. M., Fong, K. M., Wright, C. M., Yang, I. A., Klepetko, W., & Zöchbauer-Müller, S. (2013). Genome-wide CpG island methylation analyses in non-small cell lung cancer patients. *Carcinogenesis*, *34*(3), 513–521. DOI: 10.1093/carcin/bgs363 PMID: 23172663

Hellmann, M. D., Ciuleanu, T. E., Pluzanski, A., Lee, J. S., Otterson, G. A., Audigier-Valette, C., Minenza, E., Linardou, H., Burgers, S., Salman, P., Borghaei, H., Ramalingam, S. S., Brahmer, J., Reck, M., O'Byrne, K. J., Geese, W. J., Green, G., Chang, H., Szustakowski, J., & Paz-Ares, L. (2018). Nivolumab plus Ipilimumab in Lung Cancer with a High Tumor Mutational Burden. *The New England Journal of Medicine*, *378*(22), 2093–2104. DOI: 10.1056/NEJMoa1801946 PMID: 29658845

Herbst, R. S., Heymach, J. V., & Lippman, S. M. (2008). Lung cancer. *The New England Journal of Medicine*, *359*(13), 1367–1380. DOI: 10.1056/NEJMra0802714 PMID: 18815398

Hou, L. K., Zhang, L. P., Zhang, W., Huang, Y., Wu, W., Dong, Z. W., & Wu, C. Y. (2017). Zhonghua bing li xue za zhi [Clinicopathologic features and genetic profile of the redefined large cell lung carcinoma]. *Chinese journal of pathology*, *46*(5), 298–302.

IARC Working Group on the Evaluation of Carcinogenic Risks to Humans. Personal Habits and Indoor Combustions. (2022). *Lyon (FR): International Agency for Research on Cancer,* (IARC Monographs on the Evaluation of Carcinogenic Risks to Humans, No. 100E).

Islami, F., Goding Sauer, A., Miller, K. D., Siegel, R. L., Fedewa, S. A., Jacobs, E. J., McCullough, M. L., Patel, A. V., Ma, J., Soerjomataram, I., Flanders, W. D., Brawley, O. W., Gapstur, S. M., & Jemal, A. (2018). Proportion and number of cancer cases and deaths attributable to potentially modifiable risk factors in the United States. *CA: a Cancer Journal for Clinicians*, *68*(1), 31–54. DOI: 10.3322/caac.21440 PMID: 29160902

Jamal, A., Phillips, E., Gentzke, A. S., Homa, D. M., Babb, S. D., King, B. A., & Neff, L. J. (2018). Current Cigarette Smoking Among Adults - United States, 2016. *MMWR. Morbidity and Mortality Weekly Report*, *67*(2), 53–59. DOI: 10.15585/mmwr.mm6702a1 PMID: 29346338

Janic, A., Valente, L., Wakefield, M., Di Stefano, L., Milla, L., Wilcox, S., Yang, H., Tai, L., Vandenberg, C., Kueh, A., Mizutani, S., Brennan, M., Schenk, R., Lindqvist, L., Papenfuss, A., O'Connor, L., Strasser, A., & Herold, M. (2018). DNA repair processes are critical mediators of p53-dependent tumor suppression letter. *Nature Medicine*, *24*(7), 947–953. DOI: 10.1038/s41591-018-0043-5 PMID: 29892060

Joseph, A. M., Muggli, M., Pearson, K. C., & Lando, H. (2005). The cigarette manufacturers' efforts to promote tobacco to the U.S. military. *Military Medicine*, *170*(10), 874–880. DOI: 10.7205/MILMED.170.10.874 PMID: 16435763

Kabbani, N. (2013). Not so Cool? Menthol's discovered actions on the nicotinic receptor and its implications for nicotine addiction. *Frontiers in Pharmacology*, *4*, 95. DOI: 10.3389/fphar.2013.00095 PMID: 23898298

Kennedy, T. C., Hirsch, F. R., Miller, Y. E., Prindiville, S., Murphy, J. R., Dempsey, E., Proudfoot, S., Bunn, P. A., & Franklin, W. A. (2000). A randomized study of fluorescence bronchoscopy versus white-light bronchoscopy for early detection of lung cancer in high-risk patients. *Lung Cancer (Amsterdam, Netherlands)*, *29*(1), 244–245. DOI: 10.1016/S0169-5002(00)80835-1

Kern, J. A., Slebos, R. J., Top, B., Rodenhuis, S., Lager, D., Robinson, R. A., Weiner, D., & Schwartz, D. A. (1994). C-erbB-2 expression and codon 12 K-ras mutations both predict shortened survival for patients with pulmonary adenocarcinomas. *The Journal of Clinical Investigation*, *93*(2), 516–520. DOI: 10.1172/JCI117001 PMID: 7906694

Kristeleit, H., Enting, D., & Lai, R. (2011). Basic science of lung cancer. *European journal of cancer (Oxford, England: 1990)*, *47 Suppl 3*, S319–S321.

Kupeli, M., & Koseoglu, R. D. (2018). Large Cell Carcinoma with Adenocarcinoma in Lung. *Journal of the College of Physicians and Surgeons—Pakistan. Journal of the College of Physicians and Surgeons—Pakistan*, *28*(3), 240–242. DOI: 10.29271/jcpsp.2018.03.240 PMID: 29544586

Kurie, J. M., Lee, J. S., Morice, R. C., Walsh, G. L., Khuri, F. R., Broxson, A., Ro, J. Y., Franklin, W. A., Yu, R., & Hong, W. K. (1998). Autofluorescence bronchoscopy in the detection of squamous metaplasia and dysplasia in current and former smokers. *Journal of the National Cancer Institute*, *90*(13), 991–995. DOI: 10.1093/jnci/90.13.991 PMID: 9665147

Lebanony, D., Benjamin, H., Gilad, S., Ezagouri, M., Dov, A., Ashkenazi, K., Gefen, N., Izraeli, S., Rechavi, G., Pass, H., Nonaka, D., Li, J., Spector, Y., Rosenfeld, N., Chajut, A., Cohen, D., Aharonov, R., & Mansukhani, M. (2009). Diagnostic assay based on hsa-miR-205 expression distinguishes squamous from nonsquamous non-small-cell lung carcinoma. *Journal of Clinical Oncology*, *27*(12), 2030–2037. DOI: 10.1200/JCO.2008.19.4134 PMID: 19273703

Lee, Y. J., Kim, J. H., Kim, S. K., Ha, S. J., Mok, T. S., Mitsudomi, T., & Cho, B. C. (2011). Lung cancer in never smokers: Change of a mindset in the molecular era. *Lung Cancer (Amsterdam, Netherlands)*, *72*(1), 9–15. DOI: 10.1016/j.lungcan.2010.12.013 PMID: 21272954

Levine, A. J. (2019). The many faces of p53: Something for everyone. *Journal of Molecular Cell Biology*, *11*(7), 524–530. DOI: 10.1093/jmcb/mjz026 PMID: 30925588

Lockwood, W. W., Wilson, I. M., Coe, B. P., Chari, R., Pikor, L. A., Thu, K. L., Solis, L. M., Nunez, M. I., Behrens, C., Yee, J., English, J., Murray, N., Tsao, M. S., Minna, J. D., Gazdar, A. F., Wistuba, I. I., MacAulay, C. E., Lam, S., & Lam, W. L. (2012). Divergent genomic and epigenomic landscapes of lung cancer subtypes underscore the selection of different oncogenic pathways during tumor development. *PLoS One*, *7*(5), e37775. DOI: 10.1371/journal.pone.0037775 PMID: 22629454

Maki, R. G. (2010). Small is beautiful: Insulin-like growth factors and their role in growth, development, and cancer. *Journal of Clinical Oncology*, *28*(33), 4985–4995. DOI: 10.1200/JCO.2009.27.5040 PMID: 20975071

Massarelli, E., Papadimitrakopoulou, V., Welsh, J., Tang, C., & Tsao, A. S. (2014). Immunotherapy in lung cancer. *Translational Lung Cancer Research*, *3*(1), 53–63. PMID: 25806281

McDoniels-Silvers, A. L., Nimri, C. F., Stoner, G. D., Lubet, R. A., & You, M. (2002). Differential gene expression in human lung adenocarcinomas and squamous cell carcinomas. *Clinical Cancer Research*, *8*(4), 1127–1138. PMID: 11948124

Meacham, C. E., & Morrison, S. J. (2013). Tumour heterogeneity and cancer cell plasticity. *Nature*, *501*(7467), 328–337. DOI: 10.1038/nature12624 PMID: 24048065

Minimo, C., Bibbo, M., Claudio, P. P., De Luca, A., & Giordano, A. (1999). The role of pRb2/p130 protein in diagnosing lung carcinoma on fine needle aspiration biopsies. *Pathology, Research and Practice*, *195*(2), 67–70. DOI: 10.1016/S0344-0338(99)80072-7 PMID: 10093823

Minucci, S., & Pelicci, P. G. (2006). Histone deacetylase inhibitors and the promise of epigenetic (and more) treatments for cancer. *Nature Reviews. Cancer*, *6*(1), 38–51. DOI: 10.1038/nrc1779 PMID: 16397526

Murray, N., Coy, P., Pater, J. L., Hodson, I., Arnold, A., Zee, B. C., Payne, D., Kostashuk, E. C., Evans, W. K., & Dixon, P.The National Cancer Institute of Canada Clinical Trials Group. (1993). Importance of timing for thoracic irradiation in the combined modality treatment of limited-stage small-cell lung cancer. The National Cancer Institute of Canada Clinical Trials Group. *Journal of Clinical Oncology*, *11*(2), 336–344. DOI: 10.1200/JCO.1993.11.2.336 PMID: 8381164

Nacht, M., Dracheva, T., Gao, Y., Fujii, T., Chen, Y., Player, A., Akmaev, V., Cook, B., Dufault, M., Zhang, M., Zhang, W., Guo, M., Curran, J., Han, S., Sidransky, D., Buetow, K., Madden, S. L., & Jen, J. (2001). Molecular characteristics of non-small cell lung cancer. *Proceedings of the National Academy of Sciences of the United States of America*, *98*(26), 15203–15208. DOI: 10.1073/pnas.261414598 PMID: 11752463

Nemunaitis, J., Dillman, R. O., Schwarzenberger, P. O., Senzer, N., Cunningham, C., Cutler, J., Tong, A., Kumar, P., Pappen, B., Hamilton, C., DeVol, E., Maples, P. B., Liu, L., Chamberlin, T., Shawler, D. L., & Fakhrai, H. (2006). Phase II study of belagenpumatucel-L, a transforming growth factor beta-2 antisense gene-modified allogeneic tumor cell vaccine in non-small-cell lung cancer. *Journal of Clinical Oncology*, *24*(29), 4721–4730. DOI: 10.1200/JCO.2005.05.5335 PMID: 16966690

Nooreldeen, R., & Bach, H. (2021). Current and Future Development in Lung Cancer Diagnosis. *International Journal of Molecular Sciences*, *22*(16), 8661. DOI: 10.3390/ijms22168661 PMID: 34445366

Oberg, M., Jaakkola, M. S., Woodward, A., Peruga, A., & Prüss-Ustün, A. (2011). Worldwide burden of disease from exposure to second-hand smoke: A retrospective analysis of data from 192 countries. *Lancet*, *377*(9760), 139–146. DOI: 10.1016/S0140-6736(10)61388-8 PMID: 21112082

Oken, M. M., Creech, R. H., Tormey, D. C., Horton, J., Davis, T. E., McFadden, E. T., & Carbone, P. P. (1982). Toxicity and response criteria of the Eastern Cooperative Oncology Group. *American Journal of Clinical Oncology*, *5*(6), 649–655. DOI: 10.1097/00000421-198212000-00014 PMID: 7165009

Pardoll, D. M. (2012). The blockade of immune checkpoints in cancer immunotherapy. *Nature Reviews. Cancer*, *12*(4), 252–264. DOI: 10.1038/nrc3239 PMID: 22437870

Parkin, D. M., Bray, F., Ferlay, J., & Pisani, P. (2005). Global cancer statistics, 2002. *CA: a Cancer Journal for Clinicians*, *55*(2), 74–108. DOI: 10.3322/canjclin.55.2.74 PMID: 15761078

Paz-Ares, L., de Marinis, F., Dediu, M., Thomas, M., Pujol, J. L., Bidoli, P., Molinier, O., Sahoo, T. P., Laack, E., Reck, M., Corral, J., Melemed, S., John, W., Chouaki, N., Zimmermann, A. H., Visseren-Grul, C., & Gridelli, C. (2012). Maintenance therapy with pemetrexed plus best supportive care versus placebo plus best supportive care after induction therapy with pemetrexed plus cisplatin for advanced non-squamous non-small-cell lung cancer (PARAMOUNT): A double-blind, phase 3, randomised controlled trial. *The Lancet. Oncology*, *13*(3), 247–255. DOI: 10.1016/S1470-2045(12)70063-3 PMID: 22341744

Paz-Ares, L., Horn, L., Borghaei, H., Spigel, D., Steins, M., Ready, N., Chow, L., Vokes, E., Felip, E., Holgado, E., Barlesi, F., Kohlhaeufl, M., Rodriguez, O., Burgio, M., Fayette, J., Gettinger, S., Harbison, C., Dorange, C., Finckenstein, F., & Brahmer, J. (2015). Phase III, randomized trial (CheckMate 057) of nivolumab (NIVO) versus docetaxel (DOC) in advanced non-squamous cell (non-SQ) non-small cell lung cancer (NSCLC). *Journal of Clinical Oncology*, *33*(18_suppl), LBA109–LBA109. DOI: 10.1200/jco.2015.33.18_suppl.lba109

Pfeiffer, P., Clausen, P. P., Andersen, K., & Rose, C. (1996). Lack of prognostic significance of epidermal growth factor receptor and the oncoprotein p185HER-2 in patients with systemically untreated non-small-cell lung cancer: An immunohistochemical study on cryosections. *British Journal of Cancer*, *74*(1), 86–91. DOI: 10.1038/bjc.1996.320 PMID: 8679464

Planchard, D., Popat, S., Kerr, K., Novello, S., Smit, E. F., Faivre-Finn, C., Mok, T. S., Reck, M., Van Schil, P. E., Hellmann, M. D., & Peters, S.ESMO Guidelines Committee. (2018). Metastatic non-small cell lung cancer: ESMO Clinical Practice Guidelines for diagnosis, treatment and follow-up. *Annals of Oncology : Official Journal of the European Society for Medical Oncology*, *29*(Suppl 4), iv192–iv237. DOI: 10.1093/annonc/mdy275 PMID: 30285222

Rachwal, W. J., Bongiorno, P. F., Orringer, M. B., Whyte, R. I., Ethier, S. P., & Beer, D. G. (1995). Expression and activation of erbB-2 and epidermal growth factor receptor in lung adenocarcinomas. *British Journal of Cancer*, *72*(1), 56–64. DOI: 10.1038/bjc.1995.277 PMID: 7599067

Ramalingam, S. S., Maitland, M. L., Frankel, P., Argiris, A. E., Koczywas, M., Gitlitz, B., Thomas, S., Espinoza-Delgado, I., Vokes, E. E., Gandara, D. R., & Belani, C. P. (2010). Carboplatin and Paclitaxel in combination with either vorinostat or placebo for first-line therapy of advanced non-small-cell lung cancer. *Journal of Clinical Oncology*, *28*(1), 56–62. DOI: 10.1200/JCO.2009.24.9094 PMID: 19933908

Richardson, G. E., & Johnson, B. E. (1993). The biology of lung cancer. *Seminars in Oncology*, *20*(2), 105–127. PMID: 8480184

Risse, E. K., Vooijs, G. P., & van't Hof, M. A. (1987). Relationship between the cellular composition of sputum and the cytologic diagnosis of lung cancer. *Acta Cytologica*, *31*(2), 170–176. PMID: 3469850

Rudin, C. M., Avila-Tang, E., Harris, C. C., Herman, J. G., Hirsch, F. R., Pao, W., Schwartz, A. G., Vahakangas, K. H., & Samet, J. M. (2009). Lung cancer in never smokers: Molecular profiles and therapeutic implications. *Clinical Cancer Research*, *15*(18), 5646–5661. DOI: 10.1158/1078-0432.CCR-09-0377 PMID: 19755392

Sangha, R., Price, J., & Butts, C. A. (2010). Adjuvant therapy in non-small cell lung cancer: Current and future directions. *The Oncologist, 15*(8), 862–872. DOI: 10.1634/theoncologist.2009-0186 PMID: 20682608

Schottenfeld, D., & Fraumeni, J. F., Jr., (Eds.). (2006). *Cancer Epidemiology and Prevention.* Oxford University Press. 3, 638-658. DOI: 10.1093/acprof:oso/9780195149616.001.0001

Schrump, D. S. (2009). Cytotoxicity mediated by histone deacetylase inhibitors in cancer cells: Mechanisms and potential clinical implications. *Clinical Cancer Research, 15*(12), 3947–3957. DOI: 10.1158/1078-0432.CCR-08-2787 PMID: 19509170

Selamat, S. A., Chung, B. S., Girard, L., Zhang, W., Zhang, Y., Campan, M., Siegmund, K. D., Koss, M. N., Hagen, J. A., Lam, W. L., Lam, S., Gazdar, A. F., & Laird-Offringa, I. A. (2012). Genome-scale analysis of DNA methylation in lung adenocarcinoma and integration with mRNA expression. *Genome Research, 22*(7), 1197–1211. DOI: 10.1101/gr.132662.111 PMID: 22613842

Sidorchuk, A., Agardh, E. E., Aremu, O., Hallqvist, J., Allebeck, P., & Moradi, T. (2009). Socioeconomic differences in lung cancer incidence: A systematic review and meta-analysis. *Cancer causes & control. CCC, 20*(4), 459–471. PMID: 19184626

Siegel, R. L., Miller, K. D., Wagle, N. S., & Jemal, A. (2023). Cancer statistics, 2023. *CA: a Cancer Journal for Clinicians, 73*(1), 17–48. DOI: 10.3322/caac.21763 PMID: 36633525

Simons, E., To, T., Moineddin, R., Stieb, D., & Dell, S. D. (2014). Maternal second-hand smoke exposure in pregnancy is associated with childhood asthma development. *The Journal of Allergy and Clinical Immunology. In Practice, 2*(2), 201–207. DOI: 10.1016/j.jaip.2013.11.014 PMID: 24607049

Smith, E. A., & Malone, R. E. (2009). "Everywhere the soldier will be": Wartime tobacco promotion in the US military. *American Journal of Public Health, 99*(9), 1595–1602. DOI: 10.2105/AJPH.2008.152983 PMID: 19608945

Sobue, T., Moriyama, N., Kaneko, M., Kusumoto, M., Kobayashi, T., Tsuchiya, R., Kakinuma, R., Ohmatsu, H., Nagai, K., Nishiyama, H., Matsui, E., & Eguchi, K. (2002). Screening for lung cancer with low-dose helical computed tomography: Anti-lung cancer association project. *Journal of Clinical Oncology, 20*(4), 911–920. DOI: 10.1200/JCO.2002.20.4.911 PMID: 11844811

Socinski, M. A., Scappaticci, F. A., Samant, M., Kolb, M. M., & Kozloff, M. F. (2010). Safety and efficacy of combining sunitinib with bevacizumab + paclitaxel/carboplatin in non-small cell lung cancer. *Journal of thoracic oncology: official publication of the International Association for the Study of Lung Cancer, 5*(3), 354–360.

Socinski, M. A., Schell, M. J., Peterman, A., Bakri, K., Yates, S., Gitten, R., Unger, P., Lee, J., Lee, J. H., Tynan, M., Moore, M., & Kies, M. S. (2002). Phase III trial comparing a defined duration of therapy versus continuous therapy followed by second-line therapy in advanced-stage IIIB/IV non-small-cell lung cancer. *Journal of Clinical Oncology*, *20*(5), 1335–1343. PMID: 11870177

Sun, Y. H., Lin, S. W., Hsieh, C. C., Yeh, Y. C., Tu, C. C., & Chen, K. J. (2014). Treatment outcomes of patients with different subtypes of large cell carcinoma of the lung. *The Annals of Thoracic Surgery*, *98*(3), 1013–1019. DOI: 10.1016/j.athoracsur.2014.05.012 PMID: 25085555

Sundar, R., Cho, B. C., Brahmer, J. R., & Soo, R. A. (2015). Nivolumab in NSCLC: Latest evidence and clinical potential. *Therapeutic Advances in Medical Oncology*, *7*(2), 85–96. DOI: 10.1177/1758834014567470 PMID: 25755681

Sung, H., Ferlay, J., Siegel, R. L., Laversanne, M., Soerjomataram, I., Jemal, A., & Bray, F. (2021). Global Cancer Statistics 2020: GLOBOCAN Estimates of Incidence and Mortality Worldwide for 36 Cancers in 185 Countries. *CA: a Cancer Journal for Clinicians*, *71*(3), 209–249. DOI: 10.3322/caac.21660 PMID: 33538338

Takahashi, T., Nau, M. M., Chiba, I., Birrer, M. J., Rosenberg, R. K., Vinocour, M., Levitt, M., Pass, H., Gazdar, A. F., & Minna, J. D. (1989). p53: a frequent target for genetic abnormalities in lung cancer. *Science*, *246*(4929), 491–494. DOI: 10.1126/science.2554494 PMID: 2554494

Tanoue, L. T., & Detterbeck, F. C. (2009). New TNM classification for non-small-cell lung cancer. *Expert Review of Anticancer Therapy*, *9*(4), 413–423. DOI: 10.1586/era.09.11 PMID: 19374596

Tateishi, M., Ishida, T., Mitsudomi, T., Kaneko, S., & Sugimachi, K. (1990). Immunohistochemical evidence of autocrine growth factors in adenocarcinoma of the human lung. *Cancer Research*, *50*(21), 7077–7080. PMID: 2208175

Thomas, A., & Hassan, R. (2012). Immunotherapies for non-small-cell lung cancer and mesothelioma. *The Lancet. Oncology*, *13*(7), e301–e310. DOI: 10.1016/S1470-2045(12)70126-2 PMID: 22748269

Torok, S., Hegedus, B., Laszlo, V., Hoda, M. A., Ghanim, B., Berger, W., Klepetko, W., Dome, B., & Ostoros, G. (2011). Lung cancer in never smokers. *Future Oncology (London, England)*, *7*(10), 1195–1211. DOI: 10.2217/fon.11.100 PMID: 21992731

Torre, L. A., Siegel, R. L., & Jemal, A. (2016). Lung Cancer Statistics. *Advances in Experimental Medicine and Biology*, *893*, 1–19. DOI: 10.1007/978-3-319-24223-1_1 PMID: 26667336

Toyoda, Y., Nakayama, T., Kusunoki, Y., Iso, H., & Suzuki, T. (2008). Sensitivity and specificity of lung cancer screening using chest low-dose computed tomography. *British Journal of Cancer*, *98*(10), 1602–1607. DOI: 10.1038/sj.bjc.6604351 PMID: 18475292

Travis, W. D., Brambilla, E., Nicholson, A. G., Yatabe, Y., Austin, J. H. M., Beasley, M. B., Chirieac, L. R., Dacic, S., Duhig, E., Flieder, D. B., Geisinger, K., Hirsch, F. R., Ishikawa, Y., Kerr, K. M., Noguchi, M., Pelosi, G., Powell, C. A., Tsao, M. S., Wistuba, I., & WHO Panel (2015). The 2015 World Health Organization Classification of Lung Tumors: Impact of Genetic, Clinical and Radiologic Advances Since the 2004 Classification. *Journal of thoracic oncology: official publication of the International Association for the Study of Lung Cancer, 10*(9), 1243–1260.

Tylecote, F. (1927). Cancer of the Lung. *Lancet*, *210*(5422), 256–257. DOI: 10.1016/S0140-6736(01)30802-4

Vansteenkiste, J., Zielinski, M., Linder, A., Dahabreh, J., Gonzalez, E. E., Malinowski, W., Lopez-Brea, M., Vanakesa, T., Jassem, J., Kalofonos, H., Perdeus, J., Bonnet, R., Basko, J., Janilionis, R., Passlick, B., Treasure, T., Gillet, M., Lehmann, F. F., & Brichard, V. G. (2013). Adjuvant MAGE-A3 immunotherapy in resected non-small-cell lung cancer: Phase II randomized study results. *Journal of Clinical Oncology*, *31*(19), 2396–2403. DOI: 10.1200/JCO.2012.43.7103 PMID: 23715567

Varadhachary, A., Wolf, J. S., Petrak, K., O'Malley, B. W.Jr, Spadaro, M., Curcio, C., Forni, G., & Pericle, F. (2004). Oral lactoferrin inhibits growth of established tumors and potentiates conventional chemotherapy. *International Journal of Cancer*, *111*(3), 398–403. DOI: 10.1002/ijc.20271 PMID: 15221967

Voirin, N., Berthiller, J., Benhaïm-Luzon, V., Boniol, M., Straif, K., Ayoub, W. B., Ayed, F. B., & Sasco, A. J. (2006). Risk of lung cancer and past use of cannabis in Tunisia. *Journal of thoracic oncology: official publication of the International Association for the Study of Lung Cancer, 1*(6), 577–579.

Volkow, N. D., Baler, R. D., Compton, W. M., & Weiss, S. R. (2014). Adverse health effects of marijuana use. *The New England Journal of Medicine*, *370*(23), 2219–2227. DOI: 10.1056/NEJMra1402309 PMID: 24897085

Weiner, D. B., Nordberg, J., Robinson, R., Nowell, P. C., Gazdar, A., Greene, M. I., Williams, W. V., Cohen, J. A., & Kern, J. A. (1990). Expression of the neu gene-encoded protein (P185neu) in human non-small cell carcinomas of the lung. *Cancer Research, 50*(2), 421–425. PMID: 1967224

Weiss, G. J., Langer, C., Rosell, R., Hanna, N., Shepherd, F., Einhorn, L. H., Nguyen, B., Paul, S., McAndrews, P., Bunn, P. A.Jr, & Kelly, K. (2006). Elderly patients benefit from second-line cytotoxic chemotherapy: A subset analysis of a randomized phase III trial of pemetrexed compared with docetaxel in patients with previously treated advanced non-small-cell lung cancer. *Journal of Clinical Oncology, 24*(27), 4405–4411. DOI: 10.1200/JCO.2006.06.7835 PMID: 16983108

Weissferdt, A. (2014). Large cell carcinoma of lung: On the verge of extinction? *Seminars in Diagnostic Pathology, 31*(4), 278–288. DOI: 10.1053/j.semdp.2014.06.005 PMID: 25023633

Yoo, K. Y., & Shin, H. R. (2003). Cancer Epidemiology and Prevention. *Korean J Epidemiol, 25*(1), 1–15. PMID: 11850580

Zappa, C., & Mousa, S. A. (2016). Non-small cell lung cancer: Current treatment and future advances. *Translational Lung Cancer Research, 5*(3), 288–300. DOI: 10.21037/tlcr.2016.06.07 PMID: 27413711

Zhang, W., Peyton, M., Xie, Y., Soh, J., Minna, J. D., Gazdar, A. F., & Frenkel, E. P. (2009). Histone deacetylase inhibitor romidepsin enhances anti-tumor effect of erlotinib in non-small cell lung cancer (NSCLC) cell lines. *Journal of thoracic oncology: official publication of the International Association for the Study of Lung Cancer, 4*(2), 161–166.

Zhang, Y., Yang, J., Na, X., & Zhao, A. (2023). Association between β-carotene supplementation and risk of cancer: A meta-analysis of randomized controlled trials. *Nutrition Reviews, 81*(9), 1118–1130. DOI: 10.1093/nutrit/nuac110 PMID: 36715090

KEY TERMS AND DEFINITIONS

Biomarker: It is a biological molecule that indicates some biological condition within the organism and can be present in any body fluid.

Cancer: It is a complex disease characterized by abnormal cell division, growth, and tumor formation.

Chemotherapy: It is type of treatment given to cancer patients that uses a combination of drugs to destroy abnormally growing cells thereby preventing tumor growth.

Cytology: It involves studying cell structure and function to diagnose or screen any abnormality or disease such as cancer.

Mutation: Alterations occurring in the DNA sequence of an organism caused by errors in DNA replication or environmental factors such as chemicals or radiation.

Necrosis: It is a form of cell death that leads to permanent tissue damage caused due to external factors resulting in activation of inflammatory responses.

Risk factor: Any characteristic that increases the probability of developing a disease or infection.

Tumor suppressor genes: - These genes regulate cell division, proliferation and replication thereby controlling cancer development.

Chapter 2
Genetic Mutations Associated With NSCLC and Molecular Subtypes of NSCLC

Padmavathi Vijayakumar
https://orcid.org/0000-0003-4480-8813
Sacred Heart College, India

M. Mubarak
Sacred Heart College, India

Abirami Palani
Sacred Heart College, India

S. Sindhuja
Sacred Heart College, India

ABSTRACT

Non-small cell lung cancer (NSCLC) represents the greatest prevalent sort of lung cancer. NSCLC constitutes nearly eighty percent of the overall incidence of lung cancer. Squamous cell carcinoma (SCC), adenocarcinoma (ADC), and large-cell carcinoma (LCC) are among the three predominant classifications of NSCLC. NSCLC is primarily triggered by anomalies in the epithelial growth factor receptors (EGFR). The genes that encourage malignancy and are affiliated with several kinds of pathways include EGFR, BRAF, KRAS, MET, ALK, and ROS. The primary risk factor of NSCLC is mutations in these genes. The most effective therapy for NSCLC is based on histological outcomes; nevertheless, its progress, predisposition to me-

DOI: 10.4018/979-8-3373-2096-0.ch002

tastases, and possible treatment are not well recognized. Recently, there has been a considerable increase in the use of targeted medications with low toxicity and high potency for cancer treatment due to mutations in receptor tyrosine kinases such as the EGFR, ALK, MET, and BRAF genes. This chapter explore the several gene mutations, associated pathways and targeted therapies via epigenetic modification, miRNA mutation, copy number alterations in molecular subtypes of NSCLC.

1. INTRODUCTION

Globally, the occurence of malignancy is growing; in 2040, around 28.4 million people will be affected by cancer. Lung cancer is the most common among all cancers, and it's the first cancer-related cause of death (Herbst et al., 2018; Shinya, 2019). Generally, lung cancer involves two groups; small cell lung cancer and non-small cell lung cancer (NSCLC). Squamous cell carcinoma (SCC), adenocarcinoma (ADC), and large-cell carcinoma (LCC) are some of the three primary kinds into which it is commonly divided. Subtypes of NSCLC are characterized by grow and spread in different ways. It encompasses with various subgroups, which affect both the prognosis and treatment. The epidermal growth factor receptor (EGFR) is identified as a first oncogenic alteration, and it's for treating new molecular alterations (Dempke et al., 2010). The tumor node metastasis (TNM) method is often carried to estimate the morphological anomaly, including tumor size, lymph node, and distant metastatic status in NSCLC patients. Identification of molecular subtypes of NSCLC based on the tumor-infiltrated immune cells and prognosis, which is increasingly found to facilitate treatment selection and improve disease management (Herbst et al., 2018; Shinya, 2019). As of right now, lung cancer is known to have targetable molecular changes; Alex et al., 2024 stated that these changes were present in about 80% of Asian and 60% of Western populations. Numerous somatic mutation genes, including EGFR, anaplastic lymphoma kinase (ALK), v-raf murine sarcoma viral oncogene B (BRAF), ROS protooncogene 1 (ROS1), Kirstin rat sarcoma virus (KRAS), human epidermal receptor 2 (HER2), c-MET proto-oncogene (MET), rearranged neurotrophic receptor tyrosine kinase (NTRK), RET, neuregulin 1 (NRG1), phosphoinositide 3-kinase (PI3K), and fibroblast growth factor receptor (FGFR) are among the many genes implicated in NSCLC. Lung cancer mostly results from a combination of environmental and genetic variables, and each cancer cell's genetic mutation profile is completely distinct. The effectiveness of lung cancer treatment has significantly decreased, and tailored medicines are still need for successful therapy. Personalized drug treatment is specifically designed to target a particular gene alteration within an individual tumor (Dempke et al., 2010). For example, in NSCLC patients' mutations with the *EGFR* gene, specifically non-smoking women, are widely treated with erlotinib, which blocks *EGFR* signalling and slows lung cancer progressions (Hannay, 2000; Shepherd et al., 2005).

The signaling pathway is impacted by EGFR, an RTK, while occurring of cell division. If the pathways are altered, normal cells will grow and proliferate uncontrollably (Arteaga, 2000; Yarden & Sliwkowski, 2001; Wieduwilt & Moasser, 2008). Usually, cancer caused by the significantly alterations of some genetic mechanism, hence its guide to defect the DNA repair, suppressor genes, and important oncogenes. Also, in NSCLC, epigenetic factors are most (DNA methylation, histone modification, and RNA expression) high risk of cancer. Specific genetic changes are indicative of each molecular subgroup of NSCLC. Tumorigenesis and treatment response significantly influenced by these differences. For the growth of targeted therapy and pharmaceutical methods, it is imperative to comprehend the genetic profile of NSCLC. In this chapter, we will summarize the current knowledge of genetic alterations and signalling pathways in NSCLC subtypes to enable the realization of the development of the tumorigenesis of NSCLC. Furthermore, we discuss the copy number alterations, miRNAs, and epigenetic modifications for understanding and manipulating specific genetic variations, which is to improve early diagnosis and treatment of NSCLC.

2. MOLECULAR PATHOLOGY IN NSCLC

Right now, advance various methods are using, including NGS, immunohistochemistry (IHC), Whole genome exome sequencing, fluorescence in situ hybridization (FISH), and others, molecular pathology in NSCLC aims to detect genetic changes in order to find new biomarkers and potentially lead to more effective treatments. According to their anatomy and function, the lungs are divided into two sections. Different cellular components make up the terminal respiratory unit and air-conducting system. Type I and Type II alveolar cells constitute a significant epithelial component. The molecular etiology and inherent vulnerability to a particular carcinogen vary. High-grade neuroendocrine tumors, SCC, lCC, and AC are among the molecular subgroups into which the majority of lung malignancies are histologically classified. Each type of lung cancer shows different clinicopathological features. The both LUAD and LUSC cancers are driven by heterogeneous genetic with distinct molecular subtypes and histomorphological growth patterns such as, acinar, papillary, lepidic and micropapillary. LUSC is associated with a high number of genetic mutations and chromosome alterations, however, the most common driver mutations identified in LUAD, and fewer found in LUSC, and also there are some special mutations are involved in specific cases (Sanchez-Danes & Blanpain, 2018). Chromosomal alterations can be categorized into many types in

LUSC, including the upregulation of SCC differentiation pathways, upregulation of oncogenic signalling and loss of cell cycle regulation (Lau et al., 2022). Preclinical research is currently primarily studying the many molecular pathways that underlie the genesis, progression, The propagation of (NSCLC) in a drive to stumble upon novel therapies and biomarker. Oncogenic driver mutations relating to echinoderm microtubules comprise EGFR exon 19 deletions, frame deletions, point mutations, exon 19-point mutations, translocation, and splice variants in ALK, BRAF, EGFR, NTRK1-3, RET, MET, and ROS1 in lung ADCs.

Clinically approved therapeutic agents are also needed to address these mutations. Especially, KRAS and ERBB2 possess and emerging targetability agents (Chang et al., 2021). Combination or alone of other molecular mutations incudes, TP53, STK11, and Kelch-like ECH-are not yet to directly target therapy, however, these mutations may be associated with tumor progression and immune checkpoint inhibitors (ICIs) (Qian et al., 2020) in Lung ADC. The both large cell neuroendocrine carcinoma (LCNEC) and SCLC are involved with the NSCLC components characteristics such as, ADC and ADC, which as a resistant mechanism for EGFR-TKIs (Marcoux et al., 2019). SMARCA4-deficient undifferentiated lung cancers have a rhabdoid phenotype because they resemble smoking-related NSCLC the most. Additionally, 40% of patients with SMARCA4-UT have mutations linked to KEAP1, STK11, and KRAS1, which are most prevalent in NSCLC cases with smoking. But, SMARCA4-UT is a unique from SMARCA -deficient patients of NSCLC with immunohistochemical, morphological, And prognostic distinctions (Le Loarer et al., 2015).

2.1 Various Gene Mutations in Molecular Subtypes of NSCLC

2..1.1 Mutation in SCC Subtypes

Squamous cell carcinoma (SCC), is a major subtype of NSCLC, which is mainly identified in smokers, and its causes approximately 1,000,000 cases and 40000 people death each year in the United States (Derman et al., 2015). Numerous genetic changes were found in SCC by earlier research, including mutations in TP53, CDKN24A, PIK3CA, DDR2, KEAP1 MLL2, and NFE2L2. Additionally, the CDKN2A tumor suppressor was lost, and the SOX2 lineage-specific oncogene was acquired. The TP53 gene is the most common chromosomal mutation in LUSC, accounting for >60–70% of cases (Kim et al, 2014; Hammerman et al., 2011; Bass et al., 2009; Rooney 2013). Immune indicators and genetic variants have been drastically enhanced. For example, SCC has a variation in PIK3CA, that triggers the receptor PD-1 to be significantly fewer common around immune cells and the immune inhibitory checkpoint PD-L1 to be considerably less noticeable in cancer cells than in normal cells. According to this author's research, patients with earlier-stage LUSCC had their host immune systems triggered by abnormalities and copy number variations. The biggest alterations noticed in LUSCs were in glutamate receptor GRM8, CDH8, ADCY8, CALCR, GRM8, and PTPRT *(*Kan et al., 2010). Dyregulation of epigenetic factors like *MLL2* may be feasible targets in LUSC, as may the mutant *MLL2* and histone lysine N-methyltransferase (*KMT2D*), whose change is most strongly linked to a poor prognosis. Poor response to adjuvant chemotherapy due to *KEAP1* mutations (Kadara et al., 2017). Whole exome sequencing (WES) and clinicopathological procedures indicated variants in LUSC patients, and CNVs have implications for the starting point of treatment success. consequently, investigations into immunological and molecular patterns may aid in enhancing customized immunotherapy measures (Brahmer, 2014; Herbst et al., 2014). Number of mutations such as *TP53, MLL4, COL4A1 and BRCA 2* were correlated with demographic characteristics. Mutations *TP53, MLL4 TERT, NOTCH2* and *SPEN* more significantly identified in the metastatic verse localized SCCs, the silent mutations were identified more in localized SCCs than metastatic SCC, and the more nonsense mutations were found in metastatic SCC than localized SCCs patients. An additionally the mutation was not yet identified in SCC patients such as *LRP1B, TRIO, MDN1, AHNAK2, COL4A2, VPS13C, SVIL, DST* and *DYSF.* The most common mutations, such as TP53, PIK3CA, MLL4, LKB1 FGFR1 and CDKN2A in SCC. These alterations are major contributions of tumorigenesis in SCC.

2.1.2 Mutation in ADC Subtypes

In around 15–25% of Kras variations were found in lung malignancy, and 25–35% of NSCLC cases, especially, smokers with ADC. Exon 2 at codons 12 and 13 has the most prevalent mutation. ERFR-TKI resistance also results in KRAS gene mutations. (Cullis et al., 2014; Shapiro et al., 2013). Lung cancer instances have a KRAS mutation in about 15–25% of cases. 25–35% of patients with NSCLC had a KRAS mutation. High mutations were discovered that people with a smoking A KRAS mutation was found in one-third of lung cancer cases. G12C represents 40% of all KRAS mutations, making it the most prevalent mutation (Shigematsu & Gazdar, 2006; Adderley et al., 2019). Another study found that KRAS polymorphisms detected in 20–40% of ADC, and that they are more common in Western populations (26%) than Asian cultures (11%), as well as among smokers (30%) as opposed to non-smokers (10%). With the greatest number of subtypes, including G12V, G12D, and G12C, these polymorphisms gereatly seen in codons 12 and 13. In smoker LUADs patients, Kadara and colleagues found presence of several immune markers, including PD-L1, was elevated due to the mutational burden. The immunological marker with the strongest correlation to the load of somatic mutations was CD57. Additionally, the PIK3CA mutations markedly decreased the expression of peritumoral PD-1 and tumoral PD-L1, indicating that LUSCs with PIK3CA oncogene mutations had attenuated PD-L1/PD-1 immune checkpoint signaling. Since antibody atezolizumab is significantly linked to elevated tumoral PD-L1 levels, it is plausible that PIK3CA mutations could be a reliable indicator of a lower response to immunotherapies, such as antibodies that target PD-L1. An additionally KEAP1 mutations were found to be significantly associated with poor response to chemotherapy in early stage of lung adenocarcinoma (Ads) (Kadara et al., 2017). EGFR mutations are most common in NSCLC (Cullis et al., 2014), around 34% of EGFR mutations in all lung ACs patients in non-smoking and Asian populations. TP53 mutations are prevalent genetic alterations found in different lung cancers, about 43% in SCCs and 35% in Acs (Shapiro et al., 2013). transversions at codons 157, 158, 179, 248 and 273 in cases of lung cancer in tobacco users, whereas these mutations are not as common in lung cancer in non-smokers.

2.1.3 Mutations in LCLC

At 2% to 3% of NSCLC, LCLC is the most prevalent subtype of NSCLC (Howlader et al., 2016). At the molecular level, it is still not as different as other subgroups. But some studies of smaller genes are found as abnormal expression of TP53 in LCLC and LCNEC tumors, with KRAS mutations prevailing in LCLC (Iyoda et al., 2004; Rossi et al., 2014)25, 26). TP53 mutations were frequently observed in both LCLC and LCNEC, and its low frequency alterations in *EGFR, PIK3CA* and *BRAF* genes (Rekhtman et al.,2013; Rossi et al., 2014). Additionally, TP53 mutations in both LCLC and LCNEC are primarily associated with changes in the tumor suppressors of PTEN and STK11. LCLC patients did not have KRAS mutations (Karlsson et al., 2015). *TTN* mutation or *TTN/TP53* co-mutation is involved in the prognosis of LUSC (Cheng et al., 2019), similarly, other study was found high frequency 45% of a *TTN/TP53* double mutation in LCLC and LCNEC. Approximately, 35% of *FAM135B* mutations in LCLC (paper), similarly, *FAM135B* mutations have high mutations rates in other lung cancers LUSC and SCLC (Xie et al., 2021; Hu et al., 2019). Lung cancer is characterized by the inactivation of LDL receptor-associated protein 1 B *(LRP1B),* a member of the LDL family. *LRP1B* single gene mutations linked to TMB in lung cancer (Lan et al., 2019) may be connected to immune checkpoint drugs (Brown et al., 2013).

Table 1. Genetic Alteration in Molecular Subtypes of NSCLC

Gene	Molecular Alterations	Exon	Frequency	Subtypes of NSCLC	Reference
EGFR	Point Mutations	Exon 19 and 21	90%	NSCLC	Sakurada.,2006
TP53	Harbouring Mutations	Exon 5, 7, 8, G to T transversions at codon 157, 158, 179, 248, and 273	43% 35%	SCCs ACs	Forbes et al.,2008 Denissenko., 1996; Mogi and Kuwano., 2011; Ding et al., 2008.
KRAS	Mutations	Exon 2 at codon 12 (G12A and G12C) and exon 3	19% 5%	AC SCC	Forbes et al.,2008; Karachaliou et al., 2013.
PIK3CA	Harbouring Mutations	exon 1 (R88Q), exon 9 (E542K and E545K), exon 20 (H1047L) at codon 542, 545, and 1047.	6% 4%	SCC AC	Forbes et al.,2008; Samuels et al.,2004; Kang., 2005; Kawano et al., 2006;
CDKN2A	Point mutations	S33F	7% 8%	AC SCC	Forbes et al.,2008; Hongxiang et al., 2015
HER2	Insertion mutation	Exon 20	3%	NSCLC	Mazieres et al., 2019
ALK	Mutations	Mutation in Three ways, ALK-R (ALK gene rearrangement), ALK-A (ALK gene amplification), and point mutation of the ALK gene.	10%	NSCLC	Morris., 1994; Letovanec et al., 2018
BRAF	Point mutation	V600E mutation at exon 15 and exon 11	3%	NSCLC	Ritterhouse and Barletta.,2015
MET	Exon skipping altera tions	Exon 14	68.8%	AC	Yang., 2022
RET	RET fusions and RET point mutations	3`coding region for RET kinase domain on chromosome 10	1-2%	NSCLC, AC	Choudhry and Drilon., 2020; Takeuchi et al., 2012
ROS1	Chromosome Rearrangement	Exon 32-36	86%	AC	Cui et al., 2020
NTRK	Gene fusion	Different genomic rear rangement (3' sequences of the NTRK gene fused to the 5' sequence)	-	SCC	Liu., 2022
FGFR1,	Amplifications	*FGFR1*	20% 3%	SCC AC	Heist et al., 2012; Schildhaus et al., 2012; Tiseo et al., 2015.
NRG1	Gene fusion, oncogenic drivers with EGFR and KRAS mutations Rearrangement of *ALK*, *ROS1* and *RET*.	*SDC4* and *CD74-NRG1*	6%	SCC	Johna et al., 2019; Muscarella LA, Rossi., 2017.

3. RECEPTOR TYROSINE KINASE ASSOCIATED WITH SPECIFIC GENOMIC ALTERATIONS IN SUBTYPES OF NSCLC

Through the generate of the *Ras/MAPK, PI3K/Akt, and JAK/STAT* pathways, *EGFR involve* censorious character in cell growth. T790M is a very common point mutation in 60% of patients with EGFR TKI resistance in NSCLC patients (Yu et al., 2013; Yamaura et al., 2020). Several activation mutations in EGFR gene (Exon

19 deletion, L861Q, L858R, S7811, G719A, G796D, G719C, L718Q, L844 and T790M) are observed at the diagnostic (Yamaura et al., 2020; Zheng et al., 2017). In LUAD mutations were most found in the Pkinase Tyr domain, in positions 858aa (L858R) and 747-750aa (E746_A750del, L747_E749del and L747_T751del) (Liu., 2020). EGFR is highly expressed in lung, neck, head, and esophageal cancers, and targeted therapy has shown encouraging results in these three cancer types. The significance of molecular profiling and biomarker identification for a suitable therapy selection is enhanced when EGFR abnormalities and treatment are coupled (Liu, 2020). SNV is mostly observed in FGFR2, it's associated with NSCLC, GC and endometrial cancer. N375S and T992I mutation was identified in NSCLC, small cell lung cancer SCLC), and melanoma (Xu et al., 2018). The enzyme ALK is involved in a number of malignancies. ALK is activates pathways includings Ras/MAPK, PI3K/Akt, and JAK/STAT, which is contributing to its oncogenic potential, and also ALK is a target therapy for cancer especially in NSCLC, large cell lymphoma (Christova et al., 2023). ROS1 rearrangement was observed in NSCLC, and its acts like a driver in various cancers including NSCLC (Duma et al., 2019), and it activates signalling pathways like Ras/MAPK, JAK/STAT and PI3K/Akt, which is contribute to its role in oncogenesis. Specific select inhibitors illustrating promise opposed to ROS 1-driven malignancies, ROS1 has become as a key focus in cancer therapy. As a protooncogene, RET may be important in lung cancer, and RET fusion was seen in roughly 2% of NSCLC (Takahashi, 2022). EphA3 has several structural changes, including as W790C, A749D, and F152S; EphA7 has L749F; EphB1 has G685C; and EphB4 has V748A variations in NSCLC. The significance of mutations in NSCLC is still unknown, though, and each mutation requires additional functional investigation. PTK7 was identified upregulation in several cancer including gastric, esophageal, colorectal, lung carcinoma, when a downregulation of PTK7 related to lung SCC, melanomas, and ovarian cancer, and also other studies PTK7 play a potential role as a marker for tumor initiating cells in NSCLC (Damelin et al., 2017). Usually, AXL is expression as a low in adults, however it's an abnormally high in numerous cancers such as, NSCLC, breast, pancreatic, glioblastoma, etc. Furthermore, the lower prediction of individuals with NSCLC is link with overexpression of STYK1, which is primarily involved in metastasis. Signalling pathway of ALK/LTK is responsible for the changes of invasion, migration, apoptosis and cell proliferation via JAK/STAT/VEGF, RAS/Raf/MAPK, PI3K/Akt/mTOR, and PLCγ/PIP/IP3 pathway in NSCLC (Rankin & Giaccia, 2016).

Figure 1. Genetic Alterations in Various Subtypes of NSCLC

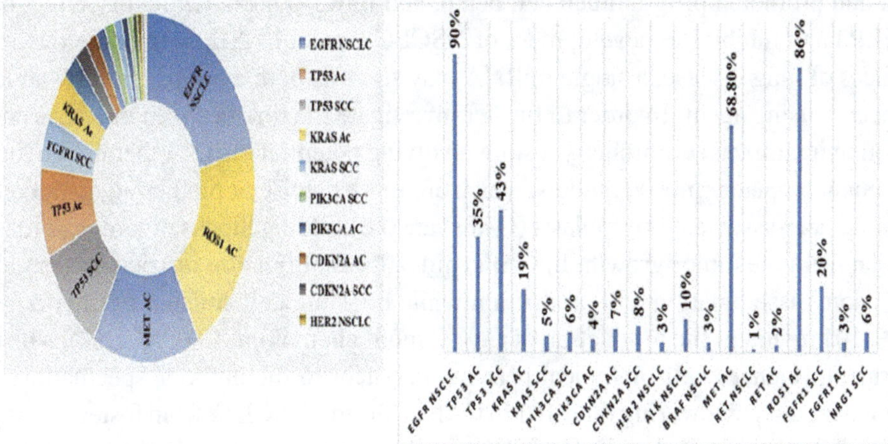

4. miRNA ALTERATIONS IN NSCLC

miRNAS are involved in both upregulated and downregulated in cancer tissues when compared to healthy tissues, its act as tumor-suppressors or oncogenes (Feng et al., 2015). Especially, each and all miRNAs show as different roles in NSCLC, including oncogenic miRNAS (miR-221miR-222, miR-21 and miR-31 and miR-17-92 cluster) and tuomr suppressors (let-7, miR-34 family, miR-200 family, miR-451, miR-126, miR-101, miR-192 and miR-545) (Feng et al., 2015). a member of the let-7 family is regularly downregulated in non-small cell lung cancer (NSCLC); if let-7 expression fails to appear in tumor tissues, the Ras GTPase communication circuit becomes impaired, which enhances the illness's propagation. Oncogenes or tumor inhibitors tied to miRNA targets reflect fluctuations in miRNA expression linked to the formation, growth and propagation of malignancies. Furthermore, miRNAs have the ability to control gene expression via several signaling pathways, such as ERK, TGF-β, AKT, MAPK, JAK-STAT, and WNT (Di Leva., 2014; Asghariazar et al., 2019). Because it directly affects the expression of EGFR, the tumor suppressor of MiR-34 may function as downregulated in NSCLC. Unfortunately, ZEBI was substantially appeared in NSCLC, while researchers discovered miR-320a bearing was decreased in NSCLC. The expression of RAD51AP1 by ZEB1, which is developed in cancer, studied by the In vivo method. The expression of miRNA -320a by the ZEB1 suppressed, it makes up-regulation of RAD51AP1 and promoted metastasis in NSCLC (Wang et al., 2021). An additionally, miR-506 is act as a tumor suppressor in NSCL by regulating of TULP3, an it also inhibited the development of cancer cell and promoted programmed cell death, and miR5-6 has a regulatory effect on TULP3 and inhibit the development of NSCLC (Li et al., 2021). In numerous instances of lung disease, a single miRNA may serve as both a tumor inhibitor and a cancer-causing agent. In order to further investigate the link between miRNAs and existing treatments, preliminary testing involving potential miRNA therapies adopt immunocompetent mouse models, which are more precise at predicting malignancies. Cancer-associated fibroblasts (CAFs) are the building blocks of tumor stomas, which facilitate tumor growth. In CAFs, miR101 amplification restricts tumor cell invasion, dissemination and production while boosting cell suicide. Furthermore, miR-101 regulates the production of C-X-C motif chemokine 12 (CXCL12), which in turn influences cell biological activity. Pursuant to the authors' speculation, a unique method of lowering miR-101 in CAFs will stop CXCL12 from fostering lung cancer growth and metastasis. NSCLC development and metastasis is lowered by restricting the PI3K/AKT signaling pathway through Metastasis-Associated Lung Adenocarcinoma Transcript 1 (MALAT-1) and MiR-101-3b. MiR-15a specifically targets and influences the levels of decapentplegic homolog3 (9Smad3) in mothers, facilitating expansion of cells, dissemination, and spreading in NSCLC (Guo et al., 2020). MiR-195 belongs to the miR-15/16 family, NSCLC is only one cancer is related to improved prognosis by expression of miR-195, and also that the miR195 directly targets Checkpoint Kinase 1 (CHEK 1), which reducing CHEK1 expression in lung cancers, based on these findings, miR-195 may inhibit NSCLC and provide as a prognostic indicator for lung cancer (Liu et al., 2015The tumor inhibitor microRNA p53 has abnormalities in many kinds of human malignancies. MiR-34 is growing more widely known due to the phase I clinical trials of MRX34, the first tumor- specific microRNA medicine. Contrary to other prior research, miR-34a and miR-34c could potentially exploited as diagnostic indicators for NSCLC. Furthermore, invasive LUAD had lower levels of miR-34b and miR-34c than non-metastatic LUAD, indicating that they might prevent LUAD cells from migrating. Multiple pathogenic processes, including swelling, apoptosis, proliferation, expansion, and cell division contribute to instability of miR-574-5p. Serum-based biomarkers miR-1254 and miR-574-5p are employed as minimally invasive screening and triage instruments for additional diagnostic examinations (Huanng et al., 2022). When miR-574-5p acts as an RNA decoy for CUGBP1, mPGES-1 facilitates the emergence of human lung tumors. meanwhile, miR-574-5p boosts NSCLC cell invasion and motility by downregulating PTPRU expression and elevating the tyrosine phosphorylation of β-catenin (Huanng et al., 2022). MiRNAs can either prevent or cause lung cancer by encouraging carcinogenesis, which includes resistance, propagation, inflammation, and growth of cells, by influencing the production of target mRNA. It is more vital to look into several miRNA activities implicated in different types of lung tumors in order to enhance screening and treatment strategies.

5. COPY NUMBER ALTERATIONS IN NSCLC

Molecular cytogenetic study was found +1q21-q24, +5p15-p14, +8q22-q24.1 and -17p13-p12 in both SqC and AdC. Based on this finding these authors were suggested that the specific chromosomal imbalance and partners found in SqC and AdC have highlighted regions for further molecular investigations into genes, which may hold importance in carcinogenesis of NSCLC (Wong et al., 2004). Another study reported that genes located in several chromosomal regions, for example, 3q25-26, may be linked with phenotypic properties that differentiate lungs SCCs from Acs, furthermore, this study reported the gains of 7q and 8q chromosome, which may be indicative of tumor aggressiveness in NSCLCs (Pei et al., 2001). The both squamous and AC cells showed the alterations in the loss of 3p and gain of 5p, and these authors were reported that the unique information generated by high resolution analysis of NSCLC genomes and uncover the presence of genetic alterations in the different subtypes of NSCLC (Cathie & William, 2006). Another study assessing copy number alteration in LUAD patients determined that the majority of defections involved spikes in 1q, 5p, 5q, 7p, 8q, 14p, 16p,17,10q, and losses in 8p, 9p, 13p, 16q,18q. Several recognized genes, such as TERT, EGFR, MYC, CDK4, MDM2, ERBB2, NKX2-1, and CCNE1, were also shown to have frequent amplifications. Telomerase reverse transcriptase (TERT), which is located on 5p15, is the gene that is typically boosted in this observation, as per past prior studies. LUAD is marked by the upregulation of oncogenes including EgFR (7p12), ERBB2 (17q12), and KRAS in the EGFR pathway, which suggests that it plays a key role in the progression of malignant cells and cell expansion (Xiaohong et al., 2019; Qiu, 2017).

6. EPIGENETIC MODIFICATION ASSOCIATED WITH PATHWAYS IN SPECIFIC ALTERATIONS

Epigenetic modification is a regulate the gene expression without alterations in the DNA sequence, which play crucial role in the development and progression of NSCLC by variety of alterations, such as, DNA methylation, histone modifications, and non-coding RNA expression (Mari-Alexandre et al., 2017; Ansari, 2016). Histone changes that may alter a gene's expression encompass phosphorylation, ubiquitination, acetylation, and epigenomics. DNA methylation, one of the most chemical epigenetic changes, is a covalent bonding of a methyl group to CPG dinucleotides for transcriptional inhibition. Tumor oncogenes and repressor genes in LSCLC had different DNA methylation patterns. These epigenetic aberrant can contribute to the development of NSCLC by promoting tumor cell proliferation, invasion, and metastasis (Mari-Alexandre et al., 2017; Ansari, 2016). In NSCLC cells, alterations of histone modifications can be implicated in the dysregulation of key signalling pathway, such as the PI3K/AKT/mTOR and Wnt/β-catenine pathway, furthermore, histone deacetylase (HDAC) inhibitors found to have anticancer activity in NSCLC via stimulate apoptosis and cell cycle arrest (Spangle, 2017; Sharma, 2021; Mamdani & Jalal, 2020). In NSCLC tissue, methylation of *DAPK1* and *TUSC3* genes were linked with increase overall survival, but in malignant pleural effusions of LUAD, the hypermethylation of P16/INK4α and BRCA1 was associated with shorter survival, when hypermethylation of RARβ was linked with longer survival (Drilon et al., 2014; Duppel et al., 2016; Botana-Rial et al., 2012). HOXA family genes composed of different classes, which were identified in primary NSCLC tissues to be downregulation. Particularly, methylation of HOXA2 and HOXA10 as a negative prognostic factor in LUSC patients (Heller et al., 2013), also the methylation of HOXA9 was linked with NSCLC in nonsmokers with poor recurrence- free survival (RFS), but the clinical significance of HOXA9 hypermethylation has not yet been reported in the early stage of LUSC (Hwang et al., 2015). In 2015, first investigated the prognostic value of PAX6 methylation in NSCLC was reported by Zhang et al., 2015 Magnolol is capable of stimulating the apoptotic signaling pathways and its suppressing *STAT3/NF- κB,* proteins and epithelial- mesenchymal transition (EMT) involved in metastasis in NSCLC (Lee et al., 2022), and it's also stimulated the G0/G1 phase cell cycle arrest, autophagy and apoptosis in NSCLC cells (Zhao et al., 2021). Although the biochemical significance of Jinfukang (JFK), an anti-NSCLC drug, has not yet been fully revealed, it has therapeutic effects of stabilizing tumor lesions, inhibiting metastases, and increasing patient survival. The JFK causes the epigenetic alterations to H3K4me3 of the promoters of tumor -related pathways genes such as *CCND2, BCL2A1, SUSD2* and *TMEM158* (Lu et al., 2016).

In lung cancer, several genes are associated with promoter methylation such as *p16INK4a, RASSF1A, APC, RARβ, CDH1, CDH13, DAPK, FHIT,* and *MGMT.* Only *p16INK4a* is most frequently methylated or deletion in NSCLC While *p16INK4a* is frequently methylated, mutated, or deleted round 60% in NSCLC, and less alteration in less than 10% in SCLC and also, p14arf encoded on the CDKN2A gens, which is commonly inactivated around 8-30% of NSCLC cells (Toyooka et al., 2011; Fischer et al., 2007). RASSF1A is methylated or deleted in 30-40% in NSCLC, and around 70-100% methylated or deleted in SCLC, an additionally, FHIT is methylated in 40-70% of NSCLC and 50-80% of NSCLC, and TSLC1 is methylated in about 85% of NSCLC (Toyooka et al., 2011). RASSF1A, APC, ESR1, ABCB1, MT1G, and HOXC9 are promoter methylation genes, which is associated with stage I NSCLC

(Lin et al., 2009), it's suggesting that they may development in early stage of cancer. Other hypermethylated genes including hDAB2IP, H-Cadherin, DAL-1, and FBN2 also linked with advanced stage in the carcinogenic process of NSCLC (Kikuchi et al., 2005; Yano et al., 2005; Chen et al., 2005). HDAC is catalyze the removal of acetyl groups on the histone tail to transcriptionally inactive of heterochromatic stage, some study reported that HDAC are overexpression in lung cancer, similarly SIN3A is a part of an HDFC repressor complex, which is downregulated in NSCLC cells (Suzuki et al., 2008). An unsaturated tetracyclic triterpenoid with antioxidant, anti-inflammatory, and anti-cancer capabilities is called cucurbitacin B (CuB). It can be recognized in a range of plants. For example, CuB inhibits the XIST/miR-let-7c/IL-6/STAT3 to regulate cell division and death in NSCLC.

Figure 2. Epigenetic Alterations for Dysregulation of Key signalling Pathway in NSCLC cells.

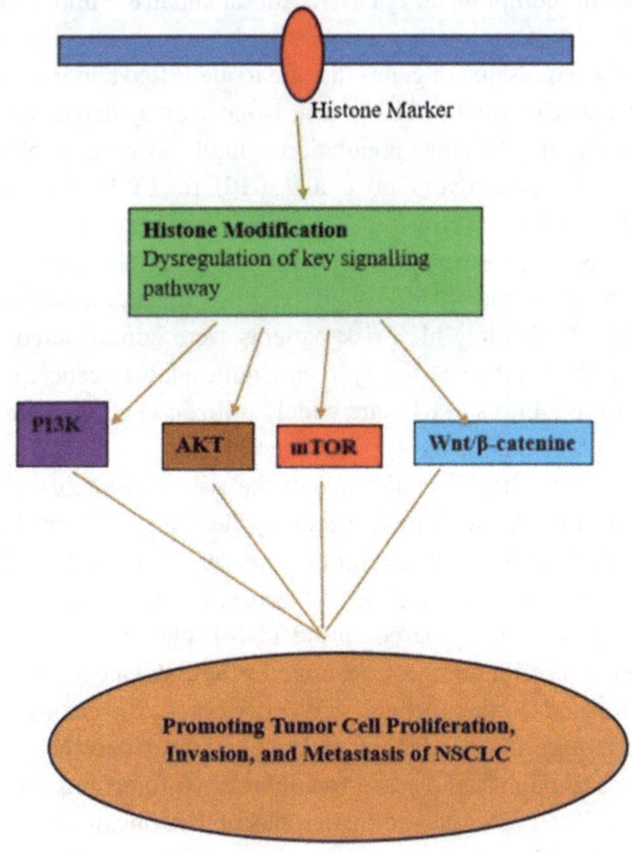

7. GENOMIC PROFILING FOR NSCLC

Genomic assessment is an emerging concept offering patients with numerous advantages and customized care for each illness. Lung cancer belongs to the most prevalent illnesses worldwide. NSCLC is the most prevalent form of lung cancer, contributing to roughly eighty percent of all cases. Patients with high-risk non-small cell lung cancer are recognized employing the Tumor Node Metastasis (TNM) method (Kratz et al., 2019). However, the To determine that this TNM system's risk classification was inadequate, external studies were conductedGenome-based screening remains the premier assay for ensuring the accurate detection of people at risk, the advantageous effects of medication, and the general well-being of patients with NSCLC. Earlier research using the microarray approach identified many genes involved in various pathways of proliferation. Later, the majority of research employed the polymerase chain reaction (PCR) to reverse-transcribe the target gene and find complimentary DNA. (Subramanian & Simon, 2010). Recently, 14- gene PCR assay (DetermaRx) is an available on commercially, which is using to quantitates the expression of genes that are to identified abnormally expresses in the NSCLC cases (DetermaRx, 2023). The 14-gene assay demonstrated its benefit in precisely identifying the target population in high-risk cases of NSCLC linked to EGFR mutations. According to Gray et al. (2019), the FLAURA trial also showed the value of EGFR mutation profiling with cobas for patient selection and treatment. Pursuant to a cohort investigations, genetic screening classified 5% of NSCLC patients as low-risk. In the absence of adjuvant treatment, the survival statistic for such people was 94%. Only high-risk patients were administered with adjuvant chemotherapy, which has a possibility to cure quite a few of cancer patients. EGFR Tyrosine Kinase Inhibitors (TKIs) are widely utilized in adjuvant immunotherapy to treat people who are not adhering to chemotherapy.

This genomic profiling is could predict the risk of mortality in the high-risk group cases of NSCLC, with more accuracy than the National Comprehensive Cancer Network (NCCN)'s clinic pathological criteria (Kratz et al., 2019; Kratz et al., 2012). Furthermore, the incidence of recurrence in patients were categorized into low and high-risk group based on the TNMB classification and it's reported that the genomic profiling is more accurate in the risk categorization of NSCLC patients as compared to others schemes (Woodard et al., 2014). In-patient treatment and prognosis require advanced molecular testing more than other traditional criteria. Woodard et al. published disease-free mortality projections for non-small cell lung cancer (NSCLC) cases according to molecular testing and the NCCN criteria. Pursuant to the NCCN criteria, the DFS estimate for intermediate-risk unresolved NSCLC cases was roughly 75.2%, while for severe-risk unresolved NSCLC cases, it was close to 61.9%. Molecular sorting, however, predicted a DFS of 48.9% for high-risk individuals and 93.8% for low-risk patients. This indicates that when evaluating participants for chemotherapy recommendations, the molecular test method of classification was more discriminative (Woodard et al., 2018). Point changes in exon 21 and exon 19 lesions of the epidermal growth factor receptor have proven to be substantial indicators of EGFR tyrosine kinase inhibitors in NSCLC. For NSCLC, genomic profiling significantly increases patient survival and delivers stronger suggested therapies. It can reduce unneeded care to those with a low risk of non-small cell lung cancer. Adjuvant chemotherapy improved 5-year overall survival and DFS rates, according to the high-risk individual. besides, genetic assessment substantially contributes to the personal treatment to people with non-small cell lung cancer.

8. CHALLENGES IN MOLECULAR SUBTYPES OF NSCLC

NSCLC is a variegated tumor which splits across multiple different variants, every one of these can be recognized by discrete genetic modifications. The main obstacles to unsuccessful therapy involve the heterogeneity of NSCLC tumors and the lack of biological characteristics since there aren't enough tumor NSCLC samples available for histological inspection. Although each tumor is known to affect the patient's outcome, nothing is known about its potential for genetic profiling. Furthermore, immune checkpoint inhibition (ICI) and molecular targeted therapy do not produce long-term results in the majority of NSCLC cases. The most common histological type of non-small cell lung cancer is lung adeno carcinoma (LUAD). Cytotoxic T-lymphocyte associated protein 4 (CTLA-4) and programmed death ligand 1 (PD-L1) respond well to ICI therapy without experiencing the negative side effects of traditional chemotherapy (Pardoll, 2012; Kris et al., 2014). Personalized medicine and ICI medication are beneficial for 20% of people with non-small cell lung cancer because they demand distinct variations in their genes. Predictive biomarkers are used in immune response in regard to malignancy deletion incidence (TMB) and microsatellite instability (MSI). TMB is responsible for a significant increase in neoantigens and non-synonymous mutations. The instability of microsatellites points to a problem with the DNA mismatch repair processes, which causes immunogenic neoantigens to build up. Many patients still do not respond to immunological treatment despite the use of these predictive indicators to raise survival rates because of resistance mechanisms such pharmacokinetic, tumor microenvironment-mediated, and epigenetic resistance (Borghaei et al., 2015; Brahmer et al., 2015; Topalian et al., 2012).

Intratumoral heterogeneity occurs for therapy resistant in LUAD associated with the distinct histomorphological growth patterns such as, acinar, papillary, lepidic and micropapillary, and these LUAD growth patterns also associated with different prognoses (Tsao et al., 2015). In the majority of cases, a single tumor with multiple growth patterns is found to be highly predictive. Nevertheless, nothing is known about the molecular variations among the LUAD patterns. LSCLC and all other lung cancer molecular subtypes are informally classified as uncommon diseases. Rare oncogene-driven lung cancer is becoming more and more difficult to detect with clinical-grade diagnostic tests and profiling algorithms. Historically, the SCC subtype has had fewer actionable molecular targets than adenocarcinoma. Advances in next generation sequencing technologies may more help to detect the rare, and novel genetic alteration within the distinct molecular subtypes of NSCLC. An additionally, liquid biopsies can help to identified genetic alterations and tumor progression. By addressing these challenges, the clinicians and researchers may studying to understating of genetic alteration with different molecular subtypes of NSCLC and develop more potential and treatment approaches for patients with NSCLC.

9. FUTURE OF TARGETED THERAPY IN NSCLC

Chemotherapy, radiation, and resection are some of the primary techniques that cancer is managed. Chemotherapy is the sole way to treat cancer with medication; it destroys tumor cells while stopping their growth and division. Chemotherapy has the characteristic of killing both healthy and malignant cells, which results in extreme toxicity and negative side effects. The first small-molecular tyrosine kinase inhibitor (TKI) approved for clinical usage was imatinib in 2001 by the Food and Drug Administration (FDA) (Savage & Antman., 2002), and its targeted drugs for cancer treatment have rapidly developed in the past 20 years. Usually, targetd drugs can be classified into two categories such as, small molecules and macromolecules (monoclonal antibodies, polypeptides, antibody-drug conjugates, and nucleic acids (Wilkes, 2018; Lee et al., 2018). likewise, medications that target smaller molecules continue to make significant strides. These tiny molecule medications engage an assortment of unique targets, notably proteasomes, DNA damage repair enzymes, kinases, and epigenetic regulatory proteins. Protein kinase is a type of enzyme inhibitor that plays an essential function in the formation of cells, proliferation, and differentiation by catalyzing the transfer of γ phosphate groups from ATP to protein residues that contain hydroxyl groups (Ardito et al., 2017). AlK inhibitor is targeting of multiple tyrosine kinase such as, ALK, cellular mesenchymal epithelial transition factor (c-Met), and proto -oncogene tyrosine-protein kinase reactive oxygen species (Cui et al., 2011), currently, ALK inhibitor is now the standard drug therapy for metastatic ALK positive NSCLC (Shaw et al., 2013; Solomon et al., 2014). EGFR TKIs possessing a quinazoline structure that are reversible inhibitors include icotinib, gefitinib, and erlotinib. These drugs respond better for NSCLC patients with EGFR mutations at exons 19 and 21 L858R (Metro et al., 2006; Gu et al., 2013; Lynch et al., 2004). The indolinone derivative nintedanib targets including VEGFR-1/2/3, FGFR1/2, and PDGFRα/β, it is the initially used as a clinically for the treatment of idiopathic pulmonary fibrosis, latterly the combination therapy of nintedanib and docetaxel as a treatment for NSCLC patients approved by the European Medicines Agency (EMA) (Alshangiti et al., 2018). Much more research study will be need to understand the epigenetic mechanism, which are involved in the beginning and progression of NSCLC, because, the epigenetic processes including DNA methylation, histone modifications, and abnormal expression of miRNAs and lncRNAs, which are contribution to protein- coding gene expression and it can be have direct implications for the progression of cancer (Yamashita et al., 2015; Xu et al., 2016). In order to diagnose NSCLC early, unique epigenetic markers have additionally been discovered. Specialized methyl sequencing, miRNA-seq, and RNA-seq are examples of next-generation sequencing technologies that are capable of discovering particular epigenetic markers and potentially influence the design of targeted assays for the rapid identification of NSCLC (Heller et al., 2013; Page et al., 2021). High-throughput technologies and AI as a powerful tool, analysis of large scale of genetic and epigenetic dataset in NSCLC. Also, these technologies able to screening of several epigenetic alterations such as histone modification, DNA methylation, miRNA and lncRNA expression, to identify the disease progression, therapeutic response, and drug sensitivity (Brasil et al., 2021; Bahado-Singh et al., 2022). Furthermore, combination of advance technologies of AI and high throughput technologies for better understanding of the molecular mechanism of underlying of disease, and it can be able to the development of novel targeted therapies (Brasil et al.,2021; Rauschert,2020). Drug resistance and adverse reactions are both problems that tiny molecules concentrated anti-cancer drugs nevertheless confront.

10. CONCLUSION

We concluded that precise molecular diagnostics, utilizing advance techniques like NGS and whole genomic sequencing, which are crucial to determine specific genetic alterations with NSCLC subtypes. Different NSCLC subtypes such as AC and SCC can exhibit distinct genomic alterations, which can directly involve therapeutic responses on currently. Also, molecular profiling can identify various alteration including EGFR, ROS1 fusions, and ALK that serve as target for specific. However, target therapies like EGFR, ALK and epigenetic factors are overcoming acquired resistance to treatments remains a major challenge, hence current research are focusing into novel drug targets and combinations therapies such as immunotherapies and cell-based approaches. Furthermore, the identifications of novel genetic alterations and signalling pathways continues to make new therapeutic drugs and novel biomarkers. Hence, Researchers and clinicians should study to characterize poor understood molecular subtypes, identify new novel markers, and explore the genetic alterations in molecular subtypes of NSCLC can develop more effective and personalized approaches, and ultimately increase the patient's outcome.

REFERENCES

Adderley, H., Blackhall, F. H., & Lindsay, C. R. (2019). KRAS-mutant non-small cell lung cancer: Converging small molecules and immune checkpoint inhibition. *EBioMedicine*, *41*, 711–716. DOI: 10.1016/j.ebiom.2019.02.049 PMID: 30852159

. Alex, F., Maurice, P., Giuseppe, L. B., Kaushal, P., & Alfredo, A. (2024). Oncogenic alterations in advanced NSCLC: a molecular super-highway. *Biomark Res*, 12, 12(1), 24.

Alshangiti, A., Chandhoke, G., & Ellis, P. M. (2018). Antiangiogenic therapies in non-small cell lung cancer. *Current Oncology (Toronto, Ont.)*, *25*(11), S45–S58. DOI: 10.3747/co.25.3747 PMID: 29910647

. Ansari, J., Shackelford, R. & El-Osta, H. (2016). Epigenetics in non-small cell lung cancer: From basics to therapeutics. Trasl. Lung Cancer Res, *5*, 155–171.

Ardito, F., Giuliani, M., Perrone, D., Troiano, G., & Muzio, L. L. (2017). The crucial role of protein phosphorylation in cell signaling and its use as targeted therapy [review]. *International Journal of Molecular Medicine*, *40*(2), 271–280. DOI: 10.3892/ijmm.2017.3036 PMID: 28656226

Arteaga, C. L. (2000). Overview of epidermal growth factor receptor biology and its role as therapeutic target in human neoplasia. *Oncol*, *29*(5, Suppl 14), 3–9. PMID: 12422308

Asghariazar, V., Sakhinia, E., Mansoori, B., Mohammadi, A., & Baradaran, B. (2019). Tumor suppressor microRNAs in Lung cancer: An insight to signaling pathways and drug resistance. *Journal of Cellular Biochemistry*, *120*(12), 19274–19289. DOI: 10.1002/jcb.29295 PMID: 31364210

Bahado-Singh, R., Vlachos, K. T., Aydas, B., Gordevicius, J., Radhakrishna, U., & Vishweswaraiah, S. (2022). Precision Oncology: Artificial Intelligence and DNA Methylation Analysis of Circulating Cell-Free DNA for Lung Cancer Detection. *Frontiers in Oncology*, *12*, 790645. DOI: 10.3389/fonc.2022.790645 PMID: 35600397

Bass, A. J., Watanabe, H., Mermel, C. H., Yu, S., Perner, S., Verhaak, R. G., Kim, S. Y., Wardwell, L., Tamayo, P., Gat-Viks, I., Ramos, A. H., Woo, M. S., Weir, B. A., Getz, G., Beroukhim, R., O'Kelly, M., Dutt, A., Rozenblatt-Rosen, O., Dziunycz, P., & Meyerson, M. (2009). SOX2. is an amplified lineage survival oncogene in lung and esophageal squamous cell carcinomas. *Nature Genetics*, *41*(11), 1238–1242. DOI: 10.1038/ng.465 PMID: 19801978

Borghaei, H., Paz-Ares, L., Horn, L., Spigel, D. R., Steins, M., Ready, N. E., Chow, L. Q., Vokes, E. E., Felip, E., Holgado, E., Barlesi, F., Kohlhäufl, M., Arrieta, O., Burgio, M. A., Fayette, J., Lena, H., Poddubskaya, E., Gerber, D. E., Gettinger, S. N., & Brahmer, J. R. (2015). Nivolumab versus Docetaxel in Advanced Nonsquamous Non- Small-Cell Lung Cancer. *The New England Journal of Medicine*, *373*(17), 1627–1639. DOI: 10.1056/NEJMoa1507643 PMID: 26412456

Botana-Rial, M., Chiara, L. D., & Valverde, D.. (2012). Prognostic value of aberrant hypermethylation in pleural effusion of lung adenocarcinoma. *Cancer Biology & Therapy*, *13*(14), 1436–1442. DOI: 10.4161/cbt.22004 PMID: 22954699

Brahmer, J., Reckamp, K. L., Baas, P., Crinò, L., Eberhardt, W. E. E., Poddubskaya, E., Antonia, S., Pluzanski, A., Vokes, E. E., Holgado, E., Waterhouse, D., Ready, N., Gainor, J., Arén Frontera, O., Havel, L., Steins, M., Garassino, M. C., Aerts, J. G., Domine, M., & Spigel, D. R. (2015). Nivolumab versus Docetaxel in Advanced Squamous-Cell Non- Small-Cell Lung Cancer. *The New England Journal of Medicine*, *373*(2), 123–135. DOI: 10.1056/NEJMoa1504627 PMID: 26028407

Brahmer, J. R. (2014). Immune check point blockade: The hope for immunotherapy as a treatment of lung cancer? *Seminars in Oncology*, *41*(1), 126–132. DOI: 10.1053/j.seminoncol.2013.12.014 PMID: 24565586

Brasil, S., Neves, C. J., Rijoff, T., Falcão, M., Valadão, G., Videira, P. A., & Ferreira, V. D. R. F. (2021). Artificial Intelligence in Epigenetic Studies: Shedding Light on Rare Diseases. *Frontiers in Molecular Biosciences*, *8*, 648012. DOI: 10.3389/fmolb.2021.648012 PMID: 34026829

Brown, L. C., Tucker, M. D., Sedhom, R., Schwartz, E. B., Zhu, J., Kao, C., Labriola, M. K., Gupta, R. T., Marin, D., Wu, Y., Gupta, S., Zhang, T., Harrison, M. R., George, D. J., Alva, A., Antonarakis, E. S., & Armstrong, A. J. (2013). LRP1B mutations are associated with favorable outcomes to immune checkpoint inhibitors across multiple cancer types. *Journal for Immunotherapy of Cancer*, *9*(3), e001792. DOI: 10.1136/jitc-2020-001792 PMID: 33653800

Cathie, G., & William, W. (2006). High resolution analysis of non-small cell lung cancer cell lines by whole genome tiling path array CGH. *International Journal of Cancer*, *118*(6), 1556–1564. DOI: 10.1002/ijc.21491 PMID: 16187286

Chang, J. C., Offin, M., Falcon, C., Brown, D., Houck-Loomis, B. R., Meng, F., Rudneva, V. A., Won, H. H., Amir, S., Montecalvo, J., Desmeules, P., Kadota, K., Adusumilli, P. S., Rusch, V. W., Teed, S., Sabari, J. K., Benayed, R., Nafa, K., Borsu, L., & Rekhtman, N. (2021). Comprehensive molecular and clinicopathologic analysis of 200 pulmonary invasive mucinous adenocarcinomas identifies distinct characteristics of molecular subtypes. *Clinical Cancer Research*, *27*(14), 4066–4076. DOI: 10.1158/1078-0432.CCR-21-0423 PMID: 33947695

Chen, H., Suzuki, M., Nakamura, Y., Ohira, M., Ando, S., Iida, T., Nakajima, T., Nakagawara, A., & Kimura, H. (2005). Aberrant methylation of FBN2 in human non-small cell lung cancer. *Lung Cancer (Amsterdam, Netherlands)*, *50*(1), 43–49. DOI: 10.1016/j.lungcan.2005.04.013 PMID: 15951052

Cheng, X., Yin, H., Fu, J., Chen, C., An, J., Guan, J., Duan, R., Li, H., & Shen, H. (2019). Aggregate analysis based on TCGA: TTN missense mutation correlates with favorable prognosis in lung squamous cell carcinoma. *Journal of Cancer Research and Clinical Oncology*, *5*(4), 1027–1035. DOI: 10.1007/s00432-019-02861-y PMID: 30810839

Christova, T., Ho, S. K., Liu, Y., Gill, M., & Attisano, L. (2023). LTK and ALK promote neuronal polarity and cortical migration by inhibiting IGF1R activity. *EMBO Reports*, *24*(7), 1–21. DOI: 10.15252/embr.202356937 PMID: 37291945

Cui, J. J., Tran-Dubé, M., Shen, H., Nambu, M., Kung, P.-P., Pairish, M., Jia, L., Meng, J., Funk, L., Botrous, I., McTigue, M., Grodsky, N., Ryan, K., Padrique, E., Alton, G., Timofeevski, S., Yamazaki, S., Li, Q., Zou, H., & Edwards, M. P. (2011). Structure based drug design of crizotinib (PF-02341066), a potent and selective dual inhibitor of mesenchymal-epithelial transition factor (c-MET) kinase and anaplastic lymphoma kinase (ALK). *Journal of Medicinal Chemistry*, *54*(18), 6342–6363. DOI: 10.1021/jm2007613 PMID: 21812414

Cullis, J., Meiri, D., Sandi, M. J., Radulovich, N., Kent, O. A., Medrano, M., Mokady, D., Normand, J., Larose, J., Marcotte, R., Marshall, C. B., Ikura, M., Ketela, T., Moffat, J., Neel, B. G., Gingras, A.-C., Tsao, M.-S., & Rottapel, R. (2014). The RhoGEF GEF-H1 is required for oncogenic RAS signalling via KSR-1. *Cancer Cell*, *25*(2), 181–195. DOI: 10.1016/j.ccr.2014.01.025 PMID: 24525234

Damelin, M.. (2017). A PTK7-targeted antibody-drug conjugated reduces tumor-initiating cells and induces sustained tumor regressions. *Science Translational Medicine*, •••, 9. PMID: 28077676

Dempke, W. C. M., Suto, T., & Reck, M. (2010). Targeted therapies for non-small cell lung cancer. *Lung Cancer (Amsterdam, Netherlands)*, *67*(3), 257–274. DOI: 10.1016/j.lungcan.2009.10.012 PMID: 19914732

Derman, B. A., Mileham, K. F., & Bonomi, P. D.. (2015). Treatment of advanced squamous cell carcinoma of the lung: A review. *Translational Lung Cancer Research*, *4*, 524–532.1. PMID: 26629421

. DetermaRx For Oncologists. (2023). Oncocyte.

Di Leva, G., Garofalo, M., & Croce, C. M. (2014). MicroRNAs in cancer. *Annual Review of Pathology*, *9*(1), 287–314. DOI: 10.1146/annurev-pathol-012513-104715 PMID: 24079833

Drilon, A., Sugita, H., Sima, C. S., Zauderer, M., Rudin, C. M., Kris, M. G., Rusch, V. W., & Azzoli, C. G. (2014). A prospective study of tumor suppressor gene methylation as a prognostic biomarker in surgically resected stage I to IIIA non-small-cell lung cancers. *Journal of Thoracic Oncology*, *9*(9), 1272–1277. DOI: 10.1097/JTO.0000000000000256 PMID: 25122424

Duma, N., Santana-Davila, R., & Molina, J. R. (2019). Non-small cell lung cancer: Epidemiology, screening, diagnosis, and treatment. *Mayo Clinic Proceedings*, *94*(8), 1623–1640. DOI: 10.1016/j.mayocp.2019.01.013 PMID: 31378236

Duppel, U., Woenckhaus, M., Schulz, C., Merk, J., & Dietmaier, W. (2016). Quantitative detection of TUSC3 promoter methylation -a potential biomarker for prognosis in lung cancer. *Oncology Letters*, *12*(4), 3004–3012. DOI: 10.3892/ol.2016.4927 PMID: 27698890

Feng, B., Zhang, K., Wang, R., & Chen, L. (2015). Non-small-cell Lung cancer and miRNAs: Novel biomarkers and promising tools for treatment. *Clinical Science (London, England)*, *128*(10), 619–634. DOI: 10.1042/CS20140530 PMID: 25760961

Fischer, J. R., Ohnmacht, U., Rieger, N., Zemaitis, M., Stoffregen, C., Manegold, C., & Lahm, H. (2007). Prognostic significance of RASSF1A promoter methylation on survival of non-small cell lung cancer patients treated with gemcitabine. *Lung Cancer (Amsterdam, Netherlands)*, *56*(1), 115–123. DOI: 10.1016/j.lungcan.2006.11.016 PMID: 17196704

Gray, J. E., Okamoto, I., Sriuranpong, V., Vansteenkiste, J., Imamura, F., Lee, J. S., Pang, Y.-K., Cobo, M., Kasahara, K., Cheng, Y., Nogami, N., Cho, E. K., Su, W. C., Zhang, G., Huang, X., Li-Sucholeiki, X., Lentrichia, B., Dearden, S., Jenkins, S., & Ramalingam, S. S. (2019). Tissue and plasma EGFR mutation analysis in the FLAURA Trial: Osimertinib versus Comparator EGFR tyrosine kinase inhibitor as first-line treatment in patients with EGFR-mutated advanced non–small cell lung cancer. *Clinical Cancer Research*, *25*(22), 6644–6652. DOI: 10.1158/1078-0432.CCR-19-1126 PMID: 31439584

Gu, A.. (2013). Efficacy and safety evaluation of icotinib in patients with advanced non-small cell lung cancer. *Chinese Journal of Cancer Research = Chung-Kuo Yen Cheng Yen Chiu*, *25*, 90–94. PMID: 23372346

Guo, S.. (2020). Inhibition mechanism of Lung cancer cell Metastasis through targeted regulation of Smad3 by miR–15a. *Oncology Letters*, *19*(2), 1516–1522. PMID: 31966076

Hammerman, P. S., Sos, M. L., Ramos, A. H., Xu, C., Dutt, A., Zhou, W., Brace, L. E., Woods, B. A., Lin, W., Zhang, J., Deng, X., Lim, S. M., Heynck, S., Peifer, M., Simard, J. R., Lawrence, M. S., Onofrio, R. C., Salvesen, H. B., Seidel, D., & Meyerson, M. (2011). Mutations in the DDR2 kin ase gene identify a novel therapeutic target in squamous cell lung cancer. *Cancer Discovery*, *1*(1), 78–89. DOI: 10.1158/2159-8274.CD-11-0005 PMID: 22328973

. Hannay, D.R. (2000). The evidence-based primary care handbook. *BMJ,* 321 (7260, 576.

Heller, G., Babinsky, V. N., Ziegler, B., Weinzierl, M., Noll, C., Altenberger, C., Müllauer, L., Dekan, G., Grin, Y., Lang, G., End-Pfützenreuter, A., Steiner, I., Zehetmayer, S., Döme, B., Arns, B.-M., Fong, K. M., Wright, C. M., Yang, I. A., Klepetko, W., & Zöchbauer-Müller, S. (2013). Genome-wide CpG island methylation analyses in non-small cell lung cancer patients. *Carcinogenesis*, *34*(3), 513–521. DOI: 10.1093/carcin/bgs363 PMID: 23172663

Heller, G., Babinsky, V. N., Ziegler, B., Weinzierl, M., Noll, C., Altenberger, C., Müllauer, L., Dekan, G., Grin, Y., Lang, G., End-Pfützenreuter, A., Steiner, I., Zehetmayer, S., Döme, B., Arns, B.-M., Fong, K. M., Wright, C. M., Yang, I. A., Klepetko, W., & Zöchbauer-Müller, S. (2013). Genome-wide CpG island methylation analyses in non-small cell lung cancer patients. *Carcinogenesis*, *34*(3), 513–521. DOI: 10.1093/carcin/bgs363 PMID: 23172663

Herbst, R. S., Morgensztern, D., & Boshoff, C. (2018). The biology and management of non- small cell lung cancer. *Nature*, *553*(7689), 446–454. DOI: 10.1038/nature25183 PMID: 29364287

Herbst, R. S., Soria, J. C., Kowanetz, M., Fine, G. D., Hamid, O., Gordon, M. S., Sosman, J. A., McDermott, D. F., Powderly, J. D., Gettinger, S. N., Kohrt, H. E. K., Horn, L., Lawrence, D. P., Rost, S., Leabman, M., Xiao, Y., Mokatrin, A., Koeppen, H., Hegde, P. S., & Hodi, F. S. (2014). Predictive correlates of response to the anti-PD-L1 antibody MPDL3280A in cancer patients. *Nature*, *515*(7528), 563–567. DOI: 10.1038/nature14011 PMID: 25428504

Howlader, N., Noone, A. M., Krapcho, M., Miller, D., Bishop, K., & Altekruse, S. F.. (2016). *SEER cancer statistics review*. National Cancer Institute.

Hu, J., Wang, Y., Zhang, Y., Yu, Y., Chen, H., Liu, K., Yao, M., Wang, K., Gu, W., & Shou, T. (2019). Comprehensive genomic profiling of small cell lung cancer in Chinese patients and the implications for therapeutic potential. *Cancer Medicine*, *8*(9), 4338–4347. DOI: 10.1002/cam4.2199 PMID: 31199602

Huanng, E.. (2022). the Regulatory mechanism of mir-574-5p expression in Cancer. *Biomolecules*, *13*(1), 40. DOI: 10.3390/biom13010040 PMID: 36671425

Hwang, J. A., Lee, B. B., Kim, Y., Hong, S.-H., Kim, Y.-H., Han, J., Shim, Y. M., Yoon, C.-Y., Lee, Y.-S., & Kim, D.-H. (2015). HOXA9 inhibits migration of lung cancer cells and its hypermethylation is associated with recurrence in non-small cell lung cancer. *Molecular Carcinogenesis*, *54*(S1), 72–80. DOI: 10.1002/mc.22180 PMID: 24817037

Iyoda, A., Hiroshima, K., Moriya, Y., Mizobuchi, T., Otsuji, M., Sekine, Y., Shibuya, K., Iizasa, T., Saitoh, Y., & Fujisawa, T. (2004). Pulmonary large cell neuroendocrine carcinoma demonstrates high proliferative activity. *The Annals of Thoracic Surgery*, *77*(6), 1891–1895. DOI: 10.1016/j.athoracsur.2003.10.119 PMID: 15172230

Kadara, H., Choi, M., Zhang, J., Parra, E. R., Rodriguez-Canales, J., Gaffney, S. G., Zhao, Z., Behrens, C., Fujimoto, J., Chow, C., Yoo, Y., Kalhor, N., Moran, C., Rimm, D., Swisher, S., Gibbons, D. L., Heymach, J., Kaftan, E., Townsend, J. P., & Herbst, R. S. (2017). Whole-exome sequencing and immune profiling of early-stage lung adenocarcinoma with fully annotated clinical follow-up. *Annals of Oncology : Official Journal of the European Society for Medical Oncology*, *28*(1), 75–82. DOI: 10.1093/annonc/mdw436 PMID: 27687306

Kan, Z., Jaiswal, B. S., Stinson, J., Janakiraman, V., Bhatt, D., Stern, H. M., Yue, P., Haverty, P. M., Bourgon, R., Zheng, J., Moorhead, M., Chaudhuri, S., Tomsho, L. P., Peters, B. A., Pujara, K., Cordes, S., Davis, D. P., Carlton, V. E. H., Yuan, W., & Seshagiri, S. (2010). Diverse somatic mutation patterns and pathway alterations in human cancers. *Nature*, *466*(7308), 869–873. DOI: 10.1038/nature09208 PMID: 20668451

Karlsson, A., Brunnstrom, H., Lindquist, K. E., Jirstrom, K., Jonsson, M., Rosengren, F., Reuterswärd, C., Cirenajwis, H., Borg, Å., Jönsson, P., Planck, M., Jönsson, G., & Staaf, J. (2015). Mutational and gene fusion analyses of primary large cell and large cell neuroendocrine lung cancer. *Oncotarget*, *6*(26), 22028–22037. DOI: 10.18632/oncotarget.4314 PMID: 26124082

Kikuchi, S., Yamada, D., Fukami, T., Masuda, M., Sakurai-Yageta, M., Williams, Y. N., Maruyama, T., Asamura, H., Matsuno, Y., Onizuka, M., & Murakami, Y. (2005). Promoter methylation of DAL-1/4.1B predicts poor prognosis in non-small cell lung cancer. *Clinical Cancer Research*, *11*(8), 2954–2961. DOI: 10.1158/1078-0432.CCR-04-2206 PMID: 15837747

Kim, Y., Hammerman, P. S., Kim, J., Yoon, J., Lee, Y., Sun, J.-M., Wilkerson, M. D., Pedamallu, C. S., Cibulskis, K., Yoo, Y. K., Lawrence, M. S., Stojanov, P., Carter, S. L., McKenna, A., Stewart, C., Sivachenko, A. Y., Oh, I.-J., Kim, H. K., Choi, Y. S., & Park, K. (2014). Integrative and comparative genomic analysis of lung squamous cell carcinomas in East Asian patients. *Journal of Clinical Oncology*, *32*(2), 121–128. DOI: 10.1200/JCO.2013.50.8556 PMID: 24323028

Kratz, J. R., Haro, G. J., Cook, N. R., He, J., Van Den Eeden, S. K., Woodard, G. A., Gubens, M. A., Jahan, T. M., Jones, K. D., Kim, I.-J., He, B., Jablons, D. M., & Mann, M. J. (2019). Incorporation of a molecular prog nostic classifier improves conventional non-small cell lung cancer staging. *Journal of Thoracic Oncology*, *14*(7), 1223–1232. DOI: 10.1016/j.jtho.2019.03.015 PMID: 30959120

Kratz, J. R., He, J., Van Den Eeden, S. K., Zhu, Z.-H., Gao, W., Pham, P. T., Mulvihill, M. S., Ziaei, F., Zhang, H., Su, B., Zhi, X., Quesenberry, C. P., Habel, L. A., Deng, Q., Wang, Z., Zhou, J., Li, H., Huang, M.-C., Yeh, C.-C., & Jablons, D. M. (2012). A practical molecular assay to pre dict survival in resected non-squamous, non-small-cell lung cancer: Devel opment and international validation studies. *Lancet*, *379*(9818), 823–832. DOI: 10.1016/S0140-6736(11)61941-7 PMID: 22285053

Kris, M. G., Johnson, B. E., Berry, L. D., Kwiatkowski, D. J., Iafrate, A. J., Wistuba, I. I., Varella-Garcia, M., Franklin, W. A., Aronson, S. L., Su, P.-F., Shyr, Y., Camidge, D. R., Sequist, L. V., Glisson, B. S., Khuri, F. R., Garon, E. B., Pao, W., Rudin, C., Schiller, J., & Bunn, P. A. (2014). Using multiplexed assays of oncogenic drivers in lung cancers to select targeted drugs. *Journal of the American Medical Association, 311*(19), 1998–2006. DOI: 10.1001/jama.2014.3741 PMID: 24846037

Lan, S., Li, H., Liu, Y., Ma, L., Liu, X., Liu, Y., Yan, S., & Cheng, Y. (2019). Somatic mutation of LRP1B is associated with tumor mutational burden in patients with lung cancer. *Lung Cancer (Amsterdam, Netherlands), 132*, 154–156. DOI: 10.1016/j.lungcan.2019.04.025 PMID: 31054778

Lau, S. C. M., Pan, Y., Velcheti, V., & Wong, K. K. (2022). Squamous cell lung cancer: Current landscape and future therapeutic options. *Cancer Cell, 40*(11), 1279–1293. DOI: 10.1016/j.ccell.2022.09.018 PMID: 36270277

Le Loarer, F., Watson, S., Pierron, G., de Montpreville, V. T., Ballet, S., Firmin, N., Auguste, A., Pissaloux, D., Boyault, S., Paindavoine, S., Dechelotte, P. J., Besse, B., Vignaud, J. M., Brevet, M., Fadel, E., Richer, W., Treilleux, I., Masliah-Planchon, J., Devouassoux-Shisheboran, M., & Tirode, F. (2015). SMARCA4 inactivation defines a group of undifferentiated thoracic malignancies transcriptionally related to BAF-deficient sarcomas. *Nature Genetics, 47*(10), 1200–1205. DOI: 10.1038/ng.3399 PMID: 26343384

Lee, Y. C., Weng, Y. S., Wang, H. Y., Hsu, F.-T., Chueh, F.-S., Wu, J.-Y., Chen, W.-L., & Chen, J.-H. (2022). Magnolol Induces Apoptosis Through Extrinsic/intrinsic Pathways and Attenuates NF-κB/STAT3 Signaling in Non-small-cell Lung Cancer Cells. *Anticancer Research, 42*(8), 3825–3833. DOI: 10.21873/anticanres.15873 PMID: 35896265

Lee, Y. T., Tan, Y. J., & Oon, C. E. (2018). Molecular targeted therapy: Treating cancer with specificity. *European Journal of Pharmacology, 834*, 188–196. DOI: 10.1016/j.ejphar.2018.07.034 PMID: 30031797

Li, Z. H., Zhou, J.-H., Chen, S.-N., Pan, L., Feng, Y., Luo, M.-Q., Li, R.-X., & Sun, G.-L. (2021). MicroRNA-506 has a suppressive effect on the tumorigenesis of nonsmall-cell Lung cancer by regulating tubby-like protein 3. *Bioengineered, 12*(2), 10176–10186. DOI: 10.1080/21655979.2021.2001216 PMID: 34874810

Lin, Q., Geng, J., Ma, K., Yu, J., Sun, J., Shen, Z., Bao, G., Chen, Y., Zhang, H., He, Y., Luo, X., Feng, X., & Zhu, J. (2009). RASSF1A, APC, ESR1, ABCB1 and HOXC9, but not p16INK4A, DAPK1, PTEN and MT1G genes were frequently methylated in the stage I non-small cell lung cancer in China. *Journal of Cancer Research and Clinical Oncology, 135*(12), 1675–1684. DOI: 10.1007/s00432-009-0614-4 PMID: 19506903

Liu, B., Qu, J., Xu, F., Guo, Y., Wang, Y., Yu, H., & Qian, B. (2015). MiR-195 suppresses non-small cell Lung cancer by targeting CHEK1. *Oncotarget, 6*(11), 9445–9456. DOI: 10.18632/oncotarget.3255 PMID: 25840419

Liu, H., Zhang, B., & Sun, Z. (2020). Spectrum of EGFR aberrations and potential clinical implications: Insights from integrative pan-cancer analysis. *Cancer Communications, 40*(1), 43–59. DOI: 10.1002/cac2.12005 PMID: 32067422

. Lu, J., Zhang, X., Shen, T., *et al.* (2016). Epigenetic Profiling of H3K4Me3 Reveals Herbal Medicine Jinfukang-Induced Epigenetic Alteration Is Involved in Anti-Lung Cancer Activity. Evidence-Based Complement. *Altern. Med,* 7276161.

Lynch, T. J., Bell, D. W., Sordella, R., Gurubhagavatula, S., Okimoto, R. A., Brannigan, B. W., Harris, P. L., Haserlat, S. M., Supko, J. G., Haluska, F. G., Louis, D. N., Christiani, D. C., Settleman, J., & Haber, D. A. (2004). Activating mutations in the epidermal growth factor receptor underlying responsiveness of non-small-cell lung cancer to gefitinib. *The New England Journal of Medicine, 350*(21), 2129–2139. DOI: 10.1056/NEJMoa040938 PMID: 15118073

Mamdani, H., & Jalal, S. I. (2020). Histone Deacetylase Inhibition in Non-small Cell Lung Cancer: Hype or Hope? *Frontiers in Cell and Developmental Biology, 8*, 582370. DOI: 10.3389/fcell.2020.582370 PMID: 33163495

Marcoux, N., Gettinger, S. N., O'Kane, G., Arbour, K. C., Neal, J. W., Husain, H., Evans, T. L., Brahmer, J. R., Muzikansky, A., Bonomi, P. D., del Prete, S., Wurtz, A., Farago, A. F., Dias-Santagata, D., Mino-Kenudson, M., Reckamp, K. L., Yu, H. A., Wakelee, H. A., Shepherd, F. A., & Sequist, L. V. (2019). EGFR-mutant adenocarcinomas that transform to small-cell lung cancer and other neuroendocrine carcinomas: Clinical outcomes. *Journal of Clinical Oncology, 37*(4), 278–285. DOI: 10.1200/JCO.18.01585 PMID: 30550363

Mari-Alexandre, J., Diaz-Lagares, A., Villalba, M., Juan, O., Crujeiras, A. B., Calvo, A., & Sandoval, J. (2017). Translating cancer epigenomics into the clinic: Focus on lung cancer. *Translational Research; the Journal of Laboratory and Clinical Medicine, 189*, 76–92. DOI: 10.1016/j.trsl.2017.05.008 PMID: 28644958

Metro, G., Finocchiaro, G., Toschi, L., Bartolini, S., Magrini, E., Cancellieri, A., Trisolini, R., Castaldini, L., Tallini, G., Crino, L., & Cappuzzo, F. (2006). Epidermal growth factor receptor (EGFR) targeted therapies in non-small cell lung cancer (NSCLC). *Reviews on Recent Clinical Trials*, *1*(1), 1–13. DOI: 10.2174/157488706775246157 PMID: 18393776

Page, M. J., McKenzie, J. E., & Bossuyt, P. M.. (2021). The PRISMA 2020 statement: An updated guideline for reporting systematic reviews. *BMJ (Clinical Research Ed.)*, *372*(71). PMID: 33782057

Pardoll, D. M. (2012). The blockade of immune checkpoints in cancer immunotherapy. *Nature Reviews. Cancer*, *12*(4), 252–264. DOI: 10.1038/nrc3239 PMID: 22437870

Pei, J., Balsara, B. R., Li, W., Litwin, S., Gabrielson, E., Feder, M., Jen, J., & Testa, J. R. (2001). Genomic imbalances in human lung adenocarcinomas and squamous cell carcinomas. *Genes, Chromosomes & Cancer*, *31*(3), 282–287. DOI: 10.1002/gcc.1145 PMID: 11391799

Qian, J., Zhao, S., Zou, Y., Rahman, S. M. J., Senosain, M.-F., Stricker, T., Chen, H., Powell, C. A., Borczuk, A. C., & Massion, P. P. (2020). Genomic underpinnings of tumor behavior in in situ and early lung adenocarcinoma. *American Journal of Respiratory and Critical Care Medicine*, *201*(6), 697–706. DOI: 10.1164/rccm.201902-0294OC PMID: 31747302

Qiu, Z. W., Bi, J. H., Gazdar, A. F., & Song, K. (2017). Genome-wide copy number variation pattern analysis and a classification signature for non-small cell lung cancer. *Genes, Chromosomes & Cancer*, *56*(7), 559–569. DOI: 10.1002/gcc.22460 PMID: 28379620

Rankin, E., & Giaccia, A. (2016). The receptor tyrosine kinase AXL in cancer progression. *Cancer*, •••, 8. PMID: 27834845

Rauschert, S., Raubenheimer, K., Melton, P. E., & Huang, R. C. (2020). Machine learning and clinical epigenetics: A review of challenges for diagnosis and classification. *Clinical Epigenetics*, *12*(1), 51. DOI: 10.1186/s13148-020-00842-4 PMID: 32245523

Rekhtman, N., Tafe, L. J., Chaft, J. E., Wang, L., Arcila, M. E., & Colanta, A.. (2013). Distinct profile of driver mutations and clinical features in immunomarker-defined subsets of pulmonary large-cell carcinoma. Mod. pathology official J. U. S. *Can. Acad. Pathology.*, *26*, 511–522. PMID: 23196793

Rooney, M., Devarakonda, S., & Govindan, R. (2013). Genomics of squamous cell lung cancer. *The Oncologist, 18*(6), 707–716. DOI: 10.1634/theoncologist.2013-0063 PMID: 23728941

Rossi, G., Mengoli, M. C., Cavazza, A., Nicoli, D., Barbareschi, M., Cantaloni, C., Papotti, M., Tironi, A., Graziano, P., Paci, M., Stefani, A., Migaldi, M., Sartori, G., & Pelosi, G. (2014). Large cell carcinoma of the lung: Clinically oriented classification integrating immunohistochemistry and molecular biology. *Virchows Archiv, 464*(1), 61–68. DOI: 10.1007/s00428-013-1501-6 PMID: 24221342

Sanchez-Danes, A., & Blanpain, C. (2018). Deciphering the cells of origin of squamous cell carcinomas. *Nature Reviews. Cancer, 18*(9), 549–561. DOI: 10.1038/s41568-018-0024-5 PMID: 29849070

Savage, D. G., & Antman, K. H. (2002). Imatinib mesylate–a new oral targeted therapy. *The New England Journal of Medicine, 346*(9), 683–693. DOI: 10.1056/NEJMra013339 PMID: 11870247

Shapiro, G., Rosen, L. S., Tolcher, A. W., Goldman, J. W., Gandhi, L., & Papadopoulos, K. P.. (2013). A first-inhuman phase 1 study of the CDK4/6 inhibitor, LY2835219, for patients with advanced cancer. [suppl]. *Journal of Clinical Oncology,* •••, 31.

Sharma, A., Mir, R., & Galande, S. (2021). Epigenetic Regulation of the Wnt/β-Catenin Signaling Pathway in Cancer. *Frontiers in Genetics, 12*, 681053. DOI: 10.3389/fgene.2021.681053 PMID: 34552611

Shaw, A. T., Kim, D.-W., Nakagawa, K., Seto, T., Crinó, L., Ahn, M.-J., De Pas, T., Besse, B., Solomon, B. J., Blackhall, F., Wu, Y.-L., Thomas, M., O'Byrne, K. J., Moro-Sibilot, D., Camidge, D. R., Mok, T., Hirsh, V., Riely, G. J., Iyer, S., & Jänne, P. A. (2013). Crizotinib versus chemotherapy in advanced ALK-positive lung cancer. *The New England Journal of Medicine, 368*(25), 2385–2394. DOI: 10.1056/NEJMoa1214886 PMID: 23724913

Shepherd, F. A., Rodrigues Pereira, J., Ciuleanu, T., Tan, E. H., Hirsh, V., Thongprasert, S., Campos, D., Maoleekoonpiroj, S., Smylie, M., Martins, R., van Kooten, M., Dediu, M., Findlay, B., Tu, D., Johnston, D., Bezjak, A., Clark, G., Santabárbara, P., & Seymour, L. (2005). National Cancer Institute of Canada Clinical Trials Group. Erlotinib in previously treated non-small-cell lung cancer. *The New England Journal of Medicine, 353*(2), 123–132. DOI: 10.1056/NEJMoa050753 PMID: 16014882

Shigematsu, H., & Gazdar, A. F. (2006). Somatic mutations of epidermal growth factor receptor signaling pathway in lung cancers. *International Journal of Cancer, 118*(2), 257–262. DOI: 10.1002/ijc.21496 PMID: 16231326

Shinya, K., Keiju, A., Genichiro, I., Shoko, N., & Takashi, S. (2019). Prognostic impact of the number of metastatic lymph nodes on the eighth edition of the TNM classification of non-small cell lung cancer. *J Thorac Oncol*, 14, 1408–18.

Solomon, B. J., Mok, T., Kim, D.-W., Wu, Y.-L., Nakagawa, K., Mekhail, T., Felip, E., Cappuzzo, F., Paolini, J., Usari, T., Iyer, S., Reisman, A., Wilner, K. D., Tursi, J., & Blackhall, F. (2014). First-line crizotinib versus chemotherapy in ALK-positive lung cancer. *The New England Journal of Medicine*, *371*(23), 2167–2177. DOI: 10.1056/NEJMoa1408440 PMID: 25470694

Spangle, J. M., Roberts, T. M., & Zhao, J. J. (2017). The emerging role of PI3K/AKT-mediated epigenetic regulation in cancer. *Biochimica et Biophysica Acta. Reviews on Cancer*, *1868*(1), 123–131. DOI: 10.1016/j.bbcan.2017.03.002 PMID: 28315368

Subramanian, J., & Simon, R. (2010). Gene expression–based prognostic signa tures in lung cancer: Ready for clinical use? *Journal of the National Cancer Institute*, *102*(7), 464–474. DOI: 10.1093/jnci/djq025 PMID: 20233996

Suzuki, H., Ouchida, M., Yamamoto, H., Yano, M., Toyooka, S., Aoe, M., Shimizu, N., Date, H., & Shimizu, K. (2008). Decreased expression of the SIN3A gene, a candidate tumor suppressor located at the prevalent allelic loss region 15q23 in non-small cell lung cancer. *Lung Cancer (Amsterdam, Netherlands)*, *59*(1), 24–31. DOI: 10.1016/j.lungcan.2007.08.002 PMID: 17854949

Takahashi, M. (2022). RET receptor signaling: Function in development, metabolic disease, and cancer. Proc. *J pn Acad. Ser. B Phys. Biomedical Science*, *98*, 112–125. PMID: 35283407

Topalian, S. L., Hodi, F. S., Brahmer, J. R., Gettinger, S. N., Smith, D. C., McDermott, D. F., Powderly, J. D., Carvajal, R. D., Sosman, J. A., Atkins, M. B., Leming, P. D., Spigel, D. R., Antonia, S. J., Horn, L., Drake, C. G., Pardoll, D. M., Chen, L., Sharfman, W. H., Anders, R. A., & Sznol, M. (2012). Safety, Activity, and Immune Correlates of Anti–PD-1 Antibody in Cancer. *The New England Journal of Medicine*, *366*(26), 2443–2454. DOI: 10.1056/NEJMoa1200690 PMID: 22658127

Toyooka, S., Mitsudomi, T., Soh, J., Aokage, K., Yamane, M., Oto, T., Kiura, K., & Miyoshi, S. (2011). Molecular oncology of lung cancer. *General Thoracic and Cardiovascular Surgery*, *59*(8), 527–537. DOI: 10.1007/s11748-010-0743-3 PMID: 21850578

Tsao, M. S., Marguet, S., Le Teuff, G., Lantuejoul, S., Shepherd, F. A., Seymour, L., Kratzke, R., Graziano, S. L., Popper, H. H., Rosell, R., Douillard, J.-Y., Le-Chevalier, T., Pignon, J.-P., Soria, J.-C., & Brambilla, E. M. (2015). Subtype Classification of Lung Adenocarcinoma Predicts Benefit from Adjuvant Chemotherapy in Patients Undergoing Complete Resection. *Journal of Clinical Oncology*, *33*(30), 3439–3446. DOI: 10.1200/JCO.2014.58.8335 PMID: 25918286

Wang, H., Dong, H., Qiao, L., Wu, Y., Wu, B., & Jin, X. (2021). ZEB1 induces non-small cell Lung cancer development by targeting microRNA-320a to increase the expression of RAD51AP1. *Experimental Cell Research*, *405*(2), 112687. DOI: 10.1016/j.yexcr.2021.112687 PMID: 34097859

Wieduwilt, M. J., & Moasser, M. M. (2008). The epidermal growth factor receptor family: Biology driving targeted therapeutics. *Cellular and Molecular Life Sciences : CMLS*, *65*(10), 1566–1584. DOI: 10.1007/s00018-008-7440-8 PMID: 18259690

Wilkes, G. M. (2018). Targeted therapy: Attacking cancer with molecular and immunological targeted agents. *Asia-Pacific Journal of Oncology Nursing*, *5*(2), 137–155. DOI: 10.4103/apjon.apjon_79_17 PMID: 29607374

Woodard, G. A., Gubens, M. A., Jahan, T. M., Jones, K. D., Kukreja, J., Theodore, P. R., Cardozo, S., Jew, G., Clary-Macy, C., Jablons, D. M., & Mann, M. J. (2014). Prognostic molecular assay might improve identification of patients at risk for recurrence in ear ly-stage non-small-cell lung cancer. *Clinical Lung Cancer*, *15*(6), 426–432. DOI: 10.1016/j.cllc.2014.07.004 PMID: 25258195

Woodard, G. A., Wang, S. X., Kratz, J. R., Zoon-Besselink, C. T., Chiang, C.-Y., Gubens, M. A., Jahan, T. M., Blakely, C. M., Jones, K. D., Mann, M. J., & Jablons, D. M. (2018). Adjuvant chemotherapy guided by molecular profiling and improved outcomes in early stage, non-small-cell lung cancer. *Clinical Lung Cancer*, *19*(1), 58–64. DOI: 10.1016/j.cllc.2017.05.015 PMID: 28645632

Xiaohong, H., Qiaoyun, T., Sheng, Y., Junling, L., & Yuankai, S.. (2019). Comprehensive profiling of gene copy number alterations predicts patient prognosis in resected stages I–III lung adenocarcinoma. *Frontiers in Oncology*, *9*, 556. DOI: 10.3389/fonc.2019.00556 PMID: 31448219

Xie, X., Tang, Y., Sheng, J., Shu, P., Zhu, X., Cai, X., Zhao, C., Wang, L., & Huang, X. (2021). Titin mutation is associated with tumor mutation burden and promotes antitumor immunity in lung squamous cell carcinoma. *Frontiers in Cell and Developmental Biology*, *9*, 761758. DOI: 10.3389/fcell.2021.761758 PMID: 34746153

Xu, T. X., Yu, S.-F., Ma, M., Dai, J., Chi, Z.-H., Si, L., Sheng, X.-N., Cui, C.-L., Kong, Y., & Guo, J. (2018). cMET-N375S germline mutation is associated with poor prognosis of melanoma in Chinese patients. *Translational Cancer Research, 7*(2), 248–256. DOI: 10.21037/tcr.2018.02.13

Xu, Y. J., Du, Y., & Fan, Y. (2016). Long noncoding RNAs in lung cancer: What we know in 2015. *Clinical & Translational Oncology, 18*(7), 660–665. DOI: 10.1007/s12094-015-1448-y PMID: 26680632

Yamashita, R., Sato, M., Kakumu, T., Hase, T., Yogo, N., Maruyama, E., Sekido, Y., Kondo, M., & Hasegawa, Y. (2015). Growth inhibitory effects of miR-221 and miR-222 in non-small cell lung cancer cells. *Cancer Medicine, 4*(4), 551–564. DOI: 10.1002/cam4.412 PMID: 25641933

Yamaura, T.. (2020). Genetic alterations in epidermal growth factor receptor-tyrosine kinase inhibitor-naïve non-small cell lung carcinoma. *Oncology Letters, 19*, 4169–4176. PMID: 32391110

. Yano, M., Toyooka, S., Tsukuda, K., *et al.* (2005). Aberrant promoter methylation of human DAB2 interactive protein (hDAB2IP) gene in lung cancers. *International journal of cancer Journal international du cancer,* 113, 59–66.

Yarden, Y., & Sliwkowski, M. X. (2001). Untangling the ErbB signalling network. *Nature Reviews. Molecular Cell Biology, 2*(2), 127–137. DOI: 10.1038/35052073 PMID: 11252954

Yu, H. A., Arcila, M. E., Rekhtman, N., Sima, C. S., Zakowski, M. F., Pao, W., Kris, M. G., Miller, V. A., Ladanyi, M., & Riely, G. J. (2020). Analysis of tumor specimens at the time of acquired resistance to EGFR-TKI therapy in 155 patients with *EGFR* -mutant lung cancers. *Clinical Cancer Research, 19*(8), 2240–2247. DOI: 10.1158/1078-0432.CCR-12-2246 PMID: 23470965

Zhang, X., Yang, X., Wang, J., Liang, T., Gu, Y., & Yang, D. (2015). Down-regulation of PAX6 by promoter methylation is associated with poor prognosis in non-small cell lung cancer. *International Journal of Clinical and Experimental Pathology, 8*, 11452–11457. PMID: 26617874

Zhao, M., Zheng, Y. H., Zhao, Q. Y., Zheng, W., Yang, J.-H., Pei, H.-Y., Liu, L., Liu, K.-J., Xue, L.-L., Deng, D.-X., Wang, L., Ma, X., Fu, S.-H., Peng, A.-H., Tang, M.-H., Luo, Y.-Z., Ye, H.-Y., & Chen, L.-J. (2021). Synthesis and evaluation of new compounds bearing 3-(4-aminopiperidin-1-methyl magnolol scaffold as anticancer agents for the treatment of non-small cell lung cancer via targeting autophagy. *European Journal of Medicinal Chemistry, 209*, 112922. DOI: 10.1016/j.ejmech.2020.112922 PMID: 33069436

Zheng, D., Hu, M., Bai, Y., Zhu, X., Lu, X., Wu, C., Wang, J., Liu, L., Wang, Z., Ni, J., Yang, Z., & Xu, J. (2017). EGFR G796D mutation mediates resistance to osimertinib. *Oncotarget*, *8*(30), 49671–49679. DOI: 10.18632/oncotarget.17913 PMID: 28572531

Chapter 3
Tumor Microenvironment and Immune Evasion in NSCLC

Payas Arora
Graphic Era University, India

Shiva Prasad Kollur
https://orcid.org/0000-0003-3914-3933
Amrita Vishwa Vidyapeetham, India

Arunima Nayak
https://orcid.org/0000-0002-1762-8019
Graphic Era University, India

Pallavi Singh
https://orcid.org/0000-0003-4537-4607
Graphic Era University, India

ABSTRACT

Non-small cell lung cancer makes up approximately 85% of all lung cancer diagnoses, around the globe. Despite advancements in therapeutic interventions, accurate prognosis for advanced-stage NSCLC is unsatisfactory and consequently, the 5-year survival rate in cases of metastasis is worrisome, amounting to less than 10%. This book chapter, aimed at providing a detailed review of the tumour microenvironment in NSCLC, highlights the contributions of stromal cells, immune infiltrates, metabolic reprogramming, and extracellular matrix remodelling. The authors explore the possible immunosuppressive mechanisms exploited by the tumors, including immune checkpoint activation, regulatory T-cell expansion, myeloid-derived suppressor cells,

DOI: 10.4018/979-8-3373-2096-0.ch003

and dysfunctional antigen presentation. Furthermore, current trends in immunotherapeutic strategies have been examined and challenges including resistance and the pressing need to develop effective combination regimens has also been addressed.

1. INTRODUCTION

Cancer represents one of the largest causes of deaths occurring in the United States according to data collected in 2021 and 2022, second only to heart diseases. Among the different types of cancer prevalent across the globe, lung cancer remains a significant concern with respect to estimated new cases recorded and estimated deaths. While cancer of the lungs and bronchi represents the second-highest source of estimated new cases in males (11%) and females (12%), it contributes to the largest number of estimated deaths in both sexes (20% in males and 21% in females) in 2025 (Siegel et al., 2025). Within the entire spectrum of varied forms encompassing lung cancer, the subtype non-small cell lung cancer (NSCLC) constitutes a staggering 85% of all the new recorded cases of lung cancer. With stage groupings of 0, I (a, b), II (a, b), III (a, b), and IV, NSCLC is itself divided into two categories: squamous cell carcinoma, which makes up 30% of the cases, and non-squamous cell carcinoma, which accounts for the remaining 70%, with the latter being further divided into large-cell carcinoma (10%) and adenocarcinoma (90%) (Gridelli et al., 2015). Figure 1 illustrates the extent of occurrence of cancer pertaining to different parts of the respiratory system in different parts of the world.

Figure 1. Age-standardized incidence rate (ASIR) of cancer of the trachea, bronchus, and lungs in both sexes as recorded from Northern America, Europe, Asia, Oceania, South America, and Africa in 2022. (Credit: GLOBOCAN 2022)

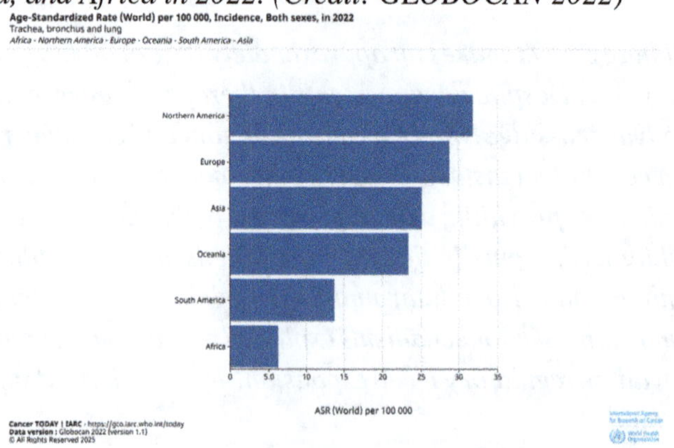

As we learn more about NSCLC biology, it has become clear that the TME is more than a passive bystander but an active driver of disease and therapeutic resistance (L. Wang et al., 2023). Within the NSCLC TME, cancer-associated fibroblasts (CAFs) restructure the extracellular matrix—cross-linking fibronectin and collagen—to increase tissue stiffness, which both prevents cytotoxic T-cell entry into the tumor and supports integrin-mediated pro-survival signalling within tumor cells (Erdogan & Webb, 2017; Shintani et al., 2023). Hypoxic niches, resulting from poor perfusion, stabilize hypoxia-inducible factor-1α (HIF-1α), in turn causing the stimulatory signals for the expression of glycolytic enzymes, for instance, lactate dehydrogenase A (LDHA). The lactate buildup generated acidifies the microenvironment, repressing the corrective functioning mechanisms associated with effector T-cells, along with stimulating Treg differentiation (Brand et al., 2016; Zhang et al., 2024). Concurrently, tumor cells redirect glutamine metabolism to fuel antioxidant defense, a process that not only increases cancer cell survival under oxidative stress but also deprives invading immune cells of essential nutrients (Jin et al., 2023; B. Wang et al., 2024). Finally, metabolic and inflammatory stress signals merge to upregulate immune checkpoint ligands on tumor and stromal cells—most notably PD-L1, thereby exerting T-cell exhaustion, functional dysregulation, and facilitation of immune escape, with all these factors ultimately contributing to the development of therapeutic resistance in NSCLC. With such adaptive mechanisms at play in NSCLC, the need to develop and deploy treatment procedures tailored to produce maximum efficacy in individual patients is gaining momentum (Huang et al., 2024).

The scientific field of study addressed in this book chapter aligns with the sustainable development goals (SDGs) presented before global nations by the 2030 Agenda for Sustainable Development. First, the elaboration of biological mechanisms responsible for the aggressive pathogenesis of NSCLC and the subsequent development of therapeutic methodologies with proven inhibition of different aspects of NSCLC contributes to the realisation of SDG 3 which underlines good health and well-being. Next, encouraging multi-disciplinary research pertaining to the advancement of knowledge associated with the prognosis, progression, and treatment of NSCLC in order to improve survivability of patients can supplement the goal of quality education and scientific learning opportunities promoted by SDG 4. Finally, SDG 9 also holds relevance with respect to the study on NSCLC owing to the potential revolution in therapeutic innovation and the pharmaceutical industry that can be favoured by positive outcomes from scientific research in the domain.

2. COMPONENTS OF THE TUMOR MICROENVIRONMENT IN NSCLC

2.1 Cellular Components

The TME in NSCLC has demonstrated remarkable heterogeneity with respect to cellular composition, especially with the development and subsequent application of advanced profiling techniques. With stage III/IV NSCLC patients included in the study group, single cell RNA (scRNA) sequencing was conducted on 42 biopsy which extensively elaborated the cellular diversity of the TME. Lung epithelial cells comprised of club cells, ciliated epithelial cells, and basal cells, while alveolar cells expressed canonical markers pertaining to Alveolar Type 2 cells (AT2), being further divided into AT2-1 and AT2-2 and AT2-1 exhibiting phenotypic shifts towards malignancy. Inside the domain of tumor-infiltrating T-cells, cellular subtypes identified were CD4+ naïve T-cells, CD8+ effector T-cells, natural killer (NK) cells, CD4+ Tregs, CD8+ exhausted T-cells, and CD4+ T-helper 17-like T-cells (Th17-like). Dendritic cells (DCs) were divided into conventional type 1 and 2 DCs (cDC1, cDC2), mature DCs, and plasmacytoid DCs (pDCs), while neutrophils were categorised into two distinct clusters, with the clusters expressing genes potentially holding association with polymorphonuclear myeloid-derived suppressor cells (PMN-MDSCs) to varying extents. Endothelial cells (ECs) were divided into five subtypes: lymphatic, venous, and arterial endothelial cells (LEC, VECs, and AECs), tip cells, and a distinct cell cluster enhanced with interferon induced genes. Fibroblasts as well as immune cells were also divided into further subtypes (F. Wu et al., 2021). From a cohort of 1,430 NSCLC patients, analysis of the immune infiltrate composition of the TME was performed using gene expression data from Gene Expression Omnibus (GEO). A total of 22 immune cell fractions were identified using CIBERSORT: M0, M1, and M2 macrophages, resting CD4 T-cells, active CD4 T-cells, CD8 T-cells, monocytes, neutrophils, eosinophils, plasma cells, naïve B-cells, B memory cells, active dendritic cells, active NK cells, resting NK cells, follicular helper cells, naïve CD4 T-cells, Tregs, resting mast cells, active mast cells, resting dendritic cells, and gamma delta T-cells (Tamminga et al., 2020). Another study produced a remarkably elaborate elucidation of the diverse immune cell infiltrates in tumors of NSCLC. The diverse cell types identified were live leukocytes, mast cells, T-cells (CD4+, CD8+, and CD4- CD8- T-cells), macrophages, B-cells (naïve B-cells, plasma cells, IgM+ IgD- B-cells, and CD27+ CD38+/- B-cells), pDCs, classical DCs (CD1c+, CD141c+, and double negative (DN) DCs), NK cells (CD16+ and CD16- NK cells), neutrophils, basophils, and eosinophils (Stankovic et al., 2019).

2.2 Non-Cellular Components

In NSCLC, the composition of the TME is not limited to only a variety of cellular components, but also a wide variety of non-cellular components that may involve tumor progression, metastasis, and resistance to therapy. Non-cellular components of the TME encompass constituents of the extracellular matrix (ECM) and soluble factors (cytokines or chemokines), along with mechanical properties (for instance, tissue stiffness). The ECM is composed of various proteins and polysaccharides existing as a dynamic and complicated mesh of interactions that give tissues an appropriate structure and influence cellular behaviour. In NSCLC, presence and configuration of the ECM is important in different aspects of tumor development and progression. A major structural protein of the ECM is collagen, particularly type I collagen. Increased accumulation and cross-linking of collagen via lysizide-oxidase (LOX) leads to increased stiffness of the ECM and allows for increased invasion and metastasis of NSCLC tumor cells. LOX is expressed in less glycolytic states which occur under hypoxia - an established environmental condition in most solid tumors and facilitates ECM remodeling and progression of the tumor. (Ramachandran et al., 2021). The mechanical properties associated with the ECM, particularly stiffness, have a significant impact on the cell behaviour in NSCLC tumors (Guo et al., 2022). Inflammation in NSCLC tumors is mediated by a number of inflammatory cytokines which exert multifaceted effects on tumor biology, proliferation, sustenance, immune escape, and metastasis. These cytokines include interleukin-1 beta (IL-1β), IL-4, IL-6, IL-8, IL-9, IL-13, IL-17C, CCL5, HIF-1α, and TNF-α (Rajasegaran et al., 2023). Several ECM bioactive fragments play crucial positive as well as negative roles with respect to the advancement of tumor biology within the TME. These bioactive fragments include collagen fragments (Type IIB procollagen NH2 propeptide, arresten, canstatin, hexastatin, vastatin, restin, tumstatin, tetrastatin, lamstatin, endostatin, NC1 XIX, 54–132 amino-acid sequence, and 185–203 amino-acid sequence), elastin fragments (VG-6 and AG-9), fibronectin fragments (Anastellin), laminin fragments (IKVAV, AG73, YIGSR, C16, A5G27, γ2 chain N-terminal fragment, and α3 chain C-terminal fragment), glypican fragments (Glypican-3 derived peptide), proteoglycans fragments (Metastatin, endorepellinLG3 fragment, versikine, lumcorin, and lumikine/lumC13), Has (HA oligosaccharides), and synstatins (SSTN 92-119, SSTN 82-130, SSTN 210-240, and SSTN87-131) (Brassart-Pasco et al., 2020).

2.3 Role of Hypoxia and Metabolic Reprogramming

Hypoxia, a defining character of the TME in NSCLC, occurs when tumor cells proliferate faster than new blood vessels can be created to provide adequate oxygen to the cells of the tumor. However, this hypoxic environment then generates a series of molecular and metabolic adaptations that promote tumor growth, immune transfusion, and/or resistance to therapy. Hypoxia promotes NSCLC progression through HIF-mediated EMT, ECM degradation, and angiogenesis, while encouraging immune escape, tumor invasion and alteration of biological pathways through exosome signaling. It reprograms tumor metabolism towards glycolysis and enhances lactate production to fuel tumor biology proliferation, adaptability, and metastatic potential. Lactate accumulation alters the TME in a way that can support immune escape and tumor growth. Hypoxia severely impairs DNA repair efficiency within the tumor cell biology, encouraging invasive phenotypes along with further development of therapeutic resistance to chemotherapy, radiotherapy, immunotherapy, and target therapy (Zhou et al., 2024). Hypoxia, in combination with metabolic reprogramming, constitutes a convoluted, multi-directional loop which possibly holds the capability to confer radio-resistance to cancer cells through various mechanisms like DNA repair, immune evasion, angiogenesis, autophagy, sustenance of cancer stem cells (CSCs), and alleviation of oxidative stress, with associated entities like HIF-1 and lactate involved in the regulation of almost all mechanisms responsible for radio-resistance. This complex loop is capable of counteracting the effects of radio-resistance by promoting cell proliferation and apoptotic blockade, along with safeguarding cancer cells against radiation by reducing oxygen supply through pathological angiogenesis or diminishing reactive oxygen species (ROS) production (Shi et al., 2024).

3. MECHANISMS OF IMMUNE EVASION IN NSCLC

3.1 Immune Checkpoints

Immune checkpoints comprise a subset of regulatory molecules which are involved in the key function of modulating the immune response, holding particularly essential relevance with respect to cancer. Checkpoint proteins such as Programmed Cell Death Protein 1 (PD-1) and Cytotoxic T-Lymphocyte Associated Protein 4 (CTLA-4) are some of the essential checkpoints that serve to sustain self-tolerance, along with effective prevention of autoimmunity through T-cell suppression. Tumors of NSCLC are able to exploit such immune checkpoints for immune escape as well as tumor growth and hence are focal points of investigation and therapeutic endeavour in cancer (Pisibon et al., 2021), such as the use of circular RNAs (circRNAs) as efficient prognostic and diagnostic markers through the regulation of immune checkpoint inhibitors (ICIs) employed for the purpose of cancer management (Meng et al., 2024). T-cells express one of the most prominent and essential immune checkpoint receptor, CTLA-4. It functions as a competitive inhibitor of the costimulatory receptor CD28 for binding to B7 molecules (CD80/CD86) present on the cells involved in antigen presentation, which provides inhibition signals and diminishes early activation of T-cells. In NSCLC, inhibition of anti-tumor responses of the immune system is the result of an upregulation of CTLA-4, thus enabling tumor growth (Mountzios et al., 2023). The binding of PD-L1 on tumor cells with PD-1 present on effector T cells brings about a state of functional exhaustion, in turn resulting in a lowered cytokine output, inhibition of proliferation, and decreased cytotoxicity, thereby enabling the cancer cells to grow without suppression (Francisco et al., 2010). In addition to PD-1 and CTLA-4, various other inhibitory receptors, including Lymphocyte Activation Gene-3 (LAG-3) and T-cell Immunoglobulin and Mucin-domain containing-3 (TIM-3), have been found to exhibit critical involvement through major contributory roles in the immune evasion observed in NSCLC. Simultaneous expression of these immune checkpoints along with PD-1 on tumor-infiltrating lymphocytes is thus indicative of a cooperative role in the enhancement of T-cell dysfunction as observed in the TME of NSCLC, further aggravating immune evasion and uncontrolled tumor proliferation (Liu, Chen, et al., 2021). These immune checkpoints, apart from being essential suppressive markers, also play the role of functional contributors to the generation of an immunologically cold TME. The blockade of these immune checkpoints through the use of immune checkpoint inhibitors (ICIs), for instance, pembrolizumab, nivolumab, and atezolizumab, has revolutionized the therapeutic procedures of NSCLC, with increased survival and durable responses being recorded in a subset of NSCLC patients (Reck et al., 2016; Herbst et al., 2020). However, sustenance of immune evasion occurs by adaptive resistance mechanisms like overexpression of alternative checkpoints like T-cell immunoreceptor with immunoglobulin and ITIM domain (TIGIT) and the other aforementioned checkpoints, or by expansion of immunosuppressive cells like Tregs and MDSCs (Sakuishi et al., 2010; Chauvin & Zarour, 2020).

3.2 Tumor-Induced Immune Suppression

Immunosuppression by tumor in NSCLC describes how NSCLC cells escape immunodetection and killing, sustaining tumor growth at the expense of patient outcomes. Key challenges to pharmacological targeting observed in NSCLC are attributed to a particular prevalence of the establishment of an immunosuppressive TME that can disrupt the efficient anti-tumor responses produced by different components of the immune system (Zhou & Yang, 2023). Various factors play an important role in this observed immunosuppression in NSCLC. These include CTLA-4 and PD-L1 pathways, the PD-1/PD-L1 pathway, tumor-associated macrophages (TAMs), defective antigen presenting cells (APCs), DCs, MDSCs, damaging expression of IDO, and activated Tregs (Munn & Bronte, 2016). Peripheral Treg cells (pTregs) with elevated expression of *FOXP3* resulting in immunosuppression through immunosuppressive receptors (like CTLA-4, TIGIT, NRP1, CD39, CD73, and LAG-3) and inhibitory cytokines, along with effector Treg cells (eTregs) producing immunosuppression by means of cell contact-dependent and cytokine-mediated pathways orchestrated by CTLA-4 and interleukin-2 receptor (IL-2R) also hold prominence in remodelling the TME and supplementing the attenuation of immune responses (Liang et al., 2022). Multiple markers directly associated with peripheral immunosuppression in NSCLC have been identified through experimental studies on brain metastatic lung tumors as well as pre-metastatic lung cancer. Up-regulated peripheral monocyte PD-L1, along with expanded populations of Tregs and MDSCs, was recorded in samples from brain metastatic lung carcinoma in comparison to these parameters recorded from healthy controls and pre-metastatic patients. Further, the elevated levels of peripheral monocyte PD-L1 were accompanied by T-cells with reduced reactivity and worse progression-free and overall survival of patients. Furthermore, stimulation of naïve monocytes with brain metastasis conditioned media obtained from tumor-derived cell cultures enhanced the PD-L1 expression on monocytes. In addition, levels of IL-6 recorded from this media demonstrated correlation with induction of PD-L1 (Li et al., 2019).

3.3 Antigen Loss and Defective Antigen Presentation

NSCLC is characterized by distinctive aberrations in processes and molecules associated with antigen presentation that holds criticality in effective elimination of cancer cells and preventing their uncontrolled proliferation. In a research focused on the investigation of a potential loss of antigen-presenting molecules, a total of 93 resection specimens of NSCLC were used for the determination of TAP-1 and MHC class I antigens. According to the results, 38% cases reported a total loss of MHC Class I molecules, with a loss of β2-microglobulin and heavy chain A locus usually accompanying this deprivation of the antigen presentation machinery. While a loss of β2-microglobulin and/or heavy chain A locus always accompanied the loss of TAP-1, selective loss of A locus and A2 allele occurred in 8.3% and 27% of the cases, respectively (Korkolopoulou et al., 1996). Out of a total of 190 primary NSCLC lesions stained with HLA class I heavy chain-specific mAb HC-10, 93.6% lesions presented defects in class I antigen of HLA. This down-regulation exhibited association with the increased survival of patients, though not significant statistically (Ramnath et al., 2006). Another study presented the application of a computational tool named loss of heterozygosity in human leukocyte antigen (LOHHLA) in an attempt to assess allele-specific copy number pertaining to HLA on the basis of sequencing data. Through the application of LOHHLA, occurrence of HLA LOH was determined in 40% of NSCLCs, with this occurrence associated with elevated cytolytic activity, presence of PD-L1, substantial burden of sub-clonal neoantigens, and APOBEC-mediated mutagenesis. In addition, HLA LOH was established as an immune escape mechanism, strongly influenced by the tumor microenvironmental selection pressures in the later stages of tumor evolution (McGranahan et al., 2017). With interferon-γ (IFNγ)-IRF1 signalling pathway contributing to the regulation of antigen presentation occurring through MHC class I, data collected from The Cancer Genome Atlas (TCGA) on lung adenocarcinoma (LuAd) and lung squamous cell carcinoma (LuSc) was analysed in an attempt to identify genetic defects pertaining to the IFNγ-IRF1 pathway that possibly hold association with the dysfunctional antigen presentation machinery of NSCLC. Loss-of-function (LOF) genetic aberrations pertaining to different IFNγ-IRF1 pathway genes were recorded in 64 out of 1,016 patients, with a primary occurrence of *JAK2* genetic defects. Upon further analysis through the utilization of wildtype as well as defective *JAK2* expressing cell lines, it was established that *JAK2* deficiency represents a critical aspect of genetic defects associated with the IFNγ-IRF1 pathway functional in the pathogenesis of NSCLC (Shen et al., 2017).

4. ROLE OF INFLAMMATION AND CYTOKINES IN NSCLC PROGRESSION

Inflammation plays an indispensable role in NSCLC, regulating various aspects of its pathogenesis and immune evasion evident in the TME. Chronic inflammation establishes a tumor microenvironment by inducing genetic mutations, enhancing angiogenesis, and suppressing anti-tumor immunity. A group of 113 patients suffering from NSCLC belonging to the People's Hospital of Pengzhou and 109 healthy volunteers (control group) were analysed for the differential expressions of IL-1, IL-6, and TNF-α occurring in the test and control groups. These pro-inflammatory cytokines existed in substantially elevated levels in the NSCLC group. Further, the NSCLC patients were divided into severe (52 cases) and mild (61 cases) groups according to the Visual Analogue Scale (VAS). The severe group reported considerably higher levels of the cytokines than the mild group. Furthermore, a combination of IL-1 + IL-6 + TNF-α provided an 81.80% sensitivity and 71.40% specificity in the poor prognosis of NSCLC, thus providing evidence for possible usage of these cytokines together for the prognosis of NSCLC (Liu, Gao, et al., 2021). Another study involving 65 tumor, adjacent tissue samples, and serum samples from NSCLC patients analysed the levels of expression of IL-6, TNF-α, E- and N-cadherin, and vimentin. From the results obtained, there was a significant up-regulation of IL-6 and TNF-α in NSCLC samples in comparison to controls of both serum and tissue.

Further, the studied cytokines reported a positive correlation with lymph node metastasis and distant metastasis. In addition, the cytokines reported a negative correlation with E-cadherin levels, while a positive correlation was observed with N-cadherin and vimentin levels. The results were thus indicative of the fact that induction of epithelial-mesenchymal transition (EMT) is possible by these cytokines, consequently promoting metastasis in NSCLC (Shang et al., 2017).

Chronic inflammation is a critical contributory factor in the development and progression of NSCLC. As a matter of fact, it is involved in every stage of tumorigenesis: initiation, promotion, invasion, and metastasis. Cancer establishes an inflammatory tumor microenvironment affecting angiogenesis, immune evasion, and growth of malignant cells (Nishida & Andoh, 2025). There are number of biological signalling pathways including nuclear factor kappa B (NF-κB), mitogen-activated protein kinase (MAPK), toll-like receptor (TLR) pathways, Janus kinase/signal transducers and activators of transcription (JAK-STAT), and cGAS/STING, along with inflammatory factors like cytokines, chemokines, growth factors, and inflammasome and inflammatory metabolites like leukotrienes, thromboxane, prostaglandins, and specialized pro-resolving mediators (SPM) hold criticality as the essential mediators of different aspects of inflammation (Zhao et al., 2021). Chronic inflammation is a major facilitator of immune escape in NSCLC, mediating a complicated relationship between pro-inflammatory signaling and immunosuppressive processes in the TME. Continually active inflammatory stimuli - including tobacco carcinogens, air pollutants, and oncogenic mutations - induce a chronic state of NF-κB and STAT3 activation, both of which are responsible for induction of transcriptional activation of pro-inflammatory cytokines, such as IL-6, IL-1β, and TNF-α (Taniguchi & Karin, 2018; Greten & Grivennikov, 2019). In addition to facilitating proliferation of tumor cells and angiogenesis, recruitment and polarization of immune cells- including TAMs and MDSCs to immunosuppressive phenotypes is also performed by these cytokines (Gabrilovich, 2017; Quail & Joyce, 2013). In this setting, Tregs are enriched and cytotoxic CD8+ cells suffer functional impairment due to chronic exposure to inhibitory cytokines and increased expression of immune checkpoints like PD-L1 and CTLA-4 on both immune and tumor cells (Togashi et al., 2019). Moreover, inflammation-mediated metabolic remodeling—which consists of the accumulation of lactate and exhaustion of important amino acids, such as tryptophan and arginine—further potentiates the bias of the immune landscape toward tolerance and exhaustion (Leone & Powell, 2020). Thus, the immunosuppressive feedback loop is what keeps tumor cells out of immune detection, subsequently fuelling uninterrupted disease progression as well as therapeutic resistance. The cognition of the bidirectional relationship between chronic inflammatory states and immune escape is an essential pillar in the development of targeted approaches to re-activate anti-tumor immunity in NSCLC.

5. THERAPEUTIC STRATEGIES TARGETING THE TME AND IMMUNE EVASION

5.1 Immune Checkpoint Inhibitors

As an effective mode of therapy, ICIs are gaining rapid prominence in the management of NSCLC, with acknowledgement from the scientific community owing to largely successful results based on experimental studies. With an approval of either the U.S. Food and Drug Administration (FDA) or in Europe by the European Medicines Agency (EMA), antibodies are being largely adopted as means to target immune checkpoints in the broad treatment regimens of NSCLC. These include three (Pembrolizumab, Nivolumab, and Cemiplimab) antibodies which have PD-1 as their target, two (Tremelimumab and Ipilimumab) with CTLA-4 as the target molecule, three (Atezolizumab, Avelumab, and Durvalumab) having PD-L1 as their target, and one (Relatlimab) targeting LAG-3 (Raskova Kafkova et al., 2024). With positive results recorded in phase I trials, these ICIs are involved in trials currently underway to evaluate their efficacy and applicability in patients afflicted with NSCLC. Among the ICIs being tested, prominent agents include nivolumab, pembrolizumab, MPDL3280A, and MEDI-4736 which have PD-1/PD-L1 as the target molecule, followed by ipilimumab and tremelimumab having CTLA-4 as the target checkpoint. These therapeutic agents, by way of inhibition of important agents which negatively influence T-cell activity, generate their respective anti-tumor responses (Johnson et al., 2014). Monoclonal antibodies nivolumab, pembrolizumab, atezolizumab, durvalumab, and ipilimumab have proven extremely effective in first-line and second-line treatment procedures employed for NSCLC patients (Borghaei et al., 2015; Faivre-Finn et al., 2020). For instance, KEYNOTE-024 and KEYNOTE-042 trials cemented pembrolizumab monotherapy as a standardized procedure of treatment in patients exhibiting high PD-L1 expression levels (TPS ≥50%), with a proven superior overall survival in patients when compared to the groups receiving treatment with platinum-containing chemotherapy regimens (Mok et al., 2019; Reck et al., 2016).

5.2 Combination Therapies

The potential oncogenic drivers that determine prognosis and define treatment plans tailored for different stages and levels of progression of NSCLC are vital to the health and survival of patients undergoing treatment. In recent years, several such oncogenic markers have come to light. In advanced NSCLC, targetable molecular oncogenic markers primarily include epidermal growth factor receptor (EGFR), v-raf murine sarcoma viral oncogene homolog B (BRAF), neuregulin 1 (NRG1), rearranged during transfection (RET), ROS proto-oncogene 1 (ROS1), anaplastic lymphoma kinase (ALK), neurotrophic receptor tyrosine kinase (NTRK), Kirstin rat sarcoma virus (KRAS), c-MET proto-oncogene (MET), and human epidermal receptor 2 (HER2), while phosphoinositide 3-kinases (PI3K) and fibroblast growth factor receptor (FGFR), though less well understood, hold considerable scientific importance in research (Friedlaender et al., 2024). ALK, KRAS, EGFR, NTRK, RET, and BRAF have also been mentioned in other pieces of scientific literature on NSCLC (Bayramova et al., 2024). The TME of NSCLC and different conventional therapeutic approaches have been illustrated in Figure 2. In an open-label, phase 3 trial with random assignment of patients suffering from NSCLC (either stage IV or recurrent) with levels of PD-L1 expression less than, equal to, or more than 1%, a therapeutic agent, consisting of nivolumab and ipilimumab in combination, was tested against nivolumab alone and chemotherapy. With patients presenting different levels of expression of PD-L1, the combination produced a significantly increased median duration of overall survival (OS) as compared to chemotherapy, with the combinational treatment presenting a remarkable 17.1 months against a duration of only 13.9 months with chemotherapy when all the trial patients were considered for both evaluations (Hellmann et al., 2019). From a massive cohort of 8,467 patients divided into 14 trials, immunotherapy + immunotherapy + chemotherapy (IO + IO + Chemo) emerged as the best possible mode of treatment with an OS probability of 68%, holding relevant OS probabilities for PD-L1-intermediate (78%) as well as PD-L1-negative (37%) cohorts. For the PD-L1-high cohort, IO + Anti-angio + Chemo, involving a combinational administration of immunotherapy, anti-angiogenic therapy, and chemotherapy, provided the most prominent results when determined for objective response rate (ORR), progression-free survival (PFS), and OS among other treatment modes (Mao et al., 2021). Evaluating the efficacy of different combinational treatment regimens for advanced NSCLC, a phase 2 umbrella HUDSON study enrolled and treated 268 patients with durvalumab (anti-PD-L1 monoclonal antibody)–ceralasertib (ATR kinase inhibitor), durvalumab–danvatirsen (STAT3 antisense oligonucleotide), durvalumab–oleclumab (anti-CD73 monoclonal antibody), or durvalumab–olaparib (PARP inhibitor). After evaluating the treatment combinations, durvalumab–ceralasertib provided the greatest clinical benefit with an acceptable safety profile. A 13.9% objective response rate was recorded with this treatment, as compared to 2.6% with the other treatments. Median PFS recorded for this particular combination also provided higher values as compared to the other combinations (5.8 vs. 2.7 months). Similarly, median overall survival also presented similar results (17.4 vs. 9.4 months). Highly positive results were also obtained with *ATM*-altered patients (Besse et al., 2024).

Figure 2. **Different components of the TME in NSCLC, the risk factors leading to its pathogenesis, associated symptoms of the disease, and the current available therapies employed in the course of treatment and management of NSCLC** *(Y. Wu et al., 2024).*

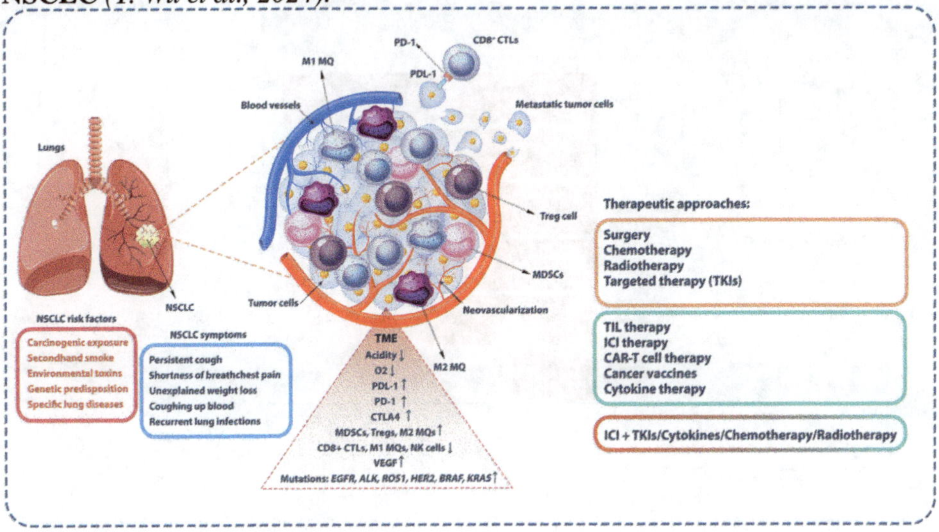

5.3 Future Perspectives

NSCLC continues to disrupt the lives of millions of people globally, with the worrisome mortality rates associated with this disease illustrated in Figure 3. As a consequence, research on different factors influencing the pathogenesis and aggressive spread of NSCLC needs to be strategically increased in a manner that befits the moderation of the current burden on healthcare settings related to poor prognosis and management of the disease. Exploration of the complex biology of the TME and immune evasion mechanisms is certain to become a growing area of study in the setting of NSCLC. Progress in next-generation technologies like single-cell RNA sequencing, spatial transcriptomics, and integrative multi-omic analysis has enabled more precise tumor-infiltrating immune and stromal cell characterization. These technologies are central to the discovery of novel spatial dynamics, signaling pathways, and cellular phenotypes underlying immunological suppression and treatment resistance. Future study findings will be used to derive predictive biomarkers to guide the design of personalized treatment approaches based on the molecular and immunologic characteristics of individual tumors, guide early detection of resistance, and guide patient stratification for immunotherapy.

Figure 3. Age-standardized mortality rate (ASMR) of cancer of the trachea, bronchus, and lungs in both sexes as recorded from Europe, Asia, Northern America, Oceania, South America, and Africa in 2022. (Credit: GLOBOCAN 2022)

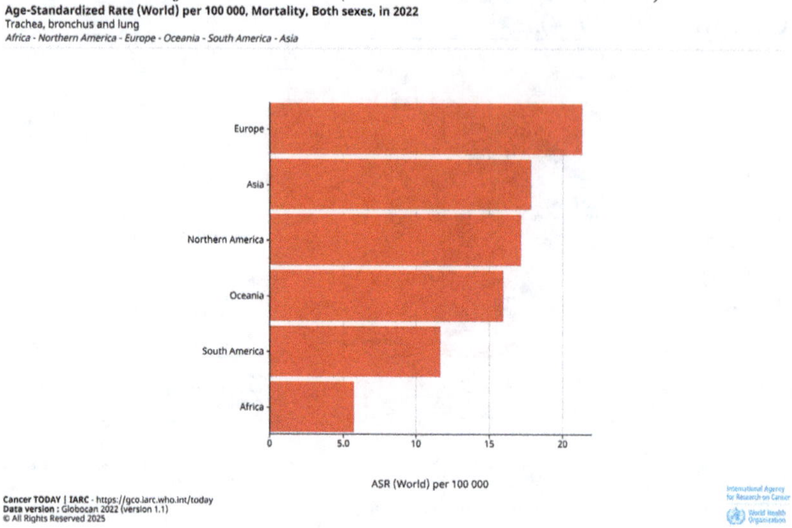

Unraveling the intricate biology of TME and the pathways through which immune evasion is achieved will be first targets of forthcoming research into NSCLC. Breakthroughs in high-throughput technologies offering ultra-high-resolution outputs for comprehensive analysis, including single-cell RNA sequencing, spatial transcriptomics, and integrative multi-omic analysis, have made it possible to precisely characterize immune and stromal cells invading tumors. These breakthrough tools will be essential in newly revealing spatial dynamics, signaling pathways, and cellular phenotypic features of immune suppression and treatment resistance. Future research will provide new avenues to delineate predictive biomarkers that guide individualized treatment options based on the molecular and immunologic features of individual tumors, enable early detection of resistance emergence, and guide patient stratification for immunotherapy.

1. Future research must prioritize high-resolution, multi-omics, single-cell profiling of the NSCLC TME. This will allow researchers to crack the code of spatial and temporal cellular and molecular interactions that govern immune evasion. Combining spatial transcriptomics with proteomics and metabolomics can provide new insights into therapeutically relevant microenvironmental niches.
2. There is a significant need for further elucidation of the mechanisms through which non-cellular components—namely, hypoxia, secreted metabolites, and stiffness of the extracellular matrix—influence the expression and activity of

immune checkpoints. Exploration of such biochemical and biophysical signals may identify new druggable targets indirectly augmenting immune responsiveness within the TME. High-tech 3D organoid and *ex-vivo* lung tissue culture systems can be exploited as model platforms to explore this.

3. As immune checkpoint inhibitors become more advanced, so do the resistance mechanisms in NSCLC. Research in the future must focus on the identification and characterization of new checkpoint molecules (e.g., VISTA, B7-H3) and the adaptive resistance loops they initiate. The development of bispecific antibodies and rational combination therapies may be central in overcoming primary and acquired resistance.
4. As a step towards connecting preclinical information and clinical applicability, follow-up studies should further refine immunocompetent models that more accurately mimic human NSCLC TME complexity. Humanized mouse models, patient-derived organoids, and tumor-on-a-chip models belong to this group. These platforms could be critical in the assessment of novel therapies aimed at TME normalization and immune reinvigoration in a clinically relevant context.
5. Complex datasets from genomics, immunophenotyping, and imaging should use machine learning and AI-driven analytics to create integrated insights. These help identify strong, composite biomarkers predictive of immune evasion and treatment outcomes. With respect to the conduct of clinical trials, AI could also help reduce the time taken for patient stratification in a strategic attempt to enable more personalised and effective treatment and regression to the mean.

6. CONCLUSION

Non-small cell lung cancer (NSCLC) cells and their tumor microenvironment (TME) maintain a complex relationship which drives multiple biological behaviors that result in disease progression, therapeutic resistance and immune evasion. The TME consists of stromal fibroblasts and immune cells and extracellular matrix and soluble factors which together create an immunosuppressive environment that allows tumor survival. The conditions become stronger because hypoxia and metabolic reprogramming modify the availability of nutrients and the function of immune cells. NSCLC tumors use various methods to evade immune surveillance including an up-regulated expression of PD-L1 along with Treg and myeloid-derived suppressor cell recruitment and antigen presentation disruption. The inflammatory environment which arises from IL-6 and TGF-β cytokines leads to immune system dysfunction that supports tumor growth. The immunological nature of the TME determines why checkpoint blockade immunotherapy produces inconsistent response rates in treatment. The future of NSCLC treatment requires molecular profiling alongside

TME remodeling and combinatorial approaches to defeat immune resistance and improve long-term clinical results in an attempt to enhance overall survivability as well as quality of life of patients suffering from NSCLC worldwide.

7. REFERENCES

Bayramova, J., Tarakci, E., Huseynova, G., Yazici, H., & Yazici, H. (2024). Genetic Alterations in Lung Cancer. *Turk Onkoloji Dergisi*, *39*(2), 234–243. DOI: 10.5505/tjo.2024.4285

Besse, B., Pons-Tostivint, E., Park, K., Hartl, S., Forde, P. M., Hochmair, M. J., Awad, M. M., Thomas, M., Goss, G., Wheatley-Price, P., Shepherd, F. A., Florescu, M., Cheema, P., Chu, Q. S. C., Kim, S.-W., Morgensztern, D., Johnson, M. L., Cousin, S., Kim, D.-W., & Heymach, J. V. (2024). Biomarker-directed targeted therapy plus durvalumab in advanced non-small-cell lung cancer: A phase 2 umbrella trial. *Nature Medicine*, *30*(3), 716–729. DOI: 10.1038/s41591-024-02808-y PMID: 38351187

Borghaei, H., Paz-Ares, L., Horn, L., Spigel, D. R., Steins, M., Ready, N. E., Chow, L. Q., Vokes, E. E., Felip, E., Holgado, E., Barlesi, F., Kohlhäufl, M., Arrieta, O., Burgio, M. A., Fayette, J., Lena, H., Poddubskaya, E., Gerber, D. E., Gettinger, S. N., & Brahmer, J. R. (2015). Nivolumab versus Docetaxel in Advanced Nonsquamous Non–Small-Cell Lung Cancer. *The New England Journal of Medicine*, *373*(17), 1627–1639. DOI: 10.1056/NEJMoa1507643 PMID: 26412456

Brand, A., Singer, K., Koehl, G. E., Kolitzus, M., Schoenhammer, G., Thiel, A., Matos, C., Bruss, C., Klobuch, S., Peter, K., Kastenberger, M., Bogdan, C., Schleicher, U., Mackensen, A., Ullrich, E., Fichtner-Feigl, S., Kesselring, R., Mack, M., Ritter, U., & Kreutz, M. (2016). LDHA-Associated Lactic Acid Production Blunts Tumor Immunosurveillance by T and NK Cells. *Cell Metabolism*, *24*(5), 657–671. DOI: 10.1016/j.cmet.2016.08.011 PMID: 27641098

Brassart-Pasco, S., Brézillon, S., Brassart, B., Ramont, L., Oudart, J.-B., & Monboisse, J. C. (2020). Tumor Microenvironment: Extracellular Matrix Alterations Influence Tumor Progression. *Frontiers in Oncology*, *10*, 397. Advance online publication. DOI: 10.3389/fonc.2020.00397 PMID: 32351878

Chauvin, J.-M., & Zarour, H. M. (2020). TIGIT in cancer immunotherapy. *Journal for Immunotherapy of Cancer*, *8*(2), e000957. DOI: 10.1136/jitc-2020-000957 PMID: 32900861

Erdogan, B., & Webb, D. J. (2017). Cancer-associated fibroblasts modulate growth factor signaling and extracellular matrix remodeling to regulate tumor metastasis. *Biochemical Society Transactions*, *45*(1), 229–236. DOI: 10.1042/BST20160387 PMID: 28202677

Faivre-Finn, C., Vicente, D., Kurata, T., Planchard, D., Paz-Ares, L., Vansteenkiste, J. F., Spigel, D. R., Garassino, M. C., Reck, M., Senan, S., Naidoo, J., Rimner, A., Wu, Y.-L., Gray, J. E., Özgüroğlu, M., Lee, K. H., Newton, M., Wang, L., Thiyagarajah, P., & Antonia, S. J. (2020). LBA49 Durvalumab after chemoradiotherapy in stage III NSCLC: 4-year survival update from the phase III PACIFIC trial. *Annals of Oncology : Official Journal of the European Society for Medical Oncology, 31*, S1178–S1179. DOI: 10.1016/j.annonc.2020.08.2281

Francisco, L. M., Sage, P. T., & Sharpe, A. H. (2010). The PD-1 pathway in tolerance and autoimmunity. *Immunological Reviews, 236*(1), 219–242. DOI: 10.1111/j.1600-065X.2010.00923.x PMID: 20636820

Friedlaender, A., Perol, M., Banna, G. L., Parikh, K., & Addeo, A. (2024). Oncogenic alterations in advanced NSCLC: A molecular super-highway. *Biomarker Research, 12*(1), 24. DOI: 10.1186/s40364-024-00566-0 PMID: 38347643

Gabrilovich, D. I. (2017). Myeloid-Derived Suppressor Cells. *Cancer Immunology Research, 5*(1), 3–8. DOI: 10.1158/2326-6066.CIR-16-0297 PMID: 28052991

Greten, F. R., & Grivennikov, S. I. (2019). Inflammation and Cancer: Triggers, Mechanisms, and Consequences. *Immunity, 51*(1), 27–41. DOI: 10.1016/j.immuni.2019.06.025 PMID: 31315034

Gridelli, C., Rossi, A., Carbone, D. P., Guarize, J., Karachaliou, N., Mok, T., Petrella, F., Spaggiari, L., & Rosell, R. (2015). Non-small-cell lung cancer. *Nature Reviews. Disease Primers, 1*(1), 15009. DOI: 10.1038/nrdp.2015.9 PMID: 27188576

Guo, T., He, C., Venado, A., & Zhou, Y. (2022). Extracellular Matrix Stiffness in Lung Health and Disease. *Comprehensive Physiology, 12*(3), 3523–3558. DOI: 10.1002/j.2040-4603.2022.tb00222.x PMID: 35766837

Hellmann, M. D., Paz-Ares, L., Bernabe Caro, R., Zurawski, B., Kim, S.-W., Carcereny Costa, E., Park, K., Alexandru, A., Lupinacci, L., de la Mora Jimenez, E., Sakai, H., Albert, I., Vergnenegre, A., Peters, S., Syrigos, K., Barlesi, F., Reck, M., Borghaei, H., Brahmer, J. R., & Ramalingam, S. S. (2019). Nivolumab plus Ipilimumab in Advanced Non–Small-Cell Lung Cancer. *The New England Journal of Medicine, 381*(21), 2020–2031. DOI: 10.1056/NEJMoa1910231 PMID: 31562796

Herbst, R. S., Giaccone, G., de Marinis, F., Reinmuth, N., Vergnenegre, A., Barrios, C. H., Morise, M., Felip, E., Andric, Z., Geater, S., Özgüroğlu, M., Zou, W., Sandler, A., Enquist, I., Komatsubara, K., Deng, Y., Kuriki, H., Wen, X., McCleland, M., & Spigel, D. R. (2020). Atezolizumab for First-Line Treatment of PD-L1–Selected Patients with NSCLC. *The New England Journal of Medicine, 383*(14), 1328–1339. DOI: 10.1056/NEJMoa1917346 PMID: 32997907

Huang, S., Chung, J. Y.-F., Li, C., Wu, Y., Qiao, G., To, K.-F., & Tang, P. M.-K. (2024). Cellular dynamics of tumor microenvironment driving immunotherapy resistance in non-small-cell lung carcinoma. *Cancer Letters*, *604*, 217272. DOI: 10.1016/j.canlet.2024.217272 PMID: 39326553

Jin, J., Byun, J.-K., Choi, Y.-K., & Park, K.-G. (2023). Targeting glutamine metabolism as a therapeutic strategy for cancer. *Experimental & Molecular Medicine*, *55*(4), 706–715. DOI: 10.1038/s12276-023-00971-9 PMID: 37009798

Johnson, D. B., Rioth, M. J., & Horn, L. (2014). Immune Checkpoint Inhibitors in NSCLC. *Current Treatment Options in Oncology*, *15*(4), 658–669. DOI: 10.1007/s11864-014-0305-5 PMID: 25096781

Korkolopoulou, P., Kaklamanis, L., Pezzella, F., Harris, A., & Gatter, K. (1996). Loss of antigen-presenting molecules (MHC class I and TAP-1) in lung cancer. *British Journal of Cancer*, *73*(2), 148–153. DOI: 10.1038/bjc.1996.28 PMID: 8546899

Li, Y. D., Lamano, J. B., Lamano, J. B., Quaggin-Smith, J., Veliceasa, D., Kaur, G., Biyashev, D., Unruh, D., & Bloch, O. (2019). Tumor-induced peripheral immunosuppression promotes brain metastasis in patients with non-small cell lung cancer. *Cancer Immunology, Immunotherapy : CII*, *68*(9), 1501–1513. DOI: 10.1007/s00262-019-02384-y PMID: 31489465

Liang, J., Bi, G., Shan, G., Jin, X., Bian, Y., & Wang, Q. (2022). Tumor-Associated Regulatory T Cells in Non-Small-Cell Lung Cancer: Current Advances and Future Perspectives. *Journal of Immunology Research*, *2022*, 1–8. DOI: 10.1155/2022/4355386 PMID: 35497874

Liu, Y., Chen, P., Wang, H., Wu, S., Zhao, S., He, Y., Zhou, C., & Hirsch, F. R. (2021). The landscape of immune checkpoints expression in non-small cell lung cancer: A narrative review. *Translational Lung Cancer Research*, *10*(2), 1029–1038. DOI: 10.21037/tlcr-20-1019 PMID: 33718041

Liu, Y., Gao, Y., & Lin, T. (2021). Expression of interleukin-1 (IL-1), IL-6, and tumor necrosis factor-α (TNF-α) in non-small cell lung cancer and its relationship with the occurrence and prognosis of cancer pain. *Annals of Palliative Medicine*, *10*(12), 12759–12766. DOI: 10.21037/apm-21-3471 PMID: 35016421

Mao, Z., Jiang, P., Zhang, Y., Li, Y., Jia, X., Wang, Q., Jiao, M., Jiang, L., Shen, Y., & Guo, H. (2021). First-line immune-based combination therapies for advanced non-small cell lung cancer: A Bayesian network meta-analysis. *Cancer Medicine*, *10*(24), 9139–9155. DOI: 10.1002/cam4.4405 PMID: 34747149

McGranahan, N., Rosenthal, R., Hiley, C. T., Rowan, A. J., Watkins, T. B. K., Wilson, G. A., Birkbak, N. J., Veeriah, S., Van Loo, P., Herrero, J., Swanton, C., Swanton, C., Jamal-Hanjani, M., Veeriah, S., Shafi, S., Czyzewska-Khan, J., Johnson, D., Laycock, J., Bosshard-Carter, L., & Dessimoz, C. (2017). Allele-Specific HLA Loss and Immune Escape in Lung Cancer Evolution. *Cell*, *171*(6), 1259–1271. DOI: 10.1016/j.cell.2017.10.001 PMID: 29107330

Meng, L., Wu, H., Wu, J., Ding, P., He, J., Sang, M., & Liu, L. (2024). Mechanisms of immune checkpoint inhibitors: Insights into the regulation of circular RNAS involved in cancer hallmarks. *Cell Death & Disease*, *15*(1), 3. DOI: 10.1038/s41419-023-06389-5 PMID: 38177102

Mok, T. S. K., Wu, Y.-L., Kudaba, I., Kowalski, D. M., Cho, B. C., Turna, H. Z., Castro, G.Jr, Srimuninnimit, V., Laktionov, K. K., Bondarenko, I., Kubota, K., Lubiniecki, G. M., Zhang, J., Kush, D., Lopes, G., Adamchuk, G., Ahn, M.-J., Alexandru, A., Altundag, O., & Zippelius, A. (2019). Pembrolizumab versus chemotherapy for previously untreated, PD-L1-expressing, locally advanced or metastatic non-small-cell lung cancer (KEYNOTE-042): A randomised, open-label, controlled, phase 3 trial. *Lancet*, *393*(10183), 1819–1830. DOI: 10.1016/S0140-6736(18)32409-7 PMID: 30955977

Mountzios, G., Remon, J., Hendriks, L. E. L., García-Campelo, R., Rolfo, C., Van Schil, P., Forde, P. M., Besse, B., Subbiah, V., Reck, M., Soria, J.-C., & Peters, S. (2023). Immune-checkpoint inhibition for resectable non-small-cell lung cancer — Opportunities and challenges. *Nature Reviews. Clinical Oncology*, *20*(10), 664–677. DOI: 10.1038/s41571-023-00794-7 PMID: 37488229

Munn, D. H., & Bronte, V. (2016). Immune suppressive mechanisms in the tumor microenvironment. *Current Opinion in Immunology*, *39*, 1–6. DOI: 10.1016/j.coi.2015.10.009 PMID: 26609943

Nishida, A., & Andoh, A. (2025). The Role of Inflammation in Cancer: Mechanisms of Tumor Initiation, Progression, and Metastasis. *Cells*, *14*(7), 488. DOI: 10.3390/cells14070488 PMID: 40214442

Pisibon, C., Ouertani, A., Bertolotto, C., Ballotti, R., & Cheli, Y. (2021). Immune Checkpoints in Cancers: From Signaling to the Clinic. *Cancers (Basel)*, *13*(18), 4573. DOI: 10.3390/cancers13184573 PMID: 34572799

Quail, D. F., & Joyce, J. A. (2013). Microenvironmental regulation of tumor progression and metastasis. *Nature Medicine*, *19*(11), 1423–1437. DOI: 10.1038/nm.3394 PMID: 24202395

Rajasegaran, T., How, C. W., Saud, A., Ali, A., & Lim, J. C. W. (2023). Targeting Inflammation in Non-Small Cell Lung Cancer through Drug Repurposing. *Pharmaceuticals (Basel, Switzerland), 16*(3), 451. DOI: 10.3390/ph16030451 PMID: 36986550

Ramachandran, S., Verma, A. K., Dev, K., Goyal, Y., Bhatt, D., Alsahli, M. A., Rahmani, A. H., Almatroudi, A., Almatroodi, S. A., Alrumaihi, F., & Khan, N. A. (2021). Role of Cytokines and Chemokines in NSCLC Immune Navigation and Proliferation. *Oxidative Medicine and Cellular Longevity, 2021*(1). DOI: 10.1155/2021/5563746

Ramnath, N., Tan, D., Li, Q., Hylander, B. L., Bogner, P., Ryes, L., & Ferrone, S. (2006). Is downregulation of MHC class I antigen expression in human non-small cell lung cancer associated with prolonged survival? *Cancer Immunology, Immunotherapy : CII, 55*(8), 891–899. DOI: 10.1007/s00262-005-0085-7 PMID: 16187081

Raskova Kafkova, L., Mierzwicka, J. M., Chakraborty, P., Jakubec, P., Fischer, O., Skarda, J., Maly, P., & Raska, M. (2024). NSCLC: From tumorigenesis, immune checkpoint misuse to current and future targeted therapy. *Frontiers in Immunology, 15*, 1342086. Advance online publication. DOI: 10.3389/fimmu.2024.1342086 PMID: 38384472

Reck, M., Rodríguez-Abreu, D., Robinson, A. G., Hui, R., Csőszi, T., Fülöp, A., Gottfried, M., Peled, N., Tafreshi, A., Cuffe, S., O'Brien, M., Rao, S., Hotta, K., Leiby, M. A., Lubiniecki, G. M., Shentu, Y., Rangwala, R., & Brahmer, J. R. (2016). Pembrolizumab versus Chemotherapy for PD-L1–Positive Non–Small-Cell Lung Cancer. *The New England Journal of Medicine, 375*(19), 1823–1833. DOI: 10.1056/NEJMoa1606774 PMID: 27718847

Sakuishi, K., Apetoh, L., Sullivan, J. M., Blazar, B. R., Kuchroo, V. K., & Anderson, A. C. (2010). Targeting Tim-3 and PD-1 pathways to reverse T cell exhaustion and restore anti-tumor immunity. *The Journal of Experimental Medicine, 207*(10), 2187–2194. DOI: 10.1084/jem.20100643 PMID: 20819927

Shang, G.-S., Liu, L., & Qin, Y.-W. (2017). IL-6 and TNF-α promote metastasis of lung cancer by inducing epithelial-mesenchymal transition. *Oncology Letters, 13*(6), 4657–4660. DOI: 10.3892/ol.2017.6048 PMID: 28599466

Shen, T., Chen, Z., Zhao, Z. J., & Wu, J. (2017). Genetic defects of the IRF1-mediated major histocompatibility complex class I antigen presentation pathway occur prevalently in the JAK2 gene in non-small cell lung cancer. *Oncotarget, 8*(37), 60975–60986. DOI: 10.18632/oncotarget.17689 PMID: 28977839

Shi, Z., Hu, C., Zheng, X., Sun, C., & Li, Q. (2024). Feedback loop between hypoxia and energy metabolic reprogramming aggravates the radioresistance of cancer cells. *Experimental Hematology & Oncology*, *13*(1), 55. DOI: 10.1186/s40164-024-00519-1 PMID: 38778409

Shintani, Y., Kimura, T., Funaki, S., Ose, N., Kanou, T., & Fukui, E. (2023). Therapeutic Targeting of Cancer-Associated Fibroblasts in the Non-Small Cell Lung Cancer Tumor Microenvironment. *Cancers (Basel)*, *15*(2), 335. DOI: 10.3390/cancers15020335 PMID: 36672284

Siegel, R. L., Kratzer, T. B., Giaquinto, A. N., Sung, H., & Jemal, A. (2025). Cancer statistics, 2025. *CA: a Cancer Journal for Clinicians*, *75*(1), 10–45. DOI: 10.3322/caac.21871 PMID: 39817679

Stankovic, B., Bjørhovde, H. A. K., Skarshaug, R., Aamodt, H., Frafjord, A., Müller, E., Hammarström, C., Beraki, K., Bækkevold, E. S., Woldbæk, P. R., Helland, Å., Brustugun, O. T., Øynebråten, I., & Corthay, A. (2019). Immune Cell Composition in Human Non-small Cell Lung Cancer. *Frontiers in Immunology*, *9*, 3101. Advance online publication. DOI: 10.3389/fimmu.2018.03101 PMID: 30774636

Tamminga, M., Hiltermann, T. J. N., Schuuring, E., Timens, W., Fehrmann, R. S., & Groen, H. J. (2020). Immune microenvironment composition in non-small cell lung cancer and its association with survival. *Clinical & Translational Immunology*, *9*(6), e1142. DOI: 10.1002/cti2.1142 PMID: 32547744

Taniguchi, K., & Karin, M. (2018). NF-κB, inflammation, immunity and cancer: Coming of age. *Nature Reviews. Immunology*, *18*(5), 309–324. DOI: 10.1038/nri.2017.142 PMID: 29379212

Togashi, Y., Shitara, K., & Nishikawa, H. (2019). Regulatory T cells in cancer immunosuppression — Implications for anticancer therapy. *Nature Reviews. Clinical Oncology*, *16*(6), 356–371. DOI: 10.1038/s41571-019-0175-7 PMID: 30705439

Wang, B., Pei, J., Xu, S., Liu, J., & Yu, J. (2024). A glutamine tug-of-war between cancer and immune cells: Recent advances in unraveling the ongoing battle. *Journal of Experimental & Clinical Cancer Research : CR*, *43*(1), 74. DOI: 10.1186/s13046-024-02994-0 PMID: 38459595

Wang, L., Jia, Q., Chu, Q., & Zhu, B. (2023). Targeting tumor microenvironment for non-small cell lung cancer immunotherapy. *Chinese Medical Journal Pulmonary and Critical Care Medicine*, *1*(1), 18–29. DOI: 10.1016/j.pccm.2022.11.001 PMID: 39170874

Wu, F., Fan, J., He, Y., Xiong, A., Yu, J., Li, Y., Zhang, Y., Zhao, W., Zhou, F., Li, W., Zhang, J., Zhang, X., Qiao, M., Gao, G., Chen, S., Chen, X., Li, X., Hou, L., Wu, C., & Zhou, C. (2021). Single-cell profiling of tumor heterogeneity and the microenvironment in advanced non-small cell lung cancer. *Nature Communications*, *12*(1), 2540. DOI: 10.1038/s41467-021-22801-0 PMID: 33953163

Wu, Y., Yu, G., Jin, K., & Qian, J. (2024). Advancing non-small cell lung cancer treatment: The power of combination immunotherapies. *Frontiers in Immunology*, *15*, 1349502. Advance online publication. DOI: 10.3389/fimmu.2024.1349502 PMID: 39015563

Zhang, H., Li, S., Wang, D., Liu, S., Xiao, T., Gu, W., Yang, H., Wang, H., Yang, M., & Chen, P. (2024). Metabolic reprogramming and immune evasion: The interplay in the tumor microenvironment. *Biomarker Research*, *12*(1), 96. DOI: 10.1186/s40364-024-00646-1 PMID: 39227970

Zhao, H., Wu, L., Yan, G., Chen, Y., Zhou, M., Wu, Y., & Li, Y. (2021). Inflammation and tumor progression: Signaling pathways and targeted intervention. *Signal Transduction and Targeted Therapy*, *6*(1), 263. DOI: 10.1038/s41392-021-00658-5 PMID: 34248142

Zhou, S., Sun, J., Zhu, W., Yang, Z., Wang, P., & Zeng, Y. (2024). Hypoxia studies in non-small cell lung cancer: Pathogenesis and clinical implications [Review]. *Oncology Reports*, *53*(2), 29. DOI: 10.3892/or.2024.8862 PMID: 39749693

Zhou, S., & Yang, H. (2023). Immunotherapy resistance in non-small-cell lung cancer: From mechanism to clinical strategies. *Frontiers in Immunology*, *14*, 1129465. DOI: 10.3389/fimmu.2023.1129465 PMID: 37090727

Chapter 4
Integration of Microbial Systems in NSCLC Emerging Paradigms in Diagnosis and Treatment

Sharmistha Sharma
https://orcid.org/0009-0006-1101-504X
Assam University, Silchar, India

Anjali Roy
https://orcid.org/0009-0001-2759-7201
Assam University, Silchar, India

Himanshu Kishore Prasad
https://orcid.org/0000-0003-0215-1323
Assam University, Silchar, India

ABSTRACT

Non-small cell lung cancer (NSCLC) remains a significant health challenge despite therapy advances. The lung and gut microbiome are crucial in NSCLC development and treatment response. This chapter reviews microbe integration in NSCLC management, focusing on: (1) identifying lung and gut microbes linked to NSCLC; (2) developing microbiome-based diagnostics using liquid biopsy and AI; (3) exploring microbiome-targeted therapies like fecal transplants to improve treatment; and (4) addressing clinical challenges of implementation. Microbial imbalances contribute to NSCLC through inflammation and immune changes via the gut-lung axis. Unique microbial profiles could serve as biomarkers for detecting and predicting NSCLC outcomes. AI helps link microbial data with clinical information for predictive

DOI: 10.4018/979-8-3373-2096-0.ch004

models. Microbiome-targeted strategies aim to improve therapy outcomes but face challenges in proving causality, standardization, and regulation. Research collaboration is needed to utilize the microbiome for personalized NSCLC care.

1. INTRODUCTION

Non-small cell lung cancer (NSCLC), the predominant form of lung cancer globally and a major contributor to the death rate from cancer, poses a substantial challenge to global health (Chakraborty et al., 2025; Lee et al., 2024). Despite considerable advances in treatment, particularly the development of biomarker-driven specific therapies and immunotherapy with immune checkpoint inhibitors (ICI), long-term survival rates for NSCLC, especially in advanced stages, remain suboptimal (Ocáriz-Díez et al., 2020). The inherent heterogeneity of NSCLC and the emergence of new treatments underscore the urgent need for innovative strategies to improve early detection, refine prognostic assessments, personalize treatment selection, and enhance therapeutic efficacy (Meyer et al., 2024).

As understanding of the human microbiome, comprising the population of microorganisms in and within the human body, including bacteria, fungi, viruses, and protozoa, has advanced, a paradigm shift has occurred in the fields of biology and medicine in recent decades (Souza et al., 2023b). Far from being passive bystanders, these microbial communities and engage with the host and perform vital roles in regulating physiological homeostasis, including metabolism, immune system development, and function. Although the profound influence of the gut (intestinal) microbiome on systemic health is well established, the conventional perspective of the lungs as a sterile environment, has been overturned by high-throughput sequencing technologies, revealing a distinct, albeit low-biomass, lung microbiome (Figure 1) (Souza et al., 2023b). The accumulation of evidence now implicates to changes in the lung and intestinal microbiomes, termed dysbiosis, in the etiology of various diseases, including cancer (Adlakha & Chhabra, 2025; Emadi et al., 2025; Ocáriz-Díez et al., 2020). Bibliometric analyses have shown a significant increase in publications on this topic since 2015 (Jia et al., 2025).

Figure 1. An illustrative representation highlighting key chronological milestones of microbiome interactions in response to NSCLC. The depiction is systematically segmented into four distinct sections that chronicle the initial investigations that led to contemporary breakthroughs, in which comparative analyses of patients with NSCLC are contrasted with those of healthy individuals. Rejecting the initial hypothesis of 'lungs are sterile', the theoretical framework of the intestinal-lung axis was posited, followed by efforts to employ advanced machine learning diagnostics and metabolomic methodologies for immunotherapeutic interventions in lung cancer. Certain breakthrough studies have proposed cutting-edge therapeutic modalities and artificial intelligence models for predicting immune checkpoint inhibitor (ICI) responses in NSCLC. Currently, clinical trials, multifaceted data integration, and implementation frameworks are being developed, which are anticipated to significantly enhance advancements in this domain (Ankudavicius et al., 2023; Li et al., 2024; Sey & Warris, 2024; Zhou et al., 2023) (created with BioGDP; Jiang et al., 2024).

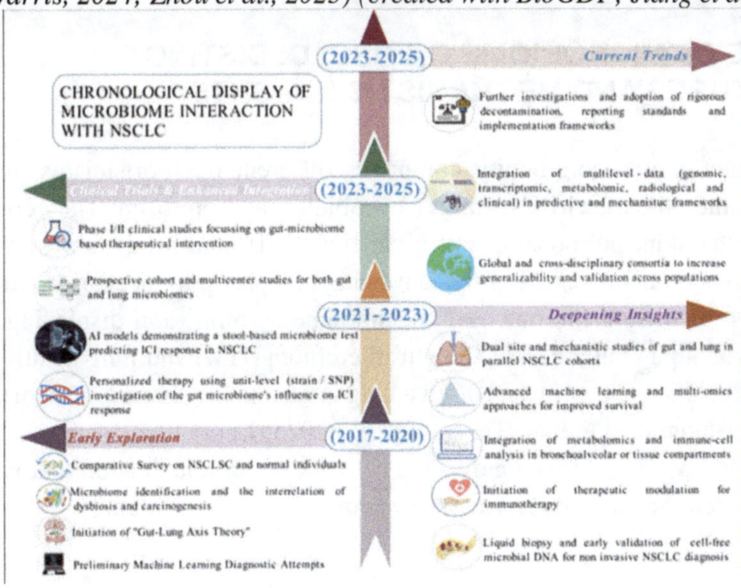

These methods have revealed a distinct, albeit low-biomass, lung microbiome, an ecosystem dynamically shaped by constant microaspiration from the oropharynx and clearance by host immune mechanisms (Ankudavicius et al., 2023; Zhou et al., 2023) (Fig. 1). This paradigm shift extends beyond the bacteriome, with emerging evidence implicating the lung's native fungal (mycobiome) and viral (virome) communities as critical, yet under-investigated players in the tripartite interactome of the host, environment, and NSCLC pathogenesis (Li et al., 2024; Moratiel-Pellitero et al., 2024). This chapter thoroughly combines the current research on integrating microbial systems into NSCLC management. Specifically, it focuses on the following four issues: (1) characterization of lung and intestinal microbial signatures associated with NSCLC and elucidation of their mechanistic links to tumorigenesis and progression; (2) development and validation of microbiome-based diagnostic and prognostic approaches, using cutting-edge technologies like liquid biopsy, metagenomics, and artificial intelligence (AI); (3) investigation of microbiome-targeted therapeutic interventions, encompassing fecal microbiota transplantation (FMT), probiotics, prebiotics, dietary modulation, and engineered microbes, as well as their impact on toxicity and effectiveness of the standard chemotherapy and immunotherapies; and (4) analysis of the challenges associated with clinical implementation and the evolving global regulatory frameworks governing these novel interventions. The scope explicitly focuses on NSCLC, aiming to provide a holistic view by incorporating perspectives from both the local lung and systemic microbial environments of the gut microbiome (GM).

2. ROLE OF MICROBIOME ON NSCLC: DISTINCT SIGNATURES AND MECHANISTIC INSIGHTS

The microbiome community comprises different microorganisms, including bacteria (microbiota), viruses, fungi (mycobiota), and protozoa. They commonly reside in the skin, pulmonary, gastrointestinal (GI), and urogenital tracts. They perform many functions, including converting complex polysaccharides to combat pathogens, regulating the mucosal and immune systems, and displaying diverse roles (Turnbaugh et al., 2007). The gut microbiota (GM) and lung health have an intriguing relationship, which is often amalgamated in the shape of a theory known as the 'gut-lung axis' theory (Deepika et al., 2025; Li et al., 2024; Sey & Warris, 2024; Zhang & Xu, 2023) (Figure 2), a network of communication that runs both ways between the gut and respiratory systems.

Figure 2. A comprehensive overview of The Lung-Gut Microbiome (LGM) and its mechanistic insights in response to NSCLC. A key factor in regulating the pathophysiology of non-small cell lung cancer (NSCLC) is the gut-lung axis (GLA). . NSCLC responsiveness to immunotherapeutic interventions is modulated through the interplay of the gut and lung microbiomes. Beneficial GMs directly influence cells of the host immune system and further disseminate along the circulatory system to stimulate pulmonary immune cells. They synthesize various metabolites, including indoles, tryptophan, and short-chain fatty acids (SCFAs), activating innate lymphoid cells (ILCs), T, and B cells. ILC activation further induces the secretion of interleukin-13 (IL-13), interleukin-22 (IL-22), and tumor necrosis factor-gamma (TNF-γ). Conversely, in response to harmful microbiomes, dendritic cells (DCs) initiate the activation of T-helper cells (Th1, Th2, Th17), regulatory T cells (Tregs), and B cells, leading to the production of antibodies and cytokines that also reach the lungs through blood and lymphatic vessels (Belaid et al., 2023; Li et al., 2024; Liu et al., 2020; Xu et al., 2024) (Created with BioGDP; Jiang et al., 2024).

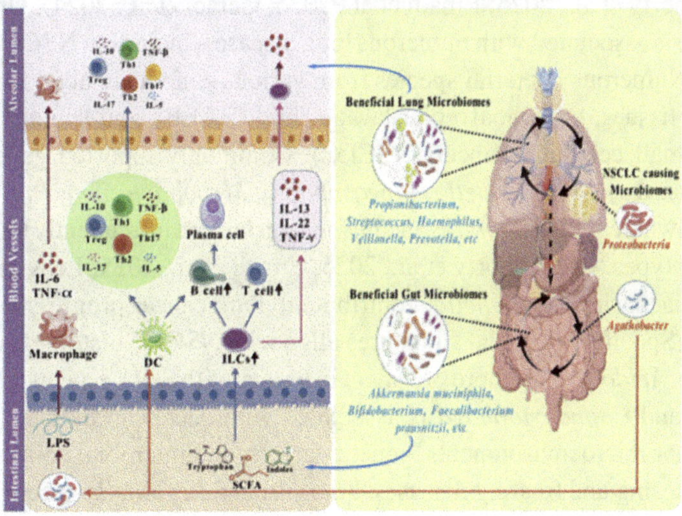

Another theory proposed by Samuelson et al. (2015), known as the 'gut lymph' theory, is based on the GLA and states that microbial communities in the gut and immune cells enter the pulmonary circulation and influence lung immunity. Therefore, microbiome imbalances, called ‘gut dysbiosis’, contribute to various lung disorders, even leading to lung cancer (Chakraborty et al., 2025; Samuelson et al., 2015). According to this axiom, dysbiosis, or imbalances in the GM, can have a major impact on lung health and exacerbate illnesses., including lung cancer, requiring the urgent need for innovative strategies to improve early detection, refine prognostic assessments, personalize treatment selection, and enhance therapeutic efficacy (Chakraborty et al., 2025; Emadi et al., 2025; Meyer et al., 2024). Elucidating the intricate relationships that exist between these microbial communities and NSCLC is necessary for advancing innovative diagnostic and therapeutic strategies. However, this understanding must transcend bacterium-centric perspectives to encompass this ecosystem's frequently neglected fungal and viral constituents, which are progressively acknowledged as significant contributors to cancer pathogenesis (Nguyen et al., 2015).

2.1 Lung Bacteriome in NSCLC

Once thought to be sterile, the lower respiratory tract is now understood to contain a unique low-biomass bacterial community (Figure 1). In healthy individuals, this community is dominated by phyla such as *Firmicutes*, *Bacteroidetes*, and *Proteobacteria*, which are maintained in a delicate balance through microaspiration and host-mediated clearance mechanisms such as coughing and mucociliary action (Figure 2) (Chakraborty et al., 2025; Emadi et al., 2025; Garaci et al., 2024). Disruption of this balance is associated with numerous lung diseases, including NSCLC (Budin et al., 2022). Numerous bacterial species from various genera are abundantly present in the lung tissues, bronchoalveolar lavage fluid (BALF), and sputum of patients with non-small cell lung cancer (NSCLC). Commonly reported genera include *Capnocytophaga*, *Granulicatella*, *Megasphaera*, *Mycobacterium*, *Prevotella*, and *Veillonella*, whereas *Haemophilus* and *Fusobacterium* are infrequently found in some NSCLC subtypes (Chakraborty et al., 2025; Emadi et al., 2025; Leng et al., 2021). Oral bacteria, such as *Veillonella*, contribute to lung cancer progression (Souza et al., 2023b). Specific microbial signatures align with NSCLC histological subtypes; for example, *Acidovorax* is more prevalent in tissues with SCC, especially with TP53 mutations, and *Capnocytophaga* is associated with adenocarcinoma (Leng et al., 2021). Tumor microenvironments, genetic factors, and microbial communities can aid in diagnosing and treating diseases. *Thermus* and *Legionella* species are linked to advanced stages of cancer, such as metastasis (Figure 2) (Souza et al., 2023b). Smoking and air pollution alter the lung microbiota (LM), increasing cancer risk, called 'gut dysbiosis' (Xu et al., 2020). The lung's microbial community is less dense than the gastrointestinal tract but maintains balance through microaspiration and coughing. *Actinobacteria* and *Bacteroidetes* are prevalent in healthy lungs and help to maintain immune homeostasis. Disruptions can cause disorders such as NSCLC. When compared to healthy people, studies have revealed notable alterations in the microbiome of patients with NSCLC (Leng et al., 2021; Souza et al., 2023b; Xu et al., 2020). This localized dysbiosis is distinct from systemic gut dysbiosis, yet frequently interacts with it, further complicating the host-microbe interactions in NSCLC.

2.2 Role of Gut Microbiota (GM) Dysbiosis in NSCLC

The GM displays systemic effects on the host, particularly on the immune system, owing to its microbial diversity and metabolic capacity (Shah & Ng, 2023). Studies have shown that, similar to the LM, dysbiosis in the GM occurs in patients with NSCLC compared to healthy individuals. Furthermore, enrichment of bacterial genera such as *Bacteroides*, *Enterococcus*, *Fusobacterium*, and *Prevotella* results in the elimination of short-chain fatty acid (SCFA)-producing genera such as *Faecalibacterium* and *Ruminococcus* (Figure 2) (Zhao et al., 2021). Thus, gut dysbiosis is not merely correlative; specific microbial signatures may be predictive biomarkers for early disease detection and may halt disease progression through anti-inflammatory and immune-boosting mechanisms (Xi et al., 2022).

2.3 Gut-Lung Axis (GLA): A Critical Analysis of the Pathway

GLA is a two-way network linking the gastrointestinal immune system to the respiratory system, highlighting the connection between gut dysbiosis and lung diseases. Despite their anatomical differences, the gut and lungs share developmental origins and structural similarities as large mucosal surfaces (Chakraborty et al., 2025). According to GLA, pulmonary health and disease risk, including NSCLC, are impacted by alterations in the gut microbiome (Li et al., 2024; Zhang & Xu, 2023). GLA involves systemic translocation, metabolite circulation, immune cell trafficking, and neurohormonal signaling. Microbe-associated patterns, such as LPS (lipopolysaccharide) and bacteria, can move from the intestine to the bloodstream, causing lung inflammation (Sha et al., 2025). The GM produces metabolites, such as SCFA (acetate, butyrate, and propionate), influencing sites such as the lungs through immunomodulation (Figure 2). The lymphatic and blood systems allow T cells, B cells, dendritic cells, and macrophages to migrate to the lungs and BALF for local immune responses, known as immune cell migration. Group 2 innate lymphoid cells migrate to the lungs, while dendritic cells stimulate T lymphocytes to migrate to the gut (Moratiel-Pellitero et al., 2024; Zhang & Xu, 2023). The GM also displays another form of signalling through neurohormones, although it is less characterized in GLA and NSCLC (Shah & Ng, 2023). Through these mechanisms, gut symbiosis contributes to a pro-inflammatory state in the lungs, regulates local lung immunity, potentially impacts the development and proliferation of NSCLC, and offers systemic therapies such as immunotherapy (Shah & Ng, 2023; Zhang & Xu, 2023).

2.4 Mechanistic Insights: Inflammation, Immunity, Metabolism, and Genotoxicity

The system through which alterations in the GM contribute to NSCLC is complex. As discussed above, chronic inflammation is exacerbated by microbial dysbiosis (Ocáriz-Díez et al., 2020). Bacterial species such as *Streptococcus* can trigger Th1 and Th17 immune responses in the lungs. *Streptococcus and Veillonella* are associated with pro-tumorigenic signaling pathways, such as ERK and PI3K (Table 1) (Leng et al., 2021). Lung flora can activate γδ T cells to produce IL-17, possibly aiding tumor growth (Souza et al., 2023b). Gut dysbiosis may cause inflammatory MAMPs to migrate to the lungs, affecting cytokine levels and pulmonary balance. Gut microbiota can alter immune responses through apoptosis, endoplasmic reticulum stress, inflammasomes, and TLR signaling (Zhang & Xu, 2023). In contrast to dysbiosis, which impairs antitumor immunity and enables cancer cells to avoid detection, a balanced microbiota promotes tumor immunosurveillance (Li et al., 2025). This is significant for immune checkpoint inhibitor (ICI) therapy, where GM composition is crucial for response (Souza et al., 2023b). Microorganisms such as *Bifidobacterium* and *Akkermansia muciniphila* can improve ICI efficacy by activating dendritic cells, priming CD8+ T cells, and modulating Treg function (Zhao et al., 2021). Microbial metabolites are frequently produced and influence host cell behavior and the progression of non-small cell lung cancer (NSCLC) (Souza et al., 2023b). Intestinal-derived short-chain fatty acids (SCFA) exhibit multifaceted roles; they are predominantly considered anti-inflammatory and immunomodulatory, potentially affecting T cell function and epigenetic regulation through mechanisms such as histone deacetylase (HDAC) inhibition (Zhang et al., 2023; Zhao et al., 2021) (Figure 2). Additionally, specific microbial metabolites have been correlated to the progression of NSCLC (e.g., 2-pentanone and tridecane of the gut microbiota (Xi et al., 2022), microcystin of lung Cyanobacteria (Xi et al., 2022), and DNA-damaging secondary bile acids produced by gut bacteria. Furthermore, the local tumor microbiome provides vital metabolites, such as methionine, directly supporting tumor growth (Souza et al., 2023b; Zhao et al., 2021).

Apart from advantageous metabolites, some bacteria generate genotoxins and virulence factors that can directly harm the host's DNA, interfere with the cell cycle, or cause cell death, all of which may lead to cancer (Zhao et al., 2021). For instance, by triggering autophagy and the TLR4/MYD88 pathway, *Fusobacterium nucleatum* increases chemoresistance in colorectal (Ting et al., 2022). Additionally, viruses can integrate their DNA into the host genome, resulting in oncogenic transformation through insertional mutagenesis or viral oncogene expression (e.g., p53/pRB inactivation by HPV E6/E7) (Sinha et al., 2024).

The mechanistic links between the microbiome and NSCLC offer viable hypotheses; however, it is important to recognize them. Evidence for microbial dysbiosis in NSCLC is predominantly correlational, and it remains difficult to prove whether it is the primary cause or consequence. An increasingly growingly feasible hypothesis, corroborated by expert consensus, posits a tripartite interactome wherein the microbiome, environmental exposures (such as smoking), and host genetic/epigenetic susceptibility collectively contribute to carcinogenesis. This intricate interplay emphasizes the requirement for comprehensive, multidimensional research methodologies (Scott et al., 2019).

2.5 The Lung and Gut Mycobiome in NSCLC: An Emerging Frontier

While bacterial communities have been the primary subject of microbiome research, the fungal kingdom, or mycobiome, appears to be a significant yet underexplored contributor in cancer (Nguyen et al., 2015; Garaci et al., 2024). Fungi are not passive colonizers but demonstrably impact host defense mechanisms and neoplastic development (Lee & Hong, 2025). Recent pan-cancer analyses have demonstrated that tumors, including NSCLC, harbor distinct tissue-specific fungal communities, with an estimated proportion of up to one fungus per 10^4 tumor cells (Wang et al., 2024). In NSCLC, specific fungal genera are enriched in tumor tissues. Metagenomic studies have identified an abundance of *Candida*, *Blastomyces*, and *Aspergillus* in lung tumors compared to adjacent non-cancerous tissues (Yuwono et al., 2024). The presence of these fungi is not merely an association, and compelling mechanistic evidence is beginning to emerge. A landmark study demonstrated that the fungus *Aspergillus sydowii* is enriched in lung adenocarcinoma (LUAD) tissues and actively promotes tumor progression (Jiang et al., 2024). The underlying mechanism is precise: β-glucan from the fungal cell wall is recognized by the Dectin-1 receptor on host myeloid cells. This engagement triggers the CARD9 signaling pathway, interleukin-1β (IL−1β). IL−1β secretion, in turn, drives the recruitment and expansion of myeloid-derived suppressor cells (MDSCs), which contain potent immunosuppressive cells that dampen the activity of cytotoxic T lymphocytes and foster a TME permissive for tumor growth (Rahal & Kadara, 2023). This provides a clear, targetable axis linking a specific intratumoral fungus to a defined immunosuppressive mechanism. The gut mycobiome also contributes to lung health and disease via the GLA (Sey & Warris, 2024). Different respiratory conditions have been associated with GM dysbiosis, and it is plausible that alterations in gut fungal communities and their metabolites could systemically influence lung immunity and NSCLC development (Lee & Hong, 2025). The dual nature of the mycobiome is highlighted by the discovery that some fungi, while potentially pathogenic, are also novel therapeutic sources. For example, *Aspergillus flavus*, a fungus known to cause respiratory infections, produces a class of molecules called asperigimycins, which have shown potent anti-leukemia activity in preclinical studies, underscoring the multifaceted, context-dependent, environment-specific role of fungi in cancer (Nie et al., 2025).

2.6 The Role of the Virome in NSCLC Pathogenesis

The virome (infectious human viruses and bacteriophages) is another critical component of the tumor microbiome (Porto, 2022). Viruses can contribute to carcinogenesis through insertional mutagenesis by integrating viral DNA and expressing viral oncoproteins that disrupt key tumor-suppressor pathways (Sinha et al., 2024). While the role of certain viruses in human cancers is well-established, their specific contribution to NSCLC remains an area of active investigation. Although most strongly associated with cervical and oropharyngeal cancers, evidence suggests a link between HPV types (high-risk HPV-16 and HPV-18) and an increased risk of NSCLC (Xiong et al., 2017). This association is more pronounced in lung adenocarcinoma and in individuals who have never smoked, suggesting that HPV may be a contributing etiological factor in a specific subset of NSCLC cases (Sequeira et al., 2024). Epstein-Barr Virus (EBV), a ubiquitous herpesvirus, is demonstrably linked with lymphoepithelioma-like carcinoma (LELC), a rare and distinct subtype of NSCLC (Chen et al., 2023). EBV DNA has also been detected in a substantial proportion of more common NSCLC types. The virus is not a passive passenger; recent studies have shown that the EBV-encoded oncoprotein BARF1 can be expressed in lung carcinoma cells, inducing tumor growth and progression *in vitro,* enhancing the proliferation, migration, and invasive capabilities of cancer cells (Osorio et al., 2024). Furthermore, discovering tumor-infiltrating T cells that recognize EBV-related antigens in lung cancer cells presents novel opportunities for focused T-cell interventions (Heslop et al., 2021). In addition to direct oncogenesis, viruses have been used for therapeutic purposes. Natural or genetically engineered oncolytic viruses (OVs) directly target and eliminate cancer cells by infecting and replicating within them or by inducing direct cell apoptosis (Dong et al., 2024). This process releases tumor-associated antigens, MAMPs, and danger signals, which can convert an immunologically "cold" TME into a "hot" TME, stimulating a potent and durable antitumor immune response. Several OVs, such as the engineered adenovirus CAN-2409, are presently undergoing clinical trials for NSCLC, along with ICIs, to leverage their synergistic immunostimulatory effects (Dong et al., 2024). The following table summarizes key microbial taxa from different kingdoms and their associations with NSCLC to provide a consolidated overview.

Table 1. Key Microbial Taxa (Bacteria, Fungi, and Viruses) Associated with NSCLC.

Species	Localization	Association with NSCLC	Association with Therapy Response	Proposed Mechanistic Insights	References
Veillonella spp.	Lung, Gut	Increased presence promotes progression	*V. dispar* increased in high-PD-L1 (ICI responder proxy)	Inflammation (ERK/PI3K activation)	(Ocáriz-Dez et al., 2020)
Streptococcus spp.	Lung, Gut	Increased presence/risk	-	Inflammation (ERK / PI3K overexpression)	(Leng et al., 2021)
Akkermansia muciniphila	Gut	Lower levels are associated with lung cancer	Increased abundance associated with good ICI response	Immune modulation (dendritic cell activation, T cell response), metabolite production (Inosine)	(Zhao et al., 2021)
Acidovorax spp.	Lung	Increase in SCC (esp. with TP53 mutation)	-	Inflammation, a Potential Biomarker	(Leng et al., 2021)
Faecalibacterium spp.	Gut	Lower levels are associated with lung cancer	Increased abundance associated with good ICI response	SCFA production (butyrate), anti-inflammatory	(Zhao et al., 2021)
Bifidobacterium spp.	Gut	-	Increased abundance associated with good ICI response	Immune modulation (DC activation, CD8+ T cell priming, NK cell activation), metabolite production (hippurate, inosine)	(Ting et al., 2022)
Ruminococcus spp.	Gut	Lower levels (butyrate producers)	Increased abundance associated with good ICI response	SCFA production, immunomodulation	(Zhao et al., 2021)
Prevotella spp.	Lung, Gut	Increased presence/risk	*P. copri* is associated with a good ICI response.	Inflammation	(Souza et al., 2023b)
Aspergillus sydowii	Lung	Enriched in LUAD; promotes tumor progression	-	Induces MDSC expansion via Dectin-1/CARD9/IL-1β pathway, suppressing T-cell activity	(Jiang et al., 2024)
Candida spp.	Lung, Gut	Enriched in lung and various GI tumors	-	Pro-inflammatory signaling, an opportunistic pathogen in immunosuppressed states	(Wang et al., 2024)
Blastomyces spp.	Lung	Enriched in lung tumors	-	Potential pro-inflammatory and immunomodulatory effects	(Wang et al., 2024)
Human Papillomavirus (HPV-16/18)	Lung	Increased risk of NSCLC, particularly adenocarcinoma, in nonsmokers.	Potential prognostic marker in adenocarcinoma.	Expression of viral oncoproteins (E6 / E7) that inactivate p53 / pRB.	(Sinha et al., 2024).
Epstein-Barr Virus (EBV)	Lung	Strongly associated with LELC subtype; present in other NSCLCs.	-	Expressing viral oncoproteins (eg, BARF1) promotes cell proliferation and invasion.	(Chen et al., 2023)

3. HARNESSING THE MICROBIOME FOR NSCLC DIAGNOSTICS

The distinct microbial alterations observed in patients with NSCLC present an opportunity to develop novel diagnostic and prognostic biomarkers for this disease.

Advanced analytical and computational techniques combined with these microbial signatures may result in an earlier, less invasive, and more precise detection of NSCLC (Table 2).

3.1. Microbial Biomarkers from Tissue and Respiratory Samples

Traditional diagnostic procedures for NSCLC often rely on invasive biopsies. Analyzing the microbial composition of more readily accessible respiratory samples, such as BALF, sputum, and even tumor tissue, provides an alternative diagnostic approach (Ocáriz-Dez et al., 2020). Studies have demonstrated that specific bacterial signatures within these samples can distinguish patients with NSCLC from healthy controls and those presenting with benign pulmonary conditions. For example, quantitative analysis using droplet digital PCR (ddPCR) identified combinations of *Acidovorax* and *Veillonella* in sputum as potential biomarkers for lung squamous cell carcinoma (SCC), achieving sensitivities of approximately 75-80% and specificities of approximately 89% in the initial and validation cohorts. Similarly, the abundance of *Capsulocytophaga* in sputum showed potential for identifying lung adenocarcinoma (AC), while *Acidovorax* levels could help delineate between subtypes (Leng et al., 2021). Analysis of BALF using 16S rRNA sequencing has also established distinct microbial profiles in patients with lung cancer compared to controls, identifying enriched species belonging to the genera *Sediminibacterium* and *Gemmiger* in cancer samples (Cheng et al., 2020). Studies have examined the diversity of respiratory microbiota as a potential prognostic indicator in advanced NSCLC, revealing that increased alpha diversity is linked to longer overall survival (OS) and progression-free survival (Zhang et al., 2025).

3.2 Liquid Biopsy Approaches for Microbial Marker Detection

In oncology, liquid biopsy has emerged as an efficacious and non-invasive technique for analyzing biomarkers in easily accessible body fluids such as blood, urine, and cerebrospinal fluid (CSF). Liquid biopsies are predominantly applied to detect circulating tumor cells (CTCs), cell-free DNA (cfDNA), and exosomes shed by tumors. It can detect tumors early, monitor therapeutic efficacy and resistance, and assess tumor heterogeneity without necessitating multiple surgical interventions (Augustus et al., 2021). This paradigm is broadening to include a microbial component. Emerging data suggest that microbial DNA and RNA can circulate in body fluids and may serve as non-invasive cancer biomarkers, including for NSCLC. Studies have detected microbe-derived cell-free RNAs (cfRNAs) in the plasma of patients across various neoplastic conditions, including lung cancer, with abundant

Proteobacteria (Zhou et al., 2023). Analysis of microbial DNA in pleural effusion has also demonstrated compositional variations related to malignancy and mortality in lung cancer patients, with enrichment of taxa such as *Rickettsiella*, *Ruminococcus*, *Enterococcus*, and *Lactobacillales* in malignant pleural effusion (Souza et al., 2023a). The ability to detect tumor-derived genetic material (ctDNA) and relevant microbial signatures from a single blood draw constitutes a notable development in this field. This integrated approach could provide a more comprehensive and non-invasive picture of the patient's disease state, facilitating personalized diagnosis and monitoring of the disease. However, this field is nascent, and challenges include the typically low abundance of microbial markers in circulation compared to host DNA, the need for highly sensitive detection methods, and the need for extensive validation in large patient cohorts (Augustus et al., 2021; Souza et al., 2023a). Establishing the ideal specimen source (e.g., whole blood versus plasma) and optimal processing methods for liquid microbial biopsy requires further investigation (Gerasimova & Nadeem, 2024).

3.3 Analytical Technologies: From Sequencing to Metabolomics

Characterizing the complex microbiome associated with NSCLC requires various analytical techniques, each with specific strengths and limitations. Sequencing methods are of prime importance in this regard. 16S rRNA gene amplicon sequencing targets conserved bacterial genes to provide taxonomic profiles, typically at the genus level. It is relatively cost-effective and widely used but suffers from PCR bias and has limited resolution for closely related species (Zhao et al., 2021). Meanwhile, whole-genome shotgun (WGS) metagenomics sequences all DNA in a sample, providing enhanced taxonomic granularity (species/strain level) and providing insights into the functional potential of the microbial community by analyzing gene content. However, it is more expensive and entails significant computational demands, and host DNA contamination can be a significant issue, particularly in low-biomass samples (Figure 3). Metatranscriptomics, another sequencing technique, analyzes RNA, providing information on gene expression and potentially distinguishing between viable and dead microbes, thereby offering a view of their functional activity. However, challenges include RNA instability and complex protocols (Fig. 3) (Gerasimova & Nadeem, 2024; Stella et al., 2022). Analytical techniques for characterizing the NSCLC-associated microbiome include quantitative PCR (qPCR), droplet digital PCR (ddPCR), and metabolomics. qPCR and ddPCR precisely quantify specific microbial genes or species, aiding in the validation of sequencing results and the development of diagnostic tests. ddPCR provides high sensitivity without the need for standard curves (Leng et al., 2021). Metabolomics primarily focuses on identifying and quantifying small-molecule metabolites produced by the microbiome (e.g., short-chain fatty acids [SCFAs] and bile acids) in various sample types (feces, serum, and tissues) (Sesma et al., 2023). This provides a direct readout of microbial functional activity but faces challenges in metabolite identification owing to incomplete databases and potential confounding by host metabolites. Other methods, such as culture (limited by bias and throughput), metaproteomics (complex interpretation), and fluorescence *in situ* hybridization (FISH) (limited throughput/resolution), also exist but are less commonly used for broad profiling (Gerasimova & Nadeem, 2024). A significant challenge in all these methods is the lack of standardization in sample collection (including minimizing contamination from collectors or the environment), processing (e.g., DNA extraction and reagent purity), data generation, and bioinformatics analysis (Stella et al., 2022). Contamination control is critical when working with low-microbial-bioburden samples from the lungs or liquid biopsies, requiring specialized practices such as protective clothing and UV treatment. Furthermore, complex data interpretation requires robust bioinformatic pipelines and curated databases that need clinical validation. Addressing these hurdles is essential for generating reproducible findings and translating microbiome analysis into clinical tools (Gerasimova & Nadeem, 2024; Stella et al., 2022).

3.4 The Role of Artificial Intelligence in Microbiome-Based Diagnostics

The sheer volume and complexity of the data generated by microbiome studies (metagenomics, metatranscriptomics, and metabolomics), often combined with clinical information, imaging data (radiomics), and other host omics data (genomics and proteomics), require advanced computational approaches for meaningful analysis (Figure 3) (Stella et al., 2022). Artificial intelligence (AI) and machine learning (ML) algorithms are indispensable for integrating these diverse datasets, identifying complex patterns, and building predictive models relevant to NSCLC (AlOsaimi et al., 2025). AI and ML have various potential applications in therapeutic interventions and disease prediction. AI models, which are intensive learning algorithms applied to medical imaging (radiomics) or other clinical data, have shown significant potential in noninvasively predicting the status of key NSCLC biomarkers, such as EGFR mutations, ALK rearrangements, PD-L1 expression, and tumor mutational burden (TMB) (AlOsaimi et al., 2025). Various data types are being combined to develop AI/ML models to predict immune response (ICI), progression-free survival (PFS), and overall survival (OS), including genomic, transcriptomic, proteomic, radiomic, and microbiomics data (Çalışkan & Tazaki, 2023). These techniques are being applied directly to microbiome data (e.g., 16S rRNA or metagenomic profiles) to classify NSCLC subtypes (e.g., AC vs. SCC) with reasonable accuracy (e.g., 71-

81% accuracy using KNN or DNN on validation data), demonstrating the potential of microbial features as diagnostic inputs for AI models (Figure 3) (Kashyap et al., 2025). AI excels at integrating microbiome data with other omics layers (radiogenomics and proteogenomics) to build more comprehensive and potentially more accurate predictive models for diagnosis, prognosis, and treatment selection (Stella et al., 2022; Wilkins et al., 2025). Standard ML techniques include deep learning (e.g., convolutional neural networks (CNNs)), Support Vector Machines (SVMs), Random Forests, K-Nearest Neighbors (KNNs), and Non-negative Matrix Factorization (NMF) (AlOsaimi et al., 2025).

Figure 3. Therapeutic interventions in NSCLC, highlighting engineered microbial and microbiome-based diagnostic approaches, and microbial methods. The traditional therapeutic approach involves understanding microbial signatures, often through high-throughput sequencing methods, followed by Artificial Intelligence (AI) and Machine Learning (ML) for data interpretation and predictive model making (AlOsaimi et al., 2025; Augustus et al., 2021). Therapy can also be performed using engineered microbes, such as Escherichia coli and Salmonella, which secrete microbe-associated molecular patterns (MAMPs) or other therapeutic agents (IL-2, Hly E) (Kim et al., 2024) (Created with BioGDP; Jiang et al., 2024).

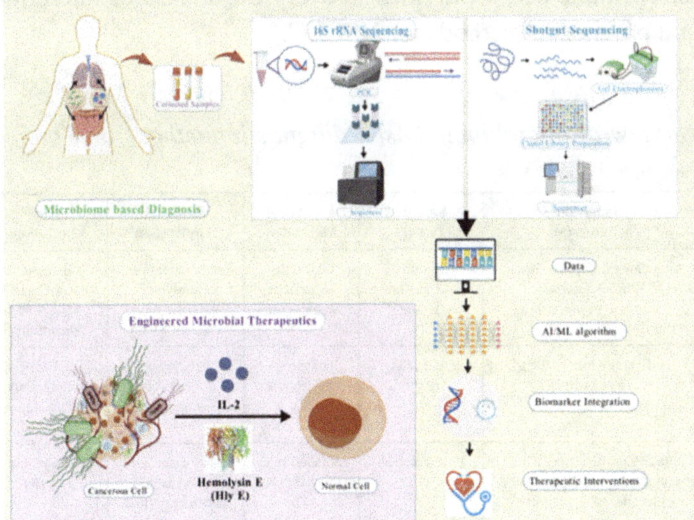

A recent study used a random forest model to analyze GM profiles from patients with lung cancer and successfully predicted their response to immunotherapy, with a receiver operating characteristic curve (AUC) with a large area of 82.1%, identifying specific species such as *Bacteroides caccae* (from responders) and *Prevotella copri*

(from non-responders) as key predictive features (Han et al., 2024). However, the true potential of AI lies in creating multimodal models that integrate various data streams. Recent systematic reviews have shown that AI models combining genomics, radiomics, and clinical data can predict lung cancer recurrence with AUCs as high as 0.92, surpassing traditional methods such as TNM staging (Table 2) (Huang et al., 2024). Although integrating microbiome data into these multi-omics models is still a nascent frontier, it represents a logical and highly promising next step (Wilkins et al., 2025).

Despite its promise, the clinical implementation of AI/ML in microbiome diagnostics faces several significant challenges. These include the need for extensive, superior, uniform datasets for training and validation, improving model interpretability and transparency (addressing the "black box" issue), and navigating regulatory hurdles, data privacy concerns, and integration into clinical workflows (Huang et al., 2024). The capacity of AI/ML to decipher complex biological patterns makes it crucial for translating microbiome research into clinical diagnostic tools for NSCLC management. However, the lack of standardization in sampling, analytical methods, and data reporting remains a bottleneck, limiting study comparability and hindering the validation of the clinical implementation of microbiome diagnostics (Stella et al., 2022). Standard protocols and reference materials are critical prerequisites for this progress. The table below provides an overview of various microbiome-based diagnostic and prognostic methods for NSCLC.

Table 2. Overview of microbiome-based diagnostic methods and biomarkers for NSCLC.

Diagnostic Approach	Key Biomarker(s)/ Signature(s)	Sample Type(s)	Analytical Method(s)	Potential Application	Key Limitations	References
Respiratory sample analysis	Abundances of *Acidovorax, Veillonella, and Capnocytophaga*)	Sputum, BALF, Lung Tissue	ddPCR, 16S rRNA sequencing	early detection, subtype classification (AC vs. SCC)	Invasive (tissue/BALF), validation, sensitivity	(Leng et al., 2021)
Respiratory microbiota diversity	α-diversity index (e.g., Shannon)	BALF, lung tissue	16S rRNA sequencing	Prognosis, ICI response prediction	Low biomass, contamination, and validation required	(Zhang et al., 2025)
Fecal/serum metabolomics	SCFA profiles, specific metabolites (e.g., 2-pentanone, tridecane, sphingolipids)	Feces, Serum	Metabolomics (LC-MS, GC-MS)	Early detection, prognosis, treatment effect monitoring	Reflects gut activity	(Moratiel-Pellitero et al., 2024)

continued on following page

Table 2. Continued

Diagnostic Approach	Key Biomarker(s)/ Signature(s)	Sample Type(s)	Analytical Method(s)	Potential Application	Key Limitations	References
AI-Integrated Multi-omics	Predictive models based on integrated data	Imaging (CT/MRI), Genomics, Proteomics, Microbiomics, Clinical Data	AI/ML algorithms (DL, SVM, RF)	Non-invasive biomarker prediction (PD-L1, TMB), and prognosis	High predictive potential, Integration capability	(AlOsaimi et al., 2025)
Gut Microbiome Profiling for ICI Response	Specific taxa (e.g., *B. caccae, P. copri*)	Feces	AI/ML on metagenomic data	Prediction of response to immunotherapy.	Correlative, requires validation in prospective trials.	(Han et al., 2024)

4. MICROBIOME-MODULATED THERAPEUTICS FOR NSCLC

As the lung and gut microbiome (GM) play a significant role in immunity and inflammation, and their relationship to NSCLC development and treatment outcomes, manipulating these communities is a compelling therapeutic strategy. Research is actively exploring various interventions, from broad ecosystem modulation using FMT to targeted approaches with specific probiotics or engineered microbes, to enhance the efficacy of standard NSCLC treatments, such as immunotherapy and chemotherapy, or to act as stand-alone therapies (Table 3).

4.1 Impact on Immunotherapy (ICI) Efficacy and Toxicity

In subsets of patients, ICIs targeting pathways such as PD-1/PD-L1 and CTLA-4 have significantly transformed NSCLC therapy. However, response rates remain variable, and many patients exhibit primary or acquired resistance to these therapies. The GM has been strongly implicated as a key modulator of patient response to ICIs in various cancers, including NSCLC (Ocáriz-Díez et al., 2020; Rother et al., 2024). Duttagupta et al. (2023) consider the microbiome a "cancer-immune set point," which influences baseline immune function and ICI-mediated anti-tumor responses (Duttagupta et al., 2023). Specific intestinal microbial signatures are consistently associated with ICI therapy outcomes. Higher microbial diversity and enrichment of specific bacterial taxa, like *Akkermansia muciniphila, Faecalibacterium* spp., *Bifidobacterium* spp., *Ruminococcus* spp., and *Alistipes* spp., are frequently linked to favourable responses (higher objective response rate (ORR), longer PFS, and OS) in patients receiving ICIs (Zhao et al., 2021). In contrast, the enrichment of other taxa, including *Enterocloster, Hungatella, Parabacteroides distasonis,* and *Bacteroides nordii*, has been correlated with suboptimal outcomes or therapeutic refractoriness

(Duttagupta et al., 2023). A recent meta-analysis confirmed that probiotic supplementation relates to enhanced OS and PFS in patients with cancer receiving ICIs (Zhao et al., 2025). While the role of the GM is well-established, emerging data suggest that the local lung microbiota (LM) may also influence ICI efficacy. For instance, higher respiratory microbiota diversity was linked to better PFS and OS in NSCLC patients on PD-1 blockade in one study (Zhang et al., 2025), and specific lung taxa have been associated with PD-L1 expression levels (Souza et al., 2023b). The multifaceted mechanisms of this modulation involve immune system interactions (Zhang & Xu, 2023). The steps involved in this mechanism include priming and activation of antigen-presenting cells (like dendritic cells), thereby promoting the activation, proliferation, and infiltration of cytotoxic CD8+ T cells and NK cells into the tumor microenvironment (TME). As a result, metabolites (such as SCFAs like butyrate or inosine) are produced that enhance antitumor T cell function or modulate the TME and activate innate immune signaling pathways, such as STING (e.g., by *Lactobacillus rhamnosus* GG); potentially providing antigens that mimic tumor antigens, leading to cross-reactive anti-tumor T cell responses (e.g., *B. breve*'s SVY antigen mimicking melanoma's SIY neoantigen, and *Enterococcus hirae* infecting bacteriophage's TMP mimicking cancer antigen PSMB4) (Figure 2, Ting et al., 2022). In addition to efficacy, the gut microbiome influences the incidence and severity of immune-related adverse events (irAEs), a common side effect of ICIs. Certain microbial profiles are linked with an increased risk of developing irAEs (e.g., *Agathobacter, Betaproteobacteria, and Enterococcus*), while others may be protective (e.g., *Akkermansia* and *Lactobacillaceae*) (Zhang & Xu, 2023). This suggests modulating the microbiome could mitigate ICI toxicity. The detrimental impact of broad-spectrum antibiotics on ICI efficacy is a consistent finding across multiple studies and cancer types, including NSCLC (Ocáriz-Díez et al., 2020). The antibiotic therapy, near to the initiation of ICI therapy, is associated with significantly lower response rates and survival outcomes, presumably due to disruption of beneficial gut microbial communities. This underscores the clinical importance of judicious antibiotic use in patients undergoing immunotherapy.

4.2 Influence on Chemotherapy Outcomes

The microbiome extends its influence on immunotherapy and conventional chemotherapy (Halley et al., 2020). Gut microbes can impact the efficacy (pharmacodynamics) and metabolism (pharmacokinetics) of chemotherapeutic agents and modulate treatment-related toxicity. Microbial enzymes can directly alter the effects of chemotherapy drugs. For example, bacterial β-glucuronidases in the gut, expressed by *Clostridium* clusters XIVa and IV, can reactivate the inactive metabolite of irinotecan (SN-38G) to its toxic form (SN-38), contributing significantly to dose-limiting diarrhea (Wang et al., 2021). Conversely, certain bacteria, including intra-tumoral Gammaproteobacteria like *Mycoplasma hyorhinis*, possess enzymes like cytidine deaminase (CDD-L) that can inactivate gemcitabine, particularly within the tumor microenvironment, leading to chemoresistance. Microbial metabolism can also influence the availability of cofactors (like B vitamins B6 and B9 produced by *E. coli*) needed for the action of drugs such as 5-fluorouracil (5-FU) (Kim et al., 2024; Ting et al., 2022). There is growing recognition that the host immune response and GM contribute to chemotherapy efficacy. For instance, cyclophosphamide (CTX) treatment alters the gut microbiota, promoting the enrichment of specific bacteria (*Enterococcus hirae* and *Lactobacillus johnsonii*) in various secondary lymphoid organs. This stimulates beneficial Th1 and Th17 immune responses crucial for CTX's anti-tumor effect, and *E. hirae* increases the intratumoral CD8+/Treg ratio. *Barnesiella intestinihominis* promotes IFN-γ-producing γδT cell infiltration during CTX treatment. Similarly, gut microbes modulate myeloid cell responses to platinum agents like oxaliplatin and cisplatin, with Gram-positive bacteria priming intratumoral myeloid cells for ROS production via MYD88 signaling. Butyrate-producing bacteria can activate CD8+ T cells via ID2-dependent IL-12 signaling, eliciting a cancer-specific immunological reaction to oxaliplatin (Ting et al., 2022). Dysbiosis and chemotherapy-associated toxicity are common side effects. These side effects may be mitigated by interventions that restore or support the gut microbiota, such as probiotics or FMT (Kim et al., 2024). Preclinical studies have revealed that *Lactobacillus acidophilus* administration enhances the antitumor effect of cisplatin in mouse models (Zhao et al., 2021). *Fusobacterium nucleatum*, often enriched in colorectal cancer, can activate the TLR4/MYD88 pathway, inhibit specific miRNAs, and cause cancer cells to transition from apoptosis to autophagy. This promotes chemoresistance against anti-cancer agents like oxaliplatin and 5-FU (Ting et al., 2022). Based on these interactions, a microbiome-based strategy to optimize conventional treatments is potentially feasible, as the microbiome can significantly affect patient response and tolerance to chemotherapy.

4.3 Therapeutic Interventions

In recent years, therapeutic approaches have developed from broad, ecosystem-level interventions to highly specific, mechanism-based approaches. In medicine, this progression reflects an increasing emphasis on precision and safety, which aims to harness the microbiome's power with reliability and consistency. Numerous strategies to modulate the microbial ecosystem are being explored based on understanding the microbiome's role in NSCLC (Elkrief et al., 2025).

4.3.1 Fecal Microbiota Transplantation (FMT)

FMT boosts microbiome diversity by transferring feces from healthy individuals (Ting et al., 2022). In cancer therapy, the aim is to transfer "responder" microbiomes to patients resistant to ICIs. Preclinical studies have shown that FMT from ICI-responsive donors can surpass resistance in other individuals (Elkrief et al., 2025). Clinical trials are assessing FMT's safety and effectiveness of FMT in NSCLC patients on ICIs, especially those who progress after prior therapy, including trials NCT03772899, NCT04951583, NCT05502913, NCT05008861, NCT04924374, and NCT03819296 (Table 3). Initial melanoma trials indicate that FMT is safe and may benefit patients previously resistant to anti-PD-1 therapy, with a significant ORR in a Canadian Phase I trial. Alternatives, such as cultured bacterial consortia (MET or RMT), are being tested in trials such as NCT03686202 and NCT04105270. The MET-4 trial (NCT03686202) showed increased taxa linked to ICI response (Duttagupta et al., 2023). However, the potential of FMT is met with challenges such as donor variability, the theoretical risk of transmitting pathogens or undesirable traits, logistical challenges associated with donor screening and material preparation, standardization of protocols, and optimal delivery methods (e.g., colonoscopy, enema, oral capsules). Moreover, a greater number of unrelated donors are being used by stool banks (Shah et al., 2024; Yadav & Chauhan, 2022).

4.3.2 Probiotics, Prebiotics, and Dietary Modulation

Alternatively, the administration of live beneficial microorganisms, known as probiotics, can be utilized to alter the existing microbiome. Furthermore, specific dietary interventions or prebiotics enhance the proliferation of beneficial bacteria (prebiotics) (Deepika et al., 2025; Elkrief et al., 2025; Shah & Ng, 2023). Specific strains, particularly from the *Bifidobacterium* and *Lactobacillus* genera, have demonstrated potential benefits for augmenting antitumor responses and potentiating ICI or chemotherapy effects (Ting et al., 2022). Clinical investigations are ongoing. A meta-analysis suggested that probiotic supplementation was associated with enhanced OS and PFS in NSCLC patients receiving ICIs (Kim et al., 2024). Studies involving *Clostridium butyricum* (CBM588) have also shown potential benefits alongside ICIs in renal cell carcinoma and NSCLC, improving PFS and OS in retrospective analyses. Numerous clinical trials are evaluating specific probiotic strains or mixtures in patients with NSCLC receiving chemotherapy or immunotherapy (e.g., NCT03642548 - Bifico for chemo side effects (Kim et al., 2024); NCT04699721 - BiFico + Nivolumab + Chemo; NCT02771470 - *C. butyricum* + Chemo; NCT03595683 - *B. longum* + Pembrolizumab in melanoma; NCT03637803 - *E. gallinarum* MRx0518 + Pembrolizumab in various cancers, including NSCLC;

NCT04601402 - *L. lactis* + Avelumab; NCT05094167 - *Lactobacillus/Bifidobacterium* V9 + Chemo + Camrelizumab (Table 3). However, the clinical evidence for probiotics in cancer therapy is not uniformly positive. Some preclinical studies have paradoxically shown that certain probiotics impair ICI efficacy (e.g., *Lactobacillus* in melanoma models), and retrospective clinical studies have yielded conflicting results, with some failing to show significant benefits. This underscores the critical importance of strain specificity, dose, timing, as well as the requirement for thorough prospective clinical trials. Although generally minimal, safety concerns include the rare risk of sepsis in immunocompromised individuals and potential horizontal transfer of antibiotic resistance genes. The lack of respiratory-specific probiotics is also a limitation (Belaid et al., 2023; Duttagupta et al., 2023; Kim et al., 2024). The complexity of the probiotic field, with conflicting results, highlights a crucial point that not all probiotics are equal, and their effects are likely context-dependent (strain, dose, host factors, concomitant therapy) (Deepika et al., 2025). A cautious, evidence-based approach focusing on well-characterized strains and rigorous clinical validation is necessary before widespread recommendations can be made, especially in vulnerable oncology patients. Diet is a powerful and accessible tool for modulating the GM (Ruban et al., 2025; Szczyrek et al., 2021). In recent years, a low-carb, high-fat diet known as the ketogenic diet has been shown to alter the body's metabolism from using glucose to ketones (Weber et al., 2018). The rationale in cancer is to starve glucose-dependent tumor cells (the Warburg effect) (Weber et al., 2018; Szczyrek et al., 2021). Exciting new preclinical research has shown that the primary ketone body, β-hydroxybutyrate (BHB), can directly enhance the function and persistence of CAR T-cells, a form of immunotherapy. BHB appears to be a superior fuel source for these engineered immune cells, improving their anti-tumor activity in mouse models (Szczyrek et al., 2021). These promising findings are now paving the way for clinical trials to test the ketogenic diet or BHB supplementation in patients receiving cellular immunotherapies.

4.3.3 Engineered Microbial Therapeutics (e.g., Bacterial Vectors)

A more sophisticated strategy involves genetically engineering bacteria—often attenuated pathogens *(Salmonella, E. coli*) or commensal strains—to function as "living medicines" or engineered Live Biotherapeutic Products (eLBPs) (Fig. 3) (Elkrief et al., 2025; Kim et al., 2024; Michán & Ramos, 2025). These engineered microbes can be programmed for various anti-cancer functions. Exploiting the natural tendency of certain bacteria (especially facultative anaerobes) to preferentially colonize the hypoxic and immunosuppressive tumor microenvironment (Kunjalwar et al., 2024) and serving as vectors to produce and deliver therapeutic agents (e.g., cytokines like IL-2, toxins, antibodies, prodrug-converting enzymes) directly within the tumor, minimizing systemic exposure and toxicity. Examples include *Salmonella* engineered to express IL-2 (Kim et al., 2024) and *E. coli* designed to secrete toxins (HlyE) specifically targeted to cancer cells (HER2+) via surface-displayed nanobodies (Shahid et al., 2024). Directly stimulating anti-tumor immune responses by releasing MAMPs or engineered immunostimulatory molecules within the TME. Some engineered strains are designed to kill cancer cells directly. Engineering bacteria to express enzymes that convert non-toxic prodrugs into active cytotoxic agents specifically at the tumor site (Kunjalwar et al., 2024; Michán & Ramos, 2025). However, significant efforts must be dedicated to generating the safety engineering process. While engineered microbial therapies offer immense potential for precision and efficacy, they are generally at an earlier stage of development. Most research is preclinical, although some candidates, like *Enterococcus gallinarum* MRx0518 (investigated in trial NCT03637803, which included NSCLC patients), are entering or have undergone early clinical testing (Kim et al., 2024). The technical complexity of designing, constructing, and controlling these living therapeutics, coupled with heightened safety and regulatory considerations (e.g., potential for horizontal gene transfer, environmental release), presents substantial hurdles that need to be overcome before they can reach widespread clinical application (Yadav & Chauhan, 2022). In systemic NSCLC treatment, the gut microbiome is a central, modifiable factor associated with immunotherapy and chemotherapy efficacy (Zhao et al., 2021). The gut, therefore, becomes a primary target for interventions that aim to improve the outcomes of overall treatment.

Table 3. Case studies of clinical trials conducted on microbiome-targeted NSCLC therapies.

Intervention	Trial Identifier	Phase	Target Population	Key Findings	References
FMT	NCT04951583	II	Advanced NSCLC & Melanoma (+ICI: Pembrolizumab, Ipilimumab, Nivolumab)	Builds on Phase I melanoma trial showing safety & efficacy	(Duttagupta et al., 2023; Duttagupta et al., 2025)
Oral Restorative Microbiota Therapy (RMT)	NCT04105270	II	Advanced NSCLC (+Durvalumab + Chemo)	Expected completion 2028	(Duttagupta et al., 2023)
Probiotic (Bifico)	NCT03642548	III	NSCLC (+ Platinum Chemo)	-	(Kim et al., 2024)
Probiotic (*Enterococcus gallinarum* MRx0518)	NCT03637803	I/II	Advanced NSCLC, RCC, Melanoma, Bladder (+Pembrolizumab)	Investigated engineered/ specific strain	(Duttagupta et al., 2023)
Probiotic (*Lactococcus lactis* CECT8666)	NCT04601402	II	Advanced Solid Tumors incl. NSCLC (+Avelumab)	-	(Duttagupta et al., 2023)

continued on following page

Table 3. Continued

Intervention	Trial Identifier	Phase	Target Population	Key Findings	References
Probiotic (*Clostridium butyricum*)	NCT02771470	I	Lung Cancer (+Chemo)	Retrospective studies suggest a benefit with ICI	(Kim et al., 2024)
Fermented Soybean Extract (MicrSoy-20, MS-20)	NCT04909034	II	Advanced Solid Tumors incl. NSCLC (+pembrolizumab)	-	(Duttagupta et al., 2023)

5. BRIDGING RESEARCH TO PRACTICE: IMPLEMENTATION AND REGULATION

Despite the exciting scientific progress and therapeutic potential, translating microbiome-based diagnostics and interventions into routine clinical practice for NSCLC faces significant hurdles. These span scientific understanding, technical standardization, clinical validation, manufacturing, cost, and navigating complex regulatory landscapes.

5.1 Challenges in Clinical Translation and Standardization

Several key challenges impede the widespread adoption of microbiome approaches in oncology. While associations abound, definitively proving causality—that specific microbial changes directly drive NSCLC or dictate therapy response—remains difficult (Elkrief et al., 2025; Scott et al., 2019). Microbiomes and immune systems interact intricately and dynamically, and we do not fully understand the interactions between individual microbes and their hosts (Yadav & Chauhan, 2022; Yaqub et al., 2025). Furthermore, the high extent of inter-individual inconsistency in microbiome composition (influenced by diet, geography, ethnicity, lifestyle, etc.) (Yaqub et al., 2025) makes it challenging to define universal "healthy" or "responder" profiles. It complicates the development of broadly applicable interventions (Gerasimova & Nadeem, 2024). A critical bottleneck across the field is the absence of standardized protocols for virtually every step: sample collection (especially for low-biomass sites like the lung, requiring sterile procedures and contamination controls), storage (e.g., impact of freeze-thaw cycle), DNA/RNA extraction, sequencing platforms and parameters, bioinformatics analysis pipelines (including robust, curated, clinical-grade databases), and data reporting. This lack of standardization severely limits the ability to compare results across studies, perform meta-analyses, and validate findings robustly. Establishing reliable reference ranges for diagnostic tests is also hampered by this variability and lack of standard methods, potentially requiring mock communities as controls (Gerasimova & Nadeem, 2024; Stella et al., 2022). Contamination control (from humans, environment, reagents, equipment, cross-contamination) is paramount, particularly for low-biomass samples, requiring specialized laboratory practices like protective clothing, UV treatment of reagents, and separating pre-/post-PCR work (Stella et al, 2022). Designing and executing rigorous clinical trials for microbiome interventions is complex. Challenges include controlling for confounding factors like diet, medication use (especially antibiotics), and host genetics; defining meaningful clinical endpoints beyond simple microbial shifts; and accounting for the inherent variability in microbiome responses (Yadav & Chauhan, 2022). Validating diagnostic biomarkers requires large, prospective, multi-center studies that adhere to standardized methodologies. More human trials are needed, as much research relies on rodent models (Rother et al., 2024; Xi et al., 2022). For therapeutic products like FMT and LBPs, safety, quality, consistency, stability, and potency present unique challenges. Donor screening for FMT must be rigorous to prevent pathogen transmission (Rother et al., 2024; Xi et al., 2022). Manufacturing live bacterial products (LBPs) requires specialized facilities and quality control measures (including rigorous cell banking and genetic monitoring) (Kim et al., 2024) to ensure batch-to-batch consistency and viability (Tseng et al., 2025). Engineered microbes pose additional safety concerns regarding genetic stability, adverse unintended consequences, horizontal gene transfer, and environmental containment (Rother et al., 2024; Xi et al., 2022). The costs associated with advanced sequencing, highly intricate computational analyses, AI model development, and the manufacturing of regulated therapeutic microbial products constrain availability, particularly in resource-limited settings (Gerasimova & Nadeem, 2024). However, some engineered therapies aim for a minimal unit cost per dose (e.g., <$10) (Prifti et al., 2025).

5.2 Navigating the Global Regulatory Landscape for Microbiome Interventions

As microbiome-based products move towards clinical application, navigating the regulatory landscape becomes essential. Ensuring patient safety while fostering innovation requires clear, appropriate, and ideally harmonized regulatory structures (Rodriguez et al., 2025). Although complex regulatory environments presently govern microbiome interventions, these environments are evolving, and they vary significantly from one jurisdiction to another. The rapid pace of scientific discovery has, in many ways, overshadowed the formation of targeted regulations, creating uncertainty for developers (Tomasulo et al., 2024). The United States FDA regulates microbiome products based primarily on their intended use. Products intended to treat, cure, prevent, or diagnose disease are typically regulated as drugs or biological products, requiring rigorous clinical trials and marketing authorization (Rodriguez et al., 2025). The FDA has approved the first MMPs (Rebyota® and VOWST®) derived from human stool for preventing recurrent *Clostridioides difficile* infection (rCDI) (Almagro & Almagro, 2024). The FDA actively engages with industry groups like the Microbiome Therapeutics Innovation Group (MTIG) to address challenges in LBP development and analytics (Barberio, 2024; Ren et al., 2024). The US remains a global leader in the volume of microbiome research and clinical trials (Tomasulo et al., 2024). The regulation of FMT in the European Union has historically been fragmented, with individual member states adopting different classifications (e.g., medicinal product, tissue preparation, procedure) (Tomasulo et al., 2024). The new EU Regulation on Substances of Human Origin (SoHO), published in July 2024 and set to apply from August 2027, aims to harmonize this by explicitly including human microbiomes within its scope (Cordaillat-Simmons et al., 2020; Rodriguez et al., 2025). This regulation will establish common standards for donating, collecting, testing, processing, storing, and distributing human-derived microbiome samples intended for therapeutic application (MT) or manufacturing medicinal products. MMPs containing live microorganisms are generally considered biological medicinal products under existing EU pharmaceutical legislation (Directive 2001/83/EC), requiring marketing authorization from the EMA or national competent authorities (Rodriguez et al., 2025). The European Pharmacopoeia (Ph. Eur.) has also incorporated definitions and standards for LBPs (Liang et al., 2022; Tseng et al., 2025). The interplay between the SoHO regulation and pharmaceutical legislation for MMPs derived from human sources is an area of ongoing development (Rodriguez et al., 2025). Regulatory frameworks exhibit considerable variation across nations within the Asia-Pacific region. South Korea is distinguished by its substantial volume of microbiome research (Tomasulo et al., 2024). In China, the National Medical Products Administration (NMPA) is responsible for the evaluation of Biologics License Applications (BLA) about LBPs, with several Phase 3 trials having been documented (Almagro & Almagro, 2024). In recognition of the necessity for regional guidance, the Asia-Pacific Microbiota Consortium (APMC) was established, convening experts from countries such as Australia, Hong Kong, Japan, Malaysia, Singapore, and Taiwan to formulate consensus statements on pivotal considerations for LBP development, encompassing elements from strain selection and preclinical evaluation to clinical trial design and manufacturing (Kim et al., 2024; Tseng et al., 2025). Globally, regulators encounter the challenge of adapting existing frameworks, initially designed for conventional drugs, biologics, or tissue products, to these innovative living therapies, ensuring appropriate standards for quality, safety, and efficacy while accommodating the distinct characteristics of microbial products (Yadav & Chauhan, 2022). The collaboration between regulatory agencies, industry stakeholders, and academia is deemed essential for the progression of the field (Barberio, 2024).

5.3 Classification and Oversight of FMT, LBPs, and Engineered Microbes

Notably, the specific regulatory classifications of microbiome interventions profoundly influence the development pathway, necessary evidence, and the level of oversight. FMT involves transferring minimally processed, complex fecal communities from donor to recipient (Elkrief et al., 2025). Its regulatory status is often ambiguous, and it is treated variously as a transplant, a drug, or a procedure depending on jurisdiction. Key oversight focuses on donor screening, ethical sourcing, and processing controls to minimize infection risk (Yadav & Chauhan, 2022). Live Biotherapeutic Products (LBPs) / Microbiome-Based Medicinal Products (MMPs) are defined products containing specific live microorganisms (single strains, defined consortia, or potentially engineered strains) intended for a therapeutic purpose (prevention, treatment, or cure of a disease) (Barberio, 2024; Cordaillat-Simmons et al., 2020). They are distinct from probiotics or food supplements, which are typically intended for general health maintenance in healthy individuals and are subject to different regulations. LBPs/MMPs are generally regulated as drugs or biologics, requiring demonstration of safety, efficacy, and consistent manufacturing (Chemistry, Manufacturing, and Controls - CMC) through preclinical studies and clinical trials (Tseng et al., 2025). Engineered Microbes (eLBPs), as a category of LBPs, encompass genetic modification. They adhere to identical regulatory requirements as other LBPs, with additional scrutiny about the genetic modification, stability, potential for horizontal gene transfer, and environmental containment (Yadav & Chauhan, 2022). The principle of "intended use" as determined by product claims and marketing is crucial for classification purposes (Rodriguez et al., 2025). Products advertised with claims to treat or prevent conditions such as NSCLC are typically regulated as medicinal products, regardless of whether their microbial components are also present in food supplements. This "intended use dilemma" necessitates that therapeutic claims for microbiome products be substantiated by rigorous scientific evidence aligning with drug approval standards, thereby averting the distribution of potentially ineffective or unsafe products to vulnerable patient populations under less stringent regulatory conditions (Tseng et al., 2025). Ultimately, the efficacy of regulatory processes is contingent upon a robust scientific foundation and consistent procedures. The potential to reliably manufacture, characterize, and test these intricate living therapies is crucial for establishing their quality, safety, and efficiency to regulatory bodies (Barberio, 2024; Cordaillat-Simmons et al., 2020; Tseng et al., 2025). Therefore, confronting the previously mentioned challenges related to technical standardization is an urgent scientific necessity and a prerequisite for navigating regulatory frameworks and achieving clinical application.

6. LIMITATIONS AND CHALLENGES

Integrating microbiome science into NSCLC management holds significant potential, yet substantial constraints hinder it. Studies have identified dysbiosis of the lung and gut microbiota as a distinctive feature of NSCLC. However, a comprehensive mechanistic understanding of the complex interactions between microbes and their hosts is necessary to devise efficacious, specific interventions. Studies identify dysbiosis of lung-gut microbiota as a principal obstacle for NSCLC patients. This imbalance causes microbes to migrate from the gut to other organs like the brain, liver, and lungs, resulting in diverse pathological conditions (Ciernikova et al., 2023; Xin et al., 2024). The interaction of gut and lung microbiomes is fundamental to NSCLC-directed therapies. Environmental factors like antibiotics, diet, and lifestyle affect microbiota activity and immune response in cancer therapy. For example, diets can promote the proliferation of commensal microorganisms (Lee et al., 2024; Xin et al., 2024). Microbial metabolites impact chemotherapy and immunotherapy, improving NSCLC diagnosis via microbiome-informed interventions (Hes & Jagoe, 2023). Studying microbiome-host interactions is vital for understanding and alleviating NSCLC. Future research must prioritize mechanistic studies, leveraging advanced preclinical models (e.g., gnotobiotic mice, organoids) to delineate the specific molecular mechanisms by which single microbes and consortia affect tumorigenesis. Methodological standardization is a significant challenge; a lack of harmonized protocols for sample collection, processing, sequencing, and data analysis impedes reproducibility and comparability across studies. The development of standardized protocols and references is imperative to facilitate evidence-based clinical decision-making. While interventions like FMT have shown remarkable preliminary efficacy in the therapeutic realm, donor variability, safety, and standardization challenges must be addressed.

7. CONCLUSION

Incorporating microbiome science into managing non-small cell lung cancer (NSCLC) constitutes a rapidly advancing and potentially transformative discipline. Empirical evidence has identified distinct microbial signatures within the pulmonary and gastrointestinal systems of NSCLC patients, which markedly differ from those observed in healthy individuals. Mechanistic investigations progressively elucidate the intricate pathways through which these microbial communities influence NSCLC pathogenesis and therapeutic responses, primarily through the modulation of chronic inflammation, host immune mechanisms, and metabolic interactions, frequently mediated via the gut-lung axis. Microbiome profiles obtained from respiratory samples, feces, or liquid biopsies exhibit substantial promise as non-invasive biomarkers for the early detection of diseases, subtype classification, prognostic assessment, and prediction of therapeutic response. Artificial intelligence is becoming indispensable for integrating these complex microbial datasets with additional clinical and omics data, thereby enabling the construction of robust predictive models. Therapeutic strategies targeting microbiome modulation, which include broad-spectrum methodologies such as fecal microbiota transplantation (FMT), are actively being explored in preclinical studies and clinical trials, primarily to enhance the efficacy and diminish the toxicity of immunotherapy and chemotherapy. However, significant hurdles remain on the path initiating from research discovery to translating into clinical implementation. Establishing definitive causality, unravelling the full complexity of host-microbe interactions, and addressing the substantial inter-individual variability in human microbiomes remain ongoing scientific challenges. Methodological standardization across sample handling, analytical techniques, and bioinformatics is notably deficient. Robust clinical trial data illustrate benefits and safety for many interventions, particularly for LBPs and engineered microbes. Future research must prioritize addressing these gaps. Key directions include: conducting extensive, well-controlled longitudinal studies; developing and validating standardized methodologies for microbiome analysis; performing rigorous clinical trials with clearly defined microbial interventions and relevant clinical endpoints; advancing the engineering of safe and effective LBPs; fostering collaboration between researchers, clinicians, industry, and regulatory agencies to streamline translation; and developing harmonized global regulatory frameworks that ensure patient safety while facilitating innovation. Harnessing lung and gut microbes could significantly advance NSCLC care, offering personalized diagnostics, better outcome predictions, and new treatments. Despite clinical challenges, ongoing research and collaboration aim to translate microbiome science into real patient benefits.

REFERENCES

Adlakha, Y. K., & Chhabra, R. (2025). The human microbiome: Redefining cancer pathogenesis and therapy. *Cancer Cell International*, *25*(1), 165. Advance online publication. DOI: 10.1186/s12935-025-03787-x PMID: 40296128

Almagro, L. G. &. A., & Almagro, L. G. &. A. (2024). Microbiome Drug Development: 2023 in review - Microbiome Times Magazine. *Microbiome Times Magazine - Reporting on The Latest Microbiome Business & Scientific Developments*.https://www.microbiometimes.com/microbiome-drug-development-2023-in-review/

AlOsaimi, H. M., Alshilash, A. M., Al-Saif, L. K., Bosbait, J. M., Albeladi, R. S., Almutairi, D. R., Alhazzaa, A. A., Alluqmani, T. A., Al Qahtani, S. M., Almohammadi, S. A., Alamri, R. A., Alkurdi, A. A., Aljohani, W. K., Alraddadi, R. H., & Alshammari, M. K. (2025). AI models for identifying prognostic and predictive biomarkers in lung cancer: A systematic review and meta-analysis. *Frontiers in Oncology*, *15*, 1424647. DOI: 10.3389/fonc.2025.1424647 PMID: 40078179

Ankudavicius, V., Nikitina, D., Lukosevicius, R., Tilinde, D., Salteniene, V., Poskiene, L., Miliauskas, S., Skieceviciene, J., Zemaitis, M., & Kupcinskas, J. (2023). Detailed Characterization of the Lung–Gut Microbiome Axis Reveals the Link between PD-L1 and the Microbiome in Non-Small-Cell Lung Cancer Patients. *International Journal of Molecular Sciences*, *25*(4), 2323. DOI: 10.3390/ijms25042323 PMID: 38396998

Augustus, E., Zwaenepoel, K., Siozopoulou, V., Raskin, J., Jordaens, S., Baggerman, G., Sorber, L., Roeyen, G., Peeters, M., & Pauwels, P. (2021). Prognostic and predictive biomarkers in non-small cell lung cancer patients on immunotherapy—The role of liquid biopsy in unraveling the puzzle. *Cancers (Basel)*, *13*(7), 1675. DOI: 10.3390/cancers13071675 PMID: 33918147

Barberio, D. (2024). Navigating regulatory and analytical challenges in live biotherapeutic product development and manufacturing. *Frontiers in Microbiomes*, *3*, 1441290. DOI: 10.3389/frmbi.2024.1441290

Belaid, A., Roméo, B., Rignol, G., Benzaquen, J., Audoin, T., Brest, P., Varraso, R., Von Bergen, M., Hugo Marquette, C., Leroy, S., Mograbi, B., & Hofman, P. (2023). Impact of the Lung Microbiota on Development and Progression of Lung Cancer. *Cancers (Basel)*, *16*(19), 3342. DOI: 10.3390/cancers16193342 PMID: 39409962

Budin, C. E., Cocuz, I. G., Sárközi, H. K., Sabau, A. H., & Grigorescu, B. L. (2022). Is the pulmonary microbiome involved in lung cancer pathophysiology? *Acta Marisiensis Seria Medica*, *68*(3), 99–102. DOI: 10.2478/amma-2022-0021

Çalışkan, M., & Tazaki, K. (2023). AI/ML advances in non-small cell lung cancer biomarker discovery. *Frontiers in Oncology*, *13*, 1260374. DOI: 10.3389/fonc.2023.1260374 PMID: 38148837

Chakraborty, J., Singh, N. L., & Das, B. K. (2025). Gut microbiome and lung cancer: Mechanisms, interactions, and dietary interventions. *Gut Microbes Reports*, *2*(1), 2501313. Advance online publication. DOI: 10.1080/29933935.2025.2501313

Chen, Y., Liu, T., Xu, Z., & Dong, M. (2023). Association of Epstein-Barr virus (EBV) with lung cancer: Meta-analysis. *Frontiers in Oncology*, *13*, 1177521. Advance online publication. DOI: 10.3389/fonc.2023.1177521 PMID: 37860200

Cheng, C., Wang, Z., Wang, J., Ding, C., Sun, C., Liu, P., Xu, X., Liu, Y., Chen, B., & Gu, B. (2020). Characterization of the lung microbiome and exploration of potential bacterial biomarkers for lung cancer. *Translational Lung Cancer Research*, *9*(3), 693–704. DOI: 10.21037/tlcr-19-590 PMID: 32676331

Ciernikova, S., Sevcikova, A., Stevurkova, V., & Mego, M. (2023). Diet-driven microbiome changes and physical activity in cancer patients. *Frontiers in Nutrition*, *10*, 1285516. DOI: 10.3389/fnut.2023.1285516 PMID: 38075222

Cordaillat-Simmons, M., Rouanet, A., & Pot, B. (2020). Live biotherapeutic products: The importance of a defined regulatory framework. *Experimental & Molecular Medicine*, *52*(9), 1397–1406. DOI: 10.1038/s12276-020-0437-6 PMID: 32908212

Deepika, N., Alsharari, Z. D., Ahmad, M. F., Singh, J., Yadav, M., Kumari, A., Kumar, A., Matthews, K. R., Aluko, R. E., Raposo, A., Albaridi, N. A., Mozaffar, B., Saraiva, A., & Saxena, S. C. (2025). Gut-lung axis, probiotics, and prebiotics: Insights on dysbiosis, mechanism, and prevention of lung cancer. *Frontiers in Nutrition*, *12*, 1624803. Advance online publication. DOI: 10.3389/fnut.2025.1624803 PMID: 40808835

Dong, W., Luo, Y., He, D., Zhang, M., Zeng, J., & Chen, Y. (2024). Oncolytic virotherapy against lung cancer: Key receptors and signaling pathways of viral entry. *Frontiers in Immunology*, *15*, 1473288. Advance online publication. DOI: 10.3389/fimmu.2024.1473288 PMID: 39430750

Duttagupta, S., Hakozaki, T., Routy, B., & Messaoudene, M. (2023). The Gut Microbiome from a Biomarker to a Novel Therapeutic Strategy for Immunotherapy Response in Patients with Lung Cancer. *Current Oncology (Toronto, Ont.)*, *30*(11), 9406–9427. DOI: 10.3390/curroncol30110681 PMID: 37999101

Duttagupta, S., Messaoudene, M., Jamal, R., Mihalcioiu, C., Marcoux, N., Hunter, S., Piccinno, G., Puncochár, M., Bélanger, K., Tehfe, M., Blais, N., Owen, S., Raphael, J., Maillou, J., Hu, Y., Benlaifaoui, M., Nilli, S., Lenehan, J., Belkaid, W., & Elkrief, A. (2025). Abstract 2210: Microbiome profiling reveals that fecal microbiota transplantation (FMT) modulates response and toxicity when combined with immunotherapy in lung cancer and melanoma (FMT-LUMINate NCT04951583). *Cancer Research*, *85*(8, Supplement_1), 2210. DOI: 10.1158/1538-7445.AM2025-2210

Elkrief, A., Pidgeon, R., Vareki, S. M., Messaoudene, M., Castagner, B., & Routy, B. (2025). The gut microbiome as a target in cancer immunotherapy: Opportunities and challenges for drug development. *Nature Reviews. Drug Discovery*, *24*(9), 685–704. Advance online publication. DOI: 10.1038/s41573-025-01211-7 PMID: 40457025

Emadi, R., Saki, S., Yousefi, P., & Tabibzadeh, A. (2025). A perspective on lung cancer and lung Microbiome: Insight on Immunity. *Immunity, Inflammation and Disease*, *13*(2), e70145. Advance online publication. DOI: 10.1002/iid3.70145 PMID: 39887959

Garaci, E., Pariano, M., Nunzi, E., Costantini, C., Bellet, M. M., Antognelli, C., Russo, M. A., & Romani, L. (2024). Bacteria and fungi of the lung: Allies or enemies? *Frontiers in Pharmacology*, *15*, 1497173. DOI: 10.3389/fphar.2024.1497173 PMID: 39584143

Gerasimova, Y., Ali, H., & Nadeem, U. (2024). Challenges for pathologists in implementing clinical microbiome diagnostic testing. *The Journal of Pathology. Clinical Research*, *10*(5), e70002. DOI: 10.1002/2056-4538.70002 PMID: 39289163

Halley, A., Leonetti, A., Gregori, A., Tiseo, M., Deng, D. M., Giovannetti, E., & Peters, G. J. (2020). The role of the microbiome in cancer and therapy efficacy: Focus on lung cancer. *Anticancer Research*, *40*(9), 4807–4818. DOI: 10.21873/anticanres.14484 PMID: 32878769

Han, W., Xu, J., Sun, T., Zhou, Y., Feng, Y., Han, L., & Liu, X. (2024). Exploring gut microbiome markers in predicting efficacy of immunotherapy against lung cancer. *Journal of Clinical Oncology*, *42*(16, suppl), 8525. DOI: 10.1200/JCO.2024.42.16_suppl.8525

Hes, C., & Jagoe, R. T. (2023). Gut microbiome and nutrition-related predictors of response to immunotherapy in cancer: Making sense of the puzzle. *BJC Reports*, *1*(1), 1–9. DOI: 10.1038/s44276-023-00008-8 PMID: 39516566

Heslop, H. E., Sharma, S., & Rooney, C. M. (2021). Adoptive T-Cell therapy for Epstein-Barr Virus–Related lymphomas. *Journal of Clinical Oncology*, *39*(5), 514–524. DOI: 10.1200/JCO.20.01709 PMID: 33434061

Huang, D., Li, Z., Jiang, T., Yang, C., & Li, N. (2024). Artificial intelligence in lung cancer: Current applications, future perspectives, and challenges. *Frontiers in Oncology*, *14*, 1486310. DOI: 10.3389/fonc.2024.1486310 PMID: 39763611

Jia, H., Gong, Y., Wei, H., Zhao, C., Zang, Q., & Liew, C. S. L. (2025). Immunoregulatory role of pulmonary microbiota in lung cancer: A bibliometric analysis. *Discover. Oncology*, *16*(1), 1054. Advance online publication. DOI: 10.1007/s12672-025-02595-z PMID: 40498209

Jiang, H., Zeng, W., Zhang, X., Li, Y., Wang, Y., Peng, A., & Cao, D. (2024). Gut microbiota and its metabolites in non-small cell lung cancer and brain metastasis: From alteration to potential microbial markers and drug targets. *Frontiers in Cellular and Infection Microbiology*, *13*, 1211855. Advance online publication. DOI: 10.3389/fcimb.2023.1211855 PMID: 38304459

Jiang, S., Li, H., Zhang, L., Mu, W., Zhang, Y., Chen, T., Wu, J., Tang, H., Zheng, S., Liu, Y., Wu, Y., Luo, X., Xie, Y., & Ren, J. (2024). Generic Diagramming Platform (GDP): A comprehensive database of high-quality biomedical graphics. *Nucleic Acids Research*, *53*(D1), D1670–D1676. DOI: 10.1093/nar/gkae973 PMID: 39470721

Kashyap, P., Raj, K. V., Sharma, J., Dutt, N., & Yadav, P. (2025). Classification of NSCLC subtypes using lung microbiome from resected tissue based on machine learning methods. *NPJ Systems Biology and Applications*, *11*(1), 11. Advance online publication. DOI: 10.1038/s41540-025-00491-4 PMID: 39824879

Kim, K., Lee, M., Shin, Y., Lee, Y., & Kim, T. (2024). Optimizing Cancer Treatment Through Gut Microbiome Modulation. *Cancers (Basel)*, *17*(7), 1252. DOI: 10.3390/cancers17071252 PMID: 40227841

Kunjalwar, R., Keerti, A., Chaudhari, A., Sahoo, K., & Meshram, S. (2024). Microbial Therapeutics in Oncology: A Comprehensive Review of Bacterial role in Cancer treatment. *Cureus*. Advance online publication. DOI: 10.7759/cureus.70920 PMID: 39502977

Lee, E. H., & Hong, C. R. (2025). Composition, developmental patterns, and pathological associations of the human gut mycobiome. *Annals of Clinical Microbiology*, *28*(1), e1–e13. DOI: 10.5145/ACM.2025.28.1.2

Lee, J. B., Huang, Y., Oya, Y., Nutzinger, J., Ang, Y. L., Sooi, K., Cho, B. C., & Soo, R. A. (2024). Modulating the gut microbiome in non-small cell lung cancer: Challenges and opportunities. *Lung Cancer (Amsterdam, Netherlands)*, *194*, 107862. DOI: 10.1016/j.lungcan.2024.107862 PMID: 38959670

Leng, Q., Holden, V. K., Deepak, J., Todd, N. W., & Jiang, F. (2021). Microbiota Biomarkers for Lung Cancer. *Diagnostics (Basel)*, *11*(3), 407. DOI: 10.3390/diagnostics11030407 PMID: 33673596

Li, D., Lan, X., Xu, L., Zhou, S., Luo, H., Zhang, X., Yu, W., Yang, Y., & Fang, X. (2025). Influence of gut microbial metabolites on tumor immunotherapy: Mechanisms and potential natural products. *Frontiers in Immunology*, *16*, 1552010. DOI: 10.3389/fimmu.2025.1552010 PMID: 40066456

Li, R., Li, J., & Zhou, X. (2024). Lung microbiome: New insights into the pathogenesis of respiratory diseases. *Signal Transduction and Targeted Therapy*, *9*(1), 19. DOI: 10.1038/s41392-023-01722-y PMID: 38228603

Liang, S., Ma, J., Wang, G., Shao, J., Li, J., Deng, H., Wang, C., & Li, W. (2022). The Application of Artificial Intelligence in the Diagnosis and Drug Resistance Prediction of Pulmonary Tuberculosis. *Frontiers in Medicine*, *9*, 935080. DOI: 10.3389/fmed.2022.935080 PMID: 35966878

Liu, N. N., Ma, Q., Ge, Y., Yi, C. X., Wei, L. Q., Tan, J. C., Chu, Q., Li, J.-Q., Zhang, P., & Wang, H. (2020). Microbiome dysbiosis in lung cancer: From composition to therapy. *NPJ Precision Oncology*, *4*(1), 33. DOI: 10.1038/s41698-020-00138-z PMID: 33303906

Meyer, M., Fitzgerald, B. G., Paz-Ares, L., Cappuzzo, F., Jänne, P. A., Peters, S., & Hirsch, F. R. (2024). New promises and challenges in the treatment of advanced non-small-cell lung cancer. *Lancet*, *404*(10454), 803–822. DOI: 10.1016/S0140-6736(24)01029-8 PMID: 39121882

Michán, C., Prados, J., & Ramos, J. L. (2025). Bacteria as Precision Tools for Cancer Therapy. *Microbial Biotechnology*, *18*(1), e70090. DOI: 10.1111/1751-7915.70090 PMID: 39831778

Moratiel-Pellitero, A., Zapata-García, M., Gascón-Ruiz, M., Sesma, A., Quílez, E., Ramirez-Labrada, A., Martínez-Lostao, L., Domingo, M. P., Esteban, P., Yubero, A., Barbero-Herranz, R., Moreno-Blanco, A., Paño, J. R., Lastra, R., Pardo, J., Isla, D., Del Campo, R., & Gálvez, E. (2024). Biomarkers of Immunotherapy Response in Patients with Non-Small-Cell Lung Cancer: Microbiota Composition, Short-Chain Fatty Acids, and Intestinal Permeability. *Cancers (Basel)*, *16*(6), 1144. DOI: 10.3390/cancers16061144 PMID: 38539479

Nguyen, L. D., Viscogliosi, E., & Delhaes, L. (2015). The lung mycobiome: An emerging field of the human respiratory microbiome. *Frontiers in Microbiology*, *6*, 128165. DOI: 10.3389/fmicb.2015.00089 PMID: 25762987

Nie, Q., Zhao, F., Yu, X., Madhusudhanan, M. C., Chang, C., Li, S., Chowdhury, S. R., Kille, B., Xu, A., Sharkey, R., Sun, C., Zeng, H., Liu, S., Zhou, D., Yu, X., Yang, K., Figueiredo, S. C., Zotova, M., Hu, Z., & Gao, X. (2025). A class of benzofuranoindoline-bearing heptacyclic fungal RiPPs with anticancer activities. *Nature Chemical Biology*. Advance online publication. DOI: 10.1038/s41589-025-01946-9 PMID: 40551021

Ocáriz-Díez, M., Cruellas, M., Gascón, M., Lastra, R., Martínez-Lostao, L., Ramírez-Labrada, A., Paño, J. R., Sesma, A., Torres, I., Yubero, A., Pardo, J., Isla, D., & Gálvez, E. M. (2020). Microbiota and lung cancer. opportunities and challenges for improving immunotherapy efficacy. *Frontiers in Oncology*, *10*, 568939. DOI: 10.3389/fonc.2020.568939 PMID: 33117698

Osorio, J. C., Armijo, A., Carvajal, F. J., Corvalán, A. H., Castillo, A., Fuentes-Pananá, E. M., Moreno-León, C., Romero, C., & Aguayo, F. (2024). Epstein-Barr Virus BARF1 Is Expressed in Lung Cancer and Is Associated with Cancer Progression. *Cells*, *13*(18), 1578. DOI: 10.3390/cells13181578 PMID: 39329759

Porto, B. N. (2022). Insights into the role of the lung virome during respiratory viral infections. *Frontiers in Immunology*, *13*, 885341. Advance online publication. DOI: 10.3389/fimmu.2022.885341 PMID: 35572506

Prifti, K., Chabu, C. Y., Kobayashi, K. S., Song, J., Han, A., & De Figueiredo, P. (2025). Bacterial Therapeutics: Addressing the affordability gap in cancer therapy. *Cancer Research*, *85*(14), 2558–2560. DOI: 10.1158/0008-5472.CAN-25-0870 PMID: 40660814

Rahal, Z., & Kadara, H. (2023). Beyond bacteria: How the intratumor mycobiome modulates lung adenocarcinoma progression. *Cancer Cell*, *41*(11), 1846–1848. DOI: 10.1016/j.ccell.2023.09.002 PMID: 37774700

Ren, S., Feng, L., Liu, H., Mao, Y., & Yu, Z. (2024). Gut microbiome affects the response to immunotherapy in non-small cell lung cancer. *Thoracic Cancer*, *15*(14), 1149–1163. DOI: 10.1111/1759-7714.15303 PMID: 38572783

Rodriguez, J., Cordaillat-Simmons, M., Pot, B., & Druart, C. (2025). The regulatory framework for microbiome-based therapies: Insights into European regulatory developments. *NPJ Biofilms and Microbiomes, 11*, 53. https://doi.org/, C., John, T., & Wong, A. (2024). Biomarkers for immunotherapy resistance in non-small cell lung cancer. *Frontiers in Oncology, 14*, 1489977. https://doi.org/DOI: 10.1038/s41522-025-00683-0Rother

Ruban, M., Pozhidaeva, E., Bolotina, L., & Kaprin, A. (2025). The role of diet and nutrition in cancer development and management: From molecular mechanisms to personalized interventions. *Foods*, *14*(10), 1788. DOI: 10.3390/foods14101788 PMID: 40428567

Samuelson, D. R., Welsh, D. A., & Shellito, J. E. (2015). Regulation of lung immunity and host defense by the intestinal microbiota. *Frontiers in Microbiology*, *6*, 1085. DOI: 10.3389/fmicb.2015.01085 PMID: 26500629

Scott, A. J., Alexander, J. L., Merrifield, C. A., Cunningham, D., Jobin, C., Brown, R., Alverdy, J., O'Keefe, S. J., Gaskins, H. R., Teare, J., Yu, J., Hughes, D. J., Verstraelen, H., Burton, J., O'Toole, P. W., Rosenberg, D. W., Marchesi, J. R., & Kinross, J. M. (2019). International Cancer Microbiome Consortium consensus statement on the role of the human microbiome in carcinogenesis. *Gut*, *68*(9), 1624–1632. DOI: 10.1136/gutjnl-2019-318556 PMID: 31092590

Sequeira, T., Pinto, R., Cardoso, C., Almeida, C., Aragão, R., Almodovar, T., Bicho, M., Bicho, M. C., & Bárbara, C. (2024). HPV and Lung Cancer: A Systematic Review. *Cancers (Basel)*, *16*(19), 3325. DOI: 10.3390/cancers16193325 PMID: 39409943

Sesma, A., Quílez, E., Domingo, M. P., Esteban, P., Yubero, A., Paño, J. R., Lastra, R., Pardo, J., Isla, D., Del Campo, R., & Gálvez, E. (2023). Biomarkers of Immunotherapy Response in Patients with Non-Small-Cell Lung Cancer: Microbiota Composition, Short-Chain Fatty Acids, and Intestinal Permeability. *Cancers (Basel)*, *16*(6), 1144. DOI: 10.3390/cancers16061144 PMID: 38539479

Sey, E. A., & Warris, A. (2024). The gut-lung axis: The impact of the gut mycobiome on pulmonary diseases and infections. *Oxford Open Immunology*, *5*(1), iqae008. Advance online publication. DOI: 10.1093/oxfimm/iqae008 PMID: 39193472

Sha, G., Wu, Z., Wang, B., Ding, Y., Xiao, Z., Zhang, W., Zhou, J., Zhou, Y., Ji, G., Tian, Z., Zhang, W., & Zhao, X. (2025). Intratumorally specific microbial-derived lipopolysaccharide contributes to non-small cell lung cancer progression. *Virulence*, *16*(1), 2548626. Advance online publication. DOI: 10.1080/21505594.2025.2548626 PMID: 40817754

Shah, H., & Ng, T. L. (2023). A narrative review from gut to lungs: Non-small cell lung cancer and the gastrointestinal microbiome. *Translational Lung Cancer Research*, *12*(4), 909–926. DOI: 10.21037/tlcr-22-595 PMID: 37197624

Shah, Y. R., Ali, H., Tiwari, A., Guevara-Lazo, D., Nombera-Aznaran, N., Mohan Pinnam, B. S., Gangwani, M. K., Gopakumar, H., Sohail, A. H., Kanumilli, S., Calderon-Martinez, E., Krishnamoorthy, G., Thakral, N., & Dahiya, D. S. (2024). Role of fecal microbiota transplant in management of hepatic encephalopathy: Current trends and future directions. *World Journal of Hepatology*, *16*(1), 17–32. DOI: 10.4254/wjh.v16.i1.17 PMID: 38313244

Shahid, G. B., Ahan, R. E., Ostaku, J., & Seker, U. O. S. (2024). Bacterial Living Therapeutics with Engineered Protein Secretion Circuits to Eliminate Breast Cancer Cells. *ACS Synthetic Biology*, *13*(10), 3150–3162. DOI: 10.1021/acssynbio.3c00723 PMID: 39367855

Sinha, T., Khan, A., Awan, M., Bokhari, S. F. H., Ali, K., Amir, M., Jadhav, A. N., Bakht, D., Puli, S. T., & Burhanuddin, M. (2024). Artificial intelligence and machine learning in predicting the response to immunotherapy in non-small cell lung carcinoma: A systematic review. *Cureus*, *16*(5). Advance online publication. DOI: 10.7759/cureus.61220 PMID: 38939246

Souza, V. G., Forder, A., Brockley, L. J., Pewarchuk, M. E., Telkar, N., de Araújo, R. P., Trejo, J., Benard, K., Seneda, A. L., Minutentag, I. W., Erkan, M., Stewart, G. L., Hasimoto, E. N., Garnis, C., Lam, W. L., Martinez, V. D., & Reis, P. P. (2023a). Liquid biopsy in lung cancer: Biomarkers for the management of recurrence and metastasis. *International Journal of Molecular Sciences*, *24*(10), 8894. DOI: 10.3390/ijms24108894 PMID: 37240238

Souza, V. G. P., Forder, A., Pewarchuk, M. E., Telkar, N., de Araujo, R. P., Stewart, G. L., Vieira, J., Reis, P. P., & Lam, W. L. (2023b). The Complex Role of the Microbiome in Non-Small Cell Lung Cancer Development and Progression. *Cells*, *12*(24), 2801. DOI: 10.3390/cells12242801 PMID: 38132121

Stella, G. M., Scialò, F., Bortolotto, C., Agustoni, F., Sanci, V., Saddi, J., Casali, L., Corsico, A. G., & Bianco, A. (2022). Pragmatic Expectancy on Microbiota and Non-Small Cell Lung Cancer: A Narrative Review. *Cancers (Basel)*, *14*(13), 3131. DOI: 10.3390/cancers14133131 PMID: 35804901

Szczyrek, M., Bitkowska, P., Chunowski, P., Czuchryta, P., Krawczyk, P., & Milanowski, J. (2021). Diet, Microbiome, and Cancer Immunotherapy—A Comprehensive Review. *Nutrients*, *13*(7), 2217. DOI: 10.3390/nu13072217 PMID: 34203292

Ting, N. L., Lau, H. C., & Yu, J. (2022). Cancer pharmacomicrobiomics: Targeting microbiota to optimise cancer therapy outcomes. *Gut*, *71*(7), 1412–1425. DOI: 10.1136/gutjnl-2021-326264 PMID: 35277453

Tomasulo, A., Simionati, B., & Facchin, S. (2024). Microbiome One health model for a healthy ecosystem. *Science in One Health*, *3*, 100065. DOI: 10.1016/j.soh.2024.100065 PMID: 39077385

Tseng, C. H., Wong, S., Yu, J., Lee, Y. Y., Terauchi, J., Lai, H. C., Luo, J.-C., Kao, C. Y., Yu, S.-L., Liou, J.-M., Wu, D.-C., Hou, M.-C., Wu, M.-S., Wu, J.-J., Sung, J. J. Y., El-Omar, E. M., & Wu, C. Y. (2025). Development of live biotherapeutic products: A position statement of Asia-Pacific Microbiota Consortium. *Gut*, *74*(5), 706–713. DOI: 10.1136/gutjnl-2024-334501 PMID: 40011030

Turnbaugh, P. J., Ley, R. E., Hamady, M., Fraser-Liggett, C. M., Knight, R., & Gordon, J. I. (2007). The Human Microbiome Project. *Nature*, *449*(7164), 804–810. DOI: 10.1038/nature06244 PMID: 17943116

Wang, P., Jia, Y., Wu, R., Chen, Z., & Yan, R. (2021). Human gut bacterial β-glucuronidase inhibition: An emerging approach to manage medication therapy. *Biochemical Pharmacology*, *190*, 114566. DOI: 10.1016/j.bcp.2021.114566 PMID: 33865833

Wang, Y., Wang, Y., Zhou, Y., Feng, Y., Sun, T., & Xu, J. (2024). Tumor-related fungi and crosstalk with gut fungi in the tumor microenvironment. *Cancer Biology & Medicine*, •••, 1–18. DOI: 10.20892/j.issn.2095-3941.2024.0240 PMID: 39601429

Weber, D. D., Aminazdeh-Gohari, S., & Kofler, B. (2018). Ketogenic diet in cancer therapy. *Aging (Albany NY)*, *10*(2), 164–165. DOI: 10.18632/aging.101382 PMID: 29443693

Wilkins, B., Hartman, E., Kelley, B., Pachika, P., Bradley, J., & Bradley, J. (2025). The impact of artificial intelligence on a multi-omics approach toward predictive biomarkers for non-small cell lung cancer. *Exploration of Digital Health Technologies*, *3*, 101153. Advance online publication. DOI: 10.37349/edht.2025.101153

Xi, Y., Liu, F., Qiu, B., Li, Y., Xie, X., Guo, J., Wu, L., Liang, T., Wang, D., Wang, J., Chen, M., Xue, L., Ding, Y., Zhang, J., Wu, Q., & Liu, H. (2022). Analysis of Gut Microbiota Signature and Microbe-Disease Progression Associations in Locally Advanced Non-Small Cell Lung Cancer Patients Treated With Concurrent Chemoradiotherapy. *Frontiers in Cellular and Infection Microbiology*, *12*, 892401. DOI: 10.3389/fcimb.2022.892401 PMID: 35719339

Xin, Y., Liu, C., Zang, D., & Chen, J. (2024). Gut microbiota and dietary intervention: Affecting immunotherapy efficacy in non–small cell lung cancer. *Frontiers in Immunology*, *15*, 1343450. DOI: 10.3389/fimmu.2024.1343450 PMID: 38361936

Xiong, W., Xu, Q., Li, X., Xiao, R., Cai, L., & He, F. (2017). The association between human papillomavirus infection and lung cancer: A system review and meta-analysis. *Oncotarget*, *8*(56), 96419–96432. DOI: 10.18632/oncotarget.21682 PMID: 29221217

Xu, C., Hao, M., Zai, X., Song, J., Huang, Y., Gui, S., & Chen, J. (2024). A new perspective on gut-lung axis affected through resident microbiome and their implications on immune response in respiratory diseases. *Archives of Microbiology*, *206*(3), 107. DOI: 10.1007/s00203-024-03843-6 PMID: 38368569

Xu, N., Wang, L., Li, C., Ding, C., Li, C., Fan, W., Cheng, C., & Gu, B. (2020). Microbiota dysbiosis in lung cancer: Evidence of association and potential mechanisms. *Translational Lung Cancer Research*, *9*(4), 1554–1568. DOI: 10.21037/tlcr-20-156 PMID: 32953527

Yadav, M., & Chauhan, N. S. (2022). Microbiome therapeutics: Exploring the present scenario and challenges. *Gastroenterology Report*, *10*, goab046. Advance online publication. DOI: 10.1093/gastro/goab046 PMID: 35382166

Yaqub, M. O., Jain, A., Joseph, C. E., & Edison, L. K. (2025). Microbiome-Driven Therapeutics: From Gut Health to Precision Medicine. *Gastrointestinal Disorders (Basel, Switzerland)*, *7*(1), 7. DOI: 10.3390/gidisord7010007

Yuwono, E., Zaini, J., & Rozaliyani, A. (2024). The Cancer Mycobiome: A highlight to lung cancer. *Jurnal Respirasi*, *10*(3), 265–271. DOI: 10.20473/jr.v10-I.3.2024.265-271

Zhang, H., & Xu, Z. (2023). Gut–lung axis: Role of the gut microbiota in non-small cell lung cancer immunotherapy. *Frontiers in Oncology*, *13*, 1257515. DOI: 10.3389/fonc.2023.1257515 PMID: 38074650

Zhang, L., Li, M. J., Li, X. P., Yang, B., Xiao, T., Wang, P., & Zhang, W. D. (2025). Respiratory microbiota diversity as a predictive biomarker for the efficacy of PD-1 blockades in patients with advanced non-small cell lung cancer: A retrospective exploratory study. *Oncology Letters*, *29*(5), 251. DOI: 10.3892/ol.2025.14997 PMID: 40201032

Zhao, S., Lu, Z., Zhao, F., Tang, S., Zhang, L., & Feng, C. (2025). Assessing the impact of probiotics on immunotherapy effectiveness and antibiotic-mediated resistance in cancer: A systematic review and meta-analysis. *Frontiers in Immunology*, *16*, 1538969. Advance online publication. DOI: 10.3389/fimmu.2025.1538969 PMID: 40191197

Zhao, Y., Liu, Y., Li, S., Peng, Z., Liu, X., Chen, J., & Zheng, X. (2021). Role of lung and gut microbiota on lung cancer pathogenesis. *Journal of Cancer Research and Clinical Oncology*, *147*(8), 2177–2186. DOI: 10.1007/s00432-021-03644-0 PMID: 34018055

Zhou, X., You, L., Xin, Z., Su, H., Zhou, J., & Ma, Y. (2023). Leveraging circulating microbiome signatures to predict tumor immune microenvironment and prognosis of patients with non-small cell lung cancer. *Journal of Translational Medicine*, *21*(1), 800. DOI: 10.1186/s12967-023-04582-w PMID: 37950236

KEY TERMS AND DEFINITIONS

Biomarkers: Measurable biological indicators, such as specific microbial taxa, metabolites, or genetic signatures, found in tissues, blood, or other body fluids that are useful for clinical assessment, including diagnosis, prognosis, or prediction of treatment response.

Fecal Microbiota Transplantation (FMT): The goal of FMT is to restore a healthy microbial ecosystem by injecting feces from a healthy, screened donor into the gastrointestinal tract of the recipient.

Gut-Lung Axis: Axis between the gastrointestinal and respiratory systems involving the interaction between microbial communities, their metabolites, and the immune response of the host.

Immune Checkpoint Inhibitors (ICIs): Immunotherapy drugs that block checkpoint proteins (such as PD-1, PD-L1, CTLA-4), which normally act as brakes on the immune system. By inhibiting these checkpoints, ICIs unleash the body's own T cells to more effectively recognize and attack cancer cells.

Live Biotherapeutic Product (LBP): A bioproduct made of living microbes, such as bacteria, that can treat or prevent disease. LBPs are regulated as drugs by authorities like the FDA and EMA.

Microbiome: A collective community of microorganisms, including their genomes and the surrounding environmental conditions, which inhabit a specific environment, such as the human gut or lung.

Non-Small Cell Lung Cancer (NSCLC): Lung cancers (adenocarcinoma, squamous cell carcinoma, and large cell carcinoma) arising from epithelial cells lining the airways—from the central bronchi to the terminal alveoli—accounting for approximately 85% of Lung cancers.

Postbiotics: Physiologically beneficial preparations of inanimate microorganisms with or without their components (e.g., enzymes, metabolites, cell wall fragments). They represent a more stable and potentially safer alternative to live probiotics.

Prebiotics: Non-digestible compounds, typically dietary fibers, which are selectively utilized by beneficial host microorganisms, thereby promoting growth and activity and conferring health benefits.

Probiotics: By providing live microorganisms to the host in adequate amounts, probiotics confer health benefits on the host. In a therapeutic context, these are often specific, well-characterized strains.

Chapter 5 Different Types of Diagnostic Approaches in NSCLC

K. Gayathri
https://orcid.org/0009-0007-3786-2009
Department of Microbiology, Sacred Heart College, Tirupattur, India

Pallavi Singh
https://orcid.org/0000-0003-4537-4607
Graphic Era University, India

M. Manigandan
Department of Microbiology, Sacred Heart College, Tirupattur, India

B. Lokeshwari
https://orcid.org/0009-0005-6612-5134
Department of Microbiology, Sacred Heart College, Tirupattur, India

P. Saranraj
https://orcid.org/0000-0002-5052-6532
Department of Microbiology, Sacred Heart College, Tirupattur, India

ABSTRACT

Non-small cell lung cancer (NSCLC) is the most common type of lung cancer and accounts for about 85% of all lung cancers, and it is still a significant cause of cancer death globally. It is intimately related to environmental, genetic, and chemical exposures as well as smoking. While recent development in liquid biopsy allows for classification utilising biological fluids like blood and saliva, TNM (Tumour, Node, Metastasis) staging system plays a crucial part in prognosis and treatment. Each with

DOI: 10.4018/979-8-3373-2096-0.ch005

unique pathological traits, the disorder consists in adenocarcinoma, squamous cell carcinoma, and big cell carcinoma. Non-invasive, quick, highly specific detection is provided by methods like biosensor technology and biomarker analysis. Imaging techniques including early discovery utilising Computed Tomography (CT), Histological validation with Biopsy, Bronchoscopy to visualise and Cytology to examine the cells define diagnostic approaches for NSCLC. Recent developments in liquid biopsy let one classify utilising biological fluids such as saliva and blood. Early detection and focused treatment may be made easier by Biomarkers including Proteins linked with NSCLC and circulating tumour DNA (ctDNA). Using Nanotechnology and Electrochemical sensing, biosensors let one detect cancer-associated molecules in real time with great accuracy. Artificial intelligence (AI) will be included into future NSCLC detection to provide better image analysis of multi-analyte biomarkers as well as diagnoses. Discovery of genes and proteins is probably going to keep improving therapeutic targeting and diagnostic accuracy. Combining new technology has great power to improve early detection, patient survival in NSCLC. Along with new detection strategies, the present chapter covers epidemiology, categorisation, and diagnosis of NSCLC.

1. INTRODUCTION

Non-Small Cell Lung Cancer (NSCLC) is the most prevalent type of lung cancer, representing approximately 85% of all cases. Its biological variation and spectrum of clinical symptoms make diagnosis and therapy somewhat challenging (Gomez et al.,2016). A diagnosis determines whether successful therapy of NSCLC and patient best possible result assurance is attainable. From instruments for imaging and histology to advanced genetic profiling techniques, diagnostic testing has advanced dramatically (Shi et al.,2014). Imaging tests like Computed Tomography (CT), Positron Emission Tomography/Computed Tomography (PET-CT), and chest X-rays take front stage in case of non-small cell lung cancer. Accurate information on tumour size and architecture, involvement of adjacent structures, and lymphadenopathy (Kawaguchi et al., 2016). CT scans offer PET-CT helps one to differentiate benign from malignant tumours and raises staging accuracy (Zhou et al., 2011).

Molecular diagnostic methods have become rather important in precision medicine as a tool for target identification for treatment and genetic disorders generating cancer (Rosell et al., 2012). The tissue samples, Liquid Biopsy Techniques, Next-Generation Sequencing (NGS), Fluorescence *in situ* Hybridisation (FISH), Polymerase Chain Reaction (PCR) have all enhanced diagnosis of Non-small cell lung cancer (NSCLC) by means of Genetic profiling. In peripheral blood, liquid biopsy in circulating tumour DNA (ctDNA) or Circulating Tumours Cells (CTCs) is a less invasive method than Molecular testing whereby Tissue biopsy is not practical or in the case of an urgent need to monitor disease progression and treatment failure (Sequest et al., 2013). NGS looks for a broad spectrum of genomic abnormalities including mutations, copy number changes, fusions, and Tumours Mutational Burden (TMB). Using diagnostic modalities, one should take into account factors such the availability of the tumour, the clinical condition of the patient, and the need of molecular testing (Wu et al., 2014).

By early detection, improved risk stratification, and better medication matching, advanced technologies Radiogenomics, Artificial Intelligence - based Image Analysis, and Biomarker Identification have the potential to greatly improve NSCLC diagnosis (Mok et al., 2017). Great progress has been the challenges still exist include finding enough tissue for most investigations, managing tumour heterogeneity, and understanding complicated genomic data to support clinic decisions (Soria et al., 2018). Crucially, the standardisation of diagnostic approaches, developments in Genetic testing, and Field-based biopsy technique innovation are all under progress (Mok et al., 2018). It uses a variety of state-of- the-art diagnostic techniques utilised by doctors and to improved NSCLC care in diagnostics.

2. EPIDEMIOLOGY OF NON-SMALL CELL LUNG CANCER (NSCLC)

About 85% of all Lung cancers worldwide and one of the main causes of Cancer-related mortality worldwide is Non-small cell lung cancer (NSCLC). Elements influencing NSCLC worldwide burden are geographical, lifestyle, environmental exposure, genetic, and health differences (Wu et al., 2017). Though more and more asbestos, radon, and air pollution exposure, the causal element is still smoking, responsible for about 85% of NSCLC (Kalanjeri and Gildea, 2016). While rising trends persist in less developed countries through explosive rates of smoking and the lack of regulatory mechanisms, the trends have levelled out or reduced in countries with established Tobacco Control Programs (Lamprecht et al., 2012). About 40% of cases of NSCLC are adenocarcinoma, the most prevalent kind of the disease; typically occurring in never-smoking individuals, especially in women from Asia, this condition mainly results from environmental factors (McWilliams et al., 2013).

The other two are Squamous cell carcinoma and Giant cell carcinoma, each with unique clinical, pathogenic, and molecular profile (Patriquin et al., 2015). Over the years, the diagnosis of NSCLC has changed from application of Radiographic examinations to that which is complicated, multi-disciplinary whereby imaging modalities, histology, and molecular diagnostics were used in conjunction (Hubers et al., 2014). Imaging studies include Computed Tomography (CT) and chest X-rays (Lam et al., 2009) reveal clinical NSCLC suspicion beginning with no explanation weight loss, haemoptysis, prolonged coughing, or dyspnoea. By means of precision in diagnosis from malignant from tumours and active lesions, Positron Emission Tomography with CT (PET-CT) provides Artificial intelligence (AI) and Radiomics in imaging diagnostics with predicted imaging features-based analytics to be contrasted against genetic profiles and the pivotal importance in Personalised treatments (Uke et al., 2017).

3. TYPES OF NON-SMALL CELL LUNG CANCER AND THEIR CLASSIFICATION FOR DIAGNOSIS

Non-Small Cell Lung Cancer (NSCLC) making up approximately 85% of all Lung cancers, is typically classified into three large Histological types: Adenocarcinoma, Squamous cell carcinoma, and Large cell carcinoma, with varying diagnostic approaches for their varying Molecular and Pathological characteristics (Kremer et al., 2010). The most prevalent sub-type, Adenocarcinoma usually affects peripheral areas of the lung and is linked to Genetic mutations like EGFR, ALK, and ROS1; hence, Molecular profiling and Next-generation sequencing are used in diagnosis and treatment (Antonangelo et al., 2015). Usually, Squamous cell carcinoma is found in the central bronchi; histologically, it shows keratinisation and intercellular bridges; the diagnosis is made based on Bronchoscopy-guided biopsies and Immunohistochemistry markers p40 and CK5/6 (Kaur et al., 2017). Large cell carcinoma is a less common, undifferentiated carcinoma diagnosed by exclusion whereby there is no glandular or squamous differentiation of the Tumours and Large cell carcinomas undergo Immunohistochemistry and Molecular testing (Huss, 2015). Emphasising subtype-specific diagnostics importance to NSCLC management, diagnostic techniques in NSCLC thus combine imaging techniques like CT, PET-CT, and MRI with the procurement of Tissues using Bronchoscopy, CT-guided biopsy, or EBUS-TBNA and following histopathological and biomarker examination for the proper sub-type classification and guide Targeted therapy or Immunotherapy accordingly (Soreide, 2009).

3.1. Histological Classification of Lung Cancer

NSCLC is classified into three principal subtypes according to histology: adenocarcinoma, squamous cell carcinoma, and large cell carcinoma (Potti et al., 2006). The most prevalent sub-type is Adenocarcinoma, arises in glandular epithelial cells and tends to be peripheral in site and is characterized by secretion of mucin and glandular structures, usually validated with immunohistochemical markers like

TTF-1 and Napsin A (Seetharamu et al., 2016). More usually central in derivation, squamous cell carcinoma is defined by intercellular bridges and keratinisation and diagnosed using markers like p63, CK5/6, and p40 (Strimbu and Tavel, 2010). Diagnosed using broad-range immunohistochemistry (Zare et al., 2018), large cell carcinoma is glandular or squamous differentiation-free tumour ruled out from other subtypes. Following tissue sample from tissue obtained by bronchoscopy, image-guided biopsy, or surgical resection that is, histological classification (Villalobos and Wistuba, 2017). Histopathological analysis and immunohistochemical labelling become very important once tissues are acquired in deciding the subtypes (Wang et al., 2023). Especially in adenocarcinomas, the sub-classification guidance for targetable mutations (e.g., EGFR, ALK, KRAS) guides next molecular investigation and so forms a fundamental part of NSCLC diagnosis paths and precision (Yuan et al., 2019).

3.2. Tumor Node Metasis (TNM) Classification

TNM staging is a common technique for diagnosing non-small cell lung cancer (NSCLC) significant for predicting prognosis as well as treatment (Garcia-Robledo et al., 2022). The TNM system considers three elements are distant metastasis (M), lymph node involvement (N), and tumour size and spread (T) (Brown et al., 2018). The T category assesses the size of the main tumour and its invasion of surrounding structures from T1 (tumours of 3 cm or less limited to the lung) to T4 (tumours infiltrating major tissues such the heart or trachea). The N category looks at regional lymph node involvement from N0 (no affected lymph nodes) to N3 (contralateral mediastinal or supraclavicular lymph node metastases). The M category indicates the degree of distant metastases; M0 and M1a–M1c levels of metastatic involvement in the pleural nodules or to distant organs signalling no metastases define this amount of distant metastases (Yang et al., 2024). Essential diagnosis tools for the proper TNM staging are CT, PET-CT, Endobronchial Ultrasonic Waves (EBUS), and Mediastinoscopy (Xie et al., 2023). Apart from ascertaining the stage of the malignancy (I–IV), staging shows the sole change of NSCLC diagnosis and therapy orientation from the resection of early disease through to the treatment of late sickness systemically (Singh et al., 2021).

3.3. Classification-based on Biological Fluids

Biological fluids is the invasive diagnostic procedure in Non-Small Cell Lung Cancer (NSCLC), into Tumor Biology, especially when tissue biopsies are limited or not available in the tissues (Ghose et al., 2019). Tumor-derived biomarkers find reservoirs in biological fluids including blood, pleural effusion, sputum, and bronchal lavage (BAL), therefore enabling early discovery, mutation profiling, and treatment monitoring (Johnson et al., 2021). Liquid biopsy which examines ctDNA, CTCs, and exosomes through blood samples helps to identify important genetic mutations like EGFR mutations, ALK rearrangements, and T790M resistance mutations (Ringborg et al., 2024). It is especially used in advanced NSCLC for dynamic monitoring devoid of repetitive intrusive treatments (Mohanty et al., 2023). Usually combined with Immunocytochemistry and Molecular studies, Pleural fluid cytology also detects malignant cells in malignant pleural effusions (Ramisetty et al., 2024). Specifically in centrally situated tumours, Bronchoscopy uses BAL fluid to help identify Cytological abnormalities and Tumour markers (Gomez et al., 2018). Less sensitive, sputum cytology is used in Squamous cell cancer diagnosis (Shi et al., 2014). These liquid-based diagnostic methods enhance conventional tissue biopsies and imaging in offering real-time, complete molecular data and so support accuracy in diagnosis and treatment of NSCLC, so reducing patient suffering (Zhou et al., 2011).

4. DIAGNOSTIC TECHNIQUES FOR NON-SMALL CELL LUNG CANCER (NSCLC)

Diagnostic techniques of Non-Small Cell Lung Cancer (NSCLC) are now the process to achieve accurate detection, categorization, and to guide personalized treatment (Rosell et al., 2012). The initial evaluation most often begins with imaging examinations, such as chest X-ray and Computed Tomography (CT), to detect pulmonary nodules and assess tumor size and location (Mitsudomi et al., 2010). Positron Emission Tomography with Computed Tomography (PET-CT) provides for the detection of distant metastases and active tumors (Maemondo et al., 2010). Magnetic Resonance Imaging (MRI) is also used to detect brain metastasis in a state of advanced disease (Sequist et al., 2013). Ultimate diagnosis must be accomplished with histological proof through tissue sampling obtained by means of Bronchoscopy, CT-Guided Needle Biopsy, or Endobronchial Ultrasound-Guided Transbronchial Needle Aspiration (EBUS-TBNA) (Wu et al., 2014). All these are procedures that facilitate sample acquisition of tumors and lymph nodes by way of minimal invasiveness (Mok et al., 2017). Histopathological Examination and Immunohistochemistry (IHC) are used to identify NSCLC subtypes such as Adenocarcinoma, Squamous cell carcinoma, or Large cell carcinoma (Soria et al., 2018). High-level molecular testing including Next-Generation Sequencing (NGS) and liquid biopsy to detect Circulating tumor DNA (ctDNA) and Actionable mutations (e.g., EGFR, ALK, KRAS) are detected, and candidacy for targeted therapy is established (Mok et al., 2018). These diagnostic techniques support precise staging and molecular characterization on which individualized NSCLC therapies are established (Lee et al., 2013).

Table 1. Overview of Diagnostic Techniques for Non-Small Cell Lung Cancer (NSCLC)

Diagnostic Techniques	**Purposes**
Chest X-ray	Imaging method to evaluate lung abnormalities.
Computed Tomography (CT) Scan	Cross-sectional imaging that offers good views of lung tissue.
Magnetic Resonance Imaging (MRI)	Uses magnetic fields and radio waves to create good images.
Positron Emission Tomography (PET) Scan	Imaging method that identifies metabolic activity with a radiotracer.
Bronchoscopy	A procedure using a flexible tube to view airways and collect tissue samples.
Transthoracic Needle Biopsy	A needle is inserted through the chest wall to obtain tissue for analysis.
Sputum Cytology	Examination of sputum under a microscope for cancer cells.
Mediastinoscopy	A method to biopsy lymph nodes in the chest via a minimal incision. Uses bronchoscopy with ultrasound to take pictures of lymph nodes and lesions.
Endobronchial Ultrasound (EBUS)	Blood work testing for tumor markers like carcinoembryonic antigen (CEA) and neuron-specific enolase (NSE).
Blood Tests (e.g., CEA, NSE)	Blood tests measuring tumor markers such as carcinoembryonic antigen (CEA) and neuron-specific enolase (NSE).

4.1. Computer-based Tomography

Computed Tomography (CT) is the central theme of Non-Small Cell Lung Cancer (NSCLC) diagnostic practice through the accurate cross-sectional images of the lungs, mediastinum, and surrounding structures for the integral to early detection, tumor localisation, and staging (Kremer et al., 2010). Usually, the first high-tech modality used is high-tech imaging by CT scan; it is more sensitive in small mass and lung nodule detection than chest X-ray (Antonangelo et al., 2015). Imaging using CT helps in NSCLC to evaluate size, shape, density, and anatomical position of the primary tumour and surrounding structures including the chest wall, pleura, or vascular (Kaur et al., 2017). Additionally assessing lymph node enlargement in the mediastinum and hilar nodes for TNM staging (Huss, 2015) is additionally improving vision of vascular systems and tumour delineation is contrast-enhanced CT (Soreide, 2009). For Histological diagnosis, CT results direct Biopsy procedures include core biopsies or CT-guided Fine-needle aspiration (FNA). Low-dose CT (LDCT) has also become rather important for screening high-risk populations, including heavy smokers, to enable early NSCLC diagnosis and lower mortality (Seetharamu et al., 2016). Although CT cannot differentiate benign from malignant lesions that complement histological and molecular analyses in NSCLC diagnosis (Strimbu and Tavel, 2010).

4.2. Biopsy

Biopsy is a diagnostic tool that cannot be overlooked when evaluating Non-Small Cell Lung Cancer (NSCLC) and provides histological diagnosis along with precise tumor classification and molecular analysis (Zare et al., 2018). Biopsy refers to the excision of tissue or cellular material from a lesion where it is suspected for microscopic study and is needed to NSCLC from another lung disease or Small cell lung cancer (SCLC) (Villalobos and Wistuba, 2017). Tumour location and patients guide the application of certain biopsy methods (Wang et al., 2023). Bronchoscopic biopsy treats central tumours; they could be paired with Endobronchial Ultrasonic Guided Transbronchial Needle Aspiration (EBUS-TBNA) for mediastinal node biopsy (Yuan et al., 2019). Highly diagnostic yield CT-guided percutaneous needle biopsy is used (Garcia-Robledo et al., 2022). The complicated instances in the bigger tissue samples are handled by surgical operations including Mediastinoscopy or Video-Assisted Thoracoscopic Surgery (VATS) (Brown et al., 2018). Once obtained, biopsy samples undergo Histological investigation, Immunohistochemical (IHC) analysis to determine the sub-type (Adenocarcinoma, Squamous cell carcinoma, or Big cell carcinoma), and Molecular analysis for Mutations including EGFR, ALK, and KRAS (Kanan et al., 2024). Individualised treatment modalities, that is, targeted therapy and immunotherapy guided biopsies by helping to predict illness prognosis (Garg et al., 2023).

4.3. Bronchoscopy

Bronchoscopy is a diagnostic procedure for the evaluation of Non-Small Cell Lung Cancer (NSCLC), extremely helpful in centrally located tumors in the bronchial tree (Yang et al., 2024). Either the oral or nasal cavity is inserted a rigid or flexible bronchoscope into the respiratory system to view the tracheobronchial tree in order to collect tissue or fluid samples for analysis (Xie et al., 2023). Bronchoscopy produces biopsy of endoscopically apparent tumours, bronchial brushings, washings, and endobronchial needle aspiration for cytopathological evaluation in the diagnosis of NSCLC (Singh et al., 2021). Specifically used to identify obstructive tumours, linked with bleeding or mucosal anomalies, bronchoscopy is (Ghose et al., 2019). Bronchoscopy for sampling medastinal and hilar lymph nodes and supporting TNM staging; endobronchial ultrasonic transbronchial needle aspiration (EBUS-TBNA). With little problems, bronchoscopy treatments offer diagnostic worth (Ringborg et al., 2024) and required for targeted therapy planning, bronchoscopy for diagnosis and staging for histopathological evaluation, immunohistochemistry, and genetic tests for EGFR and ALK mutations are bronchoscopy for diagnosis and staging for histopathological assessment. Moreover, bronchoscopy can be used therapeutively for molecular invasibility and relaxation of airway blockage (Ramisetty et al., 2024).

4.4. Cytology

Cytology is a valuable diagnostic tool in the assessment of Non-Small Cell Lung Cancer (NSCLC), particularly in difficult-to-access tissue biopsies (Gomez et al., 2016). Cytological samples are used in NSCLC are sputum, bronchial washings and brushing, Bronchoalveolar lavage (BAL), and effusion fluids from Pleural effusions (Shi et al., 2014), using Fine-needle aspiration (FNA) of the lung nodule or nodes. Investigated for aberrant mitoses (Zhou et al., 2011), cytologic samples show malignant cellular characteristics including hyperchromatic nuclei. Cytology samples fit for immunocytochemistry and molecular testing (eg., EGFR, ALK, KRAS mutations) in the days of individualised medicine. In differentiated neoplasms, less costly for first diagnosis and staging and cytology could be the diagnosis yield than histology (Mitsudomi et al., 2010).

Figure 1. Diagnostic Methods for Non-Small Cell Lung Cancer (NSCLC)

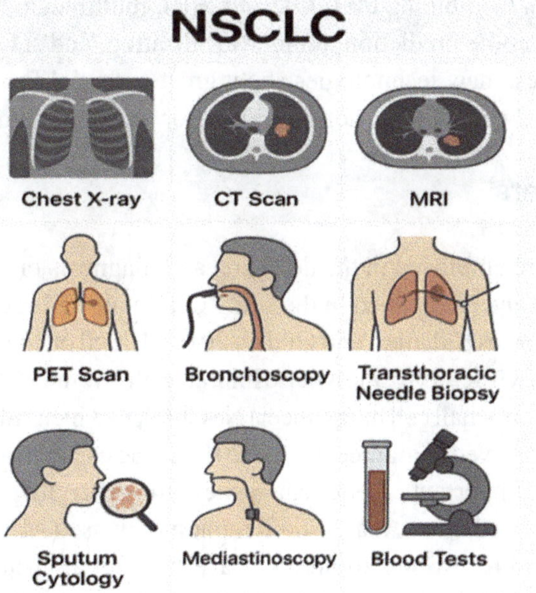

5. EMERGING TECHNIQUES FOR DETECTION OF NON-SMALL CELL LUNG CANCER (NSCLC)

Methods employed for detection of Non-Small Cell Lung Cancer (NSCLC) include early diagnosis, offering less invasive and are more accurate (Maemondo et al., 2010). Exosomes in blood, circulating tumour DNA (ctDNA), and circulating tumour cells (CTCs) are examined in liquid biopsy (Sequest et al., 2013). The non-invasive technique over conventional biopsies and enables real-time monitoring of tumour development and response to medications (Wu et al., 2014), liquid biopsy lets one evaluate genetic alterations (e.g., EGFR, ALK, and KRAS). Radiomics employs Artificial Intelligence (AI) whereby Machine Learning techniques decipher image inputs from CT and MRI scans (Mok et al., 2017).

AI systems also provide early identification and prognosis prediction (Soria et al., 2018), therefore helping radiologists to find even little tumours they might overlook. More precisely staging (Mok et al., 2018) and its potential to evaluate deep mediastinal and hilar lymph nodes make endoscopic ultrasonic with Fine-Needle Aspiration (FNA) also a desirable tool. Additionally used for the identification of molecular diagnosis to NSCLC is breath analysis or sputum biomarker detection (Lee et al., 2013). Combining PET, CT, and MRI, multimodal imaging is enhancing treatment outcome prediction, tumour localisation, and staging accuracy (Lee et al., 2015). These new technologies show great potential for early, staging, and follow-up NSCLC patient detection as well as for tracking them (Wu et al., 2017).

5.1. Biomarkers

Biomarkers are employed in the detection and diagnosis of non-small cell lung cancer (NSCLC) and are applied in the study of tumour biology, genetic mutation, and therapy response (Kalanjeri and Gildea, 2016). Based on the Epidermal Growth Factor Receptor (EGFR), Tyrosine Kinase Inhibitors (TKIs) are most typically applied Biomarketer in Non-small cell lung cancer (NSCLC), in which Adenocarcinomas are most generally observed (Lamprecht et al., 2012). One can then apply other targeted treatments in line. Important genetic changes key biomarkers for personalised therapy and personalised medicine, Anaplastic lymphoma kinase (ALK) rearrangements, ROS1 fusions, and KRAS mutations also have substantial influence (McWilliams et al., 2013). Apart from genetic components, Programmed death-ligand 1 (PD-L1) status is significant in selecting whether to treat with immunotherapy utilising PD-1/PD-L1 inhibitors (Patriquin et al., 2015). Two recently developed liquid biopsy markers that offer a non-invasive approach of track therapy and mutation discovery are Circulating cancer cells (CTCs) and Circulating Tumour DNA (ctDNA). More and more sputum, blood, and pleural fluid biomarkers will determine early diagnosis and prognosis, so Guiding therapy of Non-small cell lung cancer (Lam et al., 2009). Regular inclusion of these biomarkers into clinical practice helps NSCLC patients greatly more since they enable earlier diagnosis, better staging, and treatment choice.

5.2. Biosensors

Non-small cell lung cancer (NSCLC) can be diagnosed with biosensors, a quick, non-invasive, sensitive method for early cancer detection (Uke et al., 2017). Usually discovered in biological fluids such blood, sputum, or exhaled air, one may find the particular biomarkers of Non-small cell lung cancer (NSCLC) using biosensors that is, proteins, nucleic acids, or metabolites. Using electrochemical biosensors which may identify tumor-related proteins including cancer antigens or specific ctDNA mutations opens the most fascinating path (Antonangelo et al., 2015). By means of graphene oxide and carbon nanotubes, nanomaterial-based biosensors help to recognise very low quantities of chemicals peculiar to cancer and enhance the sensitivity and specificity of NSCLC biomarkers. Another approach to find specific markers for cancer is optical biosensing, which detects variations in light properties as fluorescence or surface plasmon resonance (Huss, 2015). For the diagnosis of Non-small cell lung cancer (NSCLC) from the distinct patterns of chemical breath (Soreide, 2009), under investigation are breath sensors based on Volatile organic compounds (VOCs). Point-of- care testing and disease monitoring among other benefits these biosensors provide help patients with Non-small cell lung cancer obtains early diagnosis, prognosis, and customised treatment plans (Potti et al., 2006).

6. FUTURE PERSPECTIVES

Non-Small Cell Lung Cancer (NSCLC) diagnosis has been revolutionised by the development of technologies that facilitate the early detection of the disease (Seetharamu et al., 2016). These consist of the exosomes from blood or bodily fluid (Strimbu and Tavel, 2010), Circulating tumour DNA (ctDNA), and Circulating tumour cells (CTCs). Reducing intrusive biopsies, this offers early diagnosis, mutation profiling, and medication response (Zare et al., 2018). Particularly in imaging and radiomics, artificial intelligence and machine learning will also enhance diagnostic accuracy by letting one identify minor trends inside CT and MRI scans (Villalobos and Wistuba, 2017). Multi-omics approaches allowing the molecular features of NSCLC in biomarkers and therapeutic targets in genomes, proteomics, and metabolomics method allowed faster, less expensive, simpler biosensors and nanotechnology early diagnosis of NSCLC will also gain from (Yuan et al., 2019). Together with Immunotherapy and Targeted treatments, these advancements create customised and successful treatment modalities that increase the future survival rates for NSCLC patients (Garcia-Robledo et al., 2022).

7. ARTIFICIAL INTELLIGENCE IN DETECTION OF NSCLC

Artificial Intelligence is fundamentally transforming the early detection of non-small cell lung cancer (NSCLC) by analyzing medical imaging with unprecedented precision. Through sophisticated deep learning algorithms, AI systems can scrutinize low-dose computed tomography (LDCT) scans to identify subtle pulmonary nodules that may be overlooked in a manual review. This capability significantly enhances the effectiveness of lung cancer screening programs by enabling diagnosis at earlier, more treatable stages, which is critical for improving patient survival rates. Beyond mere detection, AI excels in characterizing these nodules to assess their risk of malignancy. By extracting and analyzing thousands of quantitative features from a nodule's shape, density, and texture—a field known as radiomics—AI models can stratify lesions based on their likelihood of being cancerous. This advanced analysis helps reduce the number of false-positive findings, thereby minimizing unnecessary invasive procedures like biopsies for patients and alleviating the workload for radiologists (Ardila et al., 2019).

The impact of AI extends into the pathology lab, where it augments the diagnostic process. By processing digitized images of tissue samples, algorithms can assist pathologists in classifying NSCLC subtypes, such as adenocarcinoma and squamous cell carcinoma, with high accuracy. Furthermore, groundbreaking research demonstrates that AI can even predict the status of key genetic biomarkers, like EGFR and PD-L1, directly from routine pathology slides, potentially streamlining the path to personalized therapy. Despite its immense potential, the integration of AI into standard clinical practice faces challenges. These include the need for large, diverse, and high-quality datasets to train robust algorithms, ensuring patient privacy, and securing regulatory approval. Nevertheless, AI represents a powerful and evolving tool that is poised to become an indispensable ally in the fight against lung cancer, promising a future of earlier detection, more precise diagnosis, and better outcomes for patients with NSCLC (Coudray et al., 2018).

Table 2. Applications of Artificial Intelligence in NSCLC Detection and Diagnosis

Application Area	Specific Detection	AI Technology Used	Benefit	References
Radiology (CT scans)	Nodule Detection	Convolutional Neural Networks (CNNs)	Increases detection sensitivity, finds subtle nodules missed by humans, reduces oversight.	(Ardila et al., 2019)
	Nodule Characterization & Risk Stratification	Radiomics, Deep Learning	Analyzes nodule features (size, texture, growth) to predict malignancy risk, reducing false positives and unnecessary biopsies.	(Massion et al., 2022)
Pathology (Tissue Analysis)	Tumor Subtyping	CNNs on Whole-Slide Images (WSI)	Automatically classifies NSCLC subtypes (e.g., adenocarcinoma vs. squamous cell carcinoma) from H&E stains.	(Coudray et al., 2018)
	Biomarker Prediction	Deep Learning	Predicts genetic mutations (e.g., EGFR, ALK) and protein expression (PD-L1) from standard H&E slides, aiding treatment planning.	(Sha et al., 2023)
Data Integration & Prognostics	Outcome Prediction	Multimodal AI, Radiomics	Integrates imaging, pathology, genomic, and clinical data to predict patient survival, recurrence risk, and treatment response.	(Hosny et al., 2018)
Clinical Workflow	Workflow Prioritization	Deep Learning	Triages and prioritizes critical cases in a radiologist's worklist, ensuring urgent findings are reviewed quickly.	(Ramisetty et al., 2024)

8. CONCLUSION

Non-small cell lung cancer (NSCLC) is a prevalent cancer for the improved diagnostic methods for early detection, classification, and personalized treatments. Diagnostic methods have evolved from traditional imaging and histopathological strategies to advanced molecular characterization and the invasive approaches. Imaging modalities like CT, PET-CT, and MRI are crucial for initial tumor detection, localization, and staging, while low-dose CT is essential for high-risk populations. Final diagnosis relies on the tissue acquisition through biopsy methods like bronchoscopy, CT-guided needle biopsy, and surgical procedures like VATS. Next-generation sequencing and liquid biopsy have revolutionized NSCLC management by facilitating genomic profiling based on minimal tissue or blood. Biomarkers like PD-L1 expression are critical for predicting Immunotherapy responses and refining therapeutic applications. Major technologies like Biosensors and AI-driven radiomics offer potential for early detection, risk stratification, and personalized treatment strategies. Some challenges include tumor heterogeneity, sufficient tissue samples for multi-omic analysis, and standardization of diagnostics between the healthcare systems.

REFERENCES

Antonangelo, L., Sales, R. K., Corá, A. P., Acencio, M. M. P., Teixeira, L. R., & Vargas, F. S. (2015). Pleural fluid tumour markers in malignant pleural effusion with inconclusive cytologic results. *Current Oncology (Toronto, Ont.)*, *22*(5), e336. DOI: 10.3747/co.22.2563 PMID: 26628873

Ardila, D., Kiraly, A. P., Bharadwaj, S., Choi, B., Reicher, J. J., Peng, L., Tse, D., Etemadi, M., Ye, W., Corrado, G., Naidich, D. P., & Shetty, S. (2019). End-to-end lung cancer screening with three-dimensional deep learning on low-dose chest computed tomography. *Nature Medicine*, *25*(6), 954–961. DOI: 10.1038/s41591-019-0447-x PMID: 31110349

Brown, N. A., Aisner, D. L., & Oxnard, G. R. (2018). Precision medicine in non-small cell lung cancer: Current standards in pathology and biomarker interpretation. *American Society of Clinical Oncology Educational Book*, *38*(38), 708–715. DOI: 10.1200/EDBK_209089 PMID: 30231309

Coudray, N., Ocampo, P. S., Sakellaropoulos, T., Narula, N., Snuderl, M., Fenyö, D., Moreira, A. L., Razavian, N., & Tsirigos, A. (2018). Classification and mutation prediction from non-small cell lung cancer histopathology images using deep learning. *Nature Medicine*, *24*(10), 1559–1567. DOI: 10.1038/s41591-018-0177-5 PMID: 30224757

Garcia-Robledo, J. E., Rosell, R., Ruíz-Patiño, A., Sotelo, C., Arrieta, O., Zatarain-Barron, L., Ordonez, C., Jaller, E., Rojas, L., Russo, A., de Miguel-Pérez, D., Rolfo, C., & Cardona, A. F. (2022). KRAS and MET in non-small-cell lung cancer: Two of the new kids on the 'drivers' block. *Therapeutic Advances in Respiratory Disease*, *16*, 17534666211066064. DOI: 10.1177/17534666211066064 PMID: 35098800

Garg, P., Mohanty, A., Ramisetty, S., Kulkarni, P., Horne, D., Pisick, E., Salgia, R., & Singhal, S. S. (2023). Artificial intelligence and allied subsets in early detection and preclusion of gynecological cancers. *Biochimica et Biophysica Acta (BBA) -. Revisiones en Cáncer*, *1878*, 189026. PMID: 37980945

Ghose, S., Radhakrishnan, V., & Bhattacharya, S. (2019). Ethics of cancer care: Beyond biology and medicine. *Ecancermedicalscience*, *13*, 911. DOI: 10.3332/ecancer.2019.911 PMID: 31123494

Gomez, D., Tang, C., Zhang, J., Blumenschein, G. R., Hernandez, M., Lee, J. J., Ye, R., Camidge, D. R., Skoulidis, F., Doebele, R., Gaspar, L. E., Gibbons, D. L., Karam, J., Kavanagh, B. D., Palma, D. A., Louie, A. V., Tsao, A., Sepesi, B., Swisher, S. G., & Heymach, J. (2018). Local consolidative therapy (LCT) improves overall survival (OS) compared to maintenance therapy/observation in oligometastatic non-small cell lung cancer (NSCLC): Final results of a multicenter, randomized, controlled phase 2 trial. *International Journal of Radiation Oncology, Biology, Physics*, *102*(5), 1604. DOI: 10.1016/j.ijrobp.2018.08.050

Gomez, D. R., Blumenschein, G. R.Jr, Lee, J. J., Hernandez, M., Ye, R., Camidge, D. R., Doebele, R. C., Skoulidis, F., Gaspar, L. E., Gibbons, D. L., Karam, J. A., Kavanagh, B. D., Tang, C., Komaki, R., Louie, A. V., Palma, D. A., Tsao, A. S., Sepesi, B., William, W. N., & Heymach, J. V. (2016). Local consolidative therapy versus maintenance therapy or observation for patients with oligometastatic non-small-cell lung cancer without progression after first-line systemic therapy: A multicentre, randomised, controlled, phase 2 study. *The Lancet. Oncology*, *17*(12), 1672–1682. DOI: 10.1016/S1470-2045(16)30532-0 PMID: 27789196

Hubers, A. J., van der Drift, M. A., Prinsen, C. F., Witte, B. I., Wang, Y., Shivapurkar, N., Stastny, V., Bolijn, A. S., Hol, B. E., Feng, Z., Dekhuijzen, P. R., Gazdar, A. F., & Thunnissen, E. (2014). Methylation analysis in spontaneous sputum for lung cancer diagnosis. *Lung Cancer (Amsterdam, Netherlands)*, *84*(2), 127–133. DOI: 10.1016/j.lungcan.2014.01.019 PMID: 24598366

Huss, R. (2015). Biomarkers. In *Translational Regenerative Medicine* (pp. 235–241). Søreide, K. (2009). Receiver-operating characteristic curve analysis in diagnostic, prognostic and predictive biomarker research. *Journal of Clinical Pathology*, *62*(1), 1–5.

Johnson, K. B., Wei, W. Q., Weeraratne, D., Frisse, M. E., Misulis, K., Rhee, K., Zhao, J., & Snowdon, J. L. (2021). Precision medicine, AI, and the future of personalized health care. *Clinical and Translational Science*, *14*(1), 86–93. DOI: 10.1111/cts.12884 PMID: 32961010

Kalanjeri, S., & Gildea, T. R. (2016). Electromagnetic navigational bronchoscopy for peripheral pulmonary nodules. *Thoracic Surgery Clinics*, *26*(2), 203–213. DOI: 10.1016/j.thorsurg.2015.12.008 PMID: 27112259

Kanan, M., Alharbi, H., Alotaibi, N., Almasuood, L., Aljoaid, S., Alharbi, T., Albraik, L., Alothman, W., Aljohani, H., Alzahrani, A., Alqahtani, S., Kalantan, R., Althomali, R., Alameen, M., & Mufti, A. (2024). AI-driven models for diagnosing and predicting outcomes in lung cancer: A systematic review and meta-analysis. *Cancers (Basel)*, *16*(3), 674. DOI: 10.3390/cancers16030674 PMID: 38339425

Kaur, G., Nijhawan, R., Gupta, N., Singh, N., & Rajwanshi, A. (2017). Pleural fluid cytology samples in cases of suspected lung cancer: An experience from a tertiary care centre. *Diagnostic Cytopathology*, *45*(3), 195–201. DOI: 10.1002/dc.23659 PMID: 28112486

Kawaguchi, T., Koh, Y., Ando, M., Ito, N., Takeo, S., Adachi, H., Tagawa, T., Kakegawa, S., Yamashita, M., Kataoka, K., Ichinose, Y., Takeuchi, Y., Serizawa, M., Tamiya, A., Shimizu, S., Yoshimoto, N., Kubo, A., Isa, S., Saka, H., & Matsumura, A. (2016). Prospective analysis of oncogenic driver mutations and environmental factors: Japan molecular epidemiology for lung cancer study. *Journal of Clinical Oncology*, *34*(19), 2247–2257. DOI: 10.1200/JCO.2015.64.2322 PMID: 27161973

Kremer, R., Best, L. A., Savulescu, D., Gavish, M., & Nagler, R. M. (2010). Pleural fluid analysis of lung cancer vs benign inflammatory disease patients. *British Journal of Cancer*, *102*(7), 1180–1184. DOI: 10.1038/sj.bjc.6605607 PMID: 20216542

Lam, B., Lam, S. Y., Wong, M. P., Ooi, C. G., Fong, D. Y., Lam, D. C., Lai, A. Y., Tam, C. M., Pang, C. B., Ip, M. S., & Lam, W. K. (2009). Sputum cytology examination followed by autofluorescence bronchoscopy: A practical way of identifying early stage lung cancer in central airway. *Lung Cancer (Amsterdam, Netherlands)*, *64*(3), 289–294. DOI: 10.1016/j.lungcan.2008.09.016 PMID: 19010567

Lamprecht, B., Porsch, P., Wegleitner, B., Strasser, G., Kaiser, B., & Studnicka, M. (2012). Electromagnetic navigation bronchoscopy (ENB): Increasing diagnostic yield. *Respiratory Medicine*, *106*(5), 710–715. DOI: 10.1016/j.rmed.2012.02.002 PMID: 22391437

Lee, C. K., Brown, C., Gralla, R. J., Hirsh, V., Thongprasert, S., Tsai, C.-M., Tan, E. H., Ho, J. C.-M., Chu, D. T., Zaatar, A., Osorio Sanchez, J. A., Vu, V. V., Au, J. S. K., Inoue, A., Lee, S. M., Gebski, V., & Yang, J. C.-H. (2013). Impact of EGFR inhibitor in non-small cell lung cancer on progression-free and overall survival: A meta-analysis. *Journal of the National Cancer Institute*, *105*(9), 595–605. DOI: 10.1093/jnci/djt072 PMID: 23594426

Lee, C. K., Wu, Y.-L., Ding, P. N., Lord, S. J., Inoue, A., Zhou, C., Mitsudomi, T., Rosell, R., Pavlakis, N., Links, M., Gebski, V., Gralla, R. J., & Yang, J. C.-H. (2015). Impact of specific epidermal growth factor receptor (EGFR) mutations and clinical characteristics on outcomes after treatment with EGFR tyrosine kinase inhibitors versus chemotherapy in EGFR-mutant lung cancer: A meta-analysis. *Journal of Clinical Oncology*, *33*(17), 1958–1965. DOI: 10.1200/JCO.2014.58.1736 PMID: 25897154

Maemondo, M., Inoue, A., Kobayashi, K., Sugawara, S., Oizumi, S., Isobe, H., Gemma, A., Harada, M., Yoshizawa, H., Kinoshita, I., Fujita, Y., Okinaga, S., Hirano, H., Yoshimori, K., Harada, T., Ogura, T., Ando, M., Miyazawa, H., Tanaka, T., & Nukiwa, T. (2010). Gefitinib or chemotherapy for non-small-cell lung cancer with mutated EGFR. *The New England Journal of Medicine*, *362*(25), 2380–2388. DOI: 10.1056/NEJMoa0909530 PMID: 20573926

Massion, P. P., Antic, S., Ather, S., Arteta, C., Brabec, J., Chen, H., Declerck, J., Dufek, D., Hickes, W., Kadir, T., Kamen, A., Lam, S., van Ginneken, B., & Walker, P. (2022). Assessing the accuracy of a deep learning method to risk stratify indeterminate pulmonary nodules. *American Journal of Respiratory and Critical Care Medicine*, *206*(6), 699–708. PMID: 32326730

McWilliams, A., Shaipanich, T., & Lam, S. (2013). Fluorescence and navigational bronchoscopy. *Thoracic Surgery Clinics*, *23*(2), 153–161. DOI: 10.1016/j.thorsurg.2013.01.008 PMID: 23566967

Mitsudomi, T., Morita, S., Yatabe, Y., Negoro, S., Okamoto, I., Tsurutani, J., Seto, T., Satouchi, M., Tada, H., Hirashima, T., Asami, K., Katakami, N., Takada, M., Yoshioka, H., Shibata, K., Kudoh, S., Shimizu, E., Saito, H., Toyooka, S., & Fukuoka, M. (2010). Gefitinib versus cisplatin plus docetaxel in patients with non-small-cell lung cancer harbouring mutations of the epidermal growth factor receptor (WJTOG3405): An open label, randomised phase 3 trial. *The Lancet. Oncology*, *11*(2), 121–128. DOI: 10.1016/S1470-2045(09)70364-X PMID: 20022809

Mohanty, A., Nam, A., Srivastava, S., Jones, J., Lomenick, B., Singhal, S. S., Guo, L., Warden, C., Cho, H., & Li, A. (2023). Acquired resistance to KRAS G12C small molecule inhibition via genetic/non-genetic mechanisms in lung cancer. *Science Advances*, *9*(41), 3816. DOI: 10.1126/sciadv.ade3816 PMID: 37831779

Mok, T. S., Cheng, Y., Zhou, X., Lee, K. H., Nakagawa, K., Niho, S., Lee, M., Linke, R., Rosell, R., Corral, J., Migliorino, M. R., Pluzanski, A., Sbar, E. I., Wang, T., White, J. L., & Wu, Y.-L. (2018). Improvement in overall survival in a randomized study that compared dacomitinib with gefitinib in patients with advanced non-small-cell lung cancer and EGFR activating mutations. *Journal of Clinical Oncology*, *36*(22), 2244–2250. DOI: 10.1200/JCO.2018.78.7994 PMID: 29864379

Mok, T. S., Wu, Y.-L., Ahn, M.-J., Garassino, M. C., Kim, H. R., Ramalingam, S. S., Shepherd, F. A., He, Y., Akamatsu, H., Theelen, W. S. M. E., Lee, C. K., Sebastian, M., Templeton, A., Mann, H., Marotti, M., Ghiorghiu, S., & Papadimitrakopoulou, V. A. (2017). Osimertinib or platinum-pemetrexed in EGFR T790M–positive lung cancer. *The New England Journal of Medicine*, *376*(7), 629–640. DOI: 10.1056/NEJMoa1612674 PMID: 27959700

Patriquin, L., Merrick, D. T., Hill, D., Holcomb, R. G., Lemieux, M. E., Bennett, G., Karia, B., Rebel, V. I., & Bauer, T.II. (2015). Early detection of lung cancer with meso tetra (4-carboxyphenyl) porphyrin-labeled sputum. *Journal of Thoracic Oncology, 10*(9), 1311–1318. DOI: 10.1097/JTO.0000000000000627 PMID: 26200451

Potti, A., Mukherjee, S., Petersen, R., Dressman, H. K., Bild, A., Koontz, J., Kratzke, R., Watson, M. A., Kelley, M., Ginsburg, G. S., West, M., Harpole, D. H.Jr, & Nevins, J. R. (2006). A genomic strategy to refine prognosis in early-stage non–small-cell lung cancer. *The New England Journal of Medicine, 355*(6), 570–580. DOI: 10.1056/NEJMoa060467 PMID: 16899777

Ramisetty, S. R., Subbalakshmi, A. R., Pareek, S., Achuthan, S., Bhattacharya, S., Mohanty, A., Singhal, S. S., Salgia, R., & Kulkarni, P. (2024). Leveraging cancer phenotypic plasticity for novel treatment strategies. *Journal of Clinical Medicine, 13*(11), 3337. DOI: 10.3390/jcm13113337 PMID: 38893049

Ringborg, U., von Braun, J., Celis, J., Baumann, M., Berns, A., Eggermont, A., Heard, E., Heitor, M., Chandy, M., & Chen, C.-J. (2024). Strategies to decrease inequalities in cancer therapeutics, care and prevention: Proceedings on a conference organized by the Pontifical Academy of Sciences and the European Academy of Cancer Sciences, Vatican City, 2023. *Molecular Oncology, 18*, 245–279. DOI: 10.1002/1878-0261.13575 PMID: 38135904

Rosell, R., Carcereny, E., Gervais, R., Vergnenegre, A., Massuti, B., Felip, E., Palmero, R., Garcia-Gomez, R., Pallares, C., Sanchez, J. M., Porta, R., Cobo, M., Garrido, P., Longo, F., Moran, T., Insa, A., De Marinis, F., Corre, R., Bover, I., & Paz-Ares, L. (2012). Erlotinib versus standard chemotherapy as first-line treatment for European patients with advanced EGFR mutation-positive non-small-cell lung cancer (EURTAC): A multicentre, open-label, randomised phase 3 trial. *The Lancet. Oncology, 13*(3), 239–246. DOI: 10.1016/S1470-2045(11)70393-X PMID: 22285168

Seetharamu, N., Budman, D. R., & Sullivan, K. M. (2016). Immune checkpoint inhibitors in lung cancer: Past, present and future. *Future Oncology (London, England), 12*(9), 1151–1163. DOI: 10.2217/fon.16.20 PMID: 27019997

Sequist, L. V., Yang, J. C.-H., Yamamoto, N., O'Byrne, K., Hirsh, V., Mok, T., Geater, S. L., Orlov, S., Tsai, C.-M., Boyer, M., Su, W.-C., Bennouna, J., Kato, T., Gorbunova, V., Lee, K. H., Shah, R., Massey, D., Zazulina, V., Shahidi, M., & Schuler, M. (2013). Phase III study of afatinib or cisplatin plus pemetrexed in patients with metastatic lung adenocarcinoma with EGFR mutations. *Journal of Clinical Oncology, 31*(27), 3327–3334. DOI: 10.1200/JCO.2012.44.2806 PMID: 23816960

Sha, L., Osinski, B. L., Ho, I. Y., Tan, T. L., Willis, C., Weiss, H., Beaubier, N. T., & Mahon, B. M. (2023). Multi-field-of-view deep learning model predicts nonsmall cell lung cancer programmed death-ligand 1 status from whole-slide hematoxylin and eosin images. *Journal of Pathology Informatics*, *14*, 100318. PMID: 31523482

Shi, Y., Au, J. S.-K., Thongprasert, S., Srinivasan, S., Tsai, C.-M., Khoa, M. T., Heeroma, K., Itoh, Y., Cornelio, G., & Yang, P.-C. (2014). A prospective, molecular epidemiology study of EGFR mutations in Asian patients with advanced non-small-cell lung cancer of adenocarcinoma histology (PIONEER). *Journal of Thoracic Oncology*, *9*(2), 154–162. DOI: 10.1097/JTO.0000000000000033 PMID: 24419411

Singh, T., Hassanabad, M. F., & Hassanabad, A. F. (2021). Non-small cell lung cancer: Emerging molecular targeted and immunotherapeutic agents. *Biochimica et Biophysica Acta (BBA) -. Revisiones en Cáncer*, *1876*, 188636. PMID: 34655692

Soria, J.-C., Ohe, Y., Vansteenkiste, J., Reungwetwattana, T., Chewaskulyong, B., Lee, K. H., Dechaphunkul, A., Imamura, F., Nogami, N., Kurata, T., Okamoto, I., Zhou, C., Cho, B. C., Cheng, Y., Cho, E. K., Voon, P. J., Planchard, D., Su, W.-C., Gray, J. E., & Ramalingam, S. S. (2018). Osimertinib in untreated EGFR-mutated advanced non-small-cell lung cancer. *The New England Journal of Medicine*, *378*(2), 113–125. DOI: 10.1056/NEJMoa1713137 PMID: 29151359

Strimbu, K., & Tavel, J. A. (2010). What are biomarkers? *Current Opinion in HIV and AIDS*, *5*(6), 463–466. DOI: 10.1097/COH.0b013e32833ed177 PMID: 20978388

Uke, M. S., Pathuthara, S., Shaikh, A., Kumar, R., & Kane, S. (2017). Is the morning sputum sample superior to the fresh sputum sample for the detection of malignant cells? *Acta Cytologica*, *61*(3), 223–229. DOI: 10.1159/000475455 PMID: 28535501

Villalobos, P., & Wistuba, I. I. (2017). Lung cancer biomarkers. *Hematology/Oncology Clinics of North America*, *31*(1), 13–29. DOI: 10.1016/j.hoc.2016.08.006 PMID: 27912828

Wang, F., Xia, T., Li, Z., Gao, X., & Fang, X. (2023). Current status of clinical trial research and application of immune checkpoint inhibitors for non-small cell lung cancer. *Frontiers in Oncology*, *13*, 1213297. DOI: 10.3389/fonc.2023.1213297 PMID: 37727216

Wu, Y.-L., Cheng, Y., Zhou, X., Lee, K. H., Nakagawa, K., Niho, S., Tsuji, F., Linke, R., Rosell, R., Corral, J., Migliorino, M. R., Pluzanski, A., Sbar, E. I., Wang, T., White, J. L., Nadanaciva, S., Sandin, R., & Mok, T. S. (2017). Dacomitinib versus gefitinib as first-line treatment for patients with EGFR-mutation-positive non-small-cell lung cancer (ARCHER 1050): A randomised, open-label, phase 3 trial. *The Lancet. Oncology*, *18*(11), 1454–1466. DOI: 10.1016/S1470-2045(17)30608-3 PMID: 28958502

Wu, Y.-L., Zhou, C., Hu, C.-P., Feng, J., Lu, S., Huang, Y., Li, W., Hou, M., Shi, J. H., Lee, K. Y., Xu, C.-R., Massey, D., Kim, M., Shi, Y., & Geater, S. L. (2014). Afatinib versus cisplatin plus gemcitabine for first-line treatment of Asian patients with advanced non-small-cell lung cancer harbouring EGFR mutations (LUX-Lung 6): An open-label, randomised phase 3 trial. *The Lancet. Oncology*, *15*(2), 213–222. DOI: 10.1016/S1470-2045(13)70604-1 PMID: 24439929

Xie, S., Huang, G., Qian, W., Wang, X., Zhang, H., Li, Z., Liu, Y., Wang, Y., & Yu, H. (2023). Integrated analysis reveals the microenvironment of non-small cell lung cancer and a macrophage-related prognostic model. *Translational Lung Cancer Research*, *12*(2), 277–294. DOI: 10.21037/tlcr-22-866 PMID: 36895934

Yang, J., Yang, W., Zhang, J., Huang, A., Yin, S., Zhang, H., Luo, Z., Li, X., Chen, Y., Ma, L., & Wang, C. (2024). Non-small cell lung cancer and metabolism research from 2013 to 2023: A visual analysis and bibliometric study. *Frontiers in Oncology*, *14*, 1322090. DOI: 10.3389/fonc.2024.1322090 PMID: 38863621

Yuan, M., Huang, L. L., Chen, J. H., Wu, J., & Xu, Q. (2019). The emerging treatment landscape of targeted therapy in non-small-cell lung cancer. *Signal Transduction and Targeted Therapy*, *4*(1), 61. DOI: 10.1038/s41392-019-0099-9 PMID: 31871778

Zare, M., Mostafaei, S., Ahmadi, A., Jamalkandi, S. A., Abedini, A., Monfared, Z. E., Dorostkar, R., & Saadati, M. (2018). Human endogenous retrovirus env genes: Potential blood biomarkers in lung cancer. *Microbial Pathogenesis*, *115*, 189–193. DOI: 10.1016/j.micpath.2017.12.040 PMID: 29274460

Zhou, C., Wu, Y.-L., Chen, G., Feng, J., Liu, X.-Q., Wang, C., Zhang, S., Wang, J., Zhou, S., Ren, S., Lu, S., Zhang, L., Hu, C., Hu, C., Luo, Y., Chen, L., Ye, M., Huang, J., Zhi, X., & You, C. (2011). Erlotinib versus chemotherapy as first-line treatment for patients with advanced EGFR mutation-positive non-small-cell lung cancer (OPTIMAL, CTONG-0802): A multicentre, open-label, randomised, phase 3 study. *The Lancet. Oncology*, *12*(8), 735–742. DOI: 10.1016/S1470-2045(11)70184-X PMID: 21783417

Chapter 6

CAR-T Cell Therapy: Effectiveness and Limitations against NSCLC - Evaluating CAR-T Cell Therapy Outcomes

Prerna Mehta
https://orcid.org/0009-0003-1300-588X
G.D. Rungta College of Science and Technology, Bhilai, India

ABSTRACT

There is rising interest in CAR-T therapy as a potential treatment of non-small cell lung cancer (NSCLC) that comprises about 85% of all lung cancer and has a high mortality rate. This is a new technology whereby T cells are engineered to attack certain tumor-specific antigens. However, it tends to be undermined by other factors (i.e., the immunosuppressive tumor microenvironment and antigen heterogeneity). More recent data have found epidermal growth factor receptor (EGFR) and mesothelin as future targets of CAR-T therapy. The development of cars such as dual-targeting CAR improves the efficiency of treatment. However, there also exist some challenges such as safety concerns such as cytokine release syndrome (CRS). To overcome immunosuppressive barriers, CAR-T/immune checkpoint combination therapy can be used as an added advantage. Further research on new CAR-T regimens and trials is needed to improve patient treatment outcomes and survival in patients with NSCLC, a complex and advanced disease.

1. INTRODUCTION

Chimeric Antigen Receptor T-cell (CAR-T) therapy is a modern and unique method in cancer treatment that uses the body's own immune system as weapon

DOI: 10.4018/979-8-3373-2096-0.ch006

against cancer cells. This therapy is based on the manipulation of a patient's T cells to produce receptors that have ability to identify tumor-associated antigens (De Marco et al., 2023). There intervention process involves isolation of T cells from the patients through apheresis followed by genetic modification through insertion of the CAR gene by viral vectors (Jogalekar et al., 2022). The CAR is made up of an antigen-binding domain, a transmembrane domain, and a signaling domain of T cell receptor associated with CD3ζ molecules (Lindner et al., 2020) (**Figure 1**). New developments have incorporated co-stimulatory domains such as CD28 or 4-1BB which increase T cell activation and survival within the body.CAR- T therapy has shown exceptional success in the management of hematologic malignancies (Bui et al., 2024).

In NSCLC, tumor-associated immune cells including regulatory T cells, myeloid-derived suppressor cells, and the expression of cytokines including TGF-β, can directly affect the function of CAR-T cells.Moreover, the enzymatic activity of this specific microenvironment, such as IDO and arginase I,can also hinder the activity of T cells (He et al., 2023). To overcome these difficulties, new strategies, like the development of 'armored' CAR-T-cells that secrete cytokines that can alter the tumor environment in a favourable manner for T, are being investigated. Other targeting mechanisms are also in development to address the antigen heterogeneity within tumors is currently also tested to cure antigen heterogeneity within the tumor. Experience from the ongoing clinical trials analyzing these novel treatment methods is currently increasingly understanding and realization of the need to combine therapies utilizing CAR-T with traditional treatments and check point inhibitors for the improvement of outcomes when used in NSCLC and therefore increasing the overall effectiveness of this promising immunotherapeutic approach (M. Huang et al., 2020).

Figure 1. Chimeric Antigen Receptor

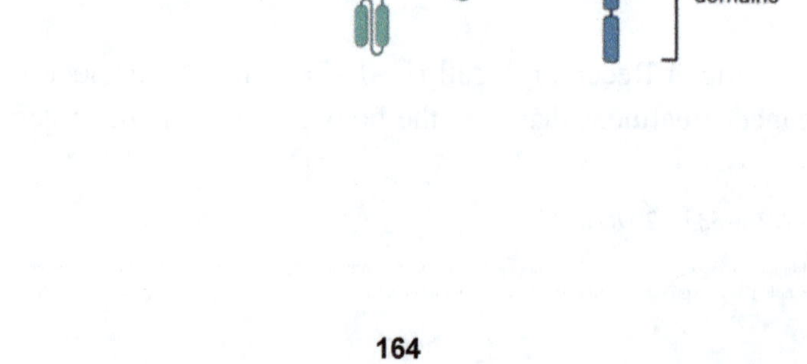

1.1 Overview of CAR-T Cell Therapy

The immunotherapy treatment that is referred to as Chimeric Antigen Receptor T-cell (CAR-T) and has become exceptional in treatment of cancer by using modified T cells to identify and destroy cancer cells (Choudhery et al., 2024). This process starts with the isolation of T cells from the patient which are further engineering to contain CARs that have specificity for certain tumor-associated antigens. CAR-T therapy has been highly successful in treating hematological malignancies with special reference to CD19 positive and has demonstrated lack of efficacy in solid tumour such as NSCLC due to problems such as Genetic variation of the tumour, low density of antigen expression and immune suppressive environment of the tumour packed with T regulatory cells and myeloid derived suppressor cells (Mohanty et al., 2019).

To address these issues, the following measures have been made by researchers as follows; Other advancement are; development of the CAR-T cell with an armored structure that can release cytokines to change tumor microenvironment in a way that enhances the functionality of CAR-T cells. The construction of CARs is changing as well, including co-stimulatory domains that increase further T-cell activation and survival. Furthermore, more work is directed toward second target CAR strategies to avoid tumour heterogeneity and understanding the interaction of CAR T with the other treatments like the checkpoint inhibitors. These are important in order to broaden the indications of CAR-T therapy from Hematological malignancies to multiple types of solid tumors (Rakhshandehroo et al., 2024).

1.2 Significance of NSCLC in Oncology

The importance of NSCLC in oncology is primary because of its prevalence, second there are numerous molecular subtypes, third there are new targeted and immunotherapy options for treatment, fourth there is constant focus on more accurate diagnostic tools, methods of prevention and improved existing treatment (Araghi et al., 2023). Finally, in **Table 1**, information about molecular subclasses, enzymes involved, and targeted therapies, immunooncology, and ongoing trials is presented.

Table 1. Overview of Non-Small Cell Lung Cancer (NSCLC): Key Features and Treatments

Aspect	Details	Molecular Targets	Enzymes and Pathways	Examples	Reference
Prevalence	NSCLC constitutes approximately 84% of lung cancer cases and is a leading cause of cancer death globally.			Significant burden on healthcare systems worldwide.	(C. Li et al., 2023)
Molecular Subtypes	NSCLC is classified into three main subtypes: adenocarcinoma, squamous cell carcinoma, and large cell carcinoma.			Subtype classification guides treatment approaches.	(Niemira et al., 2019)
Genetic Mutations	Common mutations include epidermal growth factor receptor (EGFR), anaplastic lymphoma kinase (ALK), Kirsten rat sarcoma viral oncogene homolog (KRAS), ROS proto-oncogene 1 (ROS1), and B-Raf proto-oncogene (BRAF).	EGFR, ALK, KRAS, ROS1		EGFR mutations are prevalent in adenocarcinomas; KRAS mutations are common in smokers.	(Colombino et al., 2019)
Targeted Therapy	Development of targeted therapies has revolutionized treatment for mutations identified in NSCLC.	ALK, EGFR, ROS1		Drug examples include osimertinib (EGFR), crizotinib (ALK), and entrectinib (ROS1).	(Guo et al., 2022)

continued on following page

Table 1. Continued

Aspect	Details	Molecular Targets	Enzymes and Pathways	Examples	Reference
Immunotherapy	Immune checkpoint inhibitors have significantly improved treatment outcomes for many NSCLC patients.	PD-1 (Programmed cell death protein 1), PD-L1 (Programmed death-ligand 1), CTLA-4 (Cytotoxic T-lymphocyte-associated protein 4)		Pembrolizumab (Keytruda) and nivolumab (Opdivo) have changed therapeutic landscapes for high PD-L1 tumors.	(Wojtukiewicz et al., 2021)
Biomarker Research	Biomarkers such as PD-L1 expression levels, tumor mutational burden (TMB), and circulating tumor DNA (ctDNA) are critical for personalized treatment.	PD-L1, TMB		The use of PD-L1 expression to determine eligibility for immune checkpoint inhibitors like pembrolizumab.	(Yarchoan et al., 2019)
Early Detection	Low-dose computed tomography (CT) scans have been shown to reduce mortality rates by enabling earlier diagnosis.			The National Lung Screening Trial (NLST) and NELSON trials show a 20% reduction in lung cancer deaths through screening.	(Lancaster et al., 2022)
Combination Strategies	Combining targeted therapies with immunotherapies or chemotherapy offers potential for enhanced efficacy.	Various targets	Various pathways depending on involved agents (e.g., chemotherapy affects DNA repair pathways).		(Yu et al., 2022)
Emerging Treatments	Novel approaches include next-generation sequencing (NGS) for detecting mutations and gene fusions.	NTRK (Neurotrophic tyrosine receptor kinase), BRAF	NTRK pathway: Promotes cell survival and proliferation.		(Hechtman, 2022)

continued on following page

Table 1. Continued

Aspect	Details	Molecular Targets	Enzymes and Pathways	Examples	Reference
Health Disparities	NSCLC illustrates significant disparities in outcomes based on race, socioeconomic status, and geographic factors.			Programs targeting underserved populations aim to reduce access barriers and improve outcomes.	(Sosa et al., 2021)
Clinical Trials	Ongoing clinical trials continue to explore new therapeutic combinations, novel agents, and approaches to personalized therapy.	Various targets		Examples include trials for new immunotherapies, CAR-T cell therapies, and combination drug regimens.	(Wang et al., 2023)

Abbreviations

- **NSCLC**: Non-Small Cell Lung Cancer
- **EGFR**: Epidermal Growth Factor Receptor
- **ALK**: Anaplastic Lymphoma Kinase
- **KRAS**: Kirsten Rat Sarcoma Viral Oncogene Homolog
- **ROS1**: ROS Proto-Oncogene 1
- **BRAF**: B-Raf Proto-Oncogene
- **PI3K**: Phosphoinositide 3-Kinase
- **AKT**: AKT Proto-Oncogene
- **TMB**: Tumor Mutational Burden
- **ctDNA**: Circulating Tumor DNA
- **PD-1**: Programmed Cell Death Protein 1
- **PD-L1**: Programmed Death-Ligand 1
- **CTLA-4**: Cytotoxic T-Lymphocyte-Associated Protein 4
- **CTL**: Cytotoxic T Lymphocyte
- **NLST**: National Lung Screening Trial
- **NGS**: Next-Generation Sequencing
- **NTRK**: Neurotrophic Tyrosine Receptor Kinase

2. MECHANISMS OF CAR-T CELL THERAPY

Chimeric Antigen Receptor T-cell (CAR-T) therapy marks a new era of cancer treatment especially in the setting of hematologic malignancies and now growing solid tumors like NSCLC. CAR-T therapy works based on the activating T cells from a patient and modifying them to express new receptors called chimeric antigen receptors that are able to identify and secure in a targeted manner the encompassing antigens of cancer cells (Xia et al., 2017). This sort of treatment strategy has focused on improving immune response against malignancies, and has yielded major improvements in treatment outcomes.The following are the ideas that need to be introduced: Genetic Modification and CAR DesignR-T) therapy represents a paradigm shift in cancer treatment, particularly in the context of hematologic malignancies and emerging solid tumors like non-small cell lung cancer (NSCLC) (Liu et al., 2024). The core mechanism underlying CAR-T therapy involves engineering a patient's own T cells to express chimeric antigen receptors that specifically recognize and bind to antigens present on cancer cells. This targeted approach aims to enhance the immune response against malignancies and has led to significant advancements in treatment efficacy.

- Genetic Modification and CAR Design

CAR-T therapy consists of three major steps and the first step is collection of patient's peripheral blood T cells. These cells are then genetically modified using viral vectors including lentivirus or retrovirus to incorporate sequences encoding for chimeric antigen receptors. A typical CAR consists of three main components: An extracellular antigen-binding domain – this can be most often derived from the constant regions of antibodies, a transmembrane domain and an intracellular signaling domain (Ayala Ceja et al., 2024).

Seemingly, the newer CAR constructs have developed newer forms that improve their attractiveness, specificity and effectiveness. Several novel types and designs of CARs have been developed, which are however worthy of more discussion. These constructs allow T cells to engender multiple antigens at the same time, solving the problem of tumor heterogeneity and antigen escape (Zheng et al., 2023). Thus, the application of targets such as CD19 and CD22 has been effective in B-cell malignancies, although similar strategies for solid tumor types are currently investigating targets located within the tu-mor microenvironment.Co-stimulatory signaling domains and footprint were predominantly discovered in the PDZ domain-containing proteins.(CAR-T) therapy represents a paradigm shift in cancer treatment, particularly in the context of hematologic malignancies and emerging solid tumors like non-small cell lung cancer (NSCLC). The core mechanism underlying CAR-T therapy involves engineering a patient's own T cells to express chimeric antigen receptors that specifically recognize and bind to antigens present on cancer cells. This targeted approach aims to enhance the immune response against malignancies and has led to significant advancements in treatment efficacy (Lu et al., 2021).

Figure 2. CAR T Therapy for CD19+ Cancer Cells

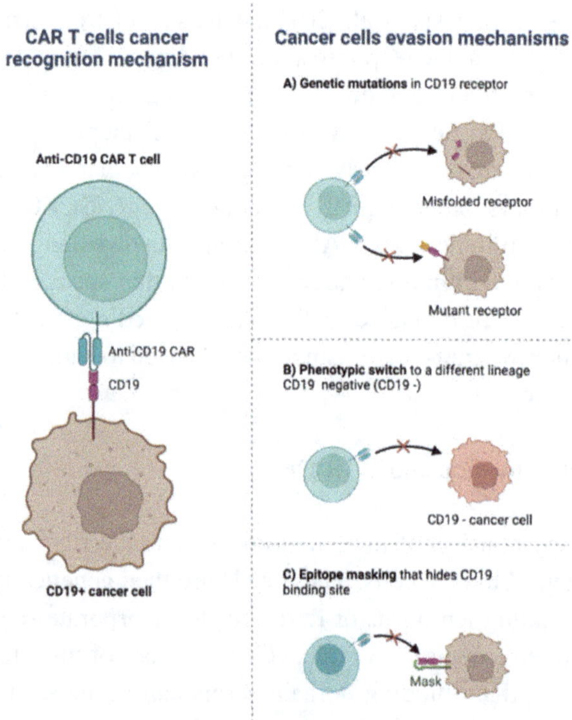

- Genetic Modification and CAR Design

The initial phase of CAR-T therapy involves the extraction of peripheral blood T cells from the patient. These cells are then genetically modified using viral vectors, such as lentivirus or retrovirus, to introduce sequences coding for chimeric antigen receptors. A typical CAR consists of three main components: an extracellular antigen-binding domain (usually derived from antibodies), a transmembrane domain, and an intracellular signaling domain (Lana & Strauss, 2020).

Recent innovations in CAR design have introduced novel constructs that enhance their specificity and efficacy. Dual-target and tandem CARs are particularly noteworthy advancements. These constructs enable T cells to recognize and bind multiple antigens simultaneously, addressing tumor heterogeneity and the potential for cancer cells to evade immune detection through antigen loss. For instance, incorporating targets like CD19 and CD22 has shown promise in B-cell malignancies, while similar strategies are being explored for solid tumors with targets identified within the tumor microenvironment (Moreno et al., 2022).

- Co-stimulatory Signaling Domains

The intracellular signalling motifs in CARs are important for T cell activation, expansion and survival. Originally the CD3ζ domain was the main part of CAR constructs, whereas at present other co-stimulatory domains are incorporated quite often (Honikel & Olejniczak, 2022). Notable examples include:

Chimeric Antigen Receptor T-cell (CAR-T) therapy marks a new era of cancer treatment especially in the setting of hematologic malignancies and now growing solid tumors like NSCLC. The basic principle of CAR-T therapy is to genetically redirect a patient's T cells for the expression of chimeric antigen receptors that selectively target cancer cell antigens. This sort of treatment strategy has focused on improving immune response against malignancies, and has yielded major improvements in treatment outcomes.The following are the ideas that need to be introduced: Genetic Modification and CAR DesignR-T) therapy represents a paradigm shift in cancer treatment, particularly in the context of hematologic malignancies and emerging solid tumors like non-small cell lung cancer (NSCLC). The core mechanism underlying CAR-T therapy involves engineering a patient's own T cells to express chimeric antigen receptors that specifically recognize and bind to antigens present on cancer cells. This targeted approach aims to enhance the immune response against malignancies and has led to significant advancements in treatment efficacy (Daei Sorkhabi et al., 2023).

- Genetic Modification and CAR Design

CAR-T therapy consists of three major steps and the first step is collection of patient's peripheral blood T cells. These cells are then tranfected using, for example, lentivirus or retrovirus to express sequences forming chimeric antigen receptors. A typical CAR consists of three main components: An extracellular antigen-binding domain – this can be most often derived from the constant regions of antibodies, a transmembrane domain and an intracellular signaling domain (Song et al., 2024).

Seemingly, the newer CAR constructs have developed newer forms that improve their attractiveness, specificity and effectiveness. Several novel types and designs of CARs have been developed, which are however worthy of more discussion. These constructs allow T cells to engender multiple antigens at the same time, solving the problem of tumor heterogeneity and antigen escape. Thus, the application of targets such as CD19 and CD22 has been effective in B-cell malignancies, although similar strategies for solid tumor types are currently investigating targets located within the tu-mor microenvironment.Co-stimulatory signaling domains and footprint were predominantly discovered in the PDZ domain-containing proteins.(CAR-T) therapy represents a paradigm shift in cancer treatment, particularly in the context of hematologic malignancies and emerging solid tumors like non-small cell lung cancer (NSCLC). The core mechanism underlying CAR-T therapy involves engineering a patient's own T cells to express chimeric antigen receptors that specifically recognize and bind to antigens present on cancer cells. This targeted approach aims to enhance the immune response against malignancies and has led to significant advancements in treatment efficacy (Colina et al., 2024).

- Genetic Modification and CAR Design

The initial phase of CAR-T therapy involves the extraction of peripheral blood T cells from the patient. These cells are then genetically modified using viral vectors, such as lentivirus or retrovirus, to introduce sequences coding for chimeric antigen receptors. A typical CAR consists of three main components: an extracellular antigen-binding domain (usually derived from antibodies), a transmembrane domain, and an intracellular signaling domain (Bulcha et al., 2021).

Recent innovations in CAR design have introduced novel constructs that enhance their specificity and efficacy. Dual-target and tandem CARs are particularly noteworthy advancements. These constructs enable T cells to recognize and bind multiple antigens simultaneously, addressing tumor heterogeneity and the potential for cancer cells to evade immune detection through antigen loss. For instance, incorporating targets like CD19 and CD22 has shown promise in B-cell malignancies, while similar strategies are being explored for solid tumors with targets identified within the tumor microenvironment (Milone et al., 2021).

- Co-stimulatory Signaling Domains

The intracellular signalling motifs in CARs are important for T cell activation, expansion and survival. Originally the CD3ζ domain was the main part of CAR constructs, whereas at present other co-stimulatory domains are incorporated quite often. Notable examples include:

FAP is also detected at high levels in many solid tumours and occupies the role of the tumor stroma; therefore, FAP is considered an optimal target for CAR-T approaches. Likewise, engaging immune checkpoints might bypass the immunosuppressive tumor-associated environment and restore T cell activity in the tumor (Castellanos-Rueda et al., 2022).

The treatment for the tumor microenvironment, comprising traits such as hypoxic environment and high immunosuppressive cytokines, affects the applicability of CAR-T therapy. Experts are currently probing such issues and choosing those antigens that stimulate a vigorous response even in such adverse conditions.

- Metabolic Considerations

There is still a lack of comprehensive knowledge about different metabolic requirements that CAR-T cells need to maintain high activity in the tumor environment. The Warburg effect which is characteristic of CAR-T cells entails enhancement of glycolysis as a leading metabolic path depending on meaningful enzymes such as HK2 and PKM2. This metabolic remodeling sustains the ATP demand required for cell activation and proliferation as well as for inflammation production (Lim et al., 2020).

Metabolic adaptation is also considered as one of the strategies intended to improve CAR-T cell stability and efficacy. Exploring mechanisms, which can stimulate biogenesis of mitochondria or oxidative phosphorylation, can result in more CAR-T cell survival and less exhaustion in the aggressive tumor micro-environment. Attempts at metabolic manipulations, the use of agents that increase glycolytic rate or decrease oxidative damages are still being considered to add on CAR-T effectiveness as well as survival (Nanjireddy et al., 2023).

Albeit the current progression of CAR-T cell therapy has many promising strategic designs and revolutionary safety strategies, improvements in the design and understanding of tumor biology and T cell metabolism could significantly change the future of cancer treatment. Thus, further development of new antigen targets and CAR-T therapy approaches are considerable and may help to control and eventually eliminate cancer, creation a personal immunotherapy for each patient based on the solid understanding of the nature of their disease (Uscanga-Palomeque et al., 2023).

2.1 Design and Engineering of CAR-T Cells

The advancements within the previous years have made an effort to increase the target identification of CAR-T cells, justify their safety, and enhance their functionality. Some notable innovations include:

- Dual-Target CARs: In order to improve the specificity and minimize the chance of tumor escape, the second generation of CARs known as dual-target CARs that targeting two distinct antigens at the same time has been designed.

This approach might enhance the treatment yields because CAR-T cells will be able to recognize the tumors that may shed one of the target antigens (Lin et al., 2024).

- Armored CAR-T Cells: These are genetically modified to release immune-modulating cytokines including the IL-15 or IL-12 upon recognition of antigen. New research demonstrates that armored CAR-T cells can improve the local immune environment and facilitate anti-tumor effects against resistant cancer states.
- iPSC-Derived CAR-T Cells: The sources of CAR-T cells are being researched for future use, including induced pluripotent stem cells (iPSCs) because of their ability to proliferate indefinitely and the fact that the cells can be designed to be used 'off the shelf'.This approach has a solution to scarcities in patient-specific CAR-T cell production, thereby lowering costs (Fang et al., 2025).
- CRISPR/Cas9 Gene Editing:This technology enables the editing of the T cell's genome to delete some genes that may hinder T cell function or increase toxicityBy for instance, deleting the PD-1 gene that codes for a checkpoint inhibitor was revealed to improve CAR-T cell survival and functionality in mice models.
- Synthetic Notch Receptors (synNotch):Rising as a way to develop CARs in the form of tumor-associated antigens,synNotch receptors enable the targeted stimulation of CAR-T cells;this enhances T cell control since they only respond to certain signals from tumors.
- Microbiome Influence on CAR-T Cell Efficacy:Some currently published studies point to the potential of how gut microbiota may affect CAR-T treatment outcomes.Specific types of bacteria have been linked to improved respon ses to the treatment,which in turn has fuelled further research on trying to manipulate microbiota as a way to improving CAR-T therapy outcomes (Charrot & Hallam, 2019).

2.2 Target Antigens in NSCLC

- In the context of NSCLC, several novel target antigens and strategies are being investigated, reflecting recent discoveries in tumor biology:
- • Neoantigens: The concept of neoantigen-based customized CAR-T treatment is emerging and attractive. The more developed tools of sequencing provide a chance to discover specific neoantigens for targeted therapy in a concrete patient. New data indicate that neoantigen-targeting CARs can trigger strong antitumor effects.

- • KRAS Mutations: KRAS is mutated in NSCLC and KRAS G12C is currently being targeted with an attempt to develop CAR-T cells. Knowledge regarding certain epitopes of a certain mutant KRAS may inform development of therapies that target the alterations that occur in this frequent oncogenic event.
- • Tumor-Associated Glycoproteins: These are glycosylated antigens that are sometimes shown to be overexpressed on the cancer cells. Ab targeting glycoproteins like MUC1 or CA-125 which can be overexpressed in NSCLC, maybe of additional utility for CAR-T strategies, as glycoproteins are likely more tumor specific than conventional cartel targets.
- • HLA Class I-Restricted Antigens: The investigation of restricted HLA class I T cell responses directed only at particular antigens is essential for NSCLC. Recognizing and lysis of cancer cells may be enhanced if the targets are tumor-specific antigens presented by HLA class I molecules.
- • NKG2D Ligands: The binding of the NKG2D receptor expressed on T cells to its targets (MICA/B) is also being investigated in terms of CAR-T targeting.... Tumor cells uniformly express ligands for NKG2D and therefore activating this receptor in CAR-T cells will improve their activation and anti-tumor responses.
- • Customized CARs Against Mesenchymal Stem Cell-Derived Pathways: Recent evidence suggests the molecular processes, which mesenchymal stem cells (MSCs) in the context of the tumor microenvironment initiate, can contribute to tumor progression. Such pathways can then be targeted in the hope of diminishing the backing that such cells offer the tumor and processes of metastasis.
- Utilization of Bispecific T Cell Engager (BiTE) Technology: BiTEs with the ability to engage both CD3 on T cells and particular antigens on NSCLC cells and thereby attract CAR-T cells to their proximity are contemplated. This approach can improve the CAR-T therapy when the conventional CAR designs are under difficulties (Xie et al., 2023).

CAR-T cell engineering and other new targets in NSCLC are the recent examples of the dynamic development of cancer therapy based on new achievements and technologies in oncology research. The above mentioned novel targets and promising approaches should be investigated in more clinical trials in treating NSCLC and possibly other cancers.

3. EFFECTIVENESS OF CAR-T THERAPY IN NSCLC

Due to the development of new clinical strategies, as well as discovering further potential targets for treatment, CAR-T therapy in NSCLC has been under profound improvement. With particular emphasis on different tumor antigens such as HER2, mesothelin, and KRAS G12C recent trials have demonstrated moderate response rates among patients with such mutations or protein production. Furthermore, combining immune checkpoint inhibitors together with CAR-T therapies is improving the therapeutic effect because immunosuppressive TME hallmark of NSCLC is counteracted. The use of superior strategies like CAR-T cell engineering involving the integration of factors that enhance the existence of the T cell including the IL-15 is being adopted to control the T cell poor persistence. In addition, the identification of the predictive biomarkers, such as TMB and specific ICI expressions, enables a better patient selection because such treatments should bring clinical benefit with minimal toxicity to the patients. These multitudinal efforts have marked a shift in strategy in using CAR-T cell therapy for NSCLC, with accumulating data of better survival rates and prominent durability across several patient populations (Ma et al., 2023).

3.1 Clinical Trials and Outcomes

New developments in CAR-T cell therapy are opening the door to innovation in the treatment of non-small cell lung cancer (NSCLC). There are even a number of clinical trials in progress on different targets and approaches to increase therapeutic efficacy. One of the most studied of these is HER2, which is an overexpressed protein in some NSCLC tumors, typically of breast cancer. Phase I preclinical evidence of HER2-targeted CAR-T cell therapy in patients with advanced NSCLC HER2-targeted CAR-T cell therapy has shown objective response rates of 30-40% based on initial clinical data. This information shows that CAR-T cells may, in fact, be used as a target in treating HER2 which has already shown promising results which need to be explored. A less specific CAR switchable system that could be used to improve safety profiles have also been developed (Dey et al., 2023).

Mesothelin is another potential target since it is overexpressed in most tumors, including NSCLC. Preclinical trials of mesothelin-targeted CAR-T therapy have shown complete to partial response in a small group of patients. These data prove the hypothesis that the expression of mesothelin has something to do with the prognosis, which is able to raise the probability of the patient surviving in long-term after the treatment (Zhai et al., 2023).

Secondly, much attention has been paid to the treatment of KRAS mutations, specifically the KRAS G12C mutation, which has been identified as an oncogene in

NSCLC. High tumor reduction rates, which is one of the steps in the development of personalized CAR-T therapy against the microenvironmental specifics of the given cancer, have already been proven by trials targeting KRAS. To make the tailored CAR-T therapy more effective, a recent trial has also found that KRAS G12C mutation patients responded to treatment with a rapid tumor response.

The other candidate is CLDN18.2 (Claudin 18.2) that is overexpressed in gastric and pancreatic cancers and found in some NSCLC patients. CAR-T cell clinical trials targeting CLDN18.2 have shown high overall response rates particularly in patients who had not previously received other lines of treatment using vorinostat. These results indicate the possibility of applying this antigen in the treatment of NSCLC.

Since the tumor microenvironment of NSCLC is immunosuppressive, researchers are considering the use of CAR-T therapy in combination with immune checkpoint inhibitors. Current trials are evaluating the safety and efficacy of CAR-T cell administration coupled with PD-1 blocking therapies such as nivolumab, and PD-L1 blocking therapies such as atezolizumab. Early co-activation approaches have been shown to be more effective in anti-tumor, and this can be due to T cell recovery enabled by checkpoint inhibitors alongside direct CAR-T targeting.

Among the main aims of such clinical trials is the improvement of the activity and survival of infused CAR-T cells. A variety of novel approaches such as IL-15 are under consideration to improve T cell survival and proliferation. The first clinical trials demonstrated engineered CAR-T cells had superior T cell survival, and tumor efficacy, and will be applied in the future to treat NSCLC (Thein et al., 2022).

As these trials continue, one of the patients who has undergone HER2-targeted CAR-T therapy can demonstrate that an individual approach to treatment is possible. A female patient having advanced NSCLC aged 68 years and who has undergone various therapies was treated with HER2-targeted CAR-T cells. After the treatment, imaging revealed a major regression of the tumour and the patient stated that his quality of life improved. The case is a good example of what the CAR-T trials can achieve and highlights the need to conduct further research on this topic.

3.2 Patient Selection and Response Predictors

The key problem in determining the role of CAR-T cells in NSCLC therapy is that accurate indicators describing the efficacy of the treatment are absent or are difficult to obtain. Genomic profiling has emerged as an important modality in this case; simply testing the patient's tumor for certain genomic alterations may predict the potential degree of benefit of any given therapy. For example, patients with high TMB have better response to immune based therapies such as CAR-T because tumor associated antigens arise from neoantigens that are detected by T cells. This implies that perhaps high TMB may be a favorable biomarker for selecting those patients who should be targeted for CAR-T therapy sessions (Zhong et al., 2020).

Another important indicator includes expression of PD-L1; since patients with high levels of PD-L1 might require better stimulation that is resulted from low endogenous immune suppression. On a related note, high expression of the molecules CD73 and IDO in the TME is associated with unfavorable treatment response thus suggesting the need for account for them in the context of patient profiling. The research published in the last couple of years has proposed that small molecular inhibitors maybe used to target these enzymes to alter the tumor microenvironment to augment the effectiveness of CAR-T therapies (Cui et al., 2024).

Also, the choice of immune checkpoint molecules such as T cell immunoglobulin and mucin-domain containing-3 (TIM-3) and LAG-3 as markers for patient selection is arising. These markers are signs of T cell exhaustion and they can help determine if a patient will undergo a poor response to CAR-T treatment. The trials are still ongoing in an attempt to mix the CAR-T therapy with inhibitors that will help to 'reactivate T cells' (Cai et al., 2023).

Till now, the immune context within the tumor is central to the success of CAR-T therapy. A differential concentration of other immune infiltrates connected to a higher baseline presence of tumor-infiltrating lymphocytes (TILs) including activated cytotoxic CD8+ T cells are identified to be favorable. On the other hand, the presence of T regulatory cells (Tregs) which are immunosuppressive impairs the ability of CAR-T therapies. Further work is dedicated to defining the factors of the immune cell infiltrate that could indicate the result of the treatment, i.e., develop the patient-tailored therapeutic strategy.

Additional studies with the focus on the metabolic contributions and conditions of CAR-T cells are needed. Research shows that CAR-T cells with high metabolic activity—characterized by functional mitochondria and well-developed glycolysis—demonstrate improved killing of target cancer cells. Scientists are still looking for metabolic targets to enhance CAR T cell metabolism and thereby increase its durability and efficacy in NSCLC's harsh tumor microenvironment.

In sum, the current state of CAR-T therapy will remain dynamic, as advances in the field remain tuned to the selection criteria of CAR-T candidate patients and the identification of evolving response determinants. Genetic profiling and immunological landscape along with metabolic studies comprise the next level in refining CAR-T therapies to improve the NSCLC patients' treatment window and to achieve the optimal therapeutic results (Zhao et al., 2021).

4. LIMITATIONS OF CAR-T THERAPY IN NSCLC

CAR-T therapy offers significant potential for treating non-small cell lung cancer (NSCLC) but faces considerable challenges. One major issue is tumor heterogeneity, which complicates CAR construction, as NSCLC exhibits diverse mutations and varied expression of tumor antigens, making it difficult to identify stable targets, unlike established targets like CD19 in hematologic malignancies (Z. Liu et al., 2024).

The immunosuppressive tumor microenvironment also hinders CAR-T efficacy, with regulatory T cells and myeloid-derived suppressor cells producing inhibitory cytokines, such as TGF-β, that diminish T cell function (Z. Liu et al., 2022). Some strategies combine CAR-T with immune checkpoint inhibitors to mitigate this challenge.

Moreover, CAR-T cells often struggle to penetrate solid tumors due to physical barriers like the extracellular matrix, which can be addressed by engineering CAR-T cells to express enzymes that degrade these barriers (Peng et al., 2024). Antigen escape, where targeted antigens are lost or mutated, further complicates treatment. Researchers are thus exploring multi-targeted CAR designs to reduce relapse risk (Bartoszewska et al., 2024).

Finally, CAR-T manufacturing remains complex, necessitating improvements in efficiency and yield (Mishra et al., 2024). Continued interdisciplinary collaboration is vital to overcoming these hurdles and enhancing CAR-T therapy's effectiveness for NSCLC.

4.1 Tumor Microenvironment Challenges

The tumor microenvironment (TME) of non-small cell lung cancer (NSCLC) presents several significant challenges for the efficacy of CAR-T cell therapy. This environment can be characterized by a dense extracellular matrix, hypoxic conditions, and high levels of immunosuppressive cytokines, all of which hinder T cell infiltration and function. Additionally, the presence of immune checkpoint molecules and a heterogeneous tumor cell population further complicates targeting efforts. Understanding and addressing these challenges is crucial for enhancing the effectiveness of CAR-T therapies in NSCLC. Below is a detailed **Table 2** outlining these Tumor Microenvironment Challenges:

Table 2. Tumor Microenvironment Challenges for CAR-T Cell Therapy in NSCLC

Tumor Microenvironment Challenge	Description	Implications for CAR-T Therapy	Potential Solutions/ Research Directions	Reference
Extracellular Matrix (ECM) Density	The TME often has a dense ECM that poses physical barriers to T-cell infiltration and access to tumor cells.	Dense ECM can limit the effectiveness of CAR-T cells in reaching and engaging with tumors, reducing therapeutic efficacy.	Research on ECM-modifying enzymes (e.g., hyaluronidase) and combining with therapies that degrade ECM structures are ongoing to improve T-cell accessibility.	(J. Huang et al., 2021)
Hypoxia	Tumors frequently exhibit hypoxic regions that impair T cell functions by altering metabolic pathways.	Hypoxia can lead to T cell exhaustion and diminished CAR-T activity, compromising patient outcomes.	Developing CAR-T cells with hypoxia-responsive elements or enhancing metabolic adaptations to function under low oxygen conditions are potential strategies.	(Zhu et al., 2024)
Immunosuppressive Cytokines	High levels of cytokines such as TGF-β and IL-10 in the TME can inhibit T cell activation and boost tumor growth.	These factors can significantly suppress CAR-T cell proliferation and cytotoxicity, decreasing therapeutic effectiveness.	Efforts to neutralize these suppressive cytokines and engineering CAR-T cells to be resistant to TGF-β signaling are promising research areas.	(Briukhovetska et al., 2021)
Immune Checkpoints	Tumor and immune cells overexpress checkpoint molecules (e.g., PD-L1, TIM-3) that inhibit T cell activity in the TME.	Interactions with immune checkpoints can induce T cell exhaustion, hindering sustained CAR-T cell responses.	Exploring combination therapies pairing CAR-T cells with immune checkpoint inhibitors (e.g., anti-PD-1/PD-L1) may enhance therapy effectiveness.	(Barrueto et al., 2020)
Tumor Heterogeneity	NSCLC exhibits significant antigenic variability, complicating the targeting of tumor cells by CAR-T cells.	Antigen variability can lead to incomplete tumor targeting and resistance, allowing some tumor cells to survive treatment.	Development of multi-targeted CAR-T cells capable of recognizing various antigens could improve efficacy against heterogeneous tumors.	(L. Zhu et al., 2021)

continued on following page

Table 2. Continued

Tumor Microenvironment Challenge	Description	Implications for CAR-T Therapy	Potential Solutions/ Research Directions	Reference
Metabolic Competition	The TME may present a hostile metabolic environment characterized by low glucose levels and high lactate, which inhibit T cell function.	Such metabolic stress can lead to reduced T cell proliferation and diminished effector functions of CAR-T cells.	Investigating metabolic modulators (e.g., metformin) to boost CAR-T cell metabolism and function in difficult environments is an area of active research.	(Castoldi et al., 2023)
Regulatory T Cells (Tregs)	Increased Tregs within the TME inhibit the activity and proliferation of CAR-T cells, further complicating the immune response against tumors.	Tregs can suppress anti-tumor activity, which poses a significant barrier for effective CAR-T cell responses.	Research focused on selectively depleting or inhibiting Tregs, as well as engineering resistant CAR-T cells, represents a crucial pathway for enhancing efficacy.	(Y. Wang et al., 2024)
Myeloid-Derived Suppressor Cells (MDSCs)	MDSCs are often elevated in the TME, contributing to immune suppression and promoting tumor survival.	MDSCs can inhibit the function of CAR-T cells, potentially leading to therapy resistance.	Strategies to deplete or block MDSC activity are under investigation to enhance CAR-T cell functionality in the TME.	(K. Li et al., 2021)

4.2 Safety Concerns and Adverse Effects

CAR-T therapy has revolutionized cancer therapy, particularly for hematological malignancies, but its use in non-small cell lung cancer (NSCLC) is fraught with significant safety issues.

Cytokine Release Syndrome (CRS): A severe side effect, CRS is caused by a systemic inflammatory reaction as a result of CAR-T cell activation against tumor antigens. Its occurrence is increased in NSCLC patients with large tumor burdens and needs careful monitoring. Effective management involves standardized grading and the administration of IL-6 inhibitors such as tocilizumab.

Neurotoxicity (ICANS): Immune effector cell-associated neurotoxicity syndrome (ICANS) is less clear in solid tumors such as NSCLC. Biomarkers, such as increased soluble CD25 and IL-10 levels, which can potentially predict ICANS risk, are the focus of current research.

On-target, Off-tumor Toxicity: Targeting antigens such as EGFR may result in toxic effects on healthy tissues, inducing skin rashes and pulmonary toxicity. Dual-targeting CAR-Ts are being investigated by researchers to improve safety.

Chronic Activation: The stability of CAR-T cells can result in extended adverse effects, thus pushing innovation such as switchable CAR technology for conditional activation.

5. ADVANCEMENTS IN CAR-T THERAPY

The field of CAR-T therapy is rapidly advancing with a focus on enhancing therapeutic efficacy and safety. Notable innovations include the development of switchable CAR constructs, which allow for the controlled activation and deactivation of CAR-T cells in response to specific signals, potentially reducing adverse effects. Researchers are also exploring the incorporation of synthetic biology techniques that enable CAR-T cells to produce therapeutic proteins on-demand, further improving their tumor-targeting capabilities. Additionally, understanding the role of the tumor microenvironment has led to new strategies such as the use of nanoparticles to deliver CAR-T cells directly to tumors, enhancing their infiltration and effectiveness. Combination strategies are also gaining traction, including the integration of CAR-T therapies with novel agents like targeted therapies and metabolic modulators that can synergistically enhance CAR-T cell function, targeting not just the tumor cells but also the supportive stromal components that contribute to cancer progression. These advancements signify a promising shift towards more personalized and effective CAR-T treatment options for a broader range of cancers.

5.1 Novel CAR Designs

Recent advancements in CAR (Chimeric Antigen Receptor) technology have led to innovative designs that enhance specificity, efficacy, and safety. Some of the notable novel CAR designs include:

- Dual-Target CARs: These CARs are engineered to recognize two different antigens simultaneously. This approach aims to improve the targeting of malignant cells while reducing off-tumor toxicity. For instance, dual-target CARs may pair an antigen frequently expressed on tumor cells with a second antigen less common on normal tissues. This strategy has shown promise in hematological malignancies and solid tumors by potentially increasing the efficacy of CAR-T cells while minimizing damage to healthy tissues.

- CARs with Enhanced T Cell Persistence: Improved CAR designs are being developed to enhance the persistence of CAR-T cells in the body. New strategies involve incorporating signaling domains from co-stimulatory receptors (e.g., 4-1BB, OX40) that promote T cell survival and memory formation. These modifications enable CAR-T cells to remain active for extended periods, potentially leading to long-lasting anti-tumor effects.
- Armored CARs: These specialized CARs are equipped with additional synthetic pathways that can secrete cytokines (e.g., IL-12, IL-15) or express co-stimulatory ligands (e.g., CD40L). Armored CARs can provide an enhanced immune response within the tumor microenvironment, leading to improved efficacy against tumors that exhibit immune evasion mechanisms.
- Self-Driving CARs: Utilizing synthetic biology, self-driving CARs are designed to autonomously respond to environmental changes in the tumor microenvironment. For example, these CARs can be engineered to express activation markers in the presence of specific tumor-associated antigens or immunosuppressive signals, allowing them to become activated only in the appropriate context. This feature aims to reduce toxicity and increase the specificity of the immune response against tumors.
- CD19 and Beyond: Initially, CAR-T therapies predominantly targeted CD19 for hematological malignancies; however, new designs are focusing on other antigens such as BCMA (B-cell maturation antigen) for multiple myeloma, and HER2 or EGFRvIII for solid tumors. These advancements reflect a growing understanding of diverse tumor antigen profiles and strategies to tackle various malignancies beyond the initial successes with CD19-targeting CARs.

5.2 Combination Therapies

Combination treatment is emerging as important strategies to enhance the efficacy of chimeric antigen receptor T-cell (CAR-T) therapy in cancer treatment, especially tumor inequality and immunosuppressive tumor to address micro-veneration. Car-Tea therapy has shown success in hematological malformations, but challenges in solid tumors include diverse tumor antigen and regulator T cells that obstruct the effectiveness.

A combination of CAR-T therapy with immune checkpoint inhibitors such as anti-PD-1 antibody, increase anti-tumor activity and improves CAR-T cell firmness. Recent studies focus on metabolic mobility; For example, obstructing pyruvet dehydrogenase can promote car-T cell glycolitis, which increases their efficacy in hypoxic conditions.

Additionally, non-six cell lung cancer (NSCLC) can increase tumor antigen appearance and T-cell reactions by combining Car-T with targeted treatments such as TKI. Cytokines such as IL-15 promote car-T cell expansion and survival, while tumors target immunospressive elements in microement-as regulators increase T cells-car-T efficacy. Optimal combinations and biomarkers will be detected to guide medical selection in ongoing clinical trials.

6. FUTURE DIRECTIONS AND RESEARCH

The future of CAR-T therapy is poised for transformative developments, with research expanding beyond traditional applications to explore innovative treatment modalities. Emerging approaches include the use of synthetic biology to design programmable CAR-T cells that can fine-tune their activity based on the tumor microenvironment, enhancing their effectiveness while minimizing off-target effects. Additionally, there is growing interest in the potential of combining CAR-T therapy with emerging gene editing technologies, such as CRISPR, to create CAR-T cells that are engineered not only to target specific antigens but also to resist immune suppression and enhance persistence in hostile tumor environments. Researchers are also investigating the role of microbiome modulation in influencing CAR-T cell efficacy, as early evidence suggests that the composition of gut bacteria may impact the immune response to therapy. Moreover, studies are underway to evaluate the safety and efficacy of CAR-T therapies in pediatric populations and across various malignancies, including rare cancers, as researchers seek to broaden the therapeutic horizon and improve outcomes for diverse patient groups. Overall, the focus on integrative, cutting-edge strategies highlights the potential for CAR-T therapies to evolve into more versatile and potent options in the oncology toolkit.

6.1 Ongoing Trials and Approaches

Car-t (chimeric antigen receptor t-call) therapy has revolutionized cancer, especially for hematological malformations, but challenges remain for solid tumors. Researchers are searching for innovative strategies to increase efficacy.

Car-T cell design adaptation is an important focus, with the next generation of construction to improve T-cell activation and perseverance, many costimulatory domains such as Ox 40 are used. Additionally, dual-goal car-TS is being developed to address tumors by recognizing different antigens simultaneously, which reduces relay risk.

Metabolic modulation strategies, such as ketogenic diet, can increase car-t cell patience in the environment of hard tumors. To retaliate immunoediting, studies are underway on car-TS targeting unique new castes for tumors.

Combination approaches with immune checkpoint inhibitors are to improve car-T functionality, while oncolytic virus can modify tumor microelement. In addition, small molecules obstructions targeting metabolic routes are being examined for their ability to increase antitumor activity. The ongoing progress promises to improve car-tee therapy results in various cancer types.

6.2 Regulatory Considerations

In the form of car-T therapy, regulatory ideas are rapidly sophisticated to solve their unique challenges. A notable development is the introduction of risk-based regulatory framework, which allows an analog approach based on the complexity of the CAR-T product. FDA and EMA are collaborating to harmonize these routes globally, increasing the approval process for developers in areas.

Increasing the use of real-world evidence (RWE), enables regulatory agencies to analyze clinical practice data for post-transformation decisions. For example, the FDA's project takes advantage of RWE for monitoring the performance of gene therapy, including the Sentinel car-T products.

In response to prolonged safety concerns, especially about neurotoxicity and cytokine release syndrome (CRS), there is a strong emphasis on post -monitoring monitoring of marketing monitoring to use risk evaluation and mitigation strategies (REMs). Additionally, regulatory structures are developed to support quick manufacturing processes, ensure moral sources of T cells and maintain the patient's consent as alogenic car-T cell products become more common. This balance facilitates innovation responsible in the medical scenario.

7. CONCLUSION

Car-t therapy represents a significant advancement in the treatment of cancer, especially for non-six cell lung cancer (NSCLC). While CAR-T has achieved remarkable success in hematological deformities, its adaptation for solid tumors faces unique challenges due to complex tumor microement and tumor inequality. Solid tumors often employ mechanisms that prevent tea cell infiltration and activity, complicating car-T efficacy.

To remove these obstacles, innovations in Car-T technology are important. Notable progresses include several receptors or engineering car-T cells with co-stimulating molecules such as CD 28 and 4-1BB, which increase T cell activation, perseverance and tumor targeting. Additionally, the development of armored CAR-T cells capable of secreting cytokines is aimed at combating the immunospressive signal generated by the tumor microement.

Clinical trials are rapidly examining the combination of car-t treatments with other treatment methods, including immune checkpoint inhibitors and targeted treatment. Initial studies indicate that CAR-T therapy pairing with agents such as pambrolizub can improve overall tumor reactions and reduce the possibility of resistance.

The regulatory landscape is developing, using adaptive test designs to facilitate rapid approval. Ethical concerns about the patient's consent and equitable access remain central as alogenic approaches receive traction. The purpose of these joint efforts is to place car-t therapy as a transformative option for NSCLC patients.

7.1 Summary of Findings

The exploration of CAR-T therapy has significantly advanced, especially in the context of hematologic malignancies, yet its application in solid tumors, particularly non-small cell lung cancer (NSCLC), presents both challenges and opportunities. Research findings indicate that while traditional CAR-T approaches have shown remarkable efficacy in blood cancers, translating these successes to solid tumors is an ongoing endeavor fraught with hurdles such as tumor heterogeneity, microenvironmental factors, and immune evasion mechanisms. Innovations in CAR-T technology, including the development of dual-targeting CARs and the incorporation of bispecific T-cell engagers, show promise in overcoming some of these barriers. Recent studies have highlighted the potential for these innovative CAR designs to improve tumor targeting specificity, enhance persistence within the tumor microenvironment, and mitigate adverse effects.

Clinical trials focused on NSCLC have underscored the need for a multidisciplinary approach to enhance treatment efficacy. For instance, some emerging strategies involve the combination of CAR-T therapy with immune checkpoint inhibitors, which can potentially bolster T-cell activation and proliferation within the tumor microenvironment. Other trials are investigating the role of oncolytic viruses in conjunction with CAR-T therapy, seeking to create a more favorable environment for CAR-T cells to thrive and attack tumor cells effectively.

As researchers continue to dissect the biology of NSCLC, findings related to specific tumor antigens are paving the way for the development of tailored CAR-T therapies. This precision medicine approach aims to address the unique molecular characteristics of each patient's tumor, leading to improved response rates and minimized risk of relapse. Furthermore, findings related to the tumor immune microenvironment in NSCLC have sparked interest in using CAR-T therapy in conjunction with other modalities, including targeted therapies, to create a synergistic effect that enhances treatment outcomes.

7.2 Final Thoughts on the Future of CAR-T Therapy in NSCLC

The ability of car-t therapy for non-sixty cell lung cancer (NSCLC) is promising, yet it comes with complications that demand ongoing innovations. Future research should prioritize to understand the mechanisms through which NSCLC detects immune to develop smart car designs capable of being adapted to immunosuppressive tumor microement.

The adaptation of patient selection based on genetic and molecular markers is also important. Complicating the broad genomic profiles with immunotheraputic strategies will probably be better results as a novel biomarker that predicts reactions to car-T treatments. This individual approach accelerates therapy effectiveness and reduces adverse effects by ensuring that only appropriate patients get treatment.

Regulatory ideas will greatly affect the scenario of car-t therapy in NSCLC. Addressing moral concerns about car-T product sourcing should be adjusted rapid progress in manufacturing to develop regulatory framework. Cooperation between researchers, physicians and policy makers will be necessary.

Additionally, the discovery of combination treatments availing CAR-T with installed methods such as chemotherapy or radiation can improve tumor reactions and increase the overall survival rate. Emerging technologies such as crispr gene editing will pave the way for the next generation car-T cells that can deal with many tumor goals. With these progressions, car-t therapy can change NSCLC treatment, setting a new standard in oncology.

STATEMENTS AND DECLARATIONS

Funding

The authors declare that no funds, grants, or other support were received during the preparation of this manuscript.

Competing Interests

The authors have no relevant financial or non-financial interests to disclose.

Author Contributions

The work reported in this study has been carried out by the author, Prerna Mehta, who has also independently written this manuscript. This contain its development and planning, sample acquisition and testing and writing and finalizing the paper for publication.

Compliance with Ethical Standards

In compliance with the standards of publishing the results of this research, the author, Prerna Mehta, hereby states that there is no conflict of interest to report. This work did not include human subjects and animals hence; no informed consent, or animal welfare statements were required. Guidelines to ethical best practice have been followed in the preparation of this manuscript.

REFERENCES

Araghi, M., Mannani, R., Heidarnejad maleki, A., Hamidi, A., Rostami, S., Safa, S. H., Faramarzi, F., Khorasani, S., Alimohammadi, M., Tahmasebi, S., & Akhavan-Sigari, R. (2023). Recent advances in non-small cell lung cancer targeted therapy; an update review. *Cancer Cell International*, *23*(1), 162. DOI: 10.1186/s12935-023-02990-y PMID: 37568193

Ayala Ceja, M., Khericha, M., Harris, C. M., Puig-Saus, C., & Chen, Y. Y. (2024). CAR-T cell manufacturing: Major process parameters and next-generation strategies. *The Journal of Experimental Medicine*, *221*(2), e20230903. Advance online publication. DOI: 10.1084/jem.20230903 PMID: 38226974

Barrueto, L., Caminero, F., Cash, L., Makris, C., Lamichhane, P., & Deshmukh, R. R. (2020). Resistance to Checkpoint Inhibition in Cancer Immunotherapy. *Translational Oncology*, *13*(3), 100738. DOI: 10.1016/j.tranon.2019.12.010 PMID: 32114384

Briukhovetska, D., Dörr, J., Endres, S., Libby, P., Dinarello, C. A., & Kobold, S. (2021). Interleukins in cancer: From biology to therapy. *Nature Reviews. Cancer*, *21*(8), 481–499. DOI: 10.1038/s41568-021-00363-z PMID: 34083781

Bui, T. A., Mei, H., Sang, R., Ortega, D. G., & Deng, W. (2024). Advancements and challenges in developing in vivo CAR T cell therapies for cancer treatment. *EBioMedicine*, *106*, 105266. DOI: 10.1016/j.ebiom.2024.105266 PMID: 39094262

Bulcha, J. T., Wang, Y., Ma, H., Tai, P. W. L., & Gao, G. (2021). Viral vector platforms within the gene therapy landscape. *Signal Transduction and Targeted Therapy*, *6*(1), 53. DOI: 10.1038/s41392-021-00487-6 PMID: 33558455

Cai, L., Li, Y., Tan, J., Xu, L., & Li, Y. (2023). Targeting LAG-3, TIM-3, and TIGIT for cancer immunotherapy. *Journal of Hematology & Oncology*, *16*(1), 101. DOI: 10.1186/s13045-023-01499-1 PMID: 37670328

Castellanos-Rueda, R., Di Roberto, R. B., Bieberich, F., Schlatter, F. S., Palianina, D., Nguyen, O. T. P., Kapetanovic, E., Läubli, H., Hierlemann, A., Khanna, N., & Reddy, S. T. (2022). speedingCARs: Accelerating the engineering of CAR T cells by signaling domain shuffling and single-cell sequencing. *Nature Communications*, *13*(1), 6555. DOI: 10.1038/s41467-022-34141-8 PMID: 36323661

Castoldi, A., Lee, J., de Siqueira Carvalho, D., & Souto, F. O. (2023). CD8+ T cell metabolic changes in breast cancer. *Biochimica et Biophysica Acta (BBA) -. Biochimica et Biophysica Acta. Molecular Basis of Disease*, *1869*(1), 166565. DOI: 10.1016/j.bbadis.2022.166565 PMID: 36220587

Charrot, S., & Hallam, S. (2019). CAR-T Cells: Future Perspectives. *HemaSphere*, *3*(2), e188. Advance online publication. DOI: 10.1097/HS9.0000000000000188 PMID: 31723827

Choudhery, M. S., Arif, T., Mahmood, R., & Harris, D. T. (2024). CAR-T-Cell-Based Cancer Immunotherapies: Potentials, Limitations, and Future Prospects. *Journal of Clinical Medicine*, *13*(11), 3202. DOI: 10.3390/jcm13113202 PMID: 38892913

Colina, A. S., Shah, V., Shah, R. K., Kozlik, T., Dash, R. K., Terhune, S., & Zamora, A. E. (2024). Current advances in experimental and computational approaches to enhance CAR T cell manufacturing protocols and improve clinical efficacy. *Frontiers in Molecular Medicine*, *4*, 1310002. Advance online publication. DOI: 10.3389/fmmed.2024.1310002 PMID: 39086435

Colombino, M., Paliogiannis, P., Cossu, A., Santeufemia, D. A., Sini, M. C., Casula, M., Palomba, G., Manca, A., Pisano, M., Doneddu, V., & Palmieri, G. (2019). EGFR, KRAS, BRAF, ALK, and cMET genetic alterations in 1440 Sardinian patients with lung adenocarcinoma. *BMC Pulmonary Medicine*, *19*(1), 209. DOI: 10.1186/s12890-019-0964-x PMID: 31711449

Cui, J.-W., Li, Y., Yang, Y., Yang, H.-K., Dong, J.-M., Xiao, Z.-H., He, X., Guo, J.-H., Wang, R.-Q., Dai, B., & Zhou, Z.-L. (2024). Tumor immunotherapy resistance: Revealing the mechanism of PD-1 / PD-L1-mediated tumor immune escape. *Biomedicine and Pharmacotherapy*, *171*, 116203. DOI: 10.1016/j.biopha.2024.116203 PMID: 38280330

Daei Sorkhabi, A., Mohamed Khosroshahi, L., Sarkesh, A., Mardi, A., Aghebati-Maleki, A., Aghebati-Maleki, L., & Baradaran, B. (2023). The current landscape of CAR T-cell therapy for solid tumors: Mechanisms, research progress, challenges, and counterstrategies. *Frontiers in Immunology*, *14*, 1113882. Advance online publication. DOI: 10.3389/fimmu.2023.1113882 PMID: 37020537

De Marco, R. C., Monzo, H. J., & Ojala, P. M. (2023). CAR T Cell Therapy: A Versatile Living Drug. *International Journal of Molecular Sciences*, *24*(7), 6300. DOI: 10.3390/ijms24076300 PMID: 37047272

Fang, Y., Chen, Y., & Li, Y.-R. (2025). Engineering the next generation of allogeneic CAR cells: iPSCs as a scalable and editable platform. *Stem Cell Reports*, *20*(7), 102515. DOI: 10.1016/j.stemcr.2025.102515 PMID: 40480218

Guo, H., Zhang, J., Qin, C., Yan, H., Liu, T., Hu, H., Tang, S., Tang, S., & Zhou, H. (2022). Biomarker-Targeted Therapies in Non–Small Cell Lung Cancer: Current Status and Perspectives. *Cells*, *11*(20), 3200. DOI: 10.3390/cells11203200 PMID: 36291069

He, Z.-N., Zhang, C.-Y., Zhao, Y.-W., He, S.-L., Li, Y., Shi, B.-L., Hu, J.-Q., Qi, R.-Z., & Hua, B.-J. (2023). Regulation of T cells by myeloid-derived suppressor cells: Emerging immunosuppressor in lung cancer. *Discover. Oncology*, *14*(1), 185. DOI: 10.1007/s12672-023-00793-1 PMID: 37857728

Hechtman, J. F. (2022). NTRK insights: Best practices for pathologists. *Modern Pathology*, *35*(3), 298–305. DOI: 10.1038/s41379-021-00913-8 PMID: 34531526

Honikel, M. M., & Olejniczak, S. H. (2022). Co-Stimulatory Receptor Signaling in CAR-T Cells. *Biomolecules*, *12*(9), 1303. DOI: 10.3390/biom12091303 PMID: 36139142

Huang, J., Zhang, L., Wan, D., Zhou, L., Zheng, S., Lin, S., & Qiao, Y. (2021). Extracellular matrix and its therapeutic potential for cancer treatment. *Signal Transduction and Targeted Therapy*, *6*(1), 153. DOI: 10.1038/s41392-021-00544-0 PMID: 33888679

Huang, M., Deng, J., Gao, L., & Zhou, J. (2020). Innovative strategies to advance CAR T cell therapy for solid tumors. *American Journal of Cancer Research*, *10*(7), 1979–1992. PMID: 32774996

Jogalekar, M. P., Rajendran, R. L., Khan, F., Dmello, C., Gangadaran, P., & Ahn, B.-C. (2022). CAR T-Cell-Based gene therapy for cancers: New perspectives, challenges, and clinical developments. *Frontiers in Immunology*, *13*, 925985. Advance online publication. DOI: 10.3389/fimmu.2022.925985 PMID: 35936003

Lana, M. G., & Strauss, B. E. (2020). *Production of Lentivirus for the Establishment of CAR-T Cells.*, DOI: 10.1007/978-1-0716-0146-4_4

Lancaster, H. L., Heuvelmans, M. A., & Oudkerk, M. (2022). Low-dose computed tomography lung cancer screening: Clinical evidence and implementation research. *Journal of Internal Medicine*, *292*(1), 68–80. DOI: 10.1111/joim.13480 PMID: 35253286

Li, C., Lei, S., Ding, L., Xu, Y., Wu, X., Wang, H., Zhang, Z., Gao, T., Zhang, Y., & Li, L. (2023). Global burden and trends of lung cancer incidence and mortality. *Chinese Medical Journal*, *136*(13), 1583–1590. Advance online publication. DOI: 10.1097/CM9.0000000000002529 PMID: 37027426

Li, K., Shi, H., Zhang, B., Ou, X., Ma, Q., Chen, Y., Shu, P., Li, D., & Wang, Y. (2021). Myeloid-derived suppressor cells as immunosuppressive regulators and therapeutic targets in cancer. *Signal Transduction and Targeted Therapy*, *6*(1), 362. DOI: 10.1038/s41392-021-00670-9 PMID: 34620838

Lim, A. R., Rathmell, W. K., & Rathmell, J. C. (2020). The tumor microenvironment as a metabolic barrier to effector T cells and immunotherapy. *eLife*, *9*, e55185. Advance online publication. DOI: 10.7554/eLife.55185 PMID: 32367803

Lin, H., Yang, X., Ye, S., Huang, L., & Mu, W. (2024). Antigen escape in CAR-T cell therapy: Mechanisms and overcoming strategies. *Biomedicine and Pharmacotherapy*, *178*, 117252. DOI: 10.1016/j.biopha.2024.117252 PMID: 39098176

Lindner, S. E., Johnson, S. M., Brown, C. E., & Wang, L. D. (2020). Chimeric antigen receptor signaling: Functional consequences and design implications. *Science Advances*, *6*(21), eaaz3223. Advance online publication. DOI: 10.1126/sciadv.aaz3223 PMID: 32637585

Liu, B., Zhou, H., Tan, L., Siu, K. T. H., & Guan, X.-Y. (2024). Exploring treatment options in cancer: Tumor treatment strategies. *Signal Transduction and Targeted Therapy*, *9*(1), 175. DOI: 10.1038/s41392-024-01856-7 PMID: 39013849

Lu, P., Hill, H. A., Navsaria, L. J., & Wang, M. L. (2021). CAR-T and other adoptive cell therapies for B cell malignancies. *Journal of the National Cancer Center*, *1*(3), 88–96. DOI: 10.1016/j.jncc.2021.07.001 PMID: 39036373

Ma, H., Das, J., Prendergast, C., De Jong, D., Braumuller, B., Paily, J., Huang, S., Liou, C., Giarratana, A., Hosseini, M., Yeh, R., & Capaccione, K. (2023). Advances in CAR T Cell Therapy for Non-Small Cell Lung Cancer. *Current Issues in Molecular Biology*, *45*(11), 9019–9038. DOI: 10.3390/cimb45110566 PMID: 37998743

Milone, M. C., Xu, J., Chen, S.-J., Collins, M. A., Zhou, J., Powell, D. J.Jr, & Melenhorst, J. J. (2021). Engineering-enhanced CAR T cells for improved cancer therapy. *Nature Cancer*, *2*(8), 780–793. DOI: 10.1038/s43018-021-00241-5 PMID: 34485921

Mohanty, R., Chowdhury, C., Arega, S., Sen, P., Ganguly, P., & Ganguly, N. (2019). CAR T cell therapy: A new era for cancer treatment [Review]. *Oncology Reports*. Advance online publication. DOI: 10.3892/or.2019.7335 PMID: 31578576

Moreno, C., Haynie, C., Cheever, A., & Weber, K. (2022). Alternative CAR Therapies: Recent Approaches in Engineering Chimeric Antigen Receptor Immune Cells to Combat Cancer. *Biomedicines*, *10*(7), 1493. DOI: 10.3390/biomedicines10071493 PMID: 35884798

Nanjireddy, P. M., Olejniczak, S. H., & Buxbaum, N. P. (2023). Targeting of chimeric antigen receptor T cell metabolism to improve therapeutic outcomes. *Frontiers in Immunology*, *14*, 1121565. Advance online publication. DOI: 10.3389/fimmu.2023.1121565 PMID: 36999013

Niemira, M., Collin, F., Szalkowska, A., Bielska, A., Chwialkowska, K., Reszec, J., Niklinski, J., Kwasniewski, M., & Kretowski, A. (2019). Molecular Signature of Subtypes of Non-Small-Cell Lung Cancer by Large-Scale Transcriptional Profiling: Identification of Key Modules and Genes by Weighted Gene Co-Expression Network Analysis (WGCNA). *Cancers (Basel), 12*(1), 37. DOI: 10.3390/cancers12010037 PMID: 31877723

Rakhshandehroo, T., Mantri, S. R., Moravej, H., Louis, B. B. V., Salehi Farid, A., Munaretto, L., Regan, K., Khan, R. M. M., Wolff, A., Farkash, Z., Cong, M., Kuhnast, A., Nili, A., Lee, U.-J., Allen, H. H., Berland, L., Simkova, E., Uslu, S. C., Tavakolpour, S., & Rashidian, M. (2024). A CAR enhancer increases the activity and persistence of CAR T cells. *Nature Biotechnology*. Advance online publication. DOI: 10.1038/s41587-024-02339-4 PMID: 39079964

Song, P., Zhang, Q., Xu, Z., Shi, Y., Jing, R., & Luo, D. (2024). CRISPR/Cas-based CAR-T cells: Production and application. *Biomarker Research, 12*(1), 54. DOI: 10.1186/s40364-024-00602-z PMID: 38816881

Sosa, E., D'Souza, G., Akhtar, A., Sur, M., Love, K., Duffels, J., Raz, D. J., Kim, J. Y., Sun, V., & Erhunmwunsee, L. (2021). Racial and socioeconomic disparities in lung cancer screening in the United States: A systematic review. *CA: a Cancer Journal for Clinicians, 71*(4), 299–314. DOI: 10.3322/caac.21671 PMID: 34015860

Uscanga-Palomeque, A. C., Chávez-Escamilla, A. K., Alvizo-Báez, C. A., Saavedra-Alonso, S., Terrazas-Armendáriz, L. D., Tamez-Guerra, R. S., Rodríguez-Padilla, C., & Alcocer-González, J. M. (2023). CAR-T Cell Therapy: From the Shop to Cancer Therapy. *International Journal of Molecular Sciences, 24*(21), 15688. DOI: 10.3390/ijms242115688 PMID: 37958672

Wang, V., Gauthier, M., Decot, V., Reppel, L., & Bensoussan, D. (2023). Systematic Review on CAR-T Cell Clinical Trials Up to 2022: Academic Center Input. *Cancers (Basel), 15*(4), 1003. DOI: 10.3390/cancers15041003 PMID: 36831349

Wang, Y., Li, J., Nakahata, S., & Iha, H. (2024). Complex Role of Regulatory T Cells (Tregs) in the Tumor Microenvironment: Their Molecular Mechanisms and Bidirectional Effects on Cancer Progression. *International Journal of Molecular Sciences, 25*(13), 7346. DOI: 10.3390/ijms25137346 PMID: 39000453

Wojtukiewicz, M. Z., Rek, M. M., Karpowicz, K., Górska, M., Polityńska, B., Wojtukiewicz, A. M., Moniuszko, M., Radziwon, P., Tucker, S. C., & Honn, K. V. (2021). Inhibitors of immune checkpoints—PD-1, PD-L1, CTLA-4—new opportunities for cancer patients and a new challenge for internists and general practitioners. *Cancer and Metastasis Reviews*, *40*(3), 949–982. DOI: 10.1007/s10555-021-09976-0 PMID: 34236546

Xia, A.-L., Wang, X.-C., Lu, Y.-J., Lu, X.-J., & Sun, B. (2017). Chimeric-antigen receptor T (CAR-T) cell therapy for solid tumors: Challenges and opportunities. *Oncotarget*, *8*(52), 90521–90531. DOI: 10.18632/oncotarget.19361 PMID: 29163850

Xie, N., Shen, G., Gao, W., Huang, Z., Huang, C., & Fu, L. (2023). Neoantigens: Promising targets for cancer therapy. *Signal Transduction and Targeted Therapy*, *8*(1), 9. DOI: 10.1038/s41392-022-01270-x PMID: 36604431

Yarchoan, M., Albacker, L. A., Hopkins, A. C., Montesion, M., Murugesan, K., Vithayathil, T. T., Zaidi, N., Azad, N. S., Laheru, D. A., Frampton, G. M., & Jaffee, E. M. (2019). PD-L1 expression and tumor mutational burden are independent biomarkers in most cancers. *JCI Insight*, *4*(6), e126908. Advance online publication. DOI: 10.1172/jci.insight.126908 PMID: 30895946

Yu, S., Wang, Y., He, P., Shao, B., Liu, F., Xiang, Z., Yang, T., Zeng, Y., He, T., Ma, J., Wang, X., & Liu, L. (2022). Effective Combinations of Immunotherapy and Radiotherapy for Cancer Treatment. *Frontiers in Oncology*, *12*, 809304. Advance online publication. DOI: 10.3389/fonc.2022.809304 PMID: 35198442

Zhao, H., Wu, L., Yan, G., Chen, Y., Zhou, M., Wu, Y., & Li, Y. (2021). Inflammation and tumor progression: Signaling pathways and targeted intervention. *Signal Transduction and Targeted Therapy*, *6*(1), 263. DOI: 10.1038/s41392-021-00658-5 PMID: 34248142

Zheng, Z., Li, S., Liu, M., Chen, C., Zhang, L., & Zhou, D. (2023). Fine-Tuning through Generations: Advances in Structure and Production of CAR-T Therapy. *Cancers (Basel)*, *15*(13), 3476. DOI: 10.3390/cancers15133476 PMID: 37444586

Zhong, S., Cui, Y., Liu, Q., & Chen, S. (2020). CAR-T cell therapy for lung cancer: A promising but challenging future. *Journal of Thoracic Disease*, *12*(8), 4516–4521. DOI: 10.21037/jtd.2020.03.118 PMID: 32944366

Zhu, L., Jiang, M., Wang, H., Sun, H., Zhu, J., Zhao, W., Fang, Q., Yu, J., Chen, P., Wu, S., Zheng, Z., & He, Y. (2021). A narrative review of tumor heterogeneity and challenges to tumor drug therapy. *Annals of Translational Medicine*, *9*(16), 1351–1351. DOI: 10.21037/atm-21-1948 PMID: 34532488

Zhu, X., Chen, J., Li, W., Xu, Y., Shan, J., Hong, J., Zhao, Y., Xu, H., Ma, J., Shen, J., & Qian, C. (2024). Hypoxia-Responsive CAR-T Cells Exhibit Reduced Exhaustion and Enhanced Efficacy in Solid Tumors. *Cancer Research*, *84*(1), 84–100. DOI: 10.1158/0008-5472.CAN-23-1038 PMID: 37874330

Chapter 7
Case Studies and Clinical Scenarios in NSCLC

Sumitha Elayaperumal
https://orcid.org/0000-0003-0740-8415
JSS Academy of Higher Education and Research, Mysuru, India

Yuvaraj Sivamani
B.S. Abdur Rahman Crescent Institute of Science and Technology, India

Raghunathan Devandiran
Martin Luther University, Germany

Chandrabose Selvaraj
https://orcid.org/0000-0002-8115-0486
CSRDD Lab, Bioinformatics Division, Department of Marine Biotechnology, AMET University, India

ABSTRACT

Lung cancer is a life threatening disease, particularly when it comes to non-small-cell lung cancer (NSCLC), and tends to have an unfortunate outlook for patients who are diagnosed with it. With surgeries and therapies such as chemotherapy, radiotherapy, targeted therapy, and immunotherapy, coupled with an enhanced grasp of genetic and molecular markers, treatment approaches can now be tailored to individuals. This chapter highlights case studies with illustrations and clinical scenarios in non-small cell lung cancer, including instances of long-term survival, disease modification, and treatment response, in an attempt to underscore the challenges in managing non-small cell lung cancer (NSCLC) and to point to areas that may be addressed in the future to improve patient outcomes. Regardless of these advances, issues remain,

DOI: 10.4018/979-8-3373-2096-0.ch007

such as financial limitations and the ethical issues of cost-effectiveness. The future of NSCLC treatments aims to deliver more effective and personalized care, thereby improving patient outcomes and quality of life.

1.NSCLC AND GLOBAL BURDEN

Lung cancers account for 100% of all cancers diagnosed every year. Among different types of lung cancer a non-small cell lung cancer (NSCLC) has the highest incidence. . Lung cancer is still the leading cause of death globally due to cancer, claiming more lives each year than breast, colorectal, and prostate cancer(Molina et al., 2008). NSCLC encompasses a variety of subtypes, of which adenocarcinoma, squamous cell carcinoma, and large cell carcinoma are the most prevalent. Adenocarcinoma, however, has become more common, particularly among nonsmokers and in areas with high rates of air pollution and environmental carcinogens. The global incidence of NSCLC continues to increase, with an estimated 2.2 million new lung cancer cases and 1.8 million deaths in 2020, according to the Global Cancer Observatory report. While incidence rates vary widely in different nations due to tobacco control, occupational exposure, socioeconomic status, and healthcare access, death from NSCLC remains high in the majority of countries because of late diagnosis and the aggressive nature of the disease(Li et al., 2023) Figure 1.. The major risk factor for NSCLC is tobacco smoking, accounting for approximately 85–90% of the cases in developed countries, with the remaining cases being mostly due to secondhand smoke, radon, industrial air pollution, and chronic lung disease. In LMICs, the situation is further worsened by weak screening modalities, delayed diagnoses, a paucity of molecular testing centers, and even fewer centers that provide access to drug treatments. The genomic heterogeneity and fluctuating mechanisms of resistance exhibited by NSCLC biology add to the difficulty of its management(Piña-Sánchez et al., 2021). On the other hand, with the maturation of molecular pathology, the treatment axis of NSCLC has changed 360 degrees, and in particular, targeted therapy for actionable driver mutations such as EGFR, ALK, ROS1, BRAF, and MET has developed. The integration of NGS into diagnostic practice has refined tumor profiling to allow a shift from empirical treatment to more tailored therapeutic regimens. Despite the progress made thus far, the striking differences in access to these technologies between high-income nations and LMICs translate into poor treatment outcomes in LMICs(Grodzka et al., 2023).

Figure 1. Global burden of lung cance-Non-Small Cell Lung Cancer (NSCLC)

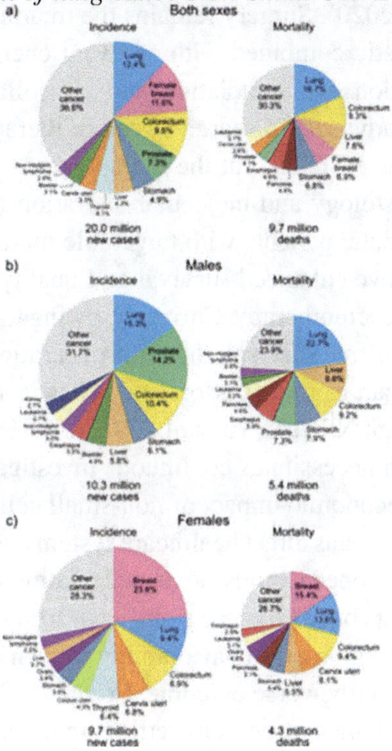

NSCLC has a significantly high mortality rate if not detected early. In such cases, immunotherapy techniques have demonstrated significant survival benefits, especially in cases with high PD-L1 expression. Both monotherapy and combination therapy with checkpoint inhibitors, being pembrolizumab, nivolumab, and atezolizumab, are signified as standard care given their lasting effects(Gang et al., 2024). However, access to this line of treatment remains restricted in many parts of the world because of its costs, lack of insurance coverage, and regulatory problems. Screening techniques for lung cancer employing low-dose computed tomography (LDCT) offer the greatest possibility for even further reductions in mortality by earlier detection, particularly among high-risk populations such as heavy smokers(Poon et al., 2022). Trials such as the National Lung Screening Trial (NLST) and the NELSON Study have demonstrated that using LDCT screening once per year causes a reduction in lung cancer mortality of approximately 20- 24% in the target population(Field et al., 2021).

However, worldwide, adoption is still rare due to cost implications, logistical issues, and the fear of false positives and radiation exposure. With mature screening programs, early-stage diagnoses are on the rise in these societies, allowing more patients to undergo curative surgical resection or stereotactic body radiotherapy (SBRT)(Biganzoli et al., 2020). Surgery remains the treatment of choice for early-stage NSCLC and is mostly combined with adjuvant chemotherapy or immunotherapy, while combination chemoradiation and consolidation immunotherapy are used to treat locally advanced disease. Systemic therapy is still at the center of treatment for metastatic NSCLC, but the therapeutic landscape is increasingly stratified according to histology and molecular alterations(O'Reilly et al., 2023). According to real-world data, patients with targetable mutations benefit considerably from TKIs, which have enhanced survival and quality of life compared with standard platinum-based chemotherapy. Currently, owing to its intracranial activity and prolonged progression-free survival, the third-generation EGFR TKI osimertinib is considered better than its predecessors and is hence adopted as the first-line treatment for EGFR-mutant NSCLC(Yu et al., 2022). Resistance to specific drugs is a matter of time, which necessitates continuous investigation of new drugs and their combinations. The economic impact of non-small cell lung cancer (NSCLC) has been severe globally. It spans direct healthcare system costs, reduced output, and caregiver expenses. In developed nations, advanced treatments and diagnostic methods lead to improved results but also cause significant strain on healthcare systems. Contrarily, in low-income regions, the unavailability of even basic chemotherapeutic agents results in a significantly worse outcome. (Yu et al., 2022). Although stigma prevents individuals with lung cancer from getting treatment, it equally affects the availability of psycho-social care and the allocation of healthcare funds. In numerous regions, NSCLC patients encounter late-stage diagnosis because their symptoms are similar to those of other non-serious diseases of the respiratory system, such as tuberculosis and chronic obstructive pulmonary disorder (COPD). At the time of diagnosis, lung cancer stigma, which is most likely due to the association with smoking, may lead to social exclusion and the avoidance of healthcare services. Despite this, there remains a challenge with the low and middle-income countries (LMICs) concerning affordability and accessibility, which calls for the formulation of policy-driven strategies aimed at providing equitable cancer care.

This psychosocial, along with physical, burden from an advanced state of illness leads to a important decline in quality of life. Hence, measures directed at reducing the overall burden of NSCLC must be multifactorial and include primary prevention (tobacco control, pollution mitigation), screening for early detection, universal access improvement to diagnostics and therapeutics, and the mainstreaming of palliative and supportive care in standard oncologic practices(Morrison et al., 2017). Lung cancer prevention programs have proven indisputably advantageous to cigarette smoking cessation; public health interventions against tobacco advertising, taxation, and smoking bans have all been proven effective in decreasing smoking rates in different countries worldwide. Nevertheless, the increasing number of cases of NSCLC in nonsmokers, especially females and young adults, calls for the exploration of other nontobacco-related etiologies(Zeng et al., 2019). In addition, factors such as urban air pollution, the indoor use of biomass fuels, and certain occupations will have greater impacts on the environmental risk profile in developing countries, worsening the global burden of NSCLC in the coming decades.

Recently, international consortia such as the IASLC and the Global Lung Cancer Coalition (GLCC) have focused on policy integration for standardized treatment and explicated multidisciplinary approaches for lung cancer awareness differentiation, education, and policy-based healthcare to curb inequities in lung cancer care(Huber et al., 2024). Advances in artificial intelligence combined with radiomics are bound to improve the diagnostic precision, stratified risk assessment, and treatment algorithms in NSCLC, although most of these innovations involve in-depth research or well-resourced institutions. Similarly, the ability to conduct liquid biopsies offers noninvasive means of obtaining critical clinical data required for real-time mutation assessment and treatment response monitoring, significantly improving disease management for NSCLC, particularly in patients unable to undergo surgical biopsies. However, cost and access to universal adoption remain significant obstacles(Mitchell Chen et al., 2023). The COVID-19 epidemic has added challenges to NSCLC management by disrupting cancer screening programs, delaying diagnosis, and restricting access to treatment services worldwide. While the nation has fixed its post-pandemic oncology abilities, maintaining the continuity and flexibility of lung cancer treatment is the top priority. Finally, the NSCLC will depend on the determination of long-term global cooperation, investment in health care facilities, and the determination to limit inequalities in providing cancer care. This includes not only an increase in screening and treatment initiatives but also culturally appropriate education campaigns that eliminate lung cancer and encourage early detection. Furthermore the global programs including WHO and IARC highlights the need for developing standardized molecular screening approaches and policy driven measures to overcome the disparities and facilitate timely management in patients with NSCLC.

Future studies will need to continue investigating new biomarkers, mechanisms of resistance, and immunologic targets to further optimize therapeutic approaches and circumvent existing limitations. With a swiftly changing therapeutic environment and increasing recognition of the global burden of this disease, NSCLC continues to be a priority area for cancer research and policy. Concerted action by governments, healthcare professionals, researchers, and patient advocacy organizations is needed to enhance outcomes and alleviate the human and economic burdens of NSCLC globally(de Jager et al., 2024). Future studies should examine new biomarkers, mechanisms of resistance, and immunological goals to further customize medical approaches and bypass existing boundaries. With increasing recognition of the rapidly changing medical environment and the global burden of this disease, NSCLC remains a priority sector for cancer research and policy. It is necessary to increase the consequences of concrete action by governments, healthcare professionals, researchers and patient advocacy organizations and reduce the human and economic burdens of NSCLC globally(Passaro et al., 2024) Table 1.

Table 1. Treatment modalities by NSCLC stage

NSCLC Stage	Standard Treatment Modality	Key Clinical Trials/ Guidelines	Outcome/Comments
Stage I–IIA	Surgical resection ± adjuvant chemotherapy	NCCN, IASLC	High 5-year survival if completely resected
Stage IIB–IIIA	Surgery or chemoradiotherapy ± adjuvant/consolidation IO	PACIFIC Trial, NRG Oncology	Durvalumab improves survival post-CRT
Stage IIIB (Unresectable)	Concurrent chemoradiotherapy + immunotherapy	PACIFIC Trial	Median OS improved from ~16 to 29 months with durvalumab
Stage IV	Systemic therapy (targeted therapy or immunotherapy)	KEYNOTE-024, IMpower150, ALEX Trial	Based on mutation status or PD-L1, long-term survival is possible

This table describes the currently implemented biologically based stagewise treatment approaches for NSCLC and highlights clinical trials designed to change the standard of care. The integration of molecular profiling and immunotherapy has dramatically altered patient outcomes, especially in advanced stages.

2. EPIDEMIOLOGY AND RISK FACTORS

In order to brige the gap between the epidemiological data with clinical practice. The present section incorporates narrative approach to emphasize the global trends in selected studies. Non-small cell lung cancer (NSCLC) is a multifactorial disease, with a wide range of risk factors contributing to its development. Among these causes, tobacco smoking is the most prominent and well-established cause, accounting for approximately 85–90% of all lung cancer cases. Carcinogenic components of cigarette smoke inspire genetic mutations and epigenetic changes that drive oncogenesis, especially in squamous cell carcinoma and small cell lung cancer, although adenocarcinoma is also strongly connected. The risk of developing NSCLC increases with both the duration and intensity of smoking, and presmokers have a significant risk for many years after the end of smoking, although the risk decreases over time. The passive risk of environmental tobacco smoke (secondhand smoke) is also important, especially between children and nonsmoking adults. However, the global increase in NSCLC cases among nonsmokers, especially women and young individuals, has attracted attention because of other major environmental, commercial and genetic risk factors Figure 2.

Figure 2. Epidemology and Risk factors NSCLC

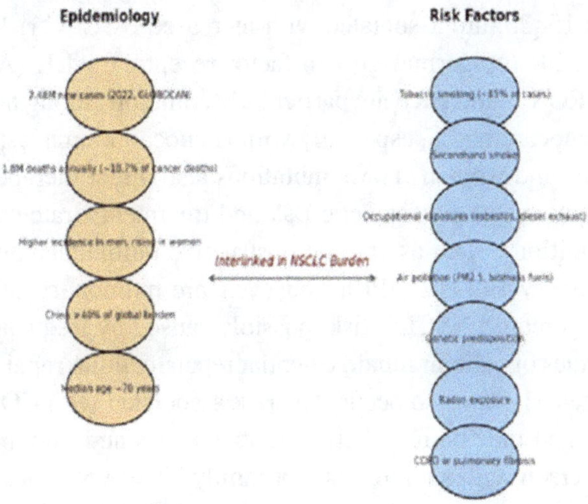

Long-term contact for air pollution, especially fine particulate matter (PM2.5), is recognized as a Class I carcinogen by the International Agency for Research on Cancer (IARC), and many large epidemic studies have demonstrated a clear relationship between the risk of urban pollution and lung cancer. Indoor air pollution, especially from biomass fuel combustion in poorly ventilated settings, is a major contributor to NSCLC in low- and medium-income countries. Radon gas, a naturally occurring radioactive gas that occurs in homes and buildings from soil and rocks, is the second major cause of lung cancer in the general population and is a major cause of nonsmoking. Professional exposure also contributes significantly to NSCLC risk, especially in industrial settings where workers are made aware of carcinogens such as asbestos, arsenic, diesel, chromium compounds, nickel, and silica dust. Prolonged risk in these environments, especially when combined with smoking, increases a collective effect that greatly increases the risk of cancer. In particular, asbestos exposure is strongly associated with adenocarcinoma of the lungs, and the delay period can reach 40 years, which complicates the initial identification. Despite the existing regulatory efforts in many high-age countries, commercial risk is not low in many parts of the world, such as mining, construction, shipbuilding, and manufacturing risks for workers in manufacturing industries.

In addition to the environment and commercial threats, an increasing body of evidence outlines the role of host-related factors and genetic sensitivity in NSCLC. Some inherited polymorphisms and a family history of lung cancer indicate a genetic tendency, even in the absence of smoking. Genome-wide association studies (GWASs) have revealed that several Loki genes, including regions on chromosomes 5p15, 6p21, and 15q25, are associated with increased NSCLC risk. Mutations in genes such as EGFR (epidermal growth factor receptor), ALK (Anaplastic lymphoma Kinase), ROS 1, and BRF are particularly common among nondisrespectful patients with adenocarcinoma, especially with adenocarcinoma, especially in East Asian populations and women. These mutations also direct therapeutic decisions, highlighting the intersection of genetic risk and treatment strategies. Old inflammatory lung conditions, such as chronic obstructive pulmonary disease (COPD), idiopathic pulmonary fibrosis (IPF), and even pre-pulmonary tuberculosis, are associated with increased NSCLC risk, possibly caused by frequent inflammation and repetitive cycles of cellular repair, calendar repair, cellular repair, and repetitive cycles. Carcinogenesis can also occur. The risk associated with COPD is independent of smoking and may be related to oxidative stress and immune dysfunction. Additionally, a person with an individual or family history of cancer, especially an inherited cancer syndrome, may be at high risk for NSCLC. Lifestyle factors such as a sedentary lifestyle, poor diet, and excessive alcohol consumption are being detected for their role in modifying the risk of cancer, although evidence is less certain than that concerning environmental or genetic factors.

Emerging research has focused on the possible role of the lung microbiome in affecting cancer sensitivity, inflammation, and immune responses. Psychological stress, socioeconomic status, and health care inequalities affect risk indirectly by affecting the level of risk, initial identification, and timely treatment. Women appear to be biologically more susceptible to the carcinogenic effects of tobacco and air pollution, possibly due to hormonal differences and the metabolic processing of toxins, which can partially explain the increasing rates of NSCLC among non-smoking women. These diverse and overlapping risk factors highlight the complex etiology of NSCLC, which emphasizes the need for comprehensive risk evaluation models incorporating the environment and genetic and lifestyle components. Public health strategies should expand beyond smoking, including indoor and external pollution, vocational safety, genetic counseling, and similar access to screening and early clinical equipment, especially in the underrepresented population. The increasing understanding of risk factors for NSCLC has important implications for individual medical and preventive strategies and global cancer control policies.

3. EARLY-STAGE NSCLC (STAGE I-IA): INSIGHTS FROM CASE SERIES AND CLINICAL PRACTICE

Beyond clinical outcomes, early-stage survivors often face long-term psychosocial distress, anxiety about recurrence, and quality-of-life challenges; therefore, integration of survivorship programs and systematic use of patient-reported outcomes (PROs) is critical in routine care.

Early-stage NSCLC, according to the AJCC 8th edition TNM system, covers localized primary tumors affecting the lung with a maximum size of 5 cm without regional lymph node involvement or distant metastasis. Although early-stage NSCLC is amenable to potential cures, it appears heterogeneous in presentation, management, and outcome, as illustrated by various case series present in the literature. Both retrospective and prospective studies undertaken through tertiary care centers and cancer institutes have revealed the clinical characteristics, approaches to surgical treatment, recurrence modes, and survival outcomes of patients afflicted with early-stage disease. For example, in a case series by Cassivi et al. from the Mayo Clinic in 2005, in which more than 100 patients with pathologic stage I NSCLC who received lobectomies were analyzed, long-term survival was greater than 70% at five years, particularly among those with tumors ≤3 cm, well-differentiated histology, and no evidence of vascular invasion. A similar series of cases at Memorial Sloan Kettering Cancer Center highlighted the effect of tumor size and completeness of resection about the higher rate of local recurrence in patients who underwent sublobar resections than in those who underwent lobectomy, especially those with surgical margins less than 2 cm in width. Although there are good clinical outcomes the patients who were treated early stage face psychosocial stress which are often long term (1) Anxiety about the chance of recurrence, how this if occours again can impact the quality of life. This highlights the need to develop structured surviourship programs and incorporate patient reported outcome(PROs) in clinical practice

Ichinose et al. (2001) published another case study on our earlier Japanese cohort. Their study focused on 123 patients with lung adenocarcinoma in stage IA. They noted that patients with mixed ground-glass opacity-predominant lesions detected on low-dose CT scans had better DFS when compared to those with solid-predominant lesions. This emphasizes the significance of radiologic features in prognostication. These findings justify the recommendation of limited surgeries like segmentectomies for select groups of patients with small and peripheral GGOs. Lee et al.'s (2014) Korean case study concurs with these findings. In his study, 57 patients with early-stage NSCLC whose tumors were <2 cm and showed CT features suggestive of lepidic-predominant histology were treated with wedge resection or segmentectomy. The patients did incredibly well since their 5-year DFS was >95%, and the authors concluded that imaging- and histology-guided surgery is useful in lung preservation in low-risk patients. Contrarily, the case series from India by Malik et al. (2019) described a more heterogeneous case mix. Their study included 86 patients with earlystage NSCLC that was amenable to resection from three different oncology centers.

. Contrasting with Western populations, where older age, smoking, and squamous cell carcinoma are predominant, a significant portion of our patients were young, never-smokers, and were diagnosed with adenocarcinoma. We lacked sufficient VATS infrastructure; therefore, open thoracotomy was our primary surgical approach. Despite this, the surgical morbidity was within an acceptable range. Recurrence after complete resection was observed in 22% of the patients within three years, especially in patients with visceral pleural invasion or poorly differentiated tumors, emphasizing the need to perform risk stratification, even during the early stage of the disease. This is in agreement with the Western findings of the CALGB 9633 trial (Strauss et al., 2008), which looked into adjuvant chemotherapy for stage IB NSCLC and concluded that tumors greater than 4 cm possibly might benefit from adjuvant cisplatin-based therapy, and the treatment of such cases remains undecided in stage IB.

Wang and colleagues (2017) conducted a case series at the Shanghai Pulmonary Hospital involving 412 patients diagnosed with stage I NSCLC who underwent either lobectomy or segmentectomy between 2010 and 2015. Patients were stratified according to adenocarcinoma histologic subtypes, and the analysis revealed that those with acinar and lepidic patterns demonstrated more favorable survival outcomes compared with patients harboring solid or micropapillary patterns, even when confined to the same stageThe study further demonstrated that, in cases of lepidic-predominant tumors, segmentectomy could achieve oncologic results comparable to lobectomy, supporting the concept of adapting surgical choices to histologic patterns. By contrast, Silva et al. (2020) reported on a Brazilian cohort of 56 patients with early-stage NSCLC managed at a tertiary public hospital. In this series, most patients presented with symptoms at diagnosis, likely reflecting the absence of adequate screening infrastructure, and squamous cell carcinoma was the predominant histology. Delays in surgical management were common and were associated with poorer disease-free survival, largely attributed to limited health-care resources. The authors emphasized the disparity in lung cancer management worldwide and underscored the urgent need for early detection programs and timely treatment in resource-constrained settings.

Several postoperative case series have investigated the expanding application of stereotactic body radiotherapy (SBRT) in patients with early-stage NSCLC who are unsuitable candidates for surgery. In a large Dutch cohort, Haasbeek and colleagues (2012) assessed 177 individuals treated with SBRT for stage I disease and found local control exceeding 90% at three years, accompanied by low treatment-related toxicity. A U.S. case series presented by Timmerman et al. in 2010 reported similar outcomes, suggesting that SBRT could be considered in place of surgery in selected high-risk patients with comorbidities such as COPD or cardiovascular diseases. For example, a 73-year-old patient with stage IA NSCLC and severe emphysema who was unfit for surgery was treated with SBRT (54 Gy in 3 fractions) and remained free of disease at 5 years while maintaining stable pulmonary function. Taken together, these studies support the notion that SBRT represents an alternative to surgery in early-stage NSCLC for patients who cannot undergo operative management, with ongoing clinical trials such as VALOR and STABLEMATES further establishing this role.

Molecular profiling is increasingly being integrated into early-stage management, with case series chronicling adjuvant targeted therapies. The real-world impact of the ADAURA trial was experienced and established within the confines of Singapore General Hospital (Tan et al., 2022), where adjuvant osimertinib was administered to EGFR-mutant stage IB–IIA NSCLC patients after resection. All patients were alive and free of recurrence at the 18-month mark, with manageable toxicities. The case series also revealed increased patient satisfaction because of decreased anxiety related to relapse. Similarly, an Italian case series suggested that adjuvant osimertinib administration in EGFR-mutant patients after lobectomy prolonged DFS, thus further cementing the paradigm shift even for stage IIA patients. However, in many parts of the world, the availability of molecular testing and the cost of targeted agents still impede this progress.

The scenario is set for exploring the role of immunotherapy in early-stage NSCLC; in fact, a small case series from Massachusetts General Hospital exemplifies one such setting, whereby patients with resected stage II tumors, with PD-L1 ≥1%, were given the adjuvant atezolizumab under a clinical protocol (on the heels of IMpower010). Three of the five patients remained disease-free for two years, whereas two patients experienced relapses despite having high PD-L1 levels, suggesting that resistance factors need better biomarkers. Interestingly, none of these patients carried EGFR or ALK alterations, which is consistent with the trial's criteria. These case series highlight other psychological and quality-of-life factors concerning early-stage NSCLC. A Canadian qualitative case study (Lamontagne et al. 2021) indicated that many patients experience anxiety about recurrence despite curative surgery, highlighting the need for survivorship programs and counseling Table 2.

The following table displays the most relevant mutations in NSCLC and the FDA-approved therapeutic agents. These targeted therapies have, in some populations, become cornerstones of treatment, greatly improving patient outcomes while reducing systemic side effects.

Table 2. Common Molecular Targets in NSCLC and Approved Therapies.

Molecular Alteration	Targeted Therapy	Drug(s) Approved	Notable Clinical Trials	Comments
EGFR Mutations	EGFR Tyrosine Kinase Inhibition	Osimertinib, Erlotinib	FLAURA, LUX-Lung	Osimertinib has CNS activity and better PFS
ALK Rearrangement	ALK Inhibition	Alectinib, Lorlatinib	ALEX, ALTA-1 L	Alectinib is preferred for first-line due to CNS efficacy
ROS1 Rearrangement	ROS1 Inhibition	Crizotinib, Entrectinib	STARTRK-2	Effective in rare subtype (~1–2% of NSCLC)
MET exon 14 Skipping	MET Inhibition	Capmatinib, Tepotinib	GEOMETRY mono-1	MET inhibitors were FDA-approved in 2020
KRAS G12C Mutation	KRAS G12C Inhibition	Sotorasib, Adagrasib	CodeBreaK 100, KRYSTAL-1	First effective therapy in KRAS-mutated NSCLC
RET Rearrangement	RET Inhibition	Selpercatinib, Pralsetinib	LIBRETTO-001	High ORR with durable responses in RET-fusion NSCLC
NTRK Fusions	TRK Inhibition	Larotrectinib, Entrectinib	NAVIGATE, STARTRK-2	Pancancer approval for NTRK fusions

Case Study 2: Locally advanced NSCLC (stage IIB--IIIB)

Locally advanced lung cancer, as defined by clinical stages IIB to IIIB of the 8th edition TNM classification, is a somewhat complex and heterogeneous group of lung malignancies mostly composed of larger primary tumors, some regional lymph node involvement, and more or less anatomic challenges. Unlike in the early stages, where surgical treatments may be curative in themselves, there is usually a need for multimodal treatment in locally advanced NSCLC; surgery-based treatments are combined with chemotherapy and radiotherapy, and in recent times, immunotherapy has also been at play. An array of case series and clinical trials across a variety of institutions have described the different treatment approaches and prognostic factors for these patients. In one of the earliest studies, Intergroup Trial 0139 (Albain et al., 2009), it was shown that concurrently administering chemoradiotherapy followed by surgical intervention in selected patients with stage IIIA-N2 disease improved survival compared with chemoradiotherapy alone, especially in those who underwent lobectomy as opposed to pneumonectomy. Findings from this trial influenced the therapeutic approach to multimodal management in certain operable stage III cases. However, the investigators emphasized the importance of careful patient selection for surgery, given the elevated risk of perioperative mortality.

Several large institutional case series have generated detailed real-world evidence on treatment outcomes. At MD Anderson Cancer Center, a retrospective review of 213 patients with stage IIIA/B NSCLC treated using concurrent chemoradiotherapy followed by durvalumab (in line with the PACIFIC regimen) demonstrated a median progression-free survival of 17.2 months, while overall survival at two years exceeded 60%. Consistent with the PACIFIC trial findings (Antonia et al., 2018), patients whose tumors expressed PD-L1 ≥1% derived greater benefit from durvalumab. Likewise, investigators at the Netherlands Cancer Institute reported outcomes in patients with unresectable stage IIIB disease managed with intensity-modulated radiotherapy combined with platinum-based chemotherapy, followed by immunotherapy. Local disease control surpassed 80% at 18 months, and only a small proportion developed grade 3 pneumonitis, underscoring the effectiveness and precision of modern radiotherapy approaches.Top of Form

Clinical outcomes in East Asian populations have shown distinctive patterns. In a study by Ohe et al. (2011), 87 patients with stage IIB–IIIA NSCLC underwent induction chemoradiotherapy followed by surgery. A pathological complete response was achieved in 22% of cases, with long-term survival observed mainly among individuals with squamous histology and mediastinal downstaging. These findings emphasize the prognostic importance of histologic subtype and nodal clearance in surgical outcomes. Similarly, a South Korean investigation by Kim et al. (2017) focused on patients with bulky N2 disease who received induction therapy with docetaxel and cisplatin prior to resection. Although the pathological complete response rate was modest at 15%, patients who achieved nodal clearance had a median overall survival approaching 40 months, reinforcing the role of nodal clearance as a predictor of favorable downstaging. These observations are consistent with German and Italian series that linked major pathological response (MPR) to improved survival. This evidence has fueled interest in neoadjuvant immunotherapy, exemplified by the CheckMate 816 trial (Forde et al., 2022), where the addition of nivolumab to chemotherapy yielded markedly higher rates of both pCR and MPR compared with chemotherapy alone in resectable stage IIIA NSCLC.

The treatment landscape for patients with inoperable stage III NSCLC has gradually advanced with improvements in radiotherapy techniques. In a Swedish cohort, Bergqvist et al. (2020) evaluated 152 individuals with unresectable stage IIIB disease who received concurrent chemoradiotherapy followed by immune checkpoint inhibitors. The study reported a 3-year overall survival of 47%, with acceptable toxicity profiles. Modern radiotherapy modalities such as intensity-modulated radiotherapy (IMRT) and proton therapy allow for reduced exposure of the esophagus and heart, thereby lowering the risk of cardiopulmonary adverse effects. By comparison, earlier studies from the 1990s, such as that of Curran et al. (1991), documented substantially higher rates of treatment-related toxicity and poorer survival outcomes when conventional radiation techniques were employed, underscoring the progress achieved in radiotherapy over recent decades.

. Importantly, some case series emphasize the radiation dose and fractionation. A study in China (Zhou et al., 2021) including 320 patients suggested that radiation doses over 60 Gy when given concurrently with chemotherapy achieve better local control of stage III NSCLC, provided that constraints on dose–volume to critical organs are fulfilled.

Operating experiences and their results have been reported from many centers following trimodality therapy. A Spanish multicenter series (Casal et al., 2016) reported a 5-year OS exceeding 45% in 96 patients with stage IIIA-N2 disease who underwent neoadjuvant CRT with lobectomy, with a lower rate of recurrence when mediastinal nodal clearance was achieved. However, the risk of postoperative complications remains fairly high, especially after pneumonectomy, with some case series reporting perioperative mortality rates between 10% and 15%. Thus, surgical indications have become more conservative, with a preference toward minimally invasive or lung-sparing operations. Robotic and VATS approaches have been attempted in certain centers for resections after CRT, with emerging case series, including those from China and Italy, showing acceptable morbidity and encouraging results in carefully selected patients.

Molecular profiling also plays a larger role in this environment, as documented in the case series. Gainor and colleagues analyzed patients with EGFR-mutated stage III NSCLC in 2018 and reported that these patients had a high rate of distant recurrence post-CRT, most often in the brain, and that durvalumab benefited them only slightly. This led to the further examination of the use of EGFR-TKIs as adjuvant or maintenance therapies. The LAURA trial is currently evaluating osimertinib post-CRT for patients with EGFR mutations. A case series from China (Wu et al., 2022) reported very promising early results when this approach was used for lower distant metastasis. From another viewpoint, ALK-positive stage III patients also appear to have very poor outcomes post-CRT, according to a case series reported by Lin et al. (2020, further stressing the need for individualized posttreatment surveillance and perhaps targeted maintenance strategies.

In qualitative case series and patient-reported outcome studies, the psychosocial burden and quality of life of patients with locally advanced cancers of the lung have been underlined. For example, a Canadian exploratory case study series (Fearon et al., 2015) investigated patient experiences after concurrent CRT and reported that fatigue, anxiety, and nutritional impairment were persistent symptoms that affected patients in their daily activities despite good oncologic outcomes. These findings necessitate the implementation of support for patients, such as pulmonary rehabilitation, dietary assistance, and mental health services, as a key component of multidisciplinary care.

Throughout the world, variability in resources determines treatment access and outcomes. An Indian case series (Ghosh et al., 2021) comprising 70 patients with stage III NSCLC treated in a public hospital highlighted the difficulties in rendering concurrent CRT with machine unavailability and high patient volumes. However, those who underwent sequential CRT had a median survival duration of 13 months despite these constraints, and survival favored completing the whole course of therapy. These findings highlight the grim gap between clinical trial standards and practice in a low-resource setting, forming a clarion call for health systems to strengthen and ensure access to essential cancer services(Spencer et al., 2021).

Case Study 3: Advanced/Metastatic NSCLC (stage IV)

Advanced or metastatic non-small cell lung cancer (NSCLC), a stage IV disease under the 8th edition of the TNM staging system, is the critical and historically fatal final-stage biological feature of lung cancer, with distant metastases to organs such as the brain, bones, liver, adrenal glands, or contralateral lung. These tumors represent a biologically and clinically very diverse group, and for more than 20 years, the treatment paradigm has evolved dramatically from palliative care with platinum-based doublets to a precision oncology paradigm of molecular-targeted therapies, immune checkpoint inhibitors, and combination regimens(Prabhash, 2019). Different case series and clinical trials from multiple centers around the globe have highlighted the diversity in presentations, genomic profiles, and outcomes of patients with metastatic NSCLC, suggesting that histological subtype, driver mutations, PD-L1 status, and performance status play roles in treatment decisions(Sayre et al., 2017). Chemotherapy has been the mainstay, and while this has been supported by early case series such as the Eastern Cooperative Oncology Group (ECOG) 1594 trial (2002), in which four platinum-based doublets were compared, the median OS was only between 8 and 10 months, with few durable responses; these treatment paradigms have undergone significant changes with further molecular discoveries.

In a rather pivotal change, actionable mutations have been identified, notably in the epidermal growth factor receptor (EGFR), anaplastic lymphoma kinase (ALK), ROS1, BRAF, RET, MET exon 14 skipping, KRAS G12C, and NTRK fusions. East Asia, especially Japan, South Korea, and China, boasts case series indicating a high frequency of EGFR mutations (up to 40–50% in adenocarcinomas), and the use of TKIs, such as gefitinib, erlotinib, afatinib, and, more recently, osimertinib, has become widespread(Chevallier et al., 2021). According to the 2018 FLAURA trial and many other real-world series, first-line osimertinib for EGFR-mutated metastatic NSCLC yielded a median OS of approximately 38.6 months, with superior CNS penetration and less toxicity. A giant Chinese real-world registry (REAL study, 2021; more than 1,000 patients) confirmed the superiority of osimertinib, especially in brain metastases, where more than 70% of patients achieved an intracranial response(Ramalingam et al., 2020). Moreover, patients with ALK-rearranged NSCLC, who tend to be younger and nonsmokers, benefit strongly from ALK inhibitors, such as alectinib, brigatinib, and lorlatinib. The ALEX trial in 2017 (Peters et al.) revealed that alectinib substantially delayed disease progression and increased quality of life relative to crizotinib. Several case series from Europe have confirmed this finding in real-world settings, with a median PFS of over 25 months(Attili et al., 2024).

Conversely, patients with no actionable mutations but with high PD-L1 expression (≥50%) seem to benefit from immune checkpoint inhibitors. The KEYNOTE-024 trial was a turning point in patient management, with pembrolizumab monotherapy resulting in significant improvements in PFS and OS over chemotherapy in this subgroup(Russano et al., 2023). A German case series of 187 patients with PD-L1 expression ≥50% reported a median OS of 22 months with pembrolizumab and durable responses in approximately 30% of patients. Combination immunotherapy (e.g., nivolumab + ipilimumab) and chemoimmunotherapy regimens have shown survival benefits in a wider population, including the PD-L1 <1% group, as seen in the CheckMate 227 and KEYNOTE-189 trials(Hellmann et al., 2019). The latter trial compared pemetrexed-platinum chemotherapy plus pembrolizumab against chemotherapy alone in nonsquamous NSCLC patients and reported a median OS of over 22 months, nearly doubling that obtained with chemotherapy alone. This, as mentioned before, has also been reflected in many case series from the U.S., Canada, and Australia, thus accentuating the real-world performance of checkpoint inhibitors(Rodríguez-Abreu et al., 2021).

Whether osseous metastatic tumors present as stage IV NSCLC, especially in patients with adenocarcinoma and in patients with EGFR mutations, poses various unique challenges for patients with SREs and hypercalcemia. A case series report from the Mayo Clinic described the roles of bone-modifying agents, including denosumab and zoledronic acid, in reducing SREs and enhancing quality of life(Garg et al., 2024). Patients with brain metastases account for nearly 30–50% of stage IV NSCLC patients and require a careful and multifaceted approach for treatment. Local control has improved with the arrival of CNS-active TKIs (e.g., osimertinib and lorlatinib) and SRS, with deferral of whole-brain radiation therapy to preserve neurocognitive functions(Nishino et al., 2019). A case series from Memorial Sloan Kettering and other academic centers suggested that patients with asymptomatic brain metastases treated with TKIs survived just as long as those receiving SRS did, highlighting the CNS-penetrant efficacy of modern systemic therapies.

Liquid biopsy has gained significance in detecting resistance mutations that guide sequential therapy. Patients who progress on first- or second-generation EGFR-TKIs frequently develop the T790M mutation, which is detectable via plasma via liquid biopsy. The AURA3 trial, in conjunction with real-world studies carried out in Taiwan and France, showed that osimertinib could effectively target T790 M-positive tumors with reduced toxicity(Bencze et al., 2022).

In a similar vein, resistance to ALK inhibitors can occur through many bypass pathways, leading to the need for next-generation agents such as lorlatinib. Currently, KRAS G12C, which was formerly considered undruggable, is being targeted by sotorasib and adagrasib, with early case series from U.S. centers showing disease control rates of >70%, particularly when it was used early(Zhang et al., 2024).

For application, at the palliative end, quality of life, symptom control, and psychological well-being always constitute. Case series and PROs from the United Kingdom and Scandinavia have shed light on the benefits of applying palliative care at an early stage for increased survival and quality of life(Mengting Chen et al., 2023). Most notably, a milestone study by Temel et al. (2010) revealed that early integration of palliative care in advanced NSCLC patients helped in the control of symptoms and prolonged survival. Nutrition, pain management, and dyspnea control form the basis of all advanced care plans, primarily for elderly or frail patients who are considered unfit for any further aggressive systemic therapies.

Real-world problems retain their paramount nature, especially in low- and middle-income countries. Cases from India, Africa, and Latin America report very limited access, if any, to molecular diagnostics and immunotherapy; thus, they are still reliant on platinum doublets and oral metronomic regimens(Mengting Chen et al., 2023). In a multicenter study in India, the median OS in metastatic NSCLC patients who were administered chemotherapy alone was approximately 10–12 months, which was much lower than that in patients in whom targeted therapy and immunotherapy were employed. This calls for health equity, cost-effective treatment, and access to molecular testing worldwide(Araghi et al., 2023).

An interesting development was the recognition of oligometastatic NSCLC, which generally offers up to limited metastatic disease (e.g., ≤5 lesions), which has given rise to curative-intent treatment paradigms, including local ablative therapy (LAT) by surgery or stereotactic body radiotherapy (SBRT)(Jongbloed et al., 2024). Since the SABR-COMET trial and follow-up studies, prolonged progression-free survival (PFS) and even overall survival (OS) benefits have been observed in patients treated with LAT along with systemic therapies. A Canadian case series reported a 3-year OS of well over 40% in patients with limited liver or adrenal metastases treated with SBRT and immunotherapy, thereby questioning the traditional palliative-only treatment approach for stage IV patients(Olson et al., 2020).

4. SPECIAL CLINICAL SCENARIOS IN NON-SMALL CELL LUNG CANCER (NSCLC)

With the introduction of personalized medicine, high-end imaging facilities, and immunotherapeutics, the management of NSCLC has undergone tremendous transformation. However, with this transformation, a few special clinical scenarios that do not fit the conventional treatment algorithms present themselves to the clinicians, thereby demanding individualized decision-making(Ramos et al., 2025). These situations include cases such as those with poor performance status, elderly people, NSCLC during pregnancy, oligometastatic disease, NSCLC with uncommon driver mutations, autoimmune disorders, and organ dysfunction (hepatic or renal). Each of these places special demands and requires a more nuanced understanding of the disease, the overall health status of the patient, and options in treatment evolving in parallel(Pavlick et al., 2023). We hereby discuss these special scenarios in light of recent clinical evidence and large case series around the world.

One of the most tricky subgroups is those with an Eastern Cooperative Oncology Group (ECOG) performance status rating of 2--3, who have historically been excluded from clinical trials. These patients commonly suffer from comorbidities or disease burdens affecting their functional status; thus, these conventional systemic treatments could pose a threat to them. A pooled analysis by Giaj-Levra et al. (2020) highlighted that PS2 patients who have been carefully selected may still benefit from targeted therapies and immunotherapy, especially when an actionable mutation is involved. For example, in an Italian case series, NSCLC patients with EGFR mutation and PS2-3 showed marked improvements clinically with first-line use of osimertinib; in a few situations, their poor performance status was reversed so that they were subsequently reclassified back to good performance status, qualifying them for further treatment. Furthermore, immunotherapy as a single entity (e.g., pembrolizumab) was found to be tolerable in frail patients with high PD-L1 expression in the PePS2 trial (2020), reaffirming its option in such a setting.

Elderly patients ($\geq$ 70 years) are considered another important patient subgroup who often suffer from polypharmacy, frailty, and physical decline. These conditions decrease the ability of the body to tolerate side effects from chemotherapy or targeted therapies. Thus, although age per se is never an absolute contraindication to aggressive treatment, elderly patients are simply more prone to experiencing treatment-related adverse events. According to some retrospective and registry-based studies from Japan and the U.S., suitably selected elderly patients with NSCLC can tolerate EGFR TKIs very well and immunotherapy in many cases. The subgroup analysis of the KEYNOTE-024 trial demonstrated that pembrolizumab was associated with a survival benefit irrespective of age, especially for patients over 75 years. Furthermore, real-world evidence from SEER-Medicare has suggested that combination chemoimmunotherapy may not be as favorable as immunotherapy monotherapy in this population for toxicity and hospitalization. Geriatric assessment and shared decision-making aid in tailoring therapy in these patients.

A very rare but clinically significant situation is in NSCLC-associated pregnancy, in which complex ethical and therapeutic dilemmas arise. Although these are rare (at an occurrence of approximately 0.1 in 1,000 pregnancies), maternal lung cancer often progresses from delayed diagnosis. The literature in case reports and small series suggests that chemotherapy with platinum-based agents (e.g., carboplatin–paclitaxel) may be considered relatively safe with close fetal monitoring if the patient is diagnosed in the second or third trimester. In a multinational review published in Cancer (2020), chemotherapy was found not to significantly increase congenital abnormalities if it was administered past the first trimester. Nevertheless, targeted therapies and immunotherapy remain contraindicated because of a lack of safety data during pregnancy. In almost all cases, if early-stage disease is diagnosed, treatment is avoided until the patient becomes postpartum. For the care of the mother and fetus, the multidisciplinary team indeed must engage in reviewing oncologic, obstetric, and neonatal matters.

Oligometastatic NSCLC, or limited metastatic disease (usually 5 or fewer lesions), represents a potentially curable condition, where the recognition of its existence undoes the traditional distinction between metastatic and localized disease. The concept of CLT, pursued via SBRT, surgery, or ablation, seems to appear more frequently in the discussion since SABR-COMET and Gomez et al. demonstrated that CLT and systemic therapy significantly improve select patients in terms of PFS and, in some cases, OS. Case series in Canada and the Netherlands reported 40% plus 2- to 5-year survival in oligometastatic patients receiving aggressive treatment. This has led to LAT being mentioned in all the relevant guidelines for selected patients, particularly those with good PS, controlled primary tumors, and limited extrathoracic spread.

Another special scenario involves NSCLC patients with uncommon or complex molecular alterations, such as HER2 insertion, RET rearrangement, NTRK fusion, MET exon 14 skipping mutation, and BRAF V600E mutation. Since these mutations are rare individually (<3% each in NSCLC), their discovery through next-generation sequencing (NGS) has offered new treatment opportunities. Drugs such as trastuzumab deruxtecan (HER2), selpercatinib (RET), entrectinib (NTRK), tepotinib (MET), and dabrafenib-trametinib (BRAF) have shown high levels of activity within these molecular subsets. Academic centers and expanded access programs have reported case series reporting a 50–70% response rate with the use of these drugs. For example, in the LIBRETTO-001 trial, selpercatinib produced a response rate greater than 60% in RET fusion-positive NSCLC with excellent CNS activity. Thus, the challenge focuses on permitting access to these therapies and implementing them in standard-of-care algorithms in various healthcare settings.

Patients with preexisting AIDs, such as rheumatoid arthritis, lupus, or inflammatory bowel disease, introduce yet another therapeutic dilemma in the immunotherapy era. These patients were excluded from the landmark ICI trials for fear of exacerbating their underlying ailment. However, real-world data imply that ICIs can be used cautiously in selected AIDS patients under close observation. One retrospective review from MD Anderson Cancer Center reported that flares occurred in 25 to 30% of cases but could be controlled with steroids and rarely required that treatment be stopped. Those with quiescent disease who did not require immunosuppression had fewer complications and better treatment outcomes. These cases demand individualized risk–benefit analyses and collaboration among rheumatologists.

The management of NSCLC in a setting of hepatic or renal dysfunction constitutes yet another layer of complexity, with systemic therapies being largely dependent on these organs for either metabolism or excretion. All platinum agents, TKIs, and immunotherapy agents have different pharmacokinetics depending on hepatic and renal function. For example, carboplatin dosing is dependent on the glomerular filtration rate (GFR), making it superior to cisplatin in patients with moderate renal impairment. TKIs such as gefitinib and osimertinib are usually metabolized by the liver and hence require dose adjustments under conditions of severe hepatic dysfunction; however, they are generally considered safe in mild-to-moderate impairment. Cases reported from tertiary cancer centers suggest that checkpoint inhibitors have been safely used with success in patients under dialysis for end-stage renal disease, which calls for larger studies. Additionally, dose modification, monitoring of drug therapy, and interdisciplinary management are needed for the safe treatment of such patients.

In the end, for post-transplant NSCLC, these end-stage disease cases constitute a unique, yet grave, subset, particularly among recipients of lung or renal transplants who are immunocompromised and at high risk for cancer. Immunotherapy is contraindicated because of the very high risk of rejection. However, case series from transplant oncology registries suggest that patients may still benefit from being subjected to cytotoxic chemotherapy or targeted therapy if molecular markers are detected. In a France-based source cohort, the use of an EGFR TKI in a post-kidney transplant NSCLC patient was demonstrated to be a valid technique without causing much compromise to the graft. On the other hand, the use of immunotherapy remains experimental within this group and should be strictly confined to cases of refractory disease with full patient consent and ethical review.

5. EMERGING THERAPEUTICS & FUTURE DIRECTIONS

Advances in the field of science and technology has paved way for targeted therapeutic innovations and immunotherapies to address challenges associated with infrastructure, cost and access to drugs with equity thereby overcoming the limitations associated with LMICs countries. In this area of medicine, a revolution is underway for non-small cell lung cancer (NSCLC) treatment, largely due to molecular biology, immunotherapy, targeted agents, and novel drug delivery systems. Once considered a death sentence, especially at later stages, vis-à-vis NSCLC is gaining interest as a chronic disease, with some subsets undergoing durable remission or even functional cures(Ali, 2024). Therefore, the treatment armamentarium again had to change from cytotoxic chemotherapy to include a wider range of newer agents that target molecular alterations, immune checkpoints, angiogenesis, and the tumor microenvironment (TME). In tandem with the continuing inclination toward uncovering the molecular and immunologic drivers of NSCLC, future trends are now defined by precision medicine, AI-driven diagnostics, combination protocols, and patient-specific treatment algorithms(Wang et al., 2023).

In recent decades, recognizing and tackling oncogenic driver mutations has become truly groundbreaking. Classic targets, including EGFR, ALK, and ROS1, among others, play the role of tyrosine kinase inhibitors (TKIs) in front-line settings. Moreover, new molecular targets, such as KRAS G12C, MET exon 14 skipping, RET fusions, NTRK fusions, and HER2 mutations, have generalized the therapeutic landscape(Duan et al., 2024). With first-in-class KRAS G12C inhibitors, sotorasib and adagrasib have produced evidence of clinical promise and manageable toxicity in the pretreated populations of the CodeBreaK 100 and KRYSTAL-1 trials, respectively. For patients with MET-altered NSCLC, capmatinib and tepotinib have been shown to have ORRs of more than 40%, with strong intracranial activity. Similarly, selpercatinib and pralsetinib for RET-rearranged NSCLC and trastuzumab deruxtecan for HER2-mutant NSCLC are poised to change treatment paradigms in rare subtypes(Singhal et al., 2024). These agents, which have superior response rates and better quality of life than chemotherapy does, underscore the need for universal comprehensive genomic profiling for all NSCLC patients, irrespective of stage.

Immunotherapy has become the other major therapeutic strategy for NSCLC alongside molecularly guided therapy. ICIs, most famously anti-PD-1/PD-L1 monoclonal antibodies such as nivolumab, pembrolizumab, and atezolizumab, have transformed the treatment landscape of metastatic and locally advanced NSCLC. Landmark clinical trials, including KEYNOTE-024, IMpower110, and CheckMate 227, have demonstrated enhanced survival with immunotherapy administered as monotherapy or in combination with chemotherapy(Marei et al., 2023). However, several issues remain: only a subset of patients achieve long-term benefit, and biomarkers such as PD-L1 expression and TMB only imperfectly predict response to such regimens. Tomorrow's immunotherapy targets will likely include dual checkpoint blockade (e.g., PD-1 + CTLA-4 inhibition), immune agonists, bispecific antibodies, and personalized cancer vaccines(Marei et al., 2023). For example, the CheckMate 9LA regimen with nivolumab and ipilimumab plus two cycles of chemotherapy improved OS and PFS in both PD-L1-high and PD-L1-low patients and may represent a very useful tool for broadening the window for immunotherapy benefit.

Another area of intense investigation is that of combination therapies. Rational combinations of targeted therapies with immunotherapy, chemotherapy, or anti-angiogenic agents are being investigated to overcome primary and acquired resistance(Marei et al., 2023). For example, the addition of bevacizumab, an anti-VEGF agent, to atezolizumab and chemotherapy (as in IMpower150) has been shown to improve outcomes, especially in patients with liver metastases. There are stimulating combinations under consideration, including the use of epigenetic modulators such as HDAC inhibitors combined with ICIs to promote T-cell infiltration within immune-excluded tumors. ADCs are gaining traction as novel therapeutic classes in NSCLC. In addition to trastuzumab deruxtecan, datopotamab deruxtecan, an ADC that targets TROP2, is under phase 3 evaluation and has demonstrated prominent activity in both squamous and nonsquamous histologies(Rebuzzi et al., 2019).

In parallel, the tumor microenvironment has surfaced as a promising therapeutic frontier. Tumor-associated macrophages (TAMs), cancer-associated fibroblasts (CAFs), and myeloid-derived suppressor cells (MDSCs) contribute to immune evasion and the development of resistance to therapy(Jia et al., 2025). Novel agents targeting these components, such as CSF1R inhibitors and TGF-β antagonists, are being tested in early-phase clinical trials. The pathway, which includes stimulator of interferon genes (STING) and a key component of innate immune sensing, is also harnessed to favor antitumor immunity. The combination of STING agonists with ICIs is thought to convert immunologically cold tumors into responsive tumors, hence broadening the applicability of immunotherapy(Akram et al., 2025).

Liquid biopsy and real-time molecular monitoring constitute another promising field, allowing for dynamic treatment adaptation and resistance tracking. Circulating tumor DNA (ctDNA) profiling permits noninvasive mutation detection, minimal residual disease (MRD) monitoring, and early resistance mutation identification, such as EGFR T790M or MET amplification(Pandey and Yadav, 2025). The integration of liquid biopsy within clinical trials such as BFAST and NILE is shaping a potential shift toward precision-guided therapy before any form of radiologic progression can take place.

Radiation oncology has developed in areas such as stereotactic ablative radiotherapy and proton beam therapy to offer more precise, tissue-sparing treatment for oligometastatic and localized disease. There is growing evidence to suggest synergistic effects between SABR and systemic agents. For example, the SABR-COMET and NRG-LU002 trials have indicated that adding SABR to systemic therapy may enhance local control and potentially improve survival in oligometastatic NSCLC patients(Stereotactic Ablative Radiotherapy for the Treatment of Oligometastatic Cancer: A Clinical Review as Part of a Health Technology Assessment, Version 2.0, 2022). Radiation-induced immunogenic cell death is concurrently being exploited to increase checkpoint inhibitor efficacy, thus laying the framework for radioimmunotherapy protocol development. On the technical side, artificial intelligence (AI) and machine learning (ML) have started to make imprints in NSCLC care. Predictive algorithms for risk stratification, treatment selection, and early diagnosis based on radiomic, genomic, and electronic health records are being developed(Lynch et al., 2024). AI-powered platforms can help with patient selection for clinical trials while also predicting resistance mechanisms by accounting for molecular evolution Table 3.

Patient-centric precision oncology should mark the future of NSCLC care. This involves therapies customized to the molecular and immunological profile but equally integrates other parameters: patient-reported outcomes (PROs), digital biomarkers, and wearables, potentially registering patient reports on tolerability and/or effectiveness in real time. Here, multiomics approaches involving genomics, proteomics, transcriptomics, and metabolomics can shed light on tumor biology in a holistic manner and provide further target candidates(Lynch et al., 2024). NGS and scRNA-seq present themselves as the next critical technologies unlocking the intratumoral heterogeneity and evolutionary trajectories of NSCLC, setting the scene for combination strategies designed against resistance. With further reductions in price and increased availability, such broad-panel NGS is set to become the norm at diagnosis, recurrence, and progression(Satam et al., 2023). For the sake of health equity and global access, future strategies should also aim to reduce disparities in the availability of diagnostics and therapeutics. To be of impact universally, NSCLC advances must be tested in underrepresented populations, expanded access programs for expensive new agents must be provided, and practical biomarker assays for the cheaper side must be developed.

The table below provides a list of high-impact emerging trials that are shaping the future of NSCLC care. These involve novel classes of drugs, biomarker-driven designs, and combination therapies to address resistance, tumor heterogeneity, and treatment personalization.

Table 3. Selected Emerging and Ongoing Trials in NSCLC.

Trial Name	Therapeutic Focus	Patient Population	Phase	Key Investigational Agent(s)	Objective/Endpoint
CodeBreaK 200	KRAS G12C Inhibition vs. docetaxel	Previously treated NSCLC	III	Sotorasib	PFS and OS in KRAS G12C-mutant NSCLC
CheckMate 9LA	Chemo + dual immunotherapy	Stage IV NSCLC	III	Nivolumab + Ipilimumab + Chemo	Overall survival improvement
TROPION-Lung01	ADC (TROP2 targeting)	Advanced NSCLC	III	Datopotamab deruxtecan	Comparison to docetaxel in previously treated patients

continued on following page

Table 3. Continued

Trial Name	Therapeutic Focus	Patient Population	Phase	Key Investigational Agent(s)	Objective/Endpoint
LU002 (NRG)	SABR + systemic therapy	Oligometastatic NSCLC	III	Radiotherapy + Chemo/IO	OS and local control
KEYLYNK-008	ICI + PARP inhibition	Metastatic NSCLC (no driver)	III	Pembrolizumab + Olaparib	PFS/OS in PD-L1 positive patients
BFAST	ctDNA-driven targeted therapy	Stage IV NSCLC	II	Biomarker-guided multiple agents	Feasibility of plasma genotyping in real time

6. CONCLUSION

The integration of the molecular approach will help us to understand the molecular mechanisms underlying the phenotype and gobal perspective on approach to the disease will turn foster patient centered, affordable and equitable NSCLC careNon-small cell lung cancer (NSCLC) continues to be among the top global health challenges because of its high incidence, late diagnosis, and molecular heterogeneity. The past decades have seen a paradigm shift in how the disease is understood and managed—from an all-approach model to one that is becoming precision-based, ideally focused on molecular profiling, immunology, and the patient(Hendriks et al., 2024). Early-stage NSCLC (stage I-II), as seen from case studies, is usually best treated with prompt surgery, sometimes followed by chemotherapy or radiotherapy in selected cases. The developments in imaging, minimally invasive surgical techniques, and patient stratification have improved survival. Even at this curative stage, however, recurrence is a possibility; thus, closer follow-up and, if possible, targeted treatment of molecularly defined subgroups are needed(Saw et al., 2024). Locally advanced NSCLC (stage IIB--IIIB) is another level of an even more complex puzzle. Usually, multimodality treatment is the standard-of-care consisting of concurrent chemoradiation; however, consolidation immunotherapy is increasingly being adopted. Recent approval of durvalumab after chemoradiation in unresectable Stage III disease (based on the PACIFIC trial) has set new benchmarks for progression-free and overall survival. These stages necessitate interdisciplinary collaboration, and management decisions are made based on the biology of the tumor coupled with considerations of the patient's performance status, comorbidities, and anatomical factors(Spigel et al., 2022).

In advanced and metastatic NSCLC (stage IV), the most dramatic change in the approach to therapy has occurred. From conventional platinum-based chemotherapeutics to highly specific tyrosine kinase inhibitors (TKIs) and immune checkpoint inhibitors (ICIs), survival has greatly improved, especially among those harboring actionable mutations or high PD-L1 expression(König et al., 2021). Patients with EGFR mutations, ALK rearrangements, or MET exon 14 skipping may experience long-term responses to targeted therapies, whereas patients treated with immunotherapy with or without chemotherapy can experience long-term remission. However, resistance mechanisms, immune escape, and disease heterogeneity continue to press for newer and more flexible treatment strategies(König et al., 2021). There have been occasion-specific diseases such as brain metastases, oligometastatic disease, elderly patients, and poor performance status, laying the groundwork for the necessity of individualized care(Thelen and Hennessy, 2025). With the progression of stereotactic radiosurgery, blood–brain barrier (BBB)-penetrable TKIs, and immunotherapeutic modalities with palliative intent, patients with complex presentations are allowed to benefit from therapeutic innovations, ensuring that their quality of life is not compromised. The field of NSCLC treatment will continue to expand as exploratory research continues through the emergence of novel therapeutics, combination regimens, next-generation immunomodulators, ADCs, and personalized vaccines(Papastavrou et al., 2015). Liquid biopsies and AI-guided decision-making tools integrated with multiomic data could be used to streamline treatment selection and monitor disease evolution in real time. On an equal standing is the option to eradicate inequalities in care, ensure that trials are representative, and lay down a cost-effective route to implement at a global scale.

REFERENCES

Akram, F., Ali, A. M., Akhtar, M. T., Fatima, T., Shabbir, I., & ul Haq, I. (2025). ul Haq I. The journey of antibody-drug conjugates for revolutionizing cancer therapy: A review. *Bioorganic & Medicinal Chemistry*, *117*, 118010. DOI: 10.1016/j.bmc.2024.118010 PMID: 39586174

Ali A. (2024). Advances in Non-Small Cell Lung Cancer (NSCLC) Treatment—A Paradigm Shift in Oncology. Pharm 2024, Vol 17, Page 246 17:246. .DOI: 10.3390/ph17020246

Araghi, M., Mannani, R., Heidarnejad maleki, A., Hamidi, A., Rostami, S., Safa, S. H., Faramarzi, F., Khorasani, S., Alimohammadi, M., Tahmasebi, S., & Akhavan-Sigari, R. (2023). Recent advances in non-small cell lung cancer targeted therapy; an update review. *Cancer Cell International*, *23*(1), 162. DOI: 10.1186/s12935-023-02990-y PMID: 37568193

Attili, I., Fuorivia, V., Spitaleri, G., Corvaja, C., Trillo Aliaga, P., Del Signore, E., Asnaghi, R., Carnevale Schianca, A., Passaro, A., & de Marinis, F. (2024). Alectinib vs. Lorlatinib in the Front-Line Setting for ALK-Rearranged Non-Small-Cell Lung Cancer (NSCLC): A Deep Dive into the Main Differences across ALEX and CROWN Phase 3 Trials. *Cancers (Basel)*, *16*(13), 2457. DOI: 10.3390/cancers16132457 PMID: 39001519

Bencze, E., Bogos, K., Kohánka, A., Báthory-Fülöp, L., Sárosi, V., Csernák, E., Bittner, N., Melegh, Z., & Tóth, E. (2022). EGFR T790M Mutation Detection in Patients With Non-Small Cell Lung Cancer After First Line EGFR TKI Therapy: Summary of Results in a Three-Year Period and a Comparison of Commercially Available Detection Kits. *Pathology Oncology Research : POR*, *28*, 1610607. DOI: 10.3389/pore.2022.1610607 PMID: 36277960

Biganzoli, L., Cardoso, F., Beishon, M., Cameron, D., Cataliotti, L., Coles, C. E., Delgado Bolton, R. C., Trill, M. D., Erdem, S., Fjell, M., Geiss, R., Goossens, M., Kuhl, C., Marotti, L., Naredi, P., Oberst, S., Palussière, J., Ponti, A., Rosselli Del Turco, M., & Poortmans, P. (2020). The requirements of a specialist breast centre. *The Breast : Official Journal of the European Society of Mastology*, *51*, 65–84. DOI: 10.1016/j.breast.2020.02.003 PMID: 32217457

Chen, M., Yu, H., Yang, L., Yang, H., Cao, H., Lei, L., Ma, L., Liu, S., Tian, L., & Wang, S. (2023). Combined early palliative care for non-small-cell lung cancer patients: A randomized controlled trial in Chongqing, China. *Frontiers in Oncology*, *13*, 1184961. DOI: 10.3389/fonc.2023.1184961 PMID: 37781179

Chevallier, M., Borgeaud, M., Addeo, A., & Friedlaender, A. (2021). Oncogenic driver mutations in non-small cell lung cancer: Past, present and future. *World Journal of Clinical Oncology*, *12*(4), 217–237. DOI: 10.5306/wjco.v12.i4.217 PMID: 33959476

de Jager VD, Timens W, Bayle A, Botling J, Brcic L, Büttner R, et al. (2024). Future perspective for the application of predictive biomarker testing in advanced stage non-small cell lung cancer. Lancet Reg Heal - 38:100839. .DOI: 10.1016/j.lanepe.2024.100839

Duan XP, Qin BD, Jiao XD, Liu K, Wang Z, Zang YS. (2024). New clinical trial design in precision medicine: discovery, development and direction. Signal Transduct Target Ther 2024 91 9:1–29. .DOI: 10.1038/s41392-024-01760-0

Field JK, Vulkan D, Davies MPA, Baldwin DR, Brain KE, Devaraj A, et al. Lung cancer mortality reduction by LDCT screening: UKLS randomised trial results and international meta-analysis. Lancet Reg Heal - Eur 2021;10:100179. .DOI: 10.1016/j.lanepe.2021.100179

Gang, X., Yan, J., Li, X., Shi, S., Xu, L., Liu, R., Cai, L., Li, H., & Zhao, M. (2024). Immune checkpoint inhibitors rechallenge in non-small cell lung cancer: Current evidence and future directions. *Cancer Letters*, *604*, 217241. DOI: 10.1016/j.canlet.2024.217241 PMID: 39260670

Garg P, Singhal S, Kulkarni P, Horne D, Malhotra J, Salgia R, et al. (2024). Advances in Non-Small Cell Lung Cancer: Current Insights and Future Directions. J Clin Med 2024, Vol 13, Page 4189 13:4189. .DOI: 10.3390/jcm13144189

Grodzka, A., Knopik-Skrocka, A., Kowalska, K., Kurzawa, P., Krzyżaniak, M., & Stencel, K.. (2023). Molecular alterations of driver genes in non-small cell lung cancer: From diagnostics to targeted therapy. *EXCLI Journal*, *22*, 415. DOI: 10.17179/EXCLI2023-6122 PMID: 37346803

Hellmann, M. D., Paz-Ares, L., Bernabe Caro, R., Zurawski, B., Kim, S.-W., Carcereny Costa, E., Park, K., Alexandru, A., Lupinacci, L., de la Mora Jimenez, E., Sakai, H., Albert, I., Vergnenegre, A., Peters, S., Syrigos, K., Barlesi, F., Reck, M., Borghaei, H., Brahmer, J. R., & Ramalingam, S. S. (2019). Nivolumab plus Ipilimumab in Advanced Non–Small-Cell Lung Cancer. *The New England Journal of Medicine*, *381*(21), 2020–2031. DOI: 10.1056/NEJMoa1910231 PMID: 31562796

Hendriks LEL, Remon J, Faivre-Finn C, Garassino MC, Heymach J V., Kerr KM, et al. (2024). Non-small-cell lung cancer. Nat Rev Dis Prim 2024 101 10:1–22. .DOI: 10.1038/s41572-024-00551-9

Huber, R. M., Cavic, M., Balata, H., Borondy Kitts, A., Field, J. K., Henschke, C., Kazerooni, E. A., Kerpel-Fronius, A., Smith, R. A., Taioli, E., Ventura, L., Lam, S., Yankelevitz, D., Tammemägi, M., Yang, D., Zulueta, J., Viola, L., Mohan, A., Cavic, M., & Huber, R.From the International Association for the Study of Lung Cancer Early Detection and Screening Committee. (2024). Terminology Issues in Screening and Early Detection of Lung Cancer—International Association for the Study of Lung Cancer Early Detection and Screenin. *Journal of Thoracic Oncology*, *19*(12), 1606–1617. Advance online publication. DOI: 10.1016/j.jtho.2024.07.022 PMID: 39098452

Jia H, Chen X, Zhang L, Chen M. (2025). Cancer associated fibroblasts in cancer development and therapy. J Hematol Oncol 2025 181 18:1–31. .DOI: 10.1186/s13045-025-01688-0

Jongbloed, M., Bortolot, M., Wee, L., Huijs, J. W. J., Bellezo, M., Vaes, R. D. W., Aboubakar Nana, F., Hartemink, K. J., De Ruysscher, D. K. M., & Hendriks, L. E. L. (2024). Prognostic and Predictive Biomarkers of Oligometastatic NSCLC: New Insights and Clinical Applications. *JTO Clinical and Research Reports*, *5*(12), 100740. DOI: 10.1016/j.jtocrr.2024.100740 PMID: 39735889

König, D., Prince, S. S., & Rothschild, S. I. (2021). Targeted Therapy in Advanced and Metastatic Non-Small Cell Lung Cancer. An Update on Treatment of the Most Important Actionable Oncogenic Driver Alterations. *Cancers (Basel)*, *13*(4), 804. DOI: 10.3390/cancers13040804 PMID: 33671873

Lachance, C. C., Tran, K., Carson, E., Kim, J., Palma, D., Loewen, S., & Ford, C. (2021). Stereotactic Ablative Radiotherapy for the Treatment of Oligometastatic Cancer: A Clinical Review as part of a Health Technology Assessment. *Canadian Journal of Health Technologies*, *1*(3).

Li, C., Lei, S., Ding, L., Xu, Y., Wu, X., Wang, H., Zhang, Z., Gao, T., Zhang, Y., & Li, L. (2023). Global burden and trends of lung cancer incidence and mortality. *Chinese Medical Journal*, *136*(13), 1583–1590. DOI: 10.1097/CM9.0000000000002529 PMID: 37027426

Lynch, C., Pitroda, S. P., & Weichselbaum, R. R. (2024). Radiotherapy, immunity, and immune checkpoint inhibitors. *The Lancet. Oncology*, *25*(8), e352–e362. DOI: 10.1016/S1470-2045(24)00075-5 PMID: 39089313

Marei HE, Hasan A, Pozzoli G, Cenciarelli C. (2023). Cancer immunotherapy with immune checkpoint inhibitors (ICIs): potential, mechanisms of resistance, and strategies for reinvigorating T cell responsiveness when resistance is acquired. Cancer Cell Int 2023 231 23:1–20. .DOI: 10.1186/s12935-023-02902-0

Mitchell, C., Copley, S. J., Viola, P., Lu, H., & Aboagye, E. O. (2023). Radiomics and artificial intelligence for precision medicine in lung cancer treatment. *Seminars in Cancer Biology*, *93*, 97–113. DOI: 10.1016/j.semcancer.2023.05.004 PMID: 37211292

Molina, J. R., Yang, P., Cassivi, S. D., Schild, S. E., & Adjei, A. A. (2008). Non–Small Cell Lung Cancer: Epidemiology, Risk Factors, Treatment, and Survivorship. *Mayo Clinic Proceedings*, *83*(5), 584–594. DOI: 10.1016/S0025-6196(11)60735-0 PMID: 18452692

Morrison, E. J., Novotny, P. J., Sloan, J. A., Yang, P., Patten, C. A., & Ruddy, K. J.. (2017). Emotional Problems, Quality of Life, and Symptom Burden in Lung Cancer Patients. *Clinical Lung Cancer*, *18*, 497. DOI: 10.1016/j.cllc.2017.02.008 PMID: 28412094

Nishino, M., Soejima, K., & Mitsudomi, T. (2019). Brain metastases in oncogene-driven non-small cell lung cancer. *Translational Lung Cancer Research*, *8*(S3), S298–S307. DOI: 10.21037/tlcr.2019.05.15 PMID: 31857953

O'Reilly, D., Botticella, A., Barry, S., Cotter, S., Donington, J. S., & Le Pechoux, C.. (2023). *Treatment Decisions for Resectable Non–Small-Cell Lung Cancer: Balancing Less With More?* Am Soc Clin Oncol Educ B., DOI: 10.1200/EDBK_389950/ASSET/9C4BFDDA-4450-4CD7-84CB-C73FD538182F/ASSETS/IMAGES/LARGE/EDBK_389950F2.JPG

Olson, R., Mathews, L., Liu, M., Schellenberg, D., Mou, B., Berrang, T., Harrow, S., Correa, R. J. M., Bhat, V., Pai, H., Mohamed, I., Miller, S., Schneiders, F., Laba, J., Wilke, D., Senthi, S., Louie, A. V., Swaminath, A., Chalmers, A., & Palma, D. A. (2020). Stereotactic ablative radiotherapy for the comprehensive treatment of 1-3 Oligometastatic tumors (SABR-COMET-3): Study protocol for a randomized phase III trial. *BMC Cancer*, *20*(1), 1–12. DOI: 10.1186/s12885-020-06876-4 PMID: 32370765

Pandey, S., & Yadav, P. (2025). Liquid biopsy in cancer management: Integrating diagnostics and clinical applications. *Practical Laboratory Medicine*, *43*, e00446. DOI: 10.1016/j.plabm.2024.e00446 PMID: 39839814

Papastavrou, E., Acaroglu, R., Sendir, M., Berg, A., Efstathiou, G., Idvall, E., Kalafati, M., Katajisto, J., Leino-Kilpi, H., Lemonidou, C., da Luz, M. D. A., & Suhonen, R. (2015). The relationship between individualized care and the practice environment: An international study. *International Journal of Nursing Studies*, *52*(1), 121–133. DOI: 10.1016/j.ijnurstu.2014.05.008 PMID: 24947755

Passaro, A., Al Bakir, M., Hamilton, E. G., Diehn, M., André, F., Roy-Chowdhuri, S., Mountzios, G., Wistuba, I. I., Swanton, C., & Peters, S. (2024). Cancer biomarkers: Emerging trends and clinical implications for personalized treatment. *Cell, 187*(7), 1617–1635. DOI: 10.1016/j.cell.2024.02.041 PMID: 38552610

Pavlick, A. C., Ariyan, C. E., Buchbinder, E. I., Davar, D., Gibney, G. T., Hamid, O., Hieken, T. J., Izar, B., Johnson, D. B., Kulkarni, R. P., Luke, J. J., Mitchell, T. C., Mooradian, M. J., Rubin, K. M., Salama, A. K. S., Shirai, K., Taube, J. M., Tawbi, H. A., Tolley, J. K., & Sullivan, R. J. (2023). Society for Immunotherapy of Cancer (SITC) clinical practice guideline on immunotherapy for the treatment of melanoma, version 3.0. *Journal for Immunotherapy of Cancer, 11*(10), e006947. DOI: 10.1136/jitc-2023-006947 PMID: 37852736

Piña-Sánchez, P., Chávez-González, A., Ruiz-Tachiquín, M., Vadillo, E., Monroy-García, A., Montesinos, J. J., Grajales, R., Gutiérrez de la Barrera, M., & Mayani, H. (2021). Cancer Biology, Epidemiology, and Treatment in the 21st Century: Current Status and Future Challenges From a Biomedical Perspective. *Cancer Control : Cancer Care in Emerging Health Systems, 28*, 10732748211038736. DOI: 10.1177/10732748211038735 PMID: 34565215

Poon, C., Haderi, A., Roediger, A., & Yuan, M. (2022). Should we screen for lung cancer? A 10-country analysis identifying key decision-making factors. *Health Policy (Amsterdam), 126*(9), 879–888. DOI: 10.1016/j.healthpol.2022.06.003 PMID: 35750552

Prabhash, K. (2019). Treatment of advanced nonsmall cell lung cancer: First line, maintenance and second line – Indian consensus statement update. *South Asian Journal of Cancer, 8*(1), 1. DOI: 10.4103/sajc.sajc_227_18 PMID: 30766843

Ramalingam, S. S., Vansteenkiste, J., Planchard, D., Cho, B. C., Gray, J. E., Ohe, Y., Zhou, C., Reungwetwattana, T., Cheng, Y., Chewaskulyong, B., Shah, R., Cobo, M., Lee, K. H., Cheema, P., Tiseo, M., John, T., Lin, M.-C., Imamura, F., Kurata, T., & Soria, J.-C. (2020). Overall Survival with Osimertinib in Untreated, EGFR - Mutated Advanced NSCLC. *The New England Journal of Medicine, 382*(1), 41–50. DOI: 10.1056/NEJMoa1913662 PMID: 31751012

Ramos R, Moura CS, Costa M, Lamas NJ, Correia R, Garcez D, et al. (2025). Lung Cancer Therapy: The Role of Personalized Medicine. Cancers 2025, Vol 17, Page 725 17:725. .DOI: 10.3390/cancers17050725

Rebuzzi, S. E., Facchinetti, F., & Tiseo, M. (2019). Anti-angiogenesis boosts chemo-immunotherapy in patients with EGFR mutations or baseline liver metastases: Insights from IMpower150 study. *Translational Cancer Research*, *8*(Suppl 6), S612–S617. DOI: 10.21037/tcr.2019.06.21 PMID: 35117143

Rodríguez-Abreu, D., Powell, S. F., Hochmair, M. J., Gadgeel, S., Esteban, E., Felip, E., Speranza, G., De Angelis, F., Dómine, M., Cheng, S. Y., Bischoff, H. G., Peled, N., Reck, M., Hui, R., Garon, E. B., Boyer, M., Kurata, T., Yang, J., Pietanza, M. C., & Garassino, M. C. (2021). Pemetrexed plus platinum with or without pembrolizumab in patients with previously untreated metastatic nonsquamous NSCLC: Protocol-specified final analysis from KEYNOTE-189. *Annals of Oncology : Official Journal of the European Society for Medical Oncology*, *32*(7), 881–895. DOI: 10.1016/j.annonc.2021.04.008 PMID: 33894335

Russano, M., La Cava, G., Cortellini, A., Citarella, F., Galletti, A., Di Fazio, G. R., ... (2023). Immunotherapy for Metastatic Non-Small Cell Lung Cancer: Therapeutic Advances and Biomarkers. Curr Oncol 2023, Vol 30, Pages 2366-2387 30:2366–87. DOI: 10.3390/curroncol30020181

Satam, H., Joshi, K., Mangrolia, U., Waghoo, S., Zaidi, G., Rawool, S., Thakare, R. P., Banday, S., Mishra, A. K., Das, G., & Malonia, S. K. (2023). Next-Generation Sequencing Technology: Current Trends and Advancements. *Biology (Basel)*, *12*(7), 997. DOI: 10.3390/biology12070997 PMID: 37508427

Saw, S. P. L., & Le, X. (2024). *Lizza; Hendriks EL, Remon J. New Treatment Options for Patients With Oncogene-Addicted Non-Small Cell Lung Cancer Focusing on EGFR-Mutant Tumors Citation for published version (APA)*. New Treatment Options for Patients With Oncogene-Addicted Non-Small Cell Lung Cancer Focusing on EGFR., DOI: 10.1200/EDBK_432516

Sayre, J. W., Toklu, H. Z., Ye, F., Mazza, J., & Yale, S. (2017). Case Reports, Case Series – From Clinical Practice to Evidence-Based Medicine in Graduate Medical Education. *Cureus*, *9*, e1546. DOI: 10.7759/cureus.1546 PMID: 29018643

Singhal A, Li BT, O'Reilly EM. (2024). Targeting KRAS in cancer. Nat Med 2024 304 30:969–83. .DOI: 10.1038/s41591-024-02903-0

Spencer, A., Williams, J., Samuel, R., Boon, I. S., Clarke, K., & Jain, P. (2021). Concurrent versus sequential chemoradiotherapy for unresectable locally advanced stage III non-small cell lung cancer: Retrospective analysis in a single United Kingdom cancer centre. *Cancer Treatment and Research Communications*, *29*, 100460. DOI: 10.1016/j.ctarc.2021.100460 PMID: 34598059

Spigel, D. R., Faivre-Finn, C., Gray, J. E., Vicente, D., Planchard, D., Paz-Ares, L., Vansteenkiste, J. F., Garassino, M. C., Hui, R., Quantin, X., Rimner, A., Wu, Y.-L., Özgüroğlu, M., Lee, K. H., Kato, T., de Wit, M., Kurata, T., Reck, M., Cho, B. C., & Antonia, S. J. (2022). Five-Year Survival Outcomes From the PACIFIC Trial: Durvalumab After Chemoradiotherapy in Stage III Non-Small-Cell Lung Cancer. *Journal of Clinical Oncology*, *40*(12), 1301–1311. DOI: 10.1200/JCO.21.01308 PMID: 35108059

Thelen, H., & Hennessy, S. (2025). Characterizing Treatment Effect Heterogeneity Using Real-World Data. *Clinical Pharmacology and Therapeutics*, *117*(5), 1209–1216. DOI: 10.1002/cpt.3627 PMID: 40047339

Wang, Q., Shao, X., Zhang, Y., Zhu, M., Wang, F. X. C., Mu, J., Li, J., Yao, H., & Chen, K. (2023). Role of tumor microenvironment in cancer progression and therapeutic strategy. *Cancer Medicine*, *12*(10), 11149–11165. DOI: 10.1002/cam4.5698 PMID: 36807772

Yu, X., Si, J., Wei, J., Wang, Y., Sun, Y., Jin, J., Zhang, X., Ma, T., & Song, Z. (2022). The effect of EGFR-TKIs on survival in advanced non-small-cell lung cancer with EGFR mutations: A real-world study. *Cancer Medicine*, *12*(5), 5630–5638. DOI: 10.1002/cam4.5413 PMID: 36380563

Zeng, L., Yu, X., Yu, T., Xiao, J., & Huang, Y. (2019). Interventions for smoking cessation in people diagnosed with lung cancer. *Cochrane Database of Systematic Reviews*, *2019*(6), CD011751. Advance online publication. DOI: 10.1002/14651858.CD011751.pub3 PMID: 31173336

Zhang, J., Lim, S. M., Yu, M. R., Chen, C., Wang, J., Wang, W., Rui, H., Lu, J., Lu, S., Mok, T., Chen, Z. J., & Cho, B. C. (2024). D3S-001, a KRAS G12C Inhibitor with Rapid Target Engagement Kinetics, Overcomes Nucleotide Cycling, and Demonstrates Robust Preclinical and Clinical Activities. *Cancer Discovery*, *14*(9), 1675–1698. DOI: 10.1158/2159-8290.CD-24-0006 PMID: 38717075

Chapter 8
Surgical Management of NSCLC and Postoperative Care and Complications

K. Kesavardhini
Department of Microbiology, Sacred Heart College, Tirupattur, India

K. Gayathri
https://orcid.org/0009-0007-3786-2009
Department of Microbiology, Sacred Heart College, Tirupattur, India

E. Tharani
Department of Microbiology, Sacred Heart College, Tirupattur, India

P. Saranraj
https://orcid.org/0000-0002-5052-6532
Department of Microbiology, Sacred Heart College, Tirupattur, India

ABSTRACT

Approximately 85% of lung cancer incidences are classified as non-small-cell lung cancers associated with elevated death and morbidity rates. Over the past decade, significant advancements have been made in the treatment with non-small cells lung tumours, resulting in improved early detection and therapy of pre-invasive and early-stage cancers. Surgery is the primary therapeutic modality in the initial phases of non-small cells lung cancer. Thoracoscopic lobectomy as an optimal option for early-stage non-small cell lung carcinoma patients, as it minimises the likelihood of complications, discomfort, and haemorrhage postoperatively. However, problems with thoracoscopic lobectomy, like sputum retention and decreased respiratory muscle function, ranged from 19 to 59%. The significant function of

DOI: 10.4018/979-8-3373-2096-0.ch008

pneumonectomy in managing early-stage Non-Small Cells Lung Cancer (NSCLC) is its effectiveness as a surgical therapy. Stages III and IV lung cancer are often the ones that are identified as incurable. A complicated disease, stage III lung cancer can affect some people with technically resectable Non-Small Cell Tumours in the Lungs (NSCLC), multimodal options for treatment, including chemoradiotherapy post-surgery, constitute the most efficacious strategy. Salvage therapy is the principal surgical method for unresectable stages III/IV NSCLC, entailing the removal of residual or recurring lesions following non-surgical intervention. Surgical intervention may be utilised for the treatment of oligometastatic stage IV Non-Small Cell Lung Cancer (NSCLC). The management of NSCLC frequently presents difficulties for postoperative pulmonary rehabilitation. Recent advancements in surgical lung rehabilitation for those with NSCLC were disclosed, aimed at assisting researchers in identifying more efficacious therapies.

1. INTRODUCTION

Lung cancer has the highest fatality rate worldwide and negatively impacts patient health. According to data from China's National Cancer Centers (Chen et al., 2015), there were roughly 610,200 fatalities and 733,300 new diagnoses of Non-Small Cell Lung Cancer (NSCLC) in 2015. Sung et al. (2021) state that GLOBOCAN 2020 revealed China had 820,000 total lung cancer incidences in 2020, constituting nearly 18% of all new cases of cancer. Furthermore, lung cancer accounted for around 23.8 percent of all cases deaths caused by cancer, much above the proportion of mortality from other cancer types. In the past decade, China's carcinoma of the lung mortality rate has risen more rapidly than the worldwide average. The primary histological subtype for lung cancer, which includes adenocarcinoma and carcinoma of squamous cells, is classified as Non-Small Cell Lung Cancer (NSCLC), accounting for around 85% of all cases. Surgery is the principal intervention for early-onset Non-Small Cells Cell Lung Cancer (NSCLC) (Sung et al., 2021).

Recent advancements in contemporary medicine, ongoing advocacy for lung cancer screening, and heightened health awareness have enhanced the identification of early-stage pulmonary disorders. The rates of surgical procedures and patient survival are also rising. Furthermore, there has been an increased emphasis on improving patient's quality of life following surgery (Chen et al., 2016). Thoracoscopy technology has advanced significantly in recent years, offering substantial therapeutic and diagnostic advantages in the treatment of many respiratory disorders. Thoracoscopy is the principal therapeutic approach for lung cancer due to its minimal pain and repercussions. Thoracoscopic lobectomy is recognized as the superior intervention for early-stage NSCLC (Non-Small Cell Lung Cancer) due to of its diminished intraoperative bleeding, less pain, and fewer side effects (Wang et al., 2020).

The histology, tumour stages, molecular attributes, and Assessment of the patient's comprehensive health significantly influences the therapy of lungs cancer patients. The American Society of Clinical Oncology, the European Society of the Medical Oncologists, the National Comprehensive Cancer Network (NCCN), and the Japan Lung Cancer Society delineate current guidelines for lung cancer treatment management (Wei et al., 2020). Stage I-II NSCLC patients commonly have surgery to cure. Stage 3 Non-Small Cell Lung Cancer (NSCLC) patients usually receive radiation, chemotherapy, and surgery. Stage IV or recurrent patients with non-small-cell lung cancer receive chemotherapy, TKIs, and ICIs. In the presence of a mutation within the Epidermal Growth Factors Receptor (EGFR) genes, molecular-targeted therapies such as Tyrosine Kinase Inhibitors (TKIs) are selected; otherwise, cytotoxic chemotherapy or Immune Checkpoint Inhibitors (ICIs) are employed (Palma et al., 2014).

In the last two decades, many genetic alterations in genes regulating cell division and proliferation have been identified as “driver mutations” of lung cancer. Through downstream signaling pathways, these driver mutations have the ability to alter cells that depend on particular signaling for survival and ongoing evolution. Over ten low molecular inhibitors targeting the protein product of certain driver mutations are approved for routine therapeutic usage. The comprehensive Quality of Life (or QoL) and medical outcomes of patients have markedly enhanced with the advent of these novel drugs. However, they have been linked to a wide range of toxicities because of their unique Pharmacodynamic characteristics. While maintaining these treatments is essential to attaining the greatest possible clinical benefit, managing these toxicities optimally in routine clinical practice can be difficult. Furthermore, stopping these medications may cause a disease flare, which could have negative consequences. One of the characteristics of cancer is immune evasion. The identification of molecules on the surfaces of immune system cells that function as check point inhibitors, by modifying the immune response to cancerous cells, has influenced the advancement of innovative therapeutics for non-small cell lung carcinomas (Bergetho et al., 2012).

2. STAGES OF NSCLC AND THE CURRENT STATUS OF CANCER OF THE LUNG SURGERY

2.1 Clinical Staging of Patients with NSCLC

The American Society for Clinical Oncology, the European Society of the Medical Oncology, the National Comprehensive Cancer Network (NCCN) and the Japan

Lung Cancer Society represent the authoritative guidelines for lung cancer treatment (Wei et al., 2020). Patients undergoing medical treatment Patients diagnosed with Stages I-II Non-Small Cells Cell Lung Cancer (NSCLC) sometimes necessitate surgical intervention with the objective to cure. Patients being diagnosed with stage 3 NSCLC generally undergo a multimodal treatment regimen that includes radiation therapy, chemotherapy, and surgeries (Lampridis and Scarci, 2023).

Figure 1. Non-small cell lung cancer, stage IIIA

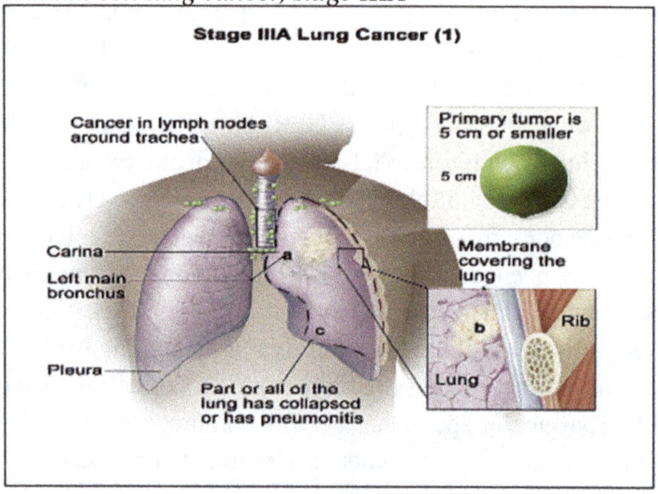

3. SURGICAL PROCEDURES FOR STAGES I–IIIA NSCLC

The surgical excision of non-small cell lung carcinomas provides the greatest likelihood of prolonged survival and the optimal opportunity for a cure. Historically, patients were offered pneumonectomy as the sole operation that consistently produced full resection, eliminating all microscopic and macroscopic signs of disease. Less invasive surgical resections for early-stage NSCLC have resulted in lower post-operative mortality and morbidity rates, as well as more exact staging and survival data (Li et al., 2024). Preoperative imaging and staging reveal that patients with Stages I, II, and a few IIIA (T3N1) NSCLC eligible for pulmonary resection, assuming no additional surgical contraindications exist (Framptom et al., 2015).

Figure 2. The Non-Small Cells Lung Carcinoma Stage 1A condition

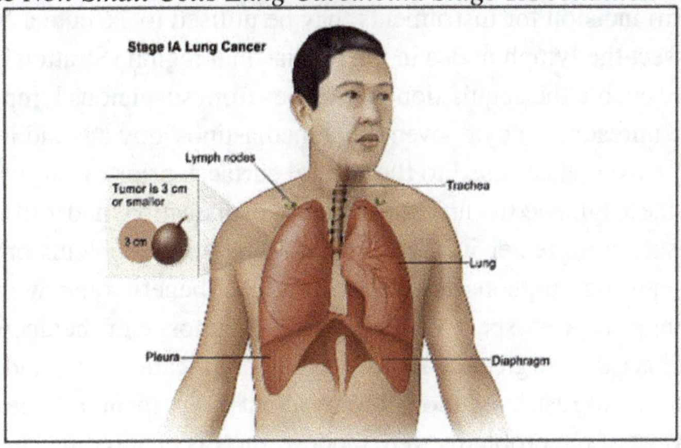

The standard treatment for N2 disease is chemotherapy, either alone or with radiotherapy in North America, whereas, in Eastern Japan and Eastern Europe, patients with proven N2 positive cancers have excision following adjuvant therapy. If a positive response is observed, a sub-group of these individuals might have further resection. In order to achieve negative surgical margins, the optimum surgical method is Thoracotomy and Total resection, depending on the tumor's load and location. This can include Lobectomy, Sleeved Lobectomy, Bilobectomy, and Pneumonectomy. A less invasive method for a typical lobectomy has recently shown comparable survival in prospective data (Wang et al., 2012).

Exact staging of non-small cell lung cancer patients is dependent on evaluation of their mediastinal lymph nodes. Thoracic vascular disease, potentially fatal hemorrhage from thoracic duct punctures (chylothorax), and also recurrent laryngeal nerve injuries necessitating prolonged surgical duration or postoperative hospitalization are among the numerous complications associated with entirely Mediastinal Lymphatic Node Dissection (MLND). The ACOSOG Z0030 experiment examines alternatives to complete dissection, involving lymph node sampling. To evaluate overall and recurrence-free overall survival, ACOSOG Z0030 was conducted randomly. Over 1,100 people with N0 or N1 non-small cell lung cancer or NSCLC have been selected for mediastinal lymph node biopsy or total lymphadenectomy. Initial data for NSCLC indicate that a comprehensive dissection on the mediastinal lymphatic nodes did not Increased morbidity or mortality associated with surgical resection relative to lymph node sampling. Sentinel lymph nodes technology has been proven for use in the mediastinum in the therapy of the melanoma and breast cancer. The clinical importance of mediastinal lymph nodes which are immuno-histochemically positive, yet hematoxylin and eosin negative is unclear. Video-Assisted Thoracoscopic Surgical (VATS) may result in reduced postoperative pain and a diminished recovery duration relative to conventional thoracotomy. A thoracoscope and two small (2–3 cm) incision for instruments may be utilised to execute a VATS lobectomy and dissect the lymph nodes in the mediastinal region (Stratton et al., 2009).

VATS may enable the acquisition of biopsies from suspicious lymph nodes that are otherwise unreachable by conventional mediastinoscopy and aid in staging tumours which have metastasised to the pleural surfaces prior to surgical resection. Nonetheless, the heightened technical complexity of dissections and restricted surgical sight may result in a greater incidence of intraoperative problems or insufficient resections, requiring surgeons to evaluate the cost-benefit ratio with minimally invasive techniques. A prospective study of 895 diagnostic or therapeutic thoracoscopies found a 1.0% surgical death rate, 14% complication rate, and an increase in conversion rate to restricted thoracotomy about 1.4 percent, all due to technical challenges. Most of the problems were modest, such as pneumonia, atelectasis that required a Bronchoscopy, Atrial Arrhythmias, and persistent air leaks that lasted more than five days. Particular patient groups demonstrated increased fatality rates, comprising the elderly Individuals with a decreased lung function (2.1 percent), patients exhibiting diminished preoperative functioning (9.8 percent), and those with a rate of 1.5 percent. The morbidity rates associated with these high-risk categories The respective percentages were 19%, 30%, and 18%. The median postoperative stay was 3 days following staged thoracoscopy and 5 days after VATS resection for many operational Non-Small Cell Lung Cancer (NSCLC) patients, especially those who is unable to tolerate conventional surgery (Stratton et al., 2009).

Prolonged monitoring of patients after VATS surgeries is crucial to address this issue; nevertheless, the recurrence on staple lines and ports remains significant issue for surgeons. Hanna et al. (2021) report that the majority of patients with Stage IA or IB cancers of the lung (T1N0 or T2N0) demonstrate 5-year survival rates ranging from 46 to 70 percent, and also lobectomy is typically adequate to secure negative surgical margins in cases of Non-Small Cell Lung Cancer. More severe surgical interventions may be required to eliminate all tumor manifestations in Stage 2 patients who have N1 metastases. Pneumonectomy may exceed lobectomy in effectiveness for individuals. Demonstrating hilar involvement of lymph nodes (at level 10), derived from an examination of 124 individuals diagnosed as having T1 or as T2, N1 disease. Patients who underwent pneumonectomy exhibited a reduced recurrence rate, hence validating this observation. But the majority of these individuals passed away due to distant recurrence, indicating that systemic therapy may be useful in treating Stage II cancer (Figure 3) (Goldstraw, 2001). Bronchial sleeve lobectomy provides a technically challenging yet viable alternative to entire pneumonectomy for the surgical resection of central bronchogenic tumours next to the carina. Airway reconstruction and immediate or phased carinal excision may be necessary if the main stem bronchus has a positive proximal border. Candidates for surgical airways reconstruction must be accurately staged with CT (Computed Tomography) and bronchoscopy. Positive N2 disease, involvement of the Superior Vena Cava, extent of fairway involvement and previous thoracic radiation are variables that may limit resectability. The 5years survival rate for this operation has been reported to be between 25 and 43 percent. Furthermore, certain evidence suggests that preoperative induction chemoradiation may diminish the necessity for a complete pneumonectomy and improve the prospects for sleeve resection in marginal candidates and those with down-staged nodal metastases (Walsh et al., 2001).

Figure 3. Stage IIA Non- Small Cell Lung Carcinoma

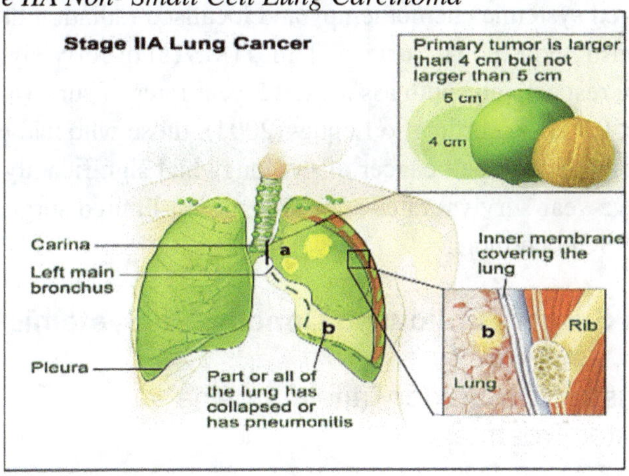

4. SURGICAL INTERVENTION WITHIN STAGE IV PULMONARY CARCINOMA

4.1. Approaches for Addressing Oligometastatic or as Non-Small Cell Lung Cancer via Surgical Intervention

The prognosis following surgical intervention with oligometastatic NSCLC is generally favourable, with a five-year Overall Survival (OS) rates between 20% and 30%, particularly in instances where metastasis has occurred in the brain and adrenal glands. According to ACCP (Advanced Critical-Care Practitioner) guidelines, cN0-1 may be utilized for localized cancer therapy and primary lesions excision in instances of single brain tumors and adrenal metastases. Furthermore, in situations of single brain metastases, the NCCN (National Comprehensive Cancer Network) recommendations advise multidisciplinary therapy, including systemic treatment, for primary lesions and local treatment for metastatic lesions. There are two main ways in which surgery can deal with oligometastasis: first, by removing the main tumor before using Radiation Therapy (RT), pharmacological intervention, or surgery to manage distant tumors; second, by combining local therapies (RT and surgery) for those whose remaining tumors are responding to drug treatment and are localized, which is called a salvage therapy (Dewey and Mack, 2000). Initial tumor excision was found to be successful in oligometastatic NSCLC (Non-Small Cell Lung Cancer) by Wang et al. (2018). Two cohort of 172 oligometastatic those with non-small-cell lung cancer were retrospectively examined: Both cohorts underwent adjuvant chemotherapy after the first surgical procedure, however only Group B received systemic chemotherapy and localised radiation therapy. Groups A and B demonstrated Median Survival Times (MSTs) of forty-eight months and also 18 months, respectively, with associated 5-year rates of survival of 21.1% and even 7.6% ($p < 0.05$). According to Leptay (2004), those who had primary oligometastatic type non-small cell cancer of the lungs had significantly better overall survival and five-year survival rates after undergoing limited surgical excision of their primary NSCLC tumors.

4.2. Rescue Surgery Following Conclusive Systemic Treatment

4.2.1. Reconstructive Surgery after Tyrosine Kinase Inhibitor Treatment

Chemotherapy enhanced one-year survival for individuals with Stage 4 (Figure 4) NSCLC by approximately 7% relative to survival with optimal supportive care. Patients having EGFR mutant-positive cancer of the lung have a favorable response to EGFR-TKI therapies, notably Osimertinib, which has an 80% response rate compared to chemotherapy. After receiving significant gains from TKI treatment, patients who have localized persistent or reoccurring lesions may be good candidates for salvage surgery (Baggstrom et al., 2007). Following gefitinib treatment, nine patients with Stage IV NSCLC had tumors removed, according to Hishida et al. (2014). Subsequent to gefitinib administration (Duration of Treatment: 2–36 months), surgical intervention was performed due to local tumour persistence, recurrence, or regrowth. The median survival rate after resection was 32 months. Reports indicate that the median interval between recurrences remained six months. Four patients who had pulmonary resection for the non-small cell lung tumors and then received gefitinib treatment for a separate study were followed up by Hishida et al. (2014) to see how they fared in the long run. Three out of four instances showed recurrence, however all of them lived for at least five years following surgery. For four years following surgery, the remaining case received TKI treatment without experiencing a recurrence of cancer. Salvage surgery of EGFR-TKI may have local control effects, despite the absence of extensive data. The application of ALK (Anaplastic Lymphoid Kinase) inhibitor for NSCLC with ALK genes translocations shown a similar significance of surgery to salvage (Imamura et al., 2018). A Phase III trial recently demonstrated that Osimertinib is an efficacious postoperative adjuvant treatment for resectable NSCLC that has an EGFR mutations (ADAURA Trials, or NCT02511106) (Hishida et al., 2010).

Figure 4. Non-small-cell lung cancer stage IV.

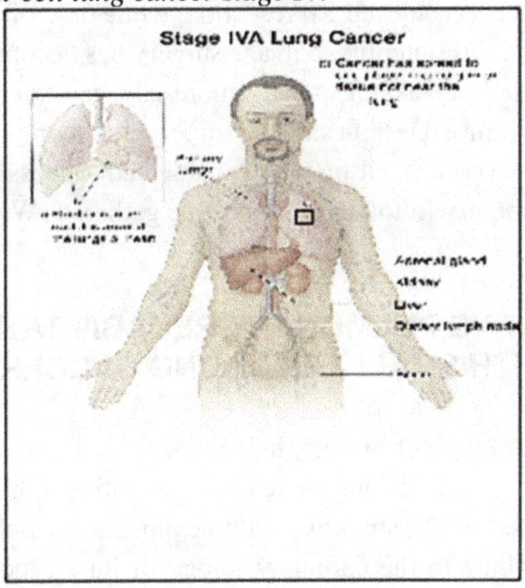

4.2.2. Rescue Surgery Following Therapy with Immune Check Point Inhibitors

Patients diagnosed with stage 4 NSCLC exhibited favourable responses to the PD-1 inhibition pembrolizumab within a trial in Phase III (KEYNOTE-407). Pembrolizumab demonstrated an anticipated overall survival rate that exceeded 80.2% at six months. The median progression-free survival (PFS) with pembrolizumab treatment has been determined 10.3 months, whereas for platinum doublet chemotherapy, it was six months. In 2014, Hishida and colleagues, [21] Moreover, patients with Stage IV non- small cells lung cancer had markedly improved overall survival and disease-free survival upon the incorporation of immune checkpoint inhibitors into chemotherapy, as seen by phase III clinical trials (KEYNOTE-189 and KEYNOTE-407). OS varied from 15 towards 22 months, PFS from 6.4 to the

8.8 months. The expression of programmable death-ligand 1 did not influence survival advantages. Evidence suggests that immune checkpoint inhibitors alone or in combination with chemotherapy should be the first line of treatment for non-small cell lung cancer patients with stage IV who do not have a driving mutation (Horio et al., 2019). Both investigations retrospectively Evaluated 19 patients who undergone lung resection following immune checkpoint inhibitor treatment for metastatic and incurable disorders, including cancer of the lungs (47%) and several metastatic illnesses. Melanoma (37%), notwithstanding the little data on salvage surgery following immune checkpoint inhibition. On average, 95% of the patients who undergone resection achieved R0 resection, while 68% of patients whose still had a live tumour had this outcome. Salvage surgery has become more common in NSCLC in recent years, and as ICI spreads, more salvage surgeries Subsequent ICI may transpire in the future. Despite salvage surgery, following immunotherapy has only been reported in one case, it may be a viable and successful treatment. More data about salvage surgery following ICI must be gathered (Wu et al., 2020).

5. POSTOPERATIVE PULMONARY REHABILITATION IN PATIENTS WITH SMALL CELL LUNG CANCER

Understanding lung cancer biology helps diagnose and treat NSCLC and also leading to enhanced prognoses and more effective patient rehabilitation. According to Kocarnik et al. (2022), smoking, radon exposure, air pollution, and genetic alterations all contribute to the pathophysiology of lung cancer. Smoking is the main cause of lung carcinoma. A global survey revealed that 63.17% of lung cancer fatalities occurred in 2017 was associated with smoking. Additionally, it was found that individuals who smoked had a higher frequency of postoperative problems. Lung cancer rates have decreased since tobacco restriction was put into place in1960s. Ongoing smoking cessation initiatives, however, use stem cells exposure to radon indoors. Radon represents a chemical radioactive gas produced by a process. Radon is a natural noble gas. The presence of uranium and also radium in crustal rocks and surrounding soil contributed significantly to lung cancer. Elevated indoor exposure to radon has been demonstrated to modify DNA and increase hazards by facilitating the deposition of decay products in epithelial cells of the lungs (Yang et al., 2021). Air pollution can indicate risk for cancer of the lungs due to the harmful impact it has on the respiratory system, particularly after coming into contact with fine particles (PM2.5). By causing inflammation, oxidative stress and apoptosis, PM2.5 exposure damages the lungs and raises the morbidity and mortality of circulatory and respiratory disorders. Lung cancer is more likely to occur and spread when exposed to PM2.5. Lung cancer has been demonstrated to manifest in mice exposed to PM2.5, as evidenced by an increased number of tumor nodules, elevated levels of the matrix metalloproteinase-1 (MP-1), and heightened concentrations of the vascular endothelial growth factors proteins compared to mice with tumors in a standard environment (Jeon et al., 2018).

Lung cancer risk is increased by chronic lung conditions including Bronchiectasis and Tuberculosis. An extensive body of research has shown that there is a substantial connection between the death rate of lung cancer and also genetic changes that are connected with respiratory issues (Kim et al., 2016). Given the swift advancement of contemporary biomedicine, researching genes with variable expression the significance of NSCLC is rising. The EGFR, or epidermal growth factor receptor, gene is one of the most frequently mutated genes in non-small cell lung tumours. In Eastern Asian populations with NSCLC, EGFR mutation genes is a predominant cause of genetic alterations. TP53 is a tumor suppressor. According to earlier research Peterson et al. (2013), TP53 mutations account for more than Mutations account for half of the frequency in cancer of the lungs and are observed in 35–60% of people having Non-Small Cells Lung Cancer. Moreover, studies into micro RNAs have advanced the investigation of the pathophysiology of cancer of the lung (Peterson et al., 2013). As a persistent ailment, NSCLC typically requires rehabilitation. Patients who get non-small-cell lung carcinoma may discontinue smoking at any point. Patients should endeavour to engage in increased physical activity in a natural environment and inhale fresh air. Further investigation is required to elucidate the molecular pathways that facilitate lung cancer metastasis, perhaps resulting in novel strategies for its eradication and guiding further research and rehabilitation efforts. It is anticipated that a multimodal approach to treatment that incorporates lifestyle changes, exercise programs, and even nutritional support will be developed in order to address the difficulties pertaining to the rehabilitation patients identified as having NSCLC. This strategy will be informed by an improved understanding of the pathophysiology of lung cancer (Ioughool and Kreski, 2009).

6. CYTOTOXIC CHEMOTHERAPY APPLIED PREOPERATIVELY AND POSTOPERATIVELY FOR NSCLC

6.1. Focused Treatment

Targeted therapies denote anticancer pharmaceuticals that obstruct the protein products produced by active oncogenes or the associated pathways. For nearly a decade, the primary therapies for advanced non-small cell lung cancer received targeted drugs and identification of driving oncogenes. Between 2013 and 2016, the population-level lung cancer-specific death rate fell, and this improvement was primarily due to the implementation of biomarker-matched targeted therapy (Martins et al., 2024). The lack of routine predictive biomarker evaluation in early-stage disease and the conventional reliance on overall survival, or OS, as an the primary endpoint within long-duration trials are the primary reasons for the slow adoption of these new therapeutic advancements in the therapy of resectable non-small-cell lung cancer, or NSCLC, (Enflo, 2022). This is not attributable to a deficiency of concern regarding the treatment. Retrospective and small one-arm trials have shown that adjuvant therapy EGFR TKIs improve outcomes relative to historical controls. Gefitinib was evaluated against cisplatin and vinorelbine within randomised Phase II studies, succeeded by Phase III trials, were done in China for individuals non-small cell lung cancer with Stage III-N2 EGFR mutations removed. DFS, Disease-Free Survival which is the primary goal of this inquiry, was successfully attained despite the lack of OS support and the failure to gain OS advantages. This trial has been criticism for the lack of a consistent preoperative stage and the omission of standard-of-care chemotherapy from the gefitinib arm. A Japanese trial with resected Stage 2 and 3 mutants EGFR NSCLC compared adjuvant gefitinib to the cisplatin plus vinorelbine did not achieve its predetermined disease-free survival target. In 2014, Phase III trials of targeted therapies for EGFR and Anaplastic Lymphoid Kinase (ALK) commenced in the United States as a component of the National Cancer Cancer Institute's ALCHEMIST trials portfolio (Howlader et al., 2020).

The investigations were designed to conform with the gold standard of stage 3 randomised controlled by placebo clinical trials, designating overall survival (OS) is the principal outcome and also Tyrosine Kinase Inhibition (TKI) administered subsequent to standard-of-care chemotherapy. The ALCHEMIST experiments were limited by a slow trial accrual rate. The high speed of pharmacological research has resulted in the availability of TKIs that are more effective and well tolerated. In 2020, the United States FDA sanctioned the inaugural perioperative medication. The EGFR TKI Osimertinib obtained a three-year approval following Phase III ADAURA standard-of-care adjuvant treatment. In comparison to the placebo, Osimertinib enhanced disease-free survival, or DFS, by 0.20 (P=.0010) in patients with resection EGFR-mutant tumors measuring 3 centimeters or with affected lymph nodes. The ADAURA OS data is several years away from maturity and serves as a secondary goal. A similar sponsored by the industry supplemental trial of Alectinib versus Chemotherapy (NCT03456076) is recruiting patients globally, however findings are probably years away (Janigian et al., 2011).

Limited trials of biomarkers-matched neoadjuvant targeted treatments have been finalised and published due to the challenges posed by low mutation incidences and prolonged biomarker testing durations in preoperative TKI studies. Initial experiments recruited participants based on clinical characteristics and subsequently aligned biomarkers. Although several single-arm EGFR TKI studies have been completed in

China, where EGFR mutations are prevalent, only one randomized research has been published (Pennell et al., 2019). With radiographic response rates as the main goal, Erlotinib, Cisplatin, and Gemcitabine were compared in the forthcoming CTONG 1103 Phase II randomised trial for EGFR-mutant non-small cells lung cancer stage IIIA-N2. Most patients responded to standard-of-care afterwards treatment with an EGFR TKI, according to data at the time of recurrence regardless of treatment arm, even though there were no clinical differences between the arms (Yue, 2018).The goal of the present initiatives is to apply targeted therapy in a neoadjuvant context. Patients with a resectable early-stage cancer of the lungs will be recruited for the LEADER trial, which is funded by the Lung Tumour Development Foundation, using centralized plasma and tumour genotyping. The predictive biomarker panel used in matched therapy studies, such as Osimertinib, chemotherapy, and the combination are being tested in Patients with EGFR-mutant non-small cell lung cancer (NCT04351555) that is resectable are also being recruited for a worldwide phase III study (Zhong et al., 2021).

6.2. Immunotherapy

6.2.1. Neoadjuvant Immunotherapy

The swift discovery and authorisation of novel therapies for advanced lung malignancies have resulted in a significant increase in anticipation for neoadjuvant clinical trials during the past decade. In a 2018 single- arm clinical trial, 21 resectable NSCLC patients received two neoadjuvant nivolumab doses that in stages IB-IIIA. Standard surgery and adjuvant therapy were then carried out. Notwithstanding the short duration of treatment, two pathological complete responses (pCR, signifying the lack of viable cancer cells) and also nine out of twenty-one resected tumours had a substantial pathological response (MPR, characterized by 10% residual viable tumour). The promise of neoadjuvant studies as a foundation for correlative science was shown by thorough correlative research. Combining chemo with PD-L1 or PD-1 blocking, single-agent PDL1 or PD-1 blockade, or combination anti-PD-1 and anti-cytotoxic T-cell lymphocyte-4 suppression are among the largest single-arm Phase II neoadjuvant trials that have since been published (Govindan et al., 2015). The median Major Pathologic Response (MPR) rate following Neoadjuvant Chemotherapy is approximately 15 percent to 20 percent. The Major Pathological Response (MPR) rates associated Using anti-PD-1 monotherapy as well as neoadjuvant anti-PD-L1 treatments have varied between 14% and 45%. The LCMC3 experiment, the largest Phase II trial to date, provided patients with resectable (NSCLC) at eight edition stages IB-IIIB with two doses of postoperative atezolizumab. Following surgery, patients who shown clinical benefit could continue taking the adjuvant medication atezolizumab for up to a year (Wu et al., 2020).

7. RESTRICTIONS ON PULMONARY REHABILITATION FOLLOWING SURGERY

There are well-established criteria for assessing the level of perceived danger and determining key components in relation to NSCLC. Nevertheless, it is still unclear how postoperative rehabilitative treatments should be implemented. Patients with NSCLC are currently trained using a variety of breathing techniques. Although there is some variation in training method, timing, and duration, the recommendations do not identify an ideal rehabilitation approach for individuals undergoing lung cancer surgery. It is still uncertain if patient's clinical prognosis is improved by short-term preoperative pulmonary rehabilitation (Rizvi et al., 2011). There are still unanswered questions, such as whether it lowers postoperative problems in high-risk lung cancer patients or encourages ineligible patients to meet surgical requirements. At the moment, thoracoscopic lung cancer surgery frequently uses accelerated rehabilitation surgery management (Hsu et al., 2024). Rehabilitation both in quantity and quality following discharge could be significantly improved, as many of these treatments are only applicable during the perioperative phase. Larger longitudinal studies are necessary because the evidence supporting the claim that physical activity improves postoperative outcomes is poor. Although the best rehabilitation program has not yet been established, a multidisciplinary team approach is essential in the treatment of lung cancer at all stages (Zhong et al., 2019).

8. INTERVENTIONS FOR COMPLICATIONS OF NSCLC

8.1. Dermatological Complications

The wild-type EGFR pathway signalling is essential for regulating keratinocyte migration, proliferation, and survival, hence preserving homeostasis within the epidermis. Keratinocytes with impaired EGFR phosphorylation exhibit growth cessation, cellular apoptosis, reduced migratory capacity, and increased production of cytokine and chemokine receptors. Consequently, subsequent to the administration with small molecule inhibitors targeting EGFR Dermatological issues are prevalent in NSCLC. According to Mendelsohn and Baselga (2003), during the clinical trials that led to the approval of Osimertinib and first- or second-generation TKIs, 80% of patients received cutaneous Adverse Events (AEs) of any grade, and 60% of patients received Osimertinib. These drugs can cause a wide range of skin problems, from xerotic dermatitis, pruritus, telangiectasias, and aberrant hair development to acneiform eruption, the classic cutaneous side effect of EGFR inhibition. The two main risk factors for rash formation are skin phototype and UV exposure. Before beginning treatment with an EGFR inhibitor, patients should be well educated so they can take certain precautions, like avoiding the sun (Albanell et al., 2002).

8.2. Gastrointestinal Complications

Although they happen less frequently with the other EGFR inhibitors, mucositis and stomatitis are frequent adverse events, particularly with afatinib. EGFR inhibitor use frequently results in diarrhea. It is essential to recognize that patients receiving concurrent radiation treatment or those with a history of radiation therapy affecting the abdomen region are at risk of growing grade 3 or higher enterotoxicity, requiring continuous monitoring. Although EGFR TKIs have been shown to elevate liver enzymes, they hardly ever result in potentially fatal liver damage (Burotto et al., 2015).

8.3. Pulmonary Complication

Compared to normal lung parenchyma, alveolar type II cells exhibit higher levels of EGFR expression in fibrotic tissues, indicating a possible function for Activation of the EGFR pathway in pulmonary regeneration. According to this theory, EGFR suppression may impair lung tissue's natural capacity for epithelial cell renewal, which could result in fibrosis (Lacouture et al., 2013). Interstitial Lung Disease (ILD) is one way that EGFR inhibitors might harm the lungs. Between 1% and 4% is the low incidence of lung toxicity. Smoking, advanced age, previous chest irradiation, and pre-existing ILD are risk factors for developing ILD following EGFR inhibitor therapy. Although the fatality rates following the development of pulmonary toxicity are modest and vary from 0% to 15% across trials, there are not enough cases to allow for the safe drawing of any conclusions. According to Ramalingam et al. (2020), the most typical manifestation of ILD brought on by EGFR inhibition is the onset or exacerbation of underlying dyspnea combined with a low-grade fever and cough.

8.4. Ocular Complications

EGFR signaling is essential for wound healing in the conjunctival and corneal epithelium, and ocular issues are often associated with EGFR TKI side effects. The incidence of ocular side effects ranges from 5% to 15%, depending on the agent employed. On the other hand, severe ocular adverse events that necessitate stopping the medication are uncommon (Kozuki 2016).

8.5. Pulmonary Complication

The development of pneumonitis has been linked to ALK TKIs. No particular risk factors have been found. Acute interstitial pneumonia and non-specific interstitial pneumonia can both show up on radiographs. It is possible and typically safe to transition to another ALK inhibitor after stopping therapy for pneumonitis, according to published case studies (Peus et al., 2000).The development of pneumonitis caused by Bragitinib does not necessitate stopping treatment because it follows a distinct pattern than other ALK TKIs. According to reports Luu et al. (2011) the incidence of pneumonitis caused by Bragitinib ranges from 4% to 9%. It usually appears within the first week of starting treatment (Luu et al., 2011).

8.6. Gastrointestinal Complications

Although upper gastrointestinal issues like nausea and vomiting are frequent, stopping a medication is rarely the result. With all ALK TKIs, diarrhea is also somewhat prevalent, however grade 3 - 4 diarrhea is uncommon. Although hepatotoxicity seldom leads to medication cessation, liver amino-transferase increase is rather common with ALK TKIs. Blood tests should be performed on patients receiving ALK TKIs atleast every two weeks for the first three months of treatment (Balagula et al., 2011).

8.7. Cardiovascular Complications

Crisotinib has been shown to cause QTc interval prolongation, albeit grade 3–4 prolongation has hardly ever been seen. There have been reports of sinus bradycardia caused by brigatinib, ceritinib, alectinib, and crizotinib. Furthermore, blood pressure should be monitored throughout treatment because hypertension is a somewhat typical side effect of Brigatinib administration (Migliore 2019).

Table 1. Common Complications and Incidence Rates of Targeted Therapies in Lung Cancer Treatment

S.No	Designated Agent	Frequent Complications	Rates	References
1	EGFR inhibitors: Gefitinib, Erlotinib, Afatinib, Dacomitinib, and Osimertinib	Interstitial pulmonary disease	1% to 3%	Vogel and Jennifer (2016)
		Acneiform eruption	Acneiform eruption occurs in 1% to 15% of cases for grade 3 rash.	Boone et al. (2007)
		Paronychia	14% of patients discontinued treatment with afatinib because to paronychia.	Sequist et al. (2013)
		Mucositis	Mucositis manifests approximately 72% of patients administered afatinib, with a reduced prevalence linked to other medicines.	Sequist et al. (2013)
		Diarrhea	Diarrhoea of grade 2 or higher occurs in 30% of patients treated with afatinib, which is lower with other medications.	Mok et al. (2017)
		Ocular complications	Ocular complications 5%–15%	Vogel and Jennifer (2016)
2	NTRK inhibitors: Larotrectinib (ROS1 inhibitors)	Elevation of liver aminotransferases	30% efficacy with Larotrectinib	Drilon et al. (2018)
		Grade 3 anaemia and neutropenia	Approximately 10% with Larotrectinib	Drilon et al. (2018)
3	RET inhibitors Selpercatinib, Pralsetinib	Hypertension (~20%)	~20%	Lee et al. (2019)
		Bone marrow toxicity	10% with Pralsetinib	Drusbosky et al. (2021)
4	KRAS inhibitors Sotorasib	Diarrhea	29%	Hong et al. (2020)
		Liver enzyme elevation	~10%–14%	Hong et al. (2020)
		Pyrexia	11%	Hong et al. (2020)

9. CURRENT RESECTABLE NSCLC CLINICAL TRIALS

Federally funded cooperative cancer organization in Northern Europe as well as America are conducting multicenter Phase II and Phase III clinical research. The NCI and Cancer Trials Supporting Units websites include more information about this research. This chapter reviews numerous surgical trials for non-small cell lung cancer. Patients with Stage I NSCLC who have been resected are eligible for randomized Phase III selenium chemoprevention research (ECOG 5597). Selenium, a glutathione-dependent peroxidase system inhibitor, was chosen for this investigation due to its antioxidant capability and lung cancer reduction in supplementing experiments. S0220 was part of the SWOG Phase II trials for Stages IIB or as III Non-Small-Cell Lung Carcinoma (NSCLC) concentrating on the more superior sulcus. This trial includes cisplatin and etoposide induction chemotherapy, surgery for resection, and docetaxel postoperatively. The survival of patients with Pancoast tumours, progression-free interval, medical response, resected rate, and toxicity will be evaluated. Participants underwent of the six week neoadjuvant therapies throughout the course of three cycles. The study objectives encompass overall survival, lifetime efficacy, resectability, relapse duration, recurrence site, and toxicity. The Phase III SWSSAKK-16/00 study conducted the Swiss Centres for the Applied Cancer Research evaluates neoadjuvant treatments with or without radiology for non-small cell lung cancer. presenting mediastinal lymph node metastases. In conjunction with preoperative docetaxel and cisplatin therapy, patients classified as T1-3, N2, and M0 are randomly assigned to surgical resection either with or without radiation therapy. The initiative evaluates event-free survival, lifespan, sickness response, and toxicity. PET scans will also be evaluated for pathological disease responses and patient outcomes (Miglior et al., 2020).

The newly formed NCI-funded American College of Surgical Surgeons Oncologist Group (ACOSOG) addresses surgical issues in solid tumour therapy. Moreover, participants with ACOSO clinical trials must engage in correlative science research and specimen banking processes. The objective of ACOSOG Z4031 is to determine if an individual's serum proteome profile might indicate presence of NSCLC. This forthcoming study will cover one thousand participants and will compare their proteome profiles of patients before and after surgery and relate them to the pathologic stage and prognosis of the patient. For high-risk NSCLC patients, two further ACOSOG studies will look at surgical options. The Z4032 study randomly allocates individuals at high risk for developing non-small cell cancer of the lungs should undergo sub-lobar resection, either accompanied by brachytherapy or not, with the primary outcome being the duration until local recurrence occurs. The goal of Z4033 is to create quality control procedures and technical recommendations for the application of High-risk patients with Stage IA non-small cell lung cancer may undergo radiofrequency ablation (Shaikha et al., 2024). One thousand people will be included in this prospective study, which will compare the proteomic profiles of patients before and after surgery and relate them to the pathologic stage and prognosis of the patient. For high-risk NSCLC patients, two further ACOSOG studies will look at surgical options. The goal of Z4033 is to create quality control procedures and technical recommendations for the application of High-risk patients with Stage IA non-small cell lung cancer may undergo radiofrequency ablation (Shaikha et al., 2024).

10. NEW DEVELOPMENTS IN NSCLC SURGICAL MANAGEMENT

The survival assessment after lobectomy and wedge excision for the stage IA and also stage II primary non-small cells of the lung cancer (SP-NSCLC) included surgical techniques (RATS, VATS, and multiportal or uniportal methods), procedural information, perioperative management, and outcomes, using Overall Survival (OS) and lung-specific cancer-related mortality as metrics endpoints individuals who had previously undergone lung cancer-directed surgery are among the topics covered in this chapter on NSCLC management (Figure 5). According to the authors Altorki et al. (2023), the 5years Overall Survival (OS) for lobectomy was 66.1%, while the OS for wedge resection was 61.3%. They came to the conclusion that for patients with stage IA SPNSCLC who have had prior lung cancer-directed surgery, wedge resection is equivalent to lobectomy in OS (Altorki et al., 2023).

A wedge resection, together with the requisite lymph node excision, is comparable to a surgical lobectomy in instances of tiny non-small cell lung tumours. Patients with ≤2 cm nodes negative for NSCLC and undergoing lobectomy or as wedge resection from 2004-2015 were identified. Patients were then evaluated based on the size of the NSCLC (less than one cm, 1-2 cm) and the surgical method (lobectomy or wedge resection). The excision of lymphatic nodes did not affect survival rates for lesions less than one cm undergoing lobectomy. Wedge resection and lobectomy were comparable when one or more nodes were removed for lesions ≤1 cm and six or more nodes were removed for lesions 1-2 cm (Migliore 2016). For Stage I non-small cell lung cancer, lobectomies are generally not a justifiable surgery, according to the authors Galetta and Spaggiari's (2018) convincing findings. Despite being retrospective, the findings are noteworthy since they resemble those of Altorki et al. (2023)prospective randomized experiment. Their findings suggest that people with limited lung Resection, including wedge resection, is sufficient for early-stage non-small cells lung cancer. achieving long-term survival; hence, more comprehensive resections, including as segmentectomy or as lobectomy, would be conducted less often.

Global practice change will take years, but it will undoubtedly occur (Govindan et al., 2015) and examined the outcomes of Open Lobectomy (OL), Propensity score-matched comparison of robotic and video-assisted thoracoscopic surgery for patients aged 75 years or older with non-small cell lung cancer, in extremely old NSCLC patients, RATS had better perioperative results than VATS and OL (Burotto et al., 2015). Enflo (2022) conducted a thorough review and meta-analysis of prospective trials contrasting video-assisted versus robot assisted thoracic surgery. Of the 614 patients, 315 received VATS treatment and 299 received RATS treatment. The RATS category had a higher quantity of dissected node locations (P less than 0.001) and a reduction in blood loss (P = 0.009). In spite of the lack of a discernible distinction between RATS and VATS regarding readmission rates, duration of hospitalisation, or patient outcomes, the researchers identified a strong correlation with the rising rate. An odds ratio of roughly 2.717 (p=0.01) for the significant adenocarcinoma patterns Multivariate analysis revealed in this outcome, 2.545 (p=0.02) represents lymph node resection. Italian research shows that nodal metastases in clinical early-stage non-small cell lung cancers are linked to the number of lymphatic nodes removed and the adenocarcinoma's histologic subtype. This outcome will undoubtedly motivate thoracic surgeons to carry out a more thorough and prolonged lymphadenectomy in the future (Enflo, 2022).

Fascinating analysis of the Artificial Intelligence (AI) applications is also used for treatment of lung cancer (Kim et al., 2025). AI improves preoperative diagnostics and molecular biomarker prediction, particularly when biopsy samples are scarce. AI revolutionizes surgery by offering real-time direction and decision help during the procedure. AI supports pathological evaluation and predictive modeling for improved treatment after surgery. AI could undoubtedly be useful in situations where interpretability is challenging and surgeons and doctors disagree on the best course of action. While 3D reconstruction in artificial intelligence and thoracic surgery is still in its infancy, there are many hopes for the future. Since there are currently no clear guidelines and misunderstanding, we think that clearer indications are necessary (Galetta and Spaggiari, 2018).

Figure 5. Operative Treatment of Non-Small Cell Lung Carcinoma

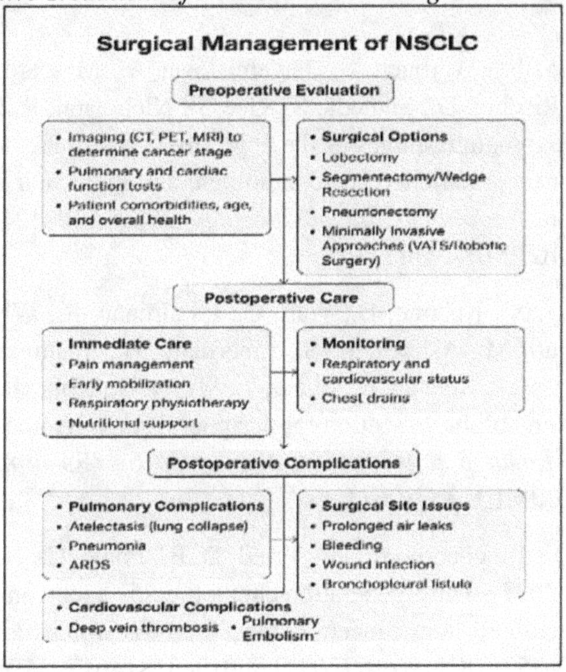

11. CONCLUSION

In summary, the clinical staging and surgical therapy of Non-Small Cell Lung Carcinoma (NSCLC) are essential for establishing suitable treatment plans and enhancing patient outcomes. Early-stage non-small cell lung cancer (categorised into stages I–II) is often amenable to surgery for resection, with lobectomy becoming the standard procedure for achieving complete tumour excision and favourable survival outcomes. In Stage IIIA cases, multimodal approaches combining Surgery combined with chemotherapy or radiation therapy yields enhanced results, particularly when negative surgery margins are attained. Video-Assisted Thoracoscopic Surgery ("VATS") with mediastinal lymphadenectomy assessments continue to evolve, offering less invasive options with reduced morbidity. Despite advancements, challenges remain in managing high-risk patients and in determining optimal approaches for those with N_2 involvement. Ultimately, precise preoperative staging, careful patient selection, and individualized surgical planning are essential to maximizing curative potential and long-term survival in NSCLC patients.

REFERENCES

Albanell, J., Rojo, F., Averbuch, S., Feyereislova, A., Mascaro, J. M., Herbst, R., LoRusso, P., Rischin, D., Sauleda, S., Gee, J., Nicholson, R. I., & Baselga, J. (2002). Pharmaco dynamic studies of the epidermal growth factor receptor inhibitor in skin from cancer patients: Histopathologic and molecular consequences of receptor inhibition. *Journal of Clinical Oncology*, *20*(1), 110–124. DOI: 10.1200/JCO.2002.20.1.110 PMID: 11773160

Altorki, N., Wang, X., Kozono, D., Watt, C., Landrenau, R., Wigle, D., Port, J., Jones, D. R., Conti, M., Ashrafi, A. S., Liberman, M., Yasufuku, K., Yang, S., Mitchell, J. D., Pass, H., Keenan, R., Bauer, T., Miller, D., Kohman, L. J., & Vokes, E. (2023). Lobar orsublobar resection for peripheral stage IA non–small-cell lung cancer. *The New England Journal of Medicine*, *388*(6), 489–498. DOI: 10.1056/NEJMoa2212083 PMID: 36780674

Baggstrom, M. Q., Stinchcombe, T. E., Fried, D. B., Poole, C., Hensing, T. A., & Socinski, M. A. (2007). Third-generation chemotherapy agents in the treatment of advanced non-small cell lung cancer: A meta-analysis. *Journal of Thoracic Oncology*, *2*(9), 845–853. DOI: 10.1097/JTO.0b013e31814617a2 PMID: 17805063

Balagula, Y., Garbe, C., Myskowski, P. L., Hauschild, A., Rapoport, B. L., Boers-Doets, C. B., & Lacouture, M. E. (2011). Boers-Doets Clinical presentation and management of dermatological toxicities of epidermal growth factor receptor inhibitors. *International Journal of Dermatology*, *50*(2), 129–146. DOI: 10.1111/j.1365-4632.2010.04791.x PMID: 21244375

Boone, S. L., Rademaker, A., Liu, D., Pfeiffer, C., Mauro, D. J., & Lacouture, M. E. (2007). Impact and management of skin toxicity associated with anti-epidermal growth factor receptor therapy: Survey Results. *Oncology*, *72*(4), 152–159. DOI: 10.1159/000112795 PMID: 18160805

Burotto, M., Manasanch, E. E., Wilkerson, J., & Fojo, T. (2015). Gefitinib and erlotinib in metastatic non–small cell lung cancer: A meta-analysis of toxicity and efficacy of randomized clinical trials. *The Oncologist*, *40*(4), 10–18. DOI: 10.1634/theoncologist.2014-0154 PMID: 25795635

Chen, W., Zheng, R., Baade, P. D., Zhang, S., Zeng, H., Bray, F., Jemal, A., Yu, X. Q., & He, J. (2016). Cancer statistics in China, 2015. *CA: a Cancer Journal for Clinicians*, *66*(2), 115–132. DOI: 10.3322/caac.21338 PMID: 26808342

Dewey, T. M., & Mack, M. J. (2000). Lung cancer: Surgical approaches and incisions. *Chest Surgery Clinics of North America, 10*(4), 803–820. DOI: 10.1016/S1052-3359(25)00543-5 PMID: 11091927

Drilon, A., Laetsch, T. W., Kummar, S., Dubois, S. G., Lassen, U. N., Demetri, G. D., Nathenson, M., Doebele, R. C., Farago, A. F., Pappo, A. S., Turpin, B., Dowlati, A., Brose, M. S., Mascarenhas, L., Federman, N., Berlin, J., El-Deiry, W. S., Baik, C., Deeken, J., & Hyman, D. M. (2018). Efficacy of larotrectinib in TRK fusion–positive cancers in adults and children. *The New England Journal of Medicine, 378*(8), 731–739. DOI: 10.1056/NEJMoa1714448 PMID: 29466156

Drusbosky, L. M., Rodriguez, E., Dawar, R., & Ikpeazu, C. V. (2021). Therapeutic strategies in RET gene rearranged non–small cell lung cancer. *Journal of Hematology & Oncology, 14*(1), 50–56. DOI: 10.1186/s13045-021-01063-9 PMID: 33771190

Enflo, A. (2022). Lung cancer risks from residential radon among smokers and non-smokers. *Journal of Radiological Protection, 22*(3A), A95–A99. DOI: 10.1088/0952-4746/22/3A/317 PMID: 12400955

Galetta, D., & Spaggiari, L. (2018). Early and long-term results of tracheal sleeve-pneumonectomy for lung cancer after induction therapy. *The Annals of Thoracic Surgery, 105*(4), 1017–1023. DOI: 10.1016/j.athoracsur.2017.11.052 PMID: 29277671

Goldstraw, P. (2001). Surgical oncologic principles. *Chest Surgery Clinics of North America, 11*(1), 1–16. DOI: 10.1016/S1052-3359(25)00550-2 PMID: 11253592

Govindan, R., Mandrekar, S. J., Gerber, D. E., Oxnard, G. R., Dahlberg, S. E., Chaft, J., Malik, S., Mooney, M., Abrams, J. S., Jänne, P. A., Gandara, D. R., Ramalingam, S. S., & Vokes, E. E. (2015). ALCHEMIST trials: A golden opportunity to transform outcomes in early-stage non-small cell lung cancer. *Clinical Cancer Research, 21*(24), 5439–5444. DOI: 10.1158/1078-0432.CCR-15-0354 PMID: 26672084

Hanna, N. H., Robinson, A. G., Temin, S., Baker, S.Jr, Brahmer, J. R., Ellis, P. M., Gaspar, L. E., Haddad, R. Y., Hesketh, P. J., Jain, D., Jaiyesimi, I., Johnson, D. H., Leighl, N. B., Moffitt, P. R., Phillips, T., Riely, G. J., Rosell, R., Schiller, J. H., Schneider, B. J., & Masters, G. (2021). Therapy for stage IV non-small-cell lung cancer with driver alterations: ASCO and OH (CCO) joint guideline update. *Journal of Clinical Oncology, 39*(9), 1040–1091. DOI: 10.1200/JCO.20.03570 PMID: 33591844

Hishida, T., Nagai, K., Mitsudomi, T., Yokoi, K., Kondo, H., Horinouchi, H., Akiyama, H., Nagayasu, T., & Tsuboi, M. (2010). Salvage surgery for advanced non-small cell lung cancer after response to gefitinib. *The Journal of Thoracic and Cardiovascular Surgery, 140*(5), e69–e71. DOI: 10.1016/j.jtcvs.2010.06.035 PMID: 20674944

Hishida, T., Yoshida, J., Aokage, K., Nagai, K., & Tsuboi, M. (2014). Long-term outcome of surgical resection for residual or regrown advanced non-small cell lung carcinomas following EGFR-TKI treatment: Report of four cases. *The Thoracic and Cardiovascular Surgeon*, *64*, 429–433. PMID: 25512091

Hong, D. S., Fakih, M. G., Strickler, J. H., Desai, J., Durm, G. A., Shapiro, G. I., Falchook, G. S., Price, T. J., Sacher, A., Denlinger, C. S., Bang, Y.-J., Dy, G. K., Krauss, J. C., Kuboki, Y., Kuo, J. C., Coveler, A. L., Park, K., Kim, T. W., Barlesi, F., & Li, B. T. (2020). KRASG12C inhibition with sotorasib in advanced solid tumors. *The New England Journal of Medicine*, *383*(13), 1207–1217. DOI: 10.1056/NEJMoa1917239 PMID: 32955176

Horio, Y., Mizuno, T., Sakao, Y., Inaba, Y., Yatabe, Y., & Hida, T. (2019). Successful salvage surgery following multimodal therapy in a patient who harboured ALK-rearranged advanced lung adenocarcinoma with multiple organ metastases. *Respirology Case Reports*, *7*(7), e00451. DOI: 10.1002/rcr2.451 PMID: 31285825

Howlader, N., Forjaz, G., Mooradian, M. J., Meza, R., Kong, C. Y., Cronin, K. A., Mariotto, A. B., Lowy, D. R., & Feuer, E. J. (2020). The effect of advances in lung-cancer treatment on population mortality. *The New England Journal of Medicine*, *383*(7), 640–649. DOI: 10.1056/NEJMoa1916623 PMID: 32786189

Hsu, C. H., Hung, C. Y., Chen, K. C., Chang, P. H., & Wu, Y. L. (2024). A narrative review on perioperative systemic therapy in non-small cell lung cancer. *Precision Cancer Medicine*, *7*, 17. PMID: 39280253

Imamura, F., Nogami, N., & Kurata, T. (2018). Osimertinib in untreated EGFR-mutated advanced non-small-cell lung cancer. *The New England Journal of Medicine*, *378*(2), 113–125. DOI: 10.1056/NEJMoa1713137 PMID: 29151359

Jeon, J., Holford, T. R., Levy, D. T., Feuer, E. J., Cao, P., Tam, J., Clarke, L., & Clarke, J. (2018). A comparative modeling approach. *Annals of Internal Medicine*, *169*, 684–693. DOI: 10.7326/M18-1250 PMID: 30304504

Kim, H., Lee, J., Park, S., Choi, Y., & Jeong, Y. (2025). A comprehensive review on the application of artificial intelligence for predicting postsurgical recurrence risk in early-stage non-small cell lung cancer using computed tomography, positron emission tomography, and clinical data. *Cancers (Basel)*, *17*(2), 215. DOI: 10.3390/cancers11020215 PMID: 39857997

Kim, S. H., Hwang, W. J., Cho, J. S., & Kang, D. R. (2016). Attributable risk of lung cancer deaths due to indoor radon exposure. *Annals of Occupational and Environmental Medicine*, *28*(1), 8–16. DOI: 10.1186/s40557-016-0093-4 PMID: 26925236

Kocarnik, J. M., Compton, K., Dean, F. E., Fu, W., Gaw, B. L., Harvey, J. D., Henrikson, H. J., Lu, D., & Pennini, A. (2022). Cancer incidence, mortality, years of life lost, years lived with disability, and disability- adjusted life years for 29 cancer groups. *JAMA Oncology*, *8*, 420–444. PMID: 34967848

Kozuki, T. (2016). Skin problems and EGFR-tyrosine kinase inhibitor. *Japanese Journal of Clinical Oncology*, *46*(4), 291–298. DOI: 10.1093/jjco/hyv207 PMID: 26826719

Lacouture, M. E., Schadendorf, D., Chu, C.-Y., Uttenreuther-Fischer, M., Stammberger, U., O'Brien, D., & Hauschild, A. (2013). Dermatologic adverse events associated with afatinib: An oral ErbB family blocker. *Expert Review of Anticancer Therapy*, *13*(6), 721–728. DOI: 10.1586/era.13.30 PMID: 23506519

Lampridis, S., & Scarci, M. (2023). Perioperative systemic therapies for non-small-cell lung cancer: Recent advances and future perspectives. *Frontiers in Surgery*, *9*, 9. DOI: 10.3389/fsurg.2022.1126486 PMID: 36743902

Lee, D. H., Subbiah, V., Gainor, J. F., Taylor, M. H., Zhu, V. W., Doebele, R. C., Lopes, G., Baik, C., Garralda, E., Gadgeel, S. M., Kim, D.-W., Turner, C. D., Palmer, M., Miller, S., & Curigliano, G. (2019). Treatment with pralsetinib (formerly BLU-667), a potent and selective RET inhibitor, provides rapid clearance of ctDNA in patients with RET-altered non–small cell lung cancer (NSCLC) and medullary thyroid cancer (MTC). *Annals of Oncology : Official Journal of the European Society for Medical Oncology*, *30*, 122–128. DOI: 10.1093/annonc/mdz431

Li, Y., Zhang, X., Chen, H., Wang, J., & Zhao, X. (2024). Survival outcomes of segmentectomy and lobectomy for early stage non-small cell lung cancer: A systematic review and meta-analysis. *Journal of Cardiothoracic Surgery*, *19*(1), 121. DOI: 10.1186/s13019-024-03210-y PMID: 38909240

Luu, M., Boone, S. L., Patel, J., Sullivan, P., Rademaker, A. W., Balagula, Y., & Lacouture, M. E. (2011). Higher severity grade of erlotinib-induced rash is associated with lower skin phototype. *Clinical and Experimental Dermatology*, *36*(7), 733–738. DOI: 10.1111/j.1365-2230.2011.04117.x PMID: 21689147

Martins, T., Santos, R., Pereira, M., Gonçalves, L., & Carvalho, L. (2024). Factors associated with safe and successful postoperative day 1 discharge after lung operations: A systematic review and meta-analysis. *Journal of Cardiothoracic Surgery*, *19*(1), 88. DOI: 10.1186/s13019-024-02505-4 PMID: 38350950

Mendelsohn, J., & Baselga, J. (2003). Status of epidermal growth factor receptor antagonists in the biology and treatment of cancer. *Journal of Clinical Oncology*, *23*(14), 2787–2799. DOI: 10.1200/JCO.2003.01.504 PMID: 12860957

Migliore, M. (2016). VATS surgery for anatomical lung resection: A different approach for every surgeon. *Video-Assisted Thoracic Surgery*, *1*, 31–40. DOI: 10.21037/vats.2016.10.01

Migliore, M., & Nardini, M. (2019). Does cytoreduction surgery and hyperthermicintrathoracic chemotherapy prolong survival in patients with N0–N1 non-small cell lung cancer and Malignant pleural effusion? *European Respiratory Review : an Official Journal of the European Respiratory Society*, *28*(151), 190018. DOI: 10.1183/16000617.0018-2019 PMID: 31366459

Mok, T. S., Wu, Y. L., Ahn, M. J., Garassino, M. C., Kim, H. R., Ramalingam, S. S., Shepherd, F. A., He, Y., Akamatsu, H., Theelen, W. S. M. E., Lee, C. K., Sebastian, M., Templeton, A., Mann, H., Marotti, M., Ghiorghiu, S., & Papadimitrakopoulou, V. A. (2017). Osimertinib or platinum-pemetrexed in EGFR T790M-positive lung cancer. *The New England Journal of Medicine*, *376*(7), 629–640. DOI: 10.1056/NEJMoa1612674 PMID: 27959700

Palma, D. A., Salama, J. K., Lo, S. S., Senan, S., Treasure, T., Govindan, R., & Weichselbaum, R. (2014). The oligometastatic state - separating truth from wishful thinking. *Nature Reviews. Clinical Oncology*, *11*(9), 549–557. DOI: 10.1038/nrclinonc.2014.96 PMID: 24958182

Pennell, N. A., Neal, J. W., Chaft, J. E., Azzoli, C. G., Jänne, P. A., Govindan, R., Evans, T. L., Costa, D. B., Wakelee, H. A., Heist, R. S., Shapiro, M. A., Muzikansky, A., Murthy, S., Lanuti, M., Rusch, V. W., Kris, M. G., & Sequist, L. V. (2019). A phase II trial of adjuvant erlotinib in patients with resected epidermal growth factor receptor-mutant non-small cell lung cancer. *Journal of Clinical Oncology*, *37*(2), 97–104. DOI: 10.1200/JCO.18.00131 PMID: 30444685

Peterson, E., Aker, A., Kim, J., Li, Y., Brand, K., & Copes, R. (2013). Lung cancer risk from radon in Ontario, Canada: How many lung cancers can we prevent? *Cancer Causes & Control*, *24*(11), 156–164. DOI: 10.1007/s10552-013-0278-x PMID: 23982909

Peus, D., Vasa, R. A., Meves, A., Beyerle, A., & Pittelkow, M. R. (2000). UVB induced epidermal growth factor receptor phosphorylation is critical for downstream signaling and keratinocyte survival. *Photochemistry and Photobiology*, *72*(1), 135–140. DOI: 10.1562/0031-8655(2000)072<0135:UIEGFR>2.0.CO;2 PMID: 10911738

Ramalingam, S. S., Vansteenkiste, J., Planchard, D., Cho, B. C., Gray, J., Ohe, Y., Zhou, C., Reungwetwattana, T., Cheng, Y., Chewaskulyong, B., Shah, R., Cobo, M., Lee, K. H., Cheema, P., Tiseo, M., John, T., Lin, M.-C., Imamura, F., Kurata, T., & Soria, J.-C. (2020). Overall survival with osimertinib in untreated, EGFR-mutated advanced NSCLC. *The New England Journal of Medicine*, *382*(1), 41–50. DOI: 10.1056/NEJMoa1913662 PMID: 31751012

Rizvi, N. A., Rusch, V., Pao, W., Chaft, J. E., Ladanyi, M., Miller, V. A., Krug, L. M., Azzoli, C. G., Bains, M., Downey, R., Flores, R., Park, B., Singh, B., Zakowski, M., Heelan, R. T., Shen, R., & Kris, M. G. (2011). Molecular characteristics predict clinical outcomes: Prospective trial correlating response to the EGFR tyrosine kinase inhibitor gefitinib with the presence of sensitizing mutations in the tyrosine binding domain of the EGFR gene. *Clinical Cancer Research*, *17*(10), 3500–3506. DOI: 10.1158/1078-0432.CCR-10-2102 PMID: 21558399

Sequist, L. V., Yang, J. C. H., Yamamoto, N., O'Byrne, K., Hirsh, V., Mok, T., Geater, S. L., Orlov, S., Tsai, C.-M., Boyer, M., Su, W.-C., Bennouna, J., Kato, T., Gorbunova, V., Lee, K. H., Shah, R., Massey, D., Zazulina, V., Shahidi, M., & Schuler, M. (2013). Phase III study of afatinib or cisplatin plus pemetrexed in patients with metastatic lung adenocarcinoma with EGFR mutations. *Journal of Clinical Oncology*, *31*(27), 3327–3334. DOI: 10.1200/JCO.2012.44.2806 PMID: 23816960

Shaikha, A., Nasar, A., Villena-Vargas, J., Harrison, S., Lee, B., & Port, J. L. (2024). Wedgeresection, segmentectomy, and lobectomy: Oncologic outcomes based on extent of surgical resection for≤ 2 cm stage IA non-small cell lung cancer. *Journal of Thoracic Disease*, *16*(3), 1875–1884. DOI: 10.21037/jtd-23-1693 PMID: 38617767

Stratton, M. R., Campbell, P. J., & Futreal, P. A. (2009). The cancer genome. *Nature*, *458*(7239), 719–724. DOI: 10.1038/nature07943 PMID: 19360079

Sung, H., Ferlay, J., Siegel, R. L., Laversanne, M., Soerjomataram, I., Jemal, A., & Bray, F. (2021). Global cancer statistics 2020: GLOBOCAN estimates of incidence and mortality worldwide for 36 cancers in 185 countries. *CA: a Cancer Journal for Clinicians*, *71*(3), 209–249. DOI: 10.3322/caac.21660 PMID: 33538338

Vogel, W. H., & Jennifer, P. (2016). Management strategies for adverse events associated with EGFR TKIs in non–small cell lung cancer. *Journal of the Advanced Practitioner in Oncology*, *7*(7), 723–735. PMID: 29670808

Walsh, G. L., Pisters, K. M. W., & Stevens, C. (2001). Treatment of stage I lung cancer. *Chest Surgery Clinics of North America*, *11*(1), 17–38. DOI: 10.1016/S1052-3359(25)00551-4 PMID: 11253597

Wang, N., Mengersen, K., Tong, S., Kimlin, M., Zhou, M., & Hu, W. (2020). Global, regional, and national burden of lung cancer and its attributable risk factors, 1990 to 2017. *Cancer, 126*(18), 4220–4234. DOI: 10.1002/cncr.33078 PMID: 32648980

Wang, R., Hu, H., Pan, Y., Li, Y., Ye, T., Li, C., Luo, X., Wang, L., Li, H., Zhang, Y., Li, F., Lu, Y., Lu, Q., Xu, J., Garfield, D., Shen, L., Ji, H., Pao, W., Sun, Y., & Chen, H. (2012). RET fusions define a unique molecular and clinicopathologic subtype of non-small-cell lung cancer. *Journal of Clinical Oncology, 30*(35), 4352–4359. DOI: 10.1200/JCO.2012.44.1477 PMID: 23150706

Wei, W., Zeng, H., Zheng, R., Zhang, S., An, L., Chen, R., Wang, S., Sun, K., Matsuda, T., Bray, F., & He, J. (2020). Cancer registration in China and its role in cancer prevention and control. *The Lancet. Oncology, 21*(7), e342–e349. DOI: 10.1016/S1470-2045(20)30073-5 PMID: 32615118

Wu, Y. L., Tsuboi, M., He, J., John, T., Grohe, C., Majem, M., Goldman, J. W., Laktionov, K., Kim, S. W., Kato, T., Vu, H.-V., Lu, S., Lee, K.-Y., Akewanlop, C., Yu, C.-J., de Marinis, F., Bonanno, L., Domine, M., Shepherd, F. A., & Herbst, R. S. (2020). Osimertinib in Resected EGFR-Mutated Non-Small-Cell Lung Cancer. *The New England Journal of Medicine, 383*(18), 1711–1723. DOI: 10.1056/NEJMoa2027071 PMID: 32955177

Yang, X., Man, J., Chen, H., Zhang, T., Yin, X., He, Q., & Lu, M. (2021). A global, regional and national analysis. *Lung Cancer (Amsterdam, Netherlands), 152*, 49–57. DOI: 10.1016/j.lungcan.2020.12.007 PMID: 33348250

Yue, D., Xu, S., Wang, Q., Li, X., Shen, Y., Zhao, H., Chen, C., Mao, W., Liu, W., Liu, J., Zhang, L., Ma, H., Li, Q., Yang, Y., Liu, Y., Chen, H., & Wang, C. (2018). Erlotinib versus vinorelbine plus cisplatin as adjuvant therapy in Chinese patients with Stage IIIA EGFR mutation-positive non-smallcell lung cancer (EVAN): A randomised, open-label, phase 2 trial. *The Lancet. Respiratory Medicine, 6*(11), 863–873. DOI: 10.1016/S2213-2600(18)30277-7 PMID: 30150014

Zhong, W. Z., Chen, K. N., Chen, C., Gu, C.-D., Wang, J., Yang, X.-N., Mao, W.-M., Wang, Q., Qiao, G.-B., Cheng, Y., Xu, L., Wang, C.-L., Chen, M.-W., Kang, X., Yan, W., Yan, H.-H., Liao, R.-Q., Yang, J.-J., Zhang, X.-C., & Wu, Y.-L. (2019). Erlotinib versus gemcitabine plus cisplatin as neoadjuvant treatment of stage IIIA-N2 EGFR-mutant non-small-cell lung cancer (EMERGING-CTONG 1103): A randomized phase II study. *Journal of Clinical Oncology, 37*(25), 2235–2245. DOI: 10.1200/JCO.19.00075 PMID: 31194613

Zhong, W. Z., Wang, Q., Mao, W. M., Xu, S.-T., Wu, L., Wei, Y.-C., Liu, Y.-Y., Chen, C., Cheng, Y., Yin, R., Yang, F., Ren, S.-X., Li, X.-F., Li, J., Huang, C., Liu, Z.-D., Xu, S., Chen, K.-N., Xu, S.-D., & Wu, Y.-L. (2021). Gefitinib versus vinorelbine plus cisplatin as adjuvant treatment for stage II-IIIA (N1-N2) EGFR-mutant NSCLC: Final overall survival analysis of CTONG1104 Phase III trial. *Journal of Clinical Oncology*, *39*(7), 713–722. DOI: 10.1200/JCO.20.01820 PMID: 33332190

Chapter 9
Role of Artificial Intelligence and Machine Learning in the Diagnosis and Treatment of NSCLC

Naveen Singh
Chitkara University School of Pharmacy, Chitkara University, India

Sonalika Bhalla
Chitkara University School of Pharmacy, Chitkara University, India

Vivek Sharma
Chitkara University School of Pharmacy, Chitkara University, India

Nitin Verma
Chitkara University School of Pharmacy, Chitkara University, India

Ankita Thakur
Chitkara University School of Pharmacy, Chitkara University, India

Rajnish Srivastava
https://orcid.org/0000-0002-5988-9858
Chitkara University School of Pharmacy, Chitkara University, India

ABSTRACT

Cancer deaths globally are most common from lung cancer. Up to 57% of patients are diagnosed late; the 5-year survival rate is 10%-16%. ML has been extensively studied to provide patient data-based solutions to improve results. ML and AI have improved non-small cell lung cancer (NSCLC) diagnosis, therapy, and prognosis. Treatment resistance has made advanced-stage NSCLC nearly incurable, despite the development of signal transduction system blockers that target driver mutations. Understanding the common molecular patterns that support targeted therapy resistance in NSCLC subtypes is essential to developing successful treatments and overcoming tumor heterogeneity. We must understand these qualities to optimize

DOI: 10.4018/979-8-3373-2096-0.ch009

treatment and overcome therapeutic challenges for squamous NSCLC patients to improve outcomes. Lung cancer imaging and early diagnosis have improved because of AI approaches like Natural language processing (NLP) and convolutional neural networks (CNNs). CNN distinguishes benign and malignant nodules to aid early detection and reduce biopsies. NLP extracts clinical information from unstructured medical texts and EHRs to improve patient histories and treatment planning. AI algorithms have shown great predictive accuracy in personalized treatment strategies. AI algorithms can help clinicians screen at-risk asymptomatic patients, investigate and triage symptomatic patients, and diagnose cancer recurrence. Possible limits and hazards include ethics, resource requirements, data security, and reporting criteria.

1. INTRODUCTION

Artificial Intelligence (AI) and Machine Learning (ML) tools demonstrate a breakthrough in cancer diagnosis, treatment procedures and detection methods in clinical oncology medicine (Iqbal et al., 2021). Data-oriented AI subsets extract knowledge to produce improved operational results through autonomous learning techniques, avoiding explicit coding practice at various stages of cancer care (Dlamini et al., 2020). These are strong analytical instruments for researchers to process the intricate datasets collected from clinical databases, imaging records, genomic records and pathological specimen analysis data (Schneider et al., 2022). Additionally, their constructive use helps in providing the prior detection, improvised diagnosis, plan of treatment, and selective medication therapy. This eventually leads to an improvement of both clinical outcome and healthcare efficiency (Khan et al., 2024). Medical imaging analysis in oncology using AI and ML algorithms is employed to detect subtle patterns that would be invisible with human vision in PET analysis, MR, and CT scans (Paudyal et al., 2023). Furthermore, the different deep learning models have demonstrated accuracy in malignancy and tumor detection, segmentation, and prediction in the therapy (Karayegen & Aksahin, 2021). Furthermore, it is often the case that genomic and proteomic data are used by the ML models for their purposes, such as finding mutations in the precision oncology domain for providing a personalized treatment approach (Xu et al., 2019). In addition, oncologists are utilizing AI-powered clinical decision support systems (CDSS) that consider the patient data with the base of evidence to provide the best treatment options (Grüger et al., 2025).

Non-Small Cell Lung Cancer (NSCLC) outlines approximately 85% of all lung cancer cases globally (Rodak et al., 2021). Consequently, it has become a major AI and ML application focus area with the high incidence and death rates (Huang et al., 2023). The histological subtypes of NSCLC include squamous cell carcinoma, adenocarcinoma, and large cell carcinoma (Qu et al., 2019). Due to its high mortality rate, the disease offers an advanced stage and recent developments in the therapy are not curative, especially for the most metastatic cases (Wang et al., 2010). NSCLC is a heterogeneous disease with EGFR mutations, ALK rearrangements, and KRAS mutations identified in cellular and molecular architectures (Fois et al., 2021). These genetic biomarkers allow for creating the road for efficient targeted therapies and immunotherapies (Khan & Zannat, 2024).

However, more advanced tools are required to forecast results and optimize treatments for tumor biology and patients' response heterogeneity. Thus, the area of development of AI and ML is increasing in this aspect (Khalighi et al., 2024). ML tools are developed for stratification of NSCLC patients based on risk, prediction of the treatment outcomes and forecasting the disease progression according to multi-omics platforms, radiomics, and electronic health records (Mei et al., 2024). Initial lung nodules analysis and the enhanced staging accuracy occur via the aid of AI-driven radiology tools (Ewals et al., 2023). Moreover, the valuable insights from unstructured clinical data to support real-time clinical decision-making are backed up by a branch of AI called natural language processing (NLP) (Hossain et al., 2024).

In conclusion, the AI and ML integration in the oncology domain is supporting the development of NSCLC management (El Sabrouty & Elouadi, 2025). It enables the diagnosis with accuracy, and personalization in the treatment strategies, and its progressive advance in novel therapeutic options research (Ho et al., 2020). The sudden increase of the complexity and size of the datasets necessitates the expanded role of AI and ML in NSCLC (Fiste et al., 2024). This will ultimately produce better patient outcomes and effective delivery of medical care.

1.1 Methodology

A systematic literature review was searched on PubMed, Scopus and Web of Science accessing the keywords as "AI", "ML", "Oncology", "NSCLC", "radiomics", "deep learning", and "clinical decision support". The search was limited to studies published from 2015 to 2025. Eligibility criteria for this review included peer-reviewed articles with those containing original research or systematic reviews on AI/ML applications on NSCLC's diagnostic, predicting prognosis, predicting treatment, and supporting clinical decision-making (**Table 1**). The dataset type, model, and external validation of the studies were assessed. Non-NSCLC cases and articles without performance measures or utilizing non-clinical data sets were excluded.

Table 1. Representative AI/ML studies in NSCLC

Study (Author, Year)	(Dataset Size)	External Validation	Key Performance Metrics
Ardila et al., 2019 (Nature Medicine)	>42,000 CT scans (NLST dataset)	Yes	AUC 0.94 for lung cancer detection
Coudray et al., 2018 (Nature Medicine) [23]	~1,000 lung cancer slides (TCGA)	Yes	Accuracy 97%; AUC 0.97 for subtype classification
Mali et al., 2025 (arXiv)	876 NSCLC patients (604 training, 272 test)	Yes (multicenter)	Clinical + foundation-model features: C-index 0.7616, t-AUC 0.8866; consensus model: t-AUC 0.92, sensitivity 97.6%, specificity 66.7%
Hosny et al., 2018 (The lancet Oncology)	350 NSCLC patients (multi-institutional radiomics dataset)	Yes	c-index 0.70 for survival prediction
Mu et al., 2020 (JAMA Network Open)	1,011 NSCLC patients (EHR + genomic data)	No	AUC 0.86 for progression prediction

The existing evidence in favour of AI and ML in the management of NSCLC is moderate to strong and growing. The strongest evidence (Level I–II) is from large multi-institutional series such as that of Ardila et al. and Coudray et al., which involve external validation and show strong diagnostic performance as well as accurate subtyping (Padinharayil et al., 2023; Coudray et al., 2018). Additionally, the study by Mali et al. (2025) provides strong evidence (Level II) for the application of AI/ML in NSCLC prognosis (Mali et al., 2025). Furthermore, a moderate level of evidence (Level III) is demonstrated by radiomics-based prognostic models and prediction of outcome studies, for example., Hosny et al, with significant potential to be validated in larger and more diverse patient cohorts (Hosny et al., 2018). Moreover, level IV evidence is provided by studies that integrate multi-omics and electronic health record (EHR) data (e.g., Mu et al.), which can offer critical insights but lack stable external validation (Mu et al., 2020). In summary, although AI and ML for NSCLC diagnosis are entering the clinical application process, their applications in prognosis and predicting therapeutic effects remain mostly investigational, requiring large datasets, verification of their clinical application, and approval from relevant regulatory authorities.

Furthermore, the recent development of AI and ML has demonstrated potential applications in NSCLC. However, clinical applications remain inconsistent across various fields. In the application of low-dose CT screening for lung cancer, AI systems have demonstrated remarkable sensitivity gains (5-20%), but at the expense of specificity and false positives, which highlights the problem of overdiagnosis and the need for integration with the workflow (Geppert et al., 2024). Deep learning histopathology methods such as CNN-Vision Transformer hybrids have high accuracy and stability for subtype classification, potentially indicating medium clinical readiness, but raising concerns about computational costs and interpretability (Liu et al., 2023). Besides imaging, transformer-based models trained on more than three million electronic health records (EHRs) have been proposed for early identification of lung cancer, but their utility needs to be validated in external cohorts (Wang et al., 2024). Furthermore, vision transformer architectures are also being increasingly used across imaging tasks such as classification and segmentation, with promising results but a lack of real-world assessment (Ali et al., 2023). Furthermore, multimodal AI-enabled CT and biomarkers-based workflows showed sensitivity >90% and specificity up to 85-90%, supporting the potential for an improved screening strategy, but also highlighting the need for strong prospective validation (Duranti et al., 2025). While these studies underscore the potential of AI for all stages of screening, molecular profiling, and treatment stratification, the majority are emerging at medium readiness levels (Table 2), hindered by challenges of generalizability and interpretability, as well as the absence of prospective clinical validation.

Table 2. Readiness of AI/ML applications in NSCLC

S.No.	Application	Recent studies	Typical Metrics	Clinical readiness	Key constraints
1.	LDCT nodule detection & screening	Systematic review: AI improves sensitivity (+5–20%), reduces specificity (−3–8%) in detection of CT lung nodules (Geppert et al., 2024)	Sensitivity +5–20%; specificity −3–8% vs. unaided reading	Medium	Increased false positives; applicability bias; workflow integration
2.	Histopathology based subtype classification	Multilayer perceptron model using CNN and Vision Transformers showed high accuracy for malignancy prediction. (Liu et al., 2023)	High accuracy and stability in classification	Emerging → Medium	Model complexity; computational cost; interpretability
3.	Transformer-based diagnosis via EHR	Transformer applied to EHR data for lung cancer early detection; built on over 3M records. (Wang et al., 2024)	Not specified; large-scale EHR-based modeling	Emerging	Validation on external cohorts; integration into clinical systems

continued on following page

Table 2. Continued

S.No.	Application	Recent studies	Typical Metrics	Clinical readiness	Key constraints
4.	Vision transformer in histopathology review	Review indicates increased use of vision transformers in lung cancer imaging tasks (diagnosis, segmentation). (Ali et al., 2023)	General improved performance in tasks like classification	Emerging	High computational needs; lacking clinical deployment testing
5.	AI + biomarker/ lung screening enhancement	Review reports AI in CT and biomarker workflows, with sensitivity >90%, specificity up to 85–90%. (Duranti et al., 2025)	Sensitivity >90%, specificity up to 85–90%	Emerging	Need clinical validation; integration of multi-modal data systems

Despite AI's promise in NSCLC diagnostics, several studies highlight limitations that can harm clinical outcomes. For instance, a study analyzing radiologist–AI interaction found that when AI outputs were incorrect, radiologists made significantly more false-negative and false-positive errors—even when previously correct—revealing a dangerous overreliance on AI results (Bernstein et al., 2023). Another radiomics model intended to predict EGFR mutation status failed in external validation, with performance (AUC $\approx$ 0.5) falling below that of a purely clinical model (AUC $\approx$ 0.74), indicating poor generalizability and limited added value (Kohan et al., 2025). Additionally, AI frequently misclassified benign lesions as malignant: in one observational study, 32 benign pulmonary lesions were initially flagged as malignant by the AI, only to be confirmed benign post-surgery; the AUC for parameters like CT value and solidity ratio was just moderate (~0.71) (Sun et al., 2023). These examples underscore the importance of robust validation, avoidance of overreliance, and careful integration into clinical workflows to prevent avoidable harm.

Lung cancer is often missed on chest radiographs, despite chest radiography typically being the first imaging modality in the diagnosis pathway. We have discussed some of the case studies that demonstrate the impact and pitfalls in lung cancer diagnosis. Firstly, a 46-year-old male with chest pain had an initial chest X-ray interpreted as normal and was discharged. Four months later, repeat imaging revealed an enlarging left perihilar mass with post-obstructive atelectasis. CT and biopsy confirmed squamous cell carcinoma. Retrospective review of the original X-ray with FDA-cleared AI software (Chest-CAD) flagged the lesion as suspicious. This case illustrates how AI support could help prevent delayed lung cancer diagnosis (Sicular et al., 2022). Secondly, in a retrospective study of 21 patients with solitary pulmonary nodules (SPNs) that were reported to be associated with

COVID-19, CT, and MR images were misclassified by AI as being high-risk nodules associated with lung cancer. While RT-PCR confirmed the diagnosis of COVID-19, abnormal patterns like burr sign, lobulation, and pleural indentation were reported by AI-generated reports. Radiologists, however, had good accuracy in recognizing them as benign. AI and radiologist diagnoses were poorly aligned ($k = 0.036$). This underlines the potential for miscalculation by AI in new disease settings such as COVID-19 (Wu et al., 2022).

2. UNDERSTANDING THE PATHOPHYSIOLOGY OF NON-SMALL CELL LUNG CANCER (NSCLC)

NSCLC develops through multiple pathophysiological factors that include mutations in epigenetic modifications, external carcinogens, genetic elements, and alterations in the surrounding tumor environment (Alduais et al., 2023). The first appearance of NSCLC usually develops in the bronchi or alveoli epithelial lining after exposure to risk factors that include tobacco smoke, air pollution, radon gas, and occupational hazards, leading to the triggering of carcinogenesis molecular pathway (Chevallier et al., 2021).

The DNA mutations in NSCLC generate active oncogenes while simultaneously disabling tumor suppressor genes at the cellular level (Mohanty et al., 2024). Furthermore, uncontrolled cell growth occurs through PI3K/AKT/mTOR and RAS/RAF/MEK/ERK signaling pathways because of mutant EGFR (Epidermal Growth Factor Receptor), KRAS, ALK (Anaplastic Lymphoma Kinase), BRAF, and ROS1 oncogenes (Dan et al., 2024). Mutations in cancer-related genes like TP53, RB1, PTEN, and LKB1 terminate essential regulatory functions, which allow cancer cells to escape

programmed death and control the cell cycle appropriately (Bhat et al., 2024). The malignant transformation of lung epithelial cells simultaneously relies on these genetic abnormalities, generating tumor heterogeneity as a major obstacle for medical diagnosis and therapy (De Visser & Joyce, 2023). The evolving tumor starts to develop new abilities to spread and grow during progression (Zhao et al., 2022). The formation of new blood vessels depends on vascular endothelial growth factor (VEGF) production by NSCLC tumors, enabling their supply with nutrients and oxygen (Stock, 2022). The tumor cells change the extracellular matrix and produce proteolytic enzymes that allow their invasion into nearby tissues, facilitating metastasis toward the brain, liver, bones, and adrenal glands (Mao et al., 2021). The tumor microenvironment, consisting of immune cells next to fibroblasts, endothelial cells, and several cytokines, actively promotes tumor expansion and immune cells to escape detection. PD-L1 overexpression by tumor cells allows them to bypass immune surveillance, making it a valid target for immune checkpoint inhibitor therapy (Xu et al., 2024). **[Figure 1]**

Figure 1. Representation of the pathogenesis of Non-Small Cell Lung Cancer (NSCLC).

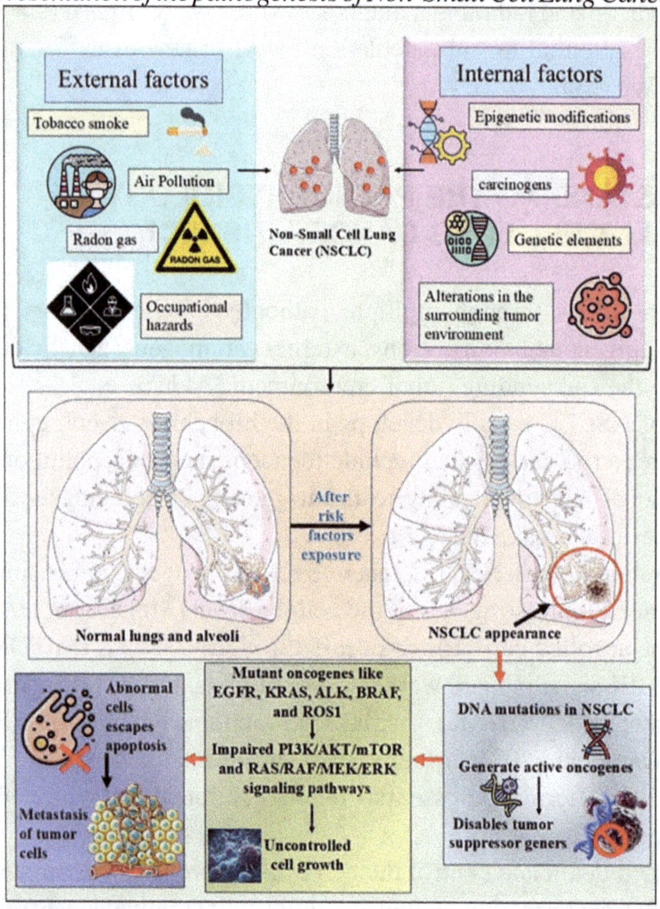

The figure illustrates the various external as well as internal risk factors responsible for causing NSCLC in the alveoli, leading to mutations in DNA. The mutant oncogenes then impair various cellular and molecular signalling pathways such as PI3K/AKT/mTOR and RAS/RAF/MEK/ERK, resulting in uncontrolled cell growth. After that, these cells escape the programmed cell death, ie. apoptosis, eventually causing metastasis of tumor cells throughout the body.

Knowledge about NSCLC pathophysiological processes leads to better development of specific therapeutic strategies and individualized treatment plans (Li et al., 2022). The driver mutation identification has created the way for precision medicine, providing selected targeted agents such as tyrosine kinase inhibitors (TKIs) and immune checkpoint inhibitors according to individual tumor profiles (Fiste et al., 2024). Lastly, by employing findings from NSCLC pathophysiology, AI-driven models provide the potential to increase diagnostic accuracy and treatment efficacy. This marks a paradigm shift in the clinical management of lung cancer.

3. AI-DRIVEN APPROACHES TO NSCLC DIAGNOSIS

Recent breakthroughs in AI present the significant potential for transforming the diagnosis of NSCLC through improved imaging analysis, data-driven decision-making, and biomarker discovery (El Sabrouty & Elouadi, 2025). AI models, particularly deep learning algorithms like convolutional neural networks (CNNs) and natural language processing (NLP) systems, are leading this diagnostic transformation (Shatnawi et al., 2025).

3.1. Imaging-Based Diagnosis: CNNs, CAD, and Radiomics

3.1.1. Convolutional neural networks

AI application in the field of NSCLC diagnosis is mainly useful for medical imaging. A class of DL models known as CNNs has been shown to have high specificity and sensitivity on analyzing X-rays and chest CT scan to distinguish benign against malignant pulmonary nodules. CNNs effectively learn spatial hierarchies in visual data, rendering them highly effective at identifying the presence of lung nodules, whether benign or malignant (Ardila et al., 2019). CNNs have the advantage of automatically extracting features such as edges, texture, density variations and values. An author employed the 3D CNN model to low dose computed tomography (LDCT) data from National lung Screening Trial (NLST) and obtained 0.94 AUC for cancer prediction. In first screenings without a preceding picture, it surpassed radiologists' performance (Quanyang et al., 2024). DenseNet, U-NeT and VGGNet, are commonly used CNN models in lung image segmentation and classification (Ladbury et al., 2023).

However, CNNs are used to analyze tumour characteristics like size and temporal growth from temporal imaging in the oncology domain. In addition, these models can accurately classify the types of tumors, for example, adenocarcinoma, squamous cell carcinoma and small cell lung cancer (SCLC). CNNs in imaging studies can also predict the spread of metastatic lymph nodes and adjacent anatomical structure involvement (Coudray et al., 2018). For example, Coudray *et al.*, trained a CNN to classify the histological type with a very high area under the curve (AUC) of 0.97. Remarkably, their model was also able to predict the presence of driver mutations (EGFR, KRAS, etc) directly from pathology slide images (Apostolopoulos et al., 2025). The CNNs are also used longitudinally to monitor treatment responses. When given multi-phase imaging data, such as data from PET/CT scans, these networks can track tumor shrinkage and changes in activity over the duration of treatment. In addition, hybrid models that combine CNNs and support vector machines (SVMs), have very high accuracy of AUCs between 0.93 - 0.98 for classifying early responders and non-responders during treatment. This facility allows real-time changes in therapeutic strategies and better patient management (Gu et al., 2021).

3.1.2. Computer-Aided Diagnosis

Computer-Aided Diagnosis (CAD) systems, usually driven by AI algorithms, are a second-level diagnostic tool for lesion appearance and characterization, among them, identification as malignant. These systems utilize different ML algorithms for automatic identification and segmentation of lung nodules and normal anatomy on lung CT, providing both the ability to act as a second opinion to the radiologist's judgement, and a source of quantitative metrics for the staging and monitoring of patients (Cellina et al., 2023). It is worth noting that these systems do not classify nodules as benign or malignant but rather highlight regions of interest. These systems indicate suspicious areas in LDCT scans by significantly reducing the burden of interpretative work and human errors (Zhang et al., 2021). Many FDA-approved systems, such as InferRead CT Lung (IRCL), which use DenseNet-based 3D CNN, have been shown to bring out diagnostic performance as well as human radiologists (Camps et al., 2025).

3.1.3. Radiomics

AI is further extended by radiomics, which provides the extraction of high–dimensional quantitative features in imaging that can subsequently be utilized with clinical and genomic data for non-invasive tumor characterization. Moreover, the use of the radiomic data by AI models has produced strong performance (AUC $\approx$ 0.93) for NSCLC classification against other types, such as small-cell lung cancer (SCLC). Radiomics gives non-invasive tumor classification, monitoring response to treatment, and gives a prediction of recurrence (Coudray et al., 2018; Lee et al., 2025).

3.2. Natural Language Processing (NLP) in Clinical Records

Natural Language Processing (NLP) in general is key for extracting and interpreting useful textual data from electronic health records (EHR) and other texts such as radiology reports, pathology findings, and clinical notes. Many times, several critical patient information, such as medical history, presenting symptoms, and radiological impressions, are stored in unstructured formats. The unstructured text is transformed through NLP techniques into structured and analyzable data, which can be used for more appropriate clinical decision making and predictive modelling (Kehl et al., 2021). A researcher developed an NLP model utilizing over 300,000 imaging results from 16,780 patients. The concordance index of this system was 0.76, and the AUC was 0.77. Such predictive capabilities provide NLP with great potential to improve prognostic assessments and guide clinical interventions (Wang et al., 2019).

NLP algorithms can evaluate historical clinical data and EHR records to identify individuals at high risk of disease development who may benefit from early screening. Furthermore, discharge summaries or follow-up notes may be analyzed for linguistic patterns to assess the likelihood of illness recurrence or metastasis (Kehl et al., 2021). Another study by Wang *et al.*, who retrieved characteristics from over 800,000 patient records via NLP. The integration of this data with an XGBoost model yielded an effective prediction model for lung cancer development during 12 months, achieving an AUC of 0.88. Furthermore, NLP may be utilized to extract patient characteristics and genetic test findings to address the challenge of individualized treatment. Additionally, the identification of patients eligible for the particular targeted treatment study is based on NSCLC molecular markers, such as ALK-positive or EGFR-mutated NSCLC. Also, NLP tools can find the patient profiles that fit the inclusion criteria from vast clinical trial databases, improving the efficiency of recruitment and supporting precision oncology efforts (Wang et al., 2019).

3.3. Liquid Biopsies & Molecular Diagnosis

In the diagnosis of NSCLC, liquid biopsies such as circulating tumor DNA (ctDNA) and microRNA profiles are processed by AI methods, including ML models to find out malignancy, monitor tumor heterogeneity, and predict mutations such as EGFR, PD-L1, and ALK. Such early detection and personalized treatment are possible since these are non-invasive methods that can predict the mutations before tissue biopsy results are available (Kumar, 2024). High accuracy of deep learning models is demonstrated to almost over 90% of precision in mutation prediction and thereby drastically reduces the need for invasive procedures and enhances patient stratification for targeted therapies. Moreover, through integration with multi-omics data (genomic, transcriptomic and proteomic), it finds biomarker patterns for the development of personalized treatment plans as well as to increase diagnostic efficiency with high sensitivity (77%) and specificity (79%) in detecting lung cancer biomarkers (Ren et al., 2024).

4. METHODS, DATA PROVENANCE & REGULATORY ETHICS

AI and ML are to be effectively translated into care in NSCLC; a clear methodological framework is required to enable translation from evidence synthesis to practice. First, the data need to be reported openly, providing both the source datasets, the steps used to clean them, and the criteria used to curate them so that others can recreate the work and test it against new data. Second, ethics must be integrated throughout the process of constructing models-including patient consent, privacy, algorithms' transparency, and bias-to prevent the possibility of inequities being baked into the AI systems. Without such safeguards, AI outputs that are already shaped to the specific circumstances of the given data collection may become even less applicable to other populations and could exacerbate existing disparities in healthcare. Employing these guidelines and implementing a stringent reporting of evidence will help to further boost the scientific credibility and support international best practices such as TRIPOD-AI and CONSORT-AI, respectively. The Data, validation, Regulatory Status, and NSCLC Relevance are shown in **Tables 3 and 4** (Huang et al., 2024; Rabbani et al., 2018; Ardila et al., 2019; Coudray et al., 2018).

Table 3. AI Models Applied to NSCLC: Data, Validation, and Outcomes (65-68).

AI Application in NSCLC	Representative Study/Model	Dataset & Size	Validation Type	Performance Metrics
Nodule classification	3D CNN (Ardila et al., 2019)	NLST LDCT (~15k scans)	External, retrospective	AUC 0.94
Histology subtype & mutation prediction	CNN (Coudray et al., 2018)	TCGA WSIs (~1k slides)	External, retrospective	AUC 0.97 (subtype), 0.85 (mutation)
NLP for incidence/ recurrence	Wang et al., 2019; Lee et al., 2025	>800k EHRs	Multi-site	AUC 0.77–0.88
Radiomics for treatment response	Trebeschi et al., 2021	Multicenter (~500 pts)	Limited prospective	AUC 0.78

Table 4. AI-Based Tools with Regulatory Status and NSCLC Relevance (69-73).

AI Tool	Indication	Regulatory Status	Relevance to NSCLC
InferRead CT Lung	Nodule detection	CE, CFDA approved	Widely used in China/EU
Arterys Lung AI	Nodule quantification, growth tracking	FDA-cleared (510k)	Supports staging & monitoring
Paige.AI Pathology	Digital histopathology	CE-IVD, FDA (for prostate; lung pipeline)	Assists NSCLC subtype classification
Qure.ai (qCT/ qXR)	CXR/CT lung disease detection	CE; FDA pending	Used in screening programs
Transpara CAD	Lesion detection	CE-marked; FDA for breast, lung in development	Expanding to lung oncology

NSCLC is a computationally expensive disease, and it is very difficult to apply AI in practice because of the economic and infrastructural constraints. Naturally, most AI systems are expensive to implement. They also need to be integrated smoothly with hospital IT systems and continuously cared for and maintained. Very little research work has been done on their cost-effectiveness. Are we OK with the costs; they say early evidence shows that AI can lower unnecessary biopsies and early diagnosis potentially layers cost. Health-economic studies can characterise actual challenges of the practical implementation of AI. They can also spell out the value they provide, the changes required, and the obstacles that need to be overcome.

5. AI-DRIVEN APPROACHES TO OPTIMIZE THE TREATMENT OF NSCLC

The rising application of AI in NSCLC treatment now plays a vital role by improving each stage, including diagnosis and selecting the most appropriate treatments (Qure.ai, 2023; CE Mark News, 2023). The most basic approaches for diagnosis and treatment incorporating the use of AI are given in **Figure 2.**

Figure 2. Basic AI integrated Approaches for Diagnosis and Treatment of NSCLC

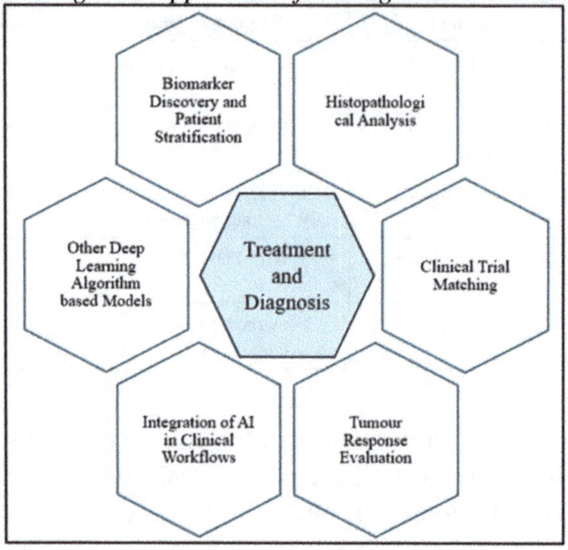

1. Biomarker Discovery and Patient Stratification

AI detective has revolutionized the discovery of biomarkers for oncology applications, specifically focused on precise medicine treatments of NSCLC cancer cases. Traditional methods fail to identify predictive biomarkers since cancer biology remains difficult to understand, while clinical data contains many dimensions. Potent AI solutions employ deep learning frameworks to detect distinctive patterns embedded in healthcare information systems comprising electronic health records (EHRs), radiology images, as well as pathology reports. The generated predictive biomarkers through these methods help doctors select proper treatments while enhancing treatment success rates for patients (Fiste et al., 2024). The Predictive Biomarker Modelling Framework (PBMF) is a revolutionary tool in healthcare that uses AI to identify biomarkers in clinical trials. This technology is crucial for developing new treatments for NSCLC patients, enabling the development of targeted therapeutic approaches (Pei et al., 2022). The PBMF uses contrastive learning to analyze predictive biomarkers, revealing information beyond genetic mutations. The integration of AI technologies and empirical data validation protocols will drive oncology practice towards efficient targeted therapeutic approaches. AI literacy training is essential for healthcare providers to effectively use these advanced tools for clinical decisions.Future oncology treatment will experience a revolutionary shift through AI-driven biomarker discovery that uses sophisticated analytical methods to combine clinical data to transform medical strategies and personalize treatment and yield better outcomes for NSCLC patients (Kaplan et al., 2021).

2. Histopathological Analysis

The application of AI in histopathological analysis leads to a transformation of cancer diagnosis procedures and treatment strategies for NSCLC. Histopathological tumour subtype analysis currently requires much time and face challenges in consistency due to pathologist dependence. The challenges of manual pathologic subtype analysis can be addressed through deep learning models which process extensive whole-slide imaging datasets to generate automated, effective classifications. Multiple scientific investigations have proven that AI algorithms achieve histological tumour classification at a level equivalent to or higher than human skill in diagnosis, so that tests become faster while enabling timely treatment choices. The processing power of AI allows it to process large datasets, which helps facilitate the integration of molecular and histological characteristics for identifying patient-specific treatment options. The specific needs in current oncology practice favour the implementation of targeted strategies because individual tumour profiles are used to match responsible treatments. AI predictive modelling achieves clinical trial patient matching and treatment outcome predictions using modern algorithms that analyse multimodal data, which combines imaging with clinical and genomic information (Shao et al., 2023; Li et al., 2022; Hu et al., 2023).

Medical diagnosis automation both decreases healthcare practitioners' workload and makes clinical workflow more efficient, which enables practitioners to focus on treating individual patients. The availability of established AI models that attained CE-IVD marking and FDA clearance makes them prepared for routine clinical practice in different cancer types. The progress of large language models (LLMs) has led to the automation of patient-trial matching through efficient processing of unstructured data found in electronic health records which optimizes clinical trial eligibility assessments. AI-based systems encounter ongoing challenges in clinical settings because of their interpretability issues, together with the need to improve robust operational stability. AI-generated classification methods require additional research to verify their efficacy against established confirmatory tests because of observed differences. Cancer research enters a critical stage because predictive biomarkers found through AI represent a major discovery area. AI-based histopathological analysis will likely play a key role in advancing precision oncology since its ongoing development will lead to better treatment decisions that yield improved patient results (Pacurari et al., 2023).

3. Clinical Trial Matching

AI technology provides essential performance improvements to clinical studies recruitment by matching suitable patients to trials during oncology research. Traditional manual clinical trial patient matching involves extensive manual record evaluation of individuals and eligibility criteria assessment that requires significant time while missing many potential patient participants (Gao et al., 2023). Large language models and GPT-4 revolutionized AI processes of unstructured electronic health record processing through their application. Automated patient identification works faster to find appropriate participants while eliminating human intervention needs to speed up exact trial matching. Extensive patient-based analysis through ML models predicts which patients fit medical trial entry requirements by processing their demographic and response and medical data. A probabilistic evaluation system within this framework enables physicians to identify participants that would receive maximum benefits from research studies. The comprehensive patient data matching becomes possible through combined analysis of genomic information and pathology reports and radiologic images (Huang et al., 2023). AI-based patient matching systems defeat heterogeneity in medical data and break down difficult clinical trial documentation so doctors can match appropriate candidates. Natural language processing analytics at an advanced level translates medical trial jargon into results that match patient data through these systems. The implementation of AI in this field accelerates patient recruiting while expanding healthcare opportunities to leading medical treatments that generate superior real-world medical results (Iqbal et al., 2021).

4. Tumour Response Evaluation

AI (AI) applications provide sophisticated tumour evaluation through simplification of cancer treatment response assessment methods. The Response Evaluation Criteria in Solid Tumours (RECIST) method requires manual expertise of radiologists to evaluate tumour size across imaging data for tracking treatment responses until today. A human-dependent standard manual evaluation process requires excessive work from radiologists and produces inconsistent results among readers, so a better method needs to be adopted. Advanced AI techniques include nnU-Net and Segment Anything Models (SAMs) for automatic segmentation, which enable robotic tumour border definition in medical imaging. The models achieve excellent accuracy when determining tumour volume modifications to provide a quantitative assessment of treatment results independent of radiologist inputs. Clinical implementation of volumetric analysis faces obstacles because contemporary practices continue to utilize diameter assessments mainly because of past protocol standards and RECIST recommendations (Yoshimi, 2025). The use of AI technology in tumour assessment has significantly improved clinical and medical practices. By integrating radiological, histopathological, and genomic information, AI systems automate the assessment of histology images, enabling better tumour type detection and treatment response evaluation. This integration reduces healthcare practitioners' workload and enhances assessment precision. AI systems also help access complex cancer treatment technology, reducing socioeconomic limitations in smaller medical facilities (Hope et al., 2021). Nintendo Game Boy Advance (NGS) is an indispensable tool in medical centres, aiding in the identification of tumour mutations and facilitating clinical trial matching and patient assessment. These advancements in oncology practice provide enhanced treatment selection systems and superior treatment results for cancer patients. AI-powered tumour response assessment development needs medical researchers to team up with clinicians who will conduct ongoing research. Oncology practice benefits from recent technological innovations, which provide enhanced treatment selection systems and superior treatment results for patients fighting cancer (Liu et al., 2023).

5. Integration of AI in Clinical Workflows

AI integration within clinical practice transforms healthcare through better decisions and individualized treatment plans that yield enhanced results. Recent discoveries in AI-based analytical systems combined with algorithms enable the efficient investigation of massive datasets that enhance drug discovery and development processes. Through their combined partnership AI systems can leverage "big data" to find new therapeutic targets and speed up the creation of personalized medicines (Johnson et al., 2022). AI automation provides healthcare practitioners with two important benefits: it reduces their workload and speeds up patient treatment. The specific automation tasks include imaging pre-screening and histological subtyping. Deep learning models that analyse histological pictures prove valuable for tumour type identification because they demonstrate results matching those of human experts in situations where expert doctors are limited. Medical research screening using AI technologies transforms the assessment process for therapeutic trial participants. Standard patient history review processes depended on manual assessment of extensive medical records while consuming a large amount of time as well as being labour intensive. GPT-4 along with Llama-3 represent leading examples of Large Language Models that process unstructured data found in electronic health records (EHRs) to carry out efficient trial-patient matching (Chiu et al., 2022). The automated recruitment process optimizes the trial recruitment workflow while improving clinical trial success through patient-prerequisite matching of their specific clinical signatures. Multimodal imaging integration with genomic data enables AI to discover predictive biomarkers, which enhances personalized medicine approaches (Trebeschi et al., 2021).

6. Other deep learning-based algorithm models:

Deep learning (DL) algorithms apply AI to revolutionize NSCLC treatment therapy via multiple applications that are part of its rapid research and development. DL technologies are instrumental in the study of predictive biomarkers since personalized medical care relies on individual biomarkers to develop personalized treatment models that consider the needs of specific patients. The AI techniques are playing vital roles in diagnosis through imaging analysis, which is typically done by pathologists to identify subtypes of tumours at the pathologist level. The AI models correlate with the evaluation of the pathologist in the patient to provide quick and effective treatments within shorter assessment time frames. By using this technology, medical professionals can make trials and patient matching easier because they would otherwise conduct manual medical record evaluations (Pei et al., 2022).

6. APPLICATIONS OF AI AND ML IN THE DIAGNOSIS AND TREATMENT OF NSCLC

AI and ML technology revolutionize healthcare practices, specifically for lung cancer treatment within oncology, while profoundly impacting various fields, particularly medicine. AI uses medical imaging analysis to detect early pulmonary nodules, thus enhancing the accuracy of diagnoses because lung cancer has high mortality and death rates. The combination of patient analysis with result prediction through ML systems helps to find optimal treatment options and presents an opportunity to enhance survival outcomes while potentially reducing mortality statistics (Huang et al., 2023). The disease that causes most cancer deaths, including lung cancer, has been significantly enhanced through the application of AI (AI) and ML (ML) for both diagnosis and disease prediction. Various AI approaches like ML, deep learning, reinforcement learning, and natural language processing (NLP) enhance diagnostic capabilities and patient outcome forecasts in medical settings. The analysis of challenging medical information with these tools leads to better lung cancer screening methods as well as therapy selection for affected patients. Survival rates increase through early detection combined with accurate treatments because AI brings great value as a medical tool during lung cancer battles (Fiste et al., 2024). Management of NSCLC is increasingly using AI (AI) and ML (ML) to improve diagnosis, therapy advice, and prognosis. These systems extract patterns and future-telling biomarkers of large datasets that may inform health decisions.

Significant applications are Pathomics (which analyzes the data of pathology to gain insights into tumour biology) and radiomics (which analyses the data of imaging to gain insights in tumour characterisation). Although the standardization and implementation of AI-driven solutions into clinical practice is challenging, their potential to change the individual approach to the treatment of NSCLC is immense, thereby offering an opportunity to improve patient outcomes (Rajesh et al., 2020). Particularly for lung cancer, which is difficult to identify early, AI (AI) and ML (ML) are used increasingly in cancer detection. Medical image analysis is improved using AI via methods like computer-aided diagnosis (CAD) and digital image processing. Although current techniques concentrate on conventional image processing for noise reduction and feature extraction, AI applications, including ML and Deep Learning, are still somewhat restricted. This work addresses the application of AI to handle CT scan images for data collecting and model training, therefore facilitating better malignant nodule prediction and detection. Furthermore, smartphone apps have been created to let patients monitor their health and remain updated about their situation (Chiu et al., 2022). Lung cancer diagnosis and treatment benefit from the increasingly used AI and ML. Several AI systems are certified by the FDA for this use, they help to analyze imaging data from CT scans and chest X-rays (CXR). Digital whole slide imaging (WSI) uses AI (AI) for annotations and combines clinical and demographic data to support decisions on EGFR mutations and PD-L1 expression. Furthermore, improving prognosis estimates is AI systems' ability to forecast therapeutic responses, tumor recurrence, and treatment adverse effects. Future developments in lung cancer treatment depend on the incorporation of AI into clinical processes, notwithstanding present obstacles (Çalışkan & Tazaki, 2023). Applications in lung cancer research using AI and ML center on biomarker finding for NSCLC. Using text-mining methods, investigators found 215 papers using AI/ML systems to document possible biomarkers. Based on BEST biomarker subtypes, these papers were arranged to show developing trends in AI/ML-driven biomarker research. This thorough study seeks to improve knowledge and enable the clinical acceptance of biomarkers produced from AI and ML in NSCLC therapy (Huang et al., 2023). Early identification of suspicious nodules through imaging (X-rays, CT, PET), differentiation between benign and malignant nodules, recognition of predictive biomarkers, help in tumour classification, and development of personalized treatment options to improve patient prognosis (Table 5) (El Arab et al., 2025).

Table 5. AI and ML applications in lung cancer management (Huang et al., 2023; Fiste et al., 2024; Rajesh et al., 2020; Chiu et al., 2022; Çalışkan & Tazaki, 2023; Huang et al., 2023; El Arab et al., 2025).

SR NO	Application in NSCLC	Role of ML (ML)	Role of AI (AI)
1.	Early Detection and Diagnosis	Trains on large imaging datasets to classify pulmonary nodules as benign or malignant; supports pattern recognition for early-stage cancer	Automates detection of lung abnormalities in CT and X-ray images; enhances diagnostic speed and accuracy
2.	Prognosis and Survival Prediction	Predicts disease progression, recurrence, and survival rates using clinical and longitudinal data	Integrates multi-source Data (clinical, genomic, imaging) to estimate patient prognosis and personalise care plans
3.	biomarker identification	Analysis of genomic, proteomic, and transcriptomic data to Discover novel predictive and prognostic biomarkers	Enables high-throughput analysis of biological data to support targeted therapy selection
4.	Radiomics and Pathomics	Extracts quantitative features from radiological And pathological images to stratify patients and predict outcomes	Automates feature extraction and interpretation for Tumour characterization and grading
5.	Drug Response and Toxicity Prediction	Predicts patient-specific response to targeted therapies and immunotherapies using Supervised learning models	Facilitates personalized treatment planning by integrating molecular, imaging, and demographic data
6.	Image Processing and Computer-Aided Diagnosis (CAD)	Enhances image clarity, removes noise, and aids in Feature extraction for accurate model training	Applies deep learning to CT, PET, and histopathological image interpretation, assisting clinicians in diagnosis
7.	Digital Health and Mobile Applications	Analyzes patient-reported data and remote monitoring inputs to detect trends or early signs of deterioration	Power patient engagement tools for symptom tracking and real-time decision support
8.	Molecular Profiling (EGFR, PD-L1, etc.)	Leams associations between molecular markers and therapeutic outcomes	Integrates molecular profiling into clinical workflows to recommend targeted treatments
9.	Treatment Planning and Optimization	Predicts optimal treatment regimens by learning from historical outcomes in similar patient profiles	Supports clinical decision-making through data integration and simulation models For personalized care
10.	Clinical Workflow Integration and Decision Support	Continuously improves from new clinical data to refine treatment recommendations	Provides real-time, evidence-based decision-making support by imaging, molecular and clinical inputs

Clinical implementation of AI in NSCLC should be based on a structured framework that goes beyond technical performance into governance, validation, training of clinicians, and reimbursement. Governance frameworks, including multidisciplinary oversight committees, have been advocated to ensure transparency, accountability and respectful use of AI before deployment (El Sabrouty & Elouadi, 2025; Kludt et al., 2024). Furthermore, robust validation practices must be applied, as recent updates to the CLAIM 2024 rules clearly state the need for external validation and standardised reporting of AI models in imaging (Chen et al., 2025; Hesso et al., 2023). Thirdly, the training of clinicians should be a priority, to support healthcare providers to build competences on how to interpret and understand AI, its limitations and its decision-supporting capabilities, thus mitigating the risks of over-reliance and misdiagnosis (Benkovszky, n.d.; Kelly et al., 2019). Finally, sustainable reimbursement models are not yet mature, but frameworks that have been proposed include tying payment to demonstrated patient outcome, cost-effectiveness, and workflow efficiency improvements (Finlayson et al., 2021). Finally, integrating the four pillars of AI adoption allows for the responsible deployment of ML tools for NSCLC diagnosis and treatment.

7. CHALLENGES, FAILURE MODES, AND MITIGATION STRATEGY IN AI APPLICATIONS FOR NSCLC

In applying AI to NSCLC, several challenges and risks need careful consideration. Overfitting and poor generalizability may lead to misdiagnosis when models are tested in new populations, which can be mitigated through multi-center external validation and domain adaptation (He et al., 2019). Model drift, caused by evolving data patterns, can reduce accuracy over time, highlighting the importance of continuous monitoring and periodic retraining (Wiens et al., 2019). A lack of interpretability often results in clinician distrust and limited adoption; this can be addressed by incorporating explainable AI methods such as saliency maps or SHAP values (Finlayson et al., 2021). Regulatory and quality assurance gaps may delay deployment and pose legal risks, underscoring the need for strict adherence to FDA, CE, and QA protocols (**Table 6**). Finally, economic barriers can hinder adoption in low-resource settings, which can be mitigated through cost-effectiveness studies and scalable cloud-based solutions (Mathew et al., 2020).

Table 6. Risks in AI Deployment for NSCLC and Mitigation Strategies (He et al., 2019; Wiens et al., 2019; Finlayson et al., 2021; Mathew et al., 2020).

Risk / Failure Mode	Potential Consequence	Mitigation Strategy	Reference
Overfitting / Poor generalizability	Misdiagnosis in new populations	Multi-center external validation, domain adaptation	10
Model drift (changing data patterns)	Declining accuracy over time	Continuous monitoring, periodic retraining	11
Lack of interpretability	Clinician distrust, non-adoption	Use explainable AI (saliency maps, SHAP values)	12
Regulatory/QA gaps	Legal liability, deployment delays	Adherence to FDA/CE frameworks, QA protocols	13
Economic barriers	Limited adoption in low-resource settings	Cost-effectiveness studies, scalable cloud solutions	14

8. FUTURE DIRECTIONS IN AI FOR NSCLC

AI is continuously evolving in its accurate predictions for oncology patients and can extend to greater benefits within the upcoming several years. New medical therapies have resulted in complex cancer treatments, which AI technology manages through transformative solutions that personalize patient care (Giaj-Levra et al., 2020). AI-based predictive biomarkers use deep learning models to analyse regular medical images and electronic health records (EHRs) with promising outcomes in their exploration as a research approach. Such biomarkers help decision-making in treatment planning since they promote better patient classification and detect who should benefit from immune checkpoint inhibitors (ICIs) and targeted treatments. AI-powered automatic histological subtyping applications speed up the entire diagnostic process and treatment initiation procedure (Xie et al., 2021). Deep learning algorithms show comparable diagnostic accuracy to pathologists in determining tumour type, eliminating the need for special health personnel to serve small hospitals. Advanced methods have since been used to integrate imaging with tissue examination findings and DNA sequences to improve on the processes of trial subject selection as well as increase our understanding of tumour traits and outcome of treatment on patients (Yang et al., 2024). AI is used in drug discovery processes at a faster rate. The implementation of deep learning systems enables researchers to analyze large chemical libraries to identify new therapy alternatives, reducing the discovery trail. Generative model-based and graph-based new drug discovery approaches help to generate optimal compounds that specifically target the NSCLC mutations, such as EGFR T790 M. AI experts are engaged in enhancing the interpretability to solve trust issues of clinical practitioners with regard to the operations of specific algorithms of black box systems (Cellina et al., 2023).

9. CONCLUSION

AI (AI) and ML (ML) integration in the diagnosis and treatment of NSCLC has been transforming the practices of oncology. The technologies enhance the accuracy of the diagnosis by becoming more sophisticated in analyzing medical pictures and can find very subtle patterns that otherwise can remain unnoticed by human eyes. With the help of these technologies, individualized treatment plans can be developed based on complex data sets (genomic data and clinical data) that are used to forecast biomarkers and eventually patient stratification. This creates good results with improved efficiency of health care delivery. Using AI software, such as Convolutional Neural Networks (CNNs), and natural language processing, which are capable of automating processes like the classification of tumors, analyzing response to treatment, and pairing clinical trials. The innovations also assist in organizing workflow; in addition, they allow the oncologists to make an informed decision using the data analysis in real-time. Standardization and clinical implementation issues do not undercut the tremendous potential of AI and ML in transforming the management of NSCLC, however. These technologies are still under development and currently could give early treatment detection, refraction, and will in the future provide the patient with an increase in the survival rates. The future of NSCLC treatment is the inclusion of AI-driven solutions within the development and integration of the NSCLC treatment that will allow the creation of an AI-driven paradigm of transformation from patient-inferior and less personalized cancer care to patient-superior and more personalized cancer care..

REFERENCES

Alduais, Y., Zhang, H., Fan, F., Chen, J., & Chen, B. (2023, February 22). Non-small cell lung cancer (NSCLC): A review of risk factors, diagnosis, and treatment. *Medicine, 102*(8), e32899. DOI: 10.1097/MD.0000000000032899 PMID: 36827002

Ali, H., Mohsen, F., & Shah, Z. (2023). Improving diagnosis and prognosis of lung cancer using vision transformers: A scoping review. *BMC Medical Imaging, 23*(1), 129. DOI: 10.1186/s12880-023-01098-z PMID: 37715137

Apostolopoulos, I. D., Papathanasiou, N. D., Apostolopoulos, D. J., Papageorgiou, E. I., & Papandrianos, N. (2025). A ML approach for determining solitary pulmonary nodule malignancy in patients undergoing PET/CT examination. *Multimedia Tools and Applications*, 1–20.

Ardila, D., Kiraly, A. P., Bharadwaj, S., Choi, B., Reicher, J. J., Peng, L., & Naidich, D. P. (2019). End-to-end lung cancer screening with three-dimensional deep learning on low-dose chest computed tomography. *Nature Medicine, 25*(6), 954–961. DOI: 10.1038/s41591-019-0447-x PMID: 31110349

Ardila, D., Kiraly, A. P., Bharadwaj, S., Choi, B., Reicher, J. J., Peng, L., Tse, D., Etemadi, M., Ye, W., Corrado, G., Naidich, D. P., & Shetty, S. (2019, June). End-to-end lung cancer screening with three-dimensional deep learning on low-dose chest computed tomography. *Nature Medicine, 25*(6), 954–961. DOI: 10.1038/s41591-019-0447-x PMID: 31110349

Arterys. (2023). Arterys Lung AI: FDA-cleared AI for chest CT interpretation. Retrieved from: https://arterys.com

Benkovszky, J. *An Analysis of Current Value-Based Payment Frameworks applied in Oncology: A Payer Perspective* (Doctoral dissertation, University of Pittsburgh).

Bernstein, M. H., Atalay, M. K., Dibble, E. H., Maxwell, A. W., Karam, A. R., Agarwal, S., Ward, R. C., Healey, T. T., & Baird, G. L. (2023). Can incorrect AI (AI) results impact radiologists, and if so, what can we do about it? A multi-reader pilot study of lung cancer detection with chest radiography. *European Radiology, 33*(11), 8263–8279. DOI: 10.1007/s00330-023-09747-1 PMID: 37266657

Bhat, G. R., Sethi, I., Sadida, H. Q., Rah, B., Mir, R., Algehainy, N., Albalawi, I. A., Masoodi, T., Subbaraj, G. K., Jamal, F., Singh, M., Kumar, R., Macha, M. A., Uddin, S., Akil, A. S. A.-S., Haris, M., & Bhat, A. A. (2024, March). Cancer cell plasticity: From cellular, molecular, and genetic mechanisms to tumor heterogeneity and drug resistance. *Cancer and Metastasis Reviews, 43*(1), 197–228. DOI: 10.1007/s10555-024-10172-z PMID: 38329598

Çalışkan, M., & Tazaki, K. (2023). AI/ML advances in non-small cell lung cancer biomarker discovery. *Frontiers in Oncology*, *13*, 1260374. DOI: 10.3389/fonc.2023.1260374 PMID: 38148837

Camps, J., Jiménez-Franco, A., García-Pablo, R., Joven, J., & Arenas, M. (2025). AI-driven integration of multi-omics and radiomics: A new hope for precision cancer diagnosis and prognosis. *Biochimica et Biophysica Acta (BBA) -. Molecular Basis ofDisease*, *1861*(6), 167841. DOI: 10.1016/j.bbadis.2025.167841 PMID: 40216368

CE Mark News. (2023). *European CE-marked AI devices in oncology*. European Medicines Agency Reports.

Cellina, M., Cacioppa, L. M., Cè, M., Chiarpenello, V., Costa, M., Vincenzo, Z., Pais, D., Bausano, M. V., Rossini, N., Bruno, A., & Floridi, C. (2023). AI in lung cancer screening: The future is now. *Cancers (Basel)*, *15*(17), 4344. DOI: 10.3390/cancers15174344 PMID: 37686619

Cellina, M., Cacioppa, L. M., Cè, M., Chiarpenello, V., Costa, M., Vincenzo, Z., Pais, D., Bausano, M. V., Rossini, N., Bruno, A., & Floridi, C. (2023). AI in lung cancer screening: The future is now. *Cancers (Basel)*, *15*(17), 4344. DOI: 10.3390/cancers15174344 PMID: 37686619

Chen HH, Wu YJ, Wu FZ. (2025) Medicine in Lung Cancer Screening: A Paradigm Shift in Early Detection—Precision Screening for Lung Cancer. Diagnostics. Jun 19;15(12):1562.

Chevallier, M., Borgeaud, M., Addeo, A., & Friedlaender, A. (2021, April 24). Oncogenic driver mutations in non-small cell lung cancer: Past, present and future. *World Journal of Clinical Oncology*, *12*(4), 217–237. DOI: 10.5306/wjco.v12.i4.217 PMID: 33959476

Chiu, H. Y., Chao, H. S., & Chen, Y. M. (2022). Application of AI in lung cancer. *Cancers (Basel)*, *14*(6), 1370. DOI: 10.3390/cancers14061370 PMID: 35326521

Coudray, N., Ocampo, P. S., Sakellaropoulos, T., Narula, N., Snuderl, M., Fenyö, D., Moreira, A. L., Razavian, N., & Tsirigos, A. (2018). Classification and mutation prediction from non–small cell lung cancer histopathology images using deep learning. *Nature Medicine*, *24*(10), 1559–1567. DOI: 10.1038/s41591-018-0177-5 PMID: 30224757

Dan, A., Burtavel, L. M., Coman, M. C., Focsa, I. O., Duta-Ion, S., Juganaru, I. R., Zaruha, A. G., Codreanu, P. C., Strugari, I. M., Hotinceanu, I. A., Bohiltea, L. C., & Radoi, V.-E. (2024, December 2). Genetic blueprints in lung cancer: Foundations for targeted therapies. *Cancers (Basel)*, *16*(23), 4048. DOI: 10.3390/cancers16234048 PMID: 39682234

De Visser, K. E., & Joyce, J. A. (2023, March 13). The evolving tumor microenvironment: From cancer initiation to metastatic outgrowth. *Cancer Cell*, *41*(3), 374–403. DOI: 10.1016/j.ccell.2023.02.016 PMID: 36917948

Dlamini, Z., Francies, F. Z., Hull, R., & Marima, R. (2020). AI (AI) and big data in cancer and precision oncology. *Computational and Structural Biotechnology Journal*, *18*, 2300–2311. DOI: 10.1016/j.csbj.2020.08.019 PMID: 32994889

Duranti, L., Tavecchio, L., Rolli, L., & Solli, P. (2025). New perspectives on lung cancer screening and AI. *Life (Chicago, Ill.)*, *15*(3), 498. PMID: 40141842

El Arab, R. A., Abu-Mahfouz, M. S., Abuadas, F. H., Alzghoul, H., Almari, M., Ghannam, A., & Seweid, M. M. (2025). *No. 7* (Vol. 13). Bridging the gap: From AI success in clinical trials to real-world healthcare implementation A narrative review. InHealthcare Mar 22. MDPI.

El Sabrouty, R., & Elouadi, A. (2025). Harnessing AI for precision oncology: Transformative advances in non-small cell lung cancer treatment. *Statistics, Optimization & Information Computing*, *13*(1), 347–367. DOI: 10.19139/soic-2310-5070-2078

Ewals, L. J., van der Wulp, K., van den Borne, B. E., Pluyter, J. R., Jacobs, I., Mavroeidis, D., van der Sommen, F., & Nederend, J. (2023). The effects of AI assistance on the radiologists' assessment of lung nodules on CT scans: A systematic review. *Journal of Clinical Medicine*, *12*(10), 3536. DOI: 10.3390/jcm12103536 PMID: 37240643

FDA. (2023). AI and ML (AI/ML) Enabled Medical Devices. *U.S. Food & Drug Administration.* Retrieved from: https://www.fda.gov/medical-devices/software-medical-device-samd/artificial-intelligence-and-machine-learning-aiml-enabled-medical-devices

Finlayson, S. G., Subbaswamy, A., Singh, K., Bowers, J., Kupke, A., Zittrain, J., & Obermeyer, Z. (2021). The clinician and dataset shift in AI. *The New England Journal of Medicine*, *385*(3), 283–286. DOI: 10.1056/NEJMc2104626 PMID: 34260843

Fiste, O., Gkiozos, I., Charpidou, A., & Syrigos, N. K. (2024, February 19). AI-based treatment decisions: A new era for NSCLC. *Cancers (Basel)*, *16*(4), 831. DOI: 10.3390/cancers16040831 PMID: 38398222

Fois, S. S., Paliogiannis, P., Zinellu, A., Fois, A. G., Cossu, A., & Palmieri, G. (2021). Molecular epidemiology of the main druggable genetic alterations in non-small cell lung cancer. *International Journal of Molecular Sciences*, *22*(2), 612. DOI: 10.3390/ijms22020612 PMID: 33435440

Gao, Q., Yang, L., Lu, M., Jin, R., Ye, H., & Ma, T. (2023). The AI and ML in lung cancer immunotherapy. *Journal of Hematology & Oncology*, *16*(1), 55. DOI: 10.1186/s13045-023-01456-y PMID: 37226190

Geppert, J., Asgharzadeh, A., Brown, A., Stinton, C., Helm, E. J., Jayakody, S., Todkill, D., Gallacher, D., Ghiasvand, H., Patel, M., & Auguste, P. (2024). Software using AI for nodule and cancer detection in CT lung cancer screening: Systematic review of test accuracy studies. *Thorax*, *79*(11), 1040–1049. DOI: 10.1136/thorax-2024-221662 PMID: 39322406

Giaj-Levra N, Borghetti P, Bruni A, Ciammella P, Cuccia F, Fozza A, Franceschini D, Scotti V, Vagge S, Alongi F (2020)Current radiotherapy techniques in NSCLC: challenges and potential solutions. Expert Review of Anticancer Therapy. May 3;20(5):387-402..

Grüger, J., Geyer, T., Brix, T., Storck, M., Leson, S., Bley, L., Weishaupt, C., Bergmann, R., & Braun, S. A. (2025). AI-driven decision support in oncology: Evaluating data readiness for skin cancer treatment. *arXiv Preprint*, arXiv:2503.09164.

Gu, Y., Chi, J., Liu, J., Yang, L., Zhang, B., Yu, D., Zhao, Y., & Lu, X. (2021). A survey of computer-aided diagnosis of lung nodules from CT scans using deep learning. *Computers in Biology and Medicine*, *137*, 104806. DOI: 10.1016/j.compbiomed.2021.104806 PMID: 34461501

He, J., Baxter, S. L., Xu, J., Xu, J., Zhou, X., & Zhang, K. (2019). The practical implementation of AI technologies in medicine. *Nature Medicine*, *25*(1), 30–36. DOI: 10.1038/s41591-018-0307-0 PMID: 30617336

Hesso I, Kayyali R, Dolton DR, Joo K, Zacharias L, Charalambous A, Lavdaniti M, Stalika E, Ajami T, Aca mpa W, Boban J (2023). Cancer care at the time of the fourth industrial revolution: an insight to healthcare professionals' perspectives on cancer care and AI. Radiation Oncology.Oct 9;18(1):167.

Ho, D., Quake, S. R., McCabe, E. R., Chng, W. J., Chow, E. K., Ding, X., Gelb, B. D., Ginsburg, G. S., Hassenstab, J., Ho, C. M., Mobley, W. C., Nolan, G. P., Rosen, S. T., Tan, P., Yen, Y., & Zarrinpar, A. (2020). Enabling technologies for personalized and precision medicine. *Trends in Biotechnology*, *38*(5), 497–518. DOI: 10.1016/j.tibtech.2019.12.021 PMID: 31980301

Hope, A., Verduin, M., Dilling, T. J., Choudhury, A., Fijten, R., Wee, L., Aerts, H. J., El Naqa, I., Mitchell, R., Vooijs, M., & Dekker, A. (2021). AI applications to improve the treatment of locally advanced non-small cell lung cancers. *Cancers (Basel)*, *13*(10), 2382. DOI: 10.3390/cancers13102382 PMID: 34069307

Hosny, A., Parmar, C., Quackenbush, J., Schwartz, L. H., & Aerts, H. J. (2018). AI in radiology. *Nature Reviews. Cancer*, *18*(8), 500–510. DOI: 10.1038/s41568-018-0016-5 PMID: 29777175

Hossain, M. R., Mahabub, S., Al Masum, A., & Jahan, I. (2024). Natural language processing (NLP) in analyzing electronic health records for better decision making. *Journal of Computer Science and Technology Studies*, *6*(5), 216–228. DOI: 10.32996/jcsts.2024.6.5.18

Hu, Q., Li, K., Yang, C., Wang, Y., Huang, R., Gu, M., Xiao, Y., Huang, Y., & Chen, L. (2023). The role of AI based on PET/CT radiomics in NSCLC: Disease management, opportunities, and challenges. *Frontiers in Oncology*, *13*, 1133164. DOI: 10.3389/fonc.2023.1133164 PMID: 36959810

Huang, D., Li, Z., Jiang, T., Yang, C., & Li, N. (2024). AI in lung cancer: Current applications, future perspectives, and challenges. *Frontiers in Oncology*, *14*, 1486310. DOI: 10.3389/fonc.2024.1486310 PMID: 39763611

Huang, L., Lin, W., & Yu, S. (2023). Application of AI technology based on deep learning in identification of lung cancer properties. *Archives of Clinical Psychiatry*, *50*(6).

Huang, S., Yang, J., Shen, N., Xu, Q., & Zhao, Q. (2023). AI in lung cancer diagnosis and prognosis: Current application and future perspective. *Seminars in Cancer Biology*, *89*, 30–37. DOI: 10.1016/j.semcancer.2023.01.006 PMID: 36682439

Iqbal, M. J., Javed, Z., Sadia, H., Qureshi, I. A., Irshad, A., Ahmed, R., Malik, K., Raza, S., Abbas, A., Pezzani, R., & Sharifi-Rad, J. (2021). Clinical applications of AI and ML in cancer diagnosis: Looking into the future. *Cancer Cell International*, *21*(1), 270. DOI: 10.1186/s12935-021-01981-1 PMID: 34020642

Johnson, M., Albizri, A., & Simsek, S. (2022). AI in healthcare operations to enhance treatment outcomes: A framework to predict lung cancer prognosis. *Annals of Operations Research*, *308*(1), 275–305. DOI: 10.1007/s10479-020-03872-6

Kaplan, A., Cao, H., FitzGerald, J. M., Iannotti, N., Yang, E., Kocks, J. W., Kostikas, K., Price, D., Reddel, H. K., Tsiligianni, I., & Vogelmeier, C. F. (2021). AI/ML in respiratory medicine and potential role in asthma and COPD diagnosis. *The Journal of Allergy and Clinical Immunology. In Practice*, *9*(6), 2255–2261. DOI: 10.1016/j.jaip.2021.02.014 PMID: 33618053

Karayegen, G., & Aksahin, M. F. (2021). Brain tumor prediction on MR images with semantic segmentation by using deep learning network and 3D imaging of tumor region. *Biomedical Signal Processing and Control*, *66*, 102458. DOI: 10.1016/j.bspc.2021.102458

Kehl, K. L., Groha, S., Lepisto, E. M., Elmarakeby, H., Lindsay, J., Gusev, A., Van Allen, E. M., Hassett, M. J., & Schrag, D. (2021). Clinical inflection point detection on the basis of EHR data to identify clinical trial–ready patients with cancer. *JCO Clinical Cancer Informatics*, *5*(5), 622–630. DOI: 10.1200/CCI.20.00184 PMID: 34097438

Kelly, C. J., Karthikesalingam, A., Suleyman, M., Corrado, G., & King, D. (2019). Key challenges for delivering clinical impact with AI. *BMC Medicine*, *17*(1), 195. DOI: 10.1186/s12916-019-1426-2 PMID: 31665002

Khalighi, S., Reddy, K., Midya, A., Pandav, K. B., Madabhushi, A., & Abedalthagafi, M. (2024). AI in neuro-oncology: Advances and challenges in brain tumor diagnosis, prognosis, and precision treatment. *NPJ Precision Oncology*, *8*(1), 80. DOI: 10.1038/s41698-024-00575-0 PMID: 38553633

Khan, M., Shiwlani, A., Qayyum, M. U., Sherani, A. M., & Hussain, H. K. (2024). Revolutionizing healthcare with AI: Innovative strategies in cancer medicine. *International Journal of Multidisciplinary Sciences and Arts*, *3*(2), 316–324. DOI: 10.47709/ijmdsa.v3i1.3922

Khan, M. A., & Zannat, N. A. (2024). Novel biomarkers and therapeutic avenues for precision oncology and effective treatment strategies. *Journal of Angiotherapy*, *8*(11), 1–8. DOI: 10.25163/angiotherapy.81110065

Kohan, A. A., Mirshahvalad, S. A., Hinzpeter, R., Kulanthaivelu, R., Avery, L., Ortega, C., Metser, U., Hope, A., & Veit-Haibach, P. (2025). External validation of a CT-based radiogenomics model for the detection of EGFR mutation in NSCLC and the impact of prevalence in model building by using synthetic minority over sampling (SMOTE): Lessons learned. *Academic Radiology*, *32*(9), 5576–5584. DOI: 10.1016/j.acra.2025.04.064 PMID: 40379588

Kumar, A. (2024). AI-driven precision oncology: Predictive biomarker discovery and personalized treatment optimization using genomic data. *International Journal of Advanced Research Publication Review*, *1*(3), 21–38. DOI: 10.55248/gengpi.5.0224.0421

Ladbury, C., Amini, A., Govindarajan, A., Mambetsariev, I., Raz, D. J., Massarelli, E., Williams, T., Rodin, A., & Salgia, R. (2023, February 21). Integration of AI in lung cancer: Rise of the machine. *Cell Reports Medicine*, *4*(2). Advance online publication. DOI: 10.1016/j.xcrm.2023.100933 PMID: 36738739

Lee, K., Liu, Z., Huang, Q., Corrigan, D., Kalsekar, I., Jun, T., Stolovitzky, G., Oh, W. K., Rajaram, R., & Wang, X. (2025). Decoding recurrence in early-stage and locoregionally advanced non–small cell lung cancer: Insights from electronic health records and natural language processing. *JCO Clinical Cancer Informatics*, *9*(9), e2400227. DOI: 10.1200/CCI-24-00227 PMID: 40249880

Li, X., Li, M., Huang, M., Lin, Q., Fang, Q., Liu, J., Chen, X., Liu, L., Zhan, X., Shan, H., Lu, D., Li, Q., Li, Z., & Zhu, X. (2022, June 1). The multi-molecular mechanisms of tumor-targeted drug resistance in precision medicine. *Biomedicine and Pharmacotherapy*, *150*, 113064. DOI: 10.1016/j.biopha.2022.113064 PMID: 35658234

Li, Y., Wu, X., Yang, P., Jiang, G., & Luo, Y. (2022). ML for lung cancer diagnosis, treatment, and prognosis. *Genomics, Proteomics & Bioinformatics*, *20*(5), 850–866. DOI: 10.1016/j.gpb.2022.11.003 PMID: 36462630

Liu, M., Li, L., Wang, H., Guo, X., Liu, Y., Li, Y., Song, K., Shao, Y., Wu, F., Zhang, J., Sun, N., Zhang, T., & Luan, L. (2023). A multilayer perceptron-based model applied to histopathology image classification of lung adenocarcinoma subtypes. *Frontiers in Oncology*, *13*, 1172234. DOI: 10.3389/fonc.2023.1172234 PMID: 37274249

Liu, M., Wu, J., Wang, N., Zhang, X., Bai, Y., Guo, J., Zhang, L., Liu, S., & Tao, K. (2023). The value of AI in the diagnosis of lung cancer: A systematic review and meta-analysis. *PLoS One*, *18*(3), e0273445. DOI: 10.1371/journal.pone.0273445 PMID: 36952523

Mali, S. A., Salahuddin, Z., Khan, D., Zhang, Y., Woodruff, H. C., Ibor-Crespo, E., Jimenez-Pastor, A., Marti-Bonmati, L., & Lambin, P. (2025, May 23). Pixels to prognosis: Harmonized multi-region CT-radiomics and foundation-model signatures across multicentre NSCLC data.

Mao, X., Xu, J., Wang, W., Liang, C., Hua, J., Liu, J., Zhang, B., Meng, Q., Yu, X., & Shi, S. (2021, December). Crosstalk between cancer-associated fibroblasts and immune cells in the tumor microenvironment: New findings and future perspectives. *Molecular Cancer, 20*(1), 1–30. DOI: 10.1186/s12943-021-01428-1 PMID: 34635121

Mathew, C. J., David, A. M., & Mathew, C. M. (2020). AI and its future potential in lung cancer screening. *EXCLI Journal, 19*, 1552. PMID: 33408594

Mei, T., Wang, T., & Zhou, Q. (2024). Multi-omics and AI predict clinical outcomes of immunotherapy in non-small cell lung cancer patients. *Clinical and Experimental Medicine, 24*(1), 60. DOI: 10.1007/s10238-024-01324-0 PMID: 38554212

Mohanty, P., Pande, B., Acharya, R., Bhaskar, L. V., & Verma, H. K. (2024, May 6). Unravelling the triad of lung cancer, drug resistance, and metabolic pathways. *Diseases (Basel, Switzerland), 12*(5), 93. DOI: 10.3390/diseases12050093 PMID: 38785748

Mu, W., Jiang, L., Zhang, J., Shi, Y., Gray, J. E., Tunali, I., Gao, C., Sun, Y., Tian, J., Zhao, X., Sun, X., Gillies, R. J., & Schabath, M. B. (2020). Non-invasive decision support for NSCLC treatment using PET/CT radiomics. *Nature Communications, 11*(1), 5228. DOI: 10.1038/s41467-020-19116-x PMID: 33067442

Pacurari, A. C., Bhattarai, S., Muhammad, A., Avram, C., Mederle, A. O., Rosca, O., Bratosin, F., Bogdan, I., Fericean, R. M., Biris, M., Olaru, F., Dumitru, C., Tapalaga, G., & Mavrea, A. (2023). Diagnostic accuracy of ML AI architectures in detection and classification of lung cancer: A systematic review. *Diagnostics (Basel), 13*(13), 2145. DOI: 10.3390/diagnostics13132145 PMID: 37443539

Padinharayil, H., Varghese, J., John, M. C., Rajanikant, G. K., Wilson, C. M., Al-Yozbaki, M., Renu, K., Dewanjee, S., Sanyal, R., Dey, A., Mukherjee, A. G., Wanjari, U. R., Gopalakrishnan, A. V., & George, A. (2023, May 1). Non-small cell lung carcinoma (NSCLC): Implications on molecular pathology and advances in early diagnostics and therapeutics. *Genes & Diseases, 10*(3), 960–989. DOI: 10.1016/j.gendis.2022.07.023 PMID: 37396553

Paige.AI. (2024). Paige Pathology AI – CE-IVD and FDA clearance updates. Retrieved from: https://paige.ai

Paudyal, R., Shah, A. D., Akin, O., Do, R. K., Konar, A. S., Hatzoglou, V., Mahmood, U., Lee, N., Wong, R. J., Banerjee, S., & Shin, J. (2023). AI in CT and MR imaging for oncological applications. *Cancers (Basel), 15*(9), 2573. DOI: 10.3390/cancers15092573 PMID: 37174039

Pei, Q., Luo, Y., Chen, Y., Li, J., Xie, D., & Ye, T. (2022). AI in clinical applications for lung cancer: Diagnosis, treatment and prognosis. *Clinical Chemistry and Laboratory Medicine*, *60*(12), 1974–1983. DOI: 10.1515/cclm-2022-0291 PMID: 35771735

Qu, Y., Emoto, K., Eguchi, T., Aly, R. G., Zheng, H., Chaft, J. E., Tan, K. S., Jones, D. R., Kris, M. G., Adusumilli, P. S., & Travis, W. D. (2019). Pathologic assessment after neoadjuvant chemotherapy for NSCLC: Importance and implications of distinguishing adenocarcinoma from squamous cell carcinoma. *Journal of Thoracic Oncology*, *14*(3), 482–493. DOI: 10.1016/j.jtho.2018.11.017 PMID: 30503889

Quanyang, W., Yao, H., Sicong, W., Linlin, Q., Zewei, Z., Donghui, H., Hongjia, L., & Shijun, Z. (2024, April). AI in lung cancer screening: Detection, classification, prediction, and prognosis. *Cancer Medicine*, *13*(7), e7140. DOI: 10.1002/cam4.7140 PMID: 38581113

Qure.ai. (2023). Qure.ai AI-driven chest X-ray and CT solutions. Retrieved from: https://qure.ai

Rabbani, M., Kanevsky, J., Kafi, K., Chandelier, F., & Giles, F. J. (2018). Role of AI in the care of patients with nonsmall cell lung cancer. *European Journal of Clinical Investigation*, *48*(4), e12901. DOI: 10.1111/eci.12901 PMID: 29405289

Rajesh, P., Murugan, A., Murugamantham, B., & Ganesh, S. (2020). Lung cancer diagnosis and treatment using AI and mobile applications. In *Proceedings* (pp. 189–203).

Ren, F., Fei, Q., Qiu, K., Zhang, Y., Zhang, H., & Sun, L. (2024). Liquid biopsy techniques and lung cancer: Diagnosis, monitoring and evaluation. *Journal of Experimental & Clinical Cancer Research : CR*, *43*(1), 96. DOI: 10.1186/s13046-024-03026-7 PMID: 38561776

Rodak, O., Peris-Díaz, M. D., Olbromski, M., Podhorska-Okołów, M., & Dzięgiel, P. (2021). Current landscape of non-small cell lung cancer: Epidemiology, histological classification, targeted therapies, and immunotherapy. *Cancers (Basel)*, *13*(18), 4705. DOI: 10.3390/cancers13184705 PMID: 34572931

Schneider, L., Laiouar-Pedari, S., Kuntz, S., Krieghoff-Henning, E., Hekler, A., Kather, J. N., Gaiser, T., Froehling, S., & Brinker, T. J. (2022). Integration of deep learning-based image analysis and genomic data in cancer pathology: A systematic review. *European Journal of Cancer*, *160*, 80–91. DOI: 10.1016/j.ejca.2021.10.007 PMID: 34810047

Shao, J., Feng, J., Li, J., Liang, S., Li, W., & Wang, C. (2023). Novel tools for early diagnosis and precision treatment based on AI. *Chinese Medical Journal Pulmonary and Critical Care Medicine*, *1*(03), 148–160. DOI: 10.1016/j.pccm.2023.05.001 PMID: 39171128

Shatnawi, M. Q., Abuein, Q., & Al-Quraan, R. (2025, January 1). Deep learning-based approach to diagnose lung cancer using CT-scan images. *Intelligence-Based Medicine*, *11*, 100188. DOI: 10.1016/j.ibmed.2024.100188

Sicular, S., Alpaslan, M., Ortega, F. A., Keathley, N., Venkatesh, S., Jones, R. M., & Lindsey, R. V. (2022). Reevaluation of missed lung cancer with AI. *Respiratory Medicine Case Reports*, *39*, 101733. DOI: 10.1016/j.rmcr.2022.101733 PMID: 36118268

Stock, C. (2022, February 10). Circulating tumor cells: Does ion transport contribute to intravascular survival, adhesion, extravasation, and metastatic organotropism? In *From Malignant Transformation to Metastasis* (pp. 139–175). Ion Transport in Tumor Biology. DOI: 10.1007/978-3-030-99800-4

Sun, H., Wei, J., Wang, J., Pang, Z., & Zhu, L. (2023). Clinical study of AI in imaging diagnosis of false positive lesions of pulmonary nodules. *The Age (Melbourne, Vic.)*, *58*(8), 44.

Trebeschi, S., Bodalal, Z., Boellaard, T. N., Tareco Bucho, T. M., Drago, S. G., Kurilova, I., Calin-Vainak, A. M., Delli Pizzi, A., Muller, M., Hummelink, K., Hartemink, K. J., Nguyen-Kim, T. D. L., Smit, E. F., Aerts, H. J. W. L., & Beets-Tan, R. G. H. (2021). Prognostic value of deep learning-mediated treatment monitoring in lung cancer patients receiving immunotherapy. *Frontiers in Oncology*, *11*, 609054. DOI: 10.3389/fonc.2021.609054 PMID: 33738253

Wang, L., Yin, Y., Glampson, B., Peach, R., Barahona, M., Delaney, B. C., & Mayer, E. K. (2024). Transformer-based deep learning model for the diagnosis of suspected lung cancer in primary care based on electronic health record data. *EBioMedicine*, *110*, 104543. DOI: 10.1016/j.ebiom.2024.105442 PMID: 39536394

Wang, T., Nelson, R. A., Bogardus, A., & Grannis, F. W.Jr. (2010). Five-year lung cancer survival: Which advanced stage nonsmall cell lung cancer patients attain long-term survival? *Cancer*, *116*(6), 1518–1525. DOI: 10.1002/cncr.24871 PMID: 20108308

Wang, X., Zhang, Y., Hao, S., Zheng, L., Liao, J., Ye, C., Xia, M., Wang, O., Liu, M., Weng, C. H., Duong, S. Q., Jin, B., Alfreds, S. T., Stearns, F., Kanov, L., Sylvester, K. G., Widen, E., McElhinney, D. B., & Ling, X. B. (2019). Prediction of the 1-year risk of incident lung cancer: Prospective study using electronic health records from the state of Maine. *Journal of Medical Internet Research*, *21*(5), e13260. DOI: 10.2196/13260 PMID: 31099339

Wiens, J., Saria, S., Sendak, M., Ghassemi, M., Liu, V. X., Doshi-Velez, F., Jung, K., Heller, K., Kale, D., Saeed, M., Ossorio, P. N., Thadaney-Israni, S., & Goldenberg, A. (2019). Do not harm: A roadmap for responsible ML for health care. *Nature Medicine*, *25*(9), 1337–1340. DOI: 10.1038/s41591-019-0548-6 PMID: 31427808

Wu, X. Y., Ding, F., Li, K., Huang, W. C., Zhang, Y., & Zhu, J. (2022). Analysis of the causes of solitary pulmonary nodule misdiagnosed as lung cancer by using AI: A retrospective study at a single center. *Diagnostics (Basel)*, *12*(9), 2218. DOI: 10.3390/diagnostics12092218 PMID: 36140618

Xie, Y., Meng, W. Y., Li, R. Z., Wang, Y. W., Qian, X., Chan, C., Yu, Z. F., Fan, X. X., Pan, H. D., Xie, C., Wu, Q. B., Yan, P.-Y., Liu, L., Tang, Y.-J., Yao, X.-J., Wang, M.-F., & Leung, E. L.-H. (2021). Early lung cancer diagnostic biomarker discovery by ML methods. *Translational Oncology*, *14*(1), 100907. DOI: 10.1016/j.tranon.2020.100907 PMID: 33217646

Xu, J., Tian, L., Qi, W., Lv, Q., & Wang, T. (2024, June 1). Advancements in NSCLC: From pathophysiological insights to targeted treatments. *American Journal of Clinical Oncology*, *47*(6), 291–303. DOI: 10.1097/COC.0000000000001088 PMID: 38375734

Xu, J., Yang, P., Xue, S., Sharma, B., Sanchez-Martin, M., Wang, F., Beaty, K. A., Dehan, E., & Parikh, B. (2019). Translating cancer genomics into precision medicine with AI: Applications, challenges and future perspectives. *Human Genetics*, *138*(2), 109–124. DOI: 10.1007/s00439-019-01970-5 PMID: 30671672

Yang, D., Miao, Y., Liu, C., Zhang, N., Zhang, D., Guo, Q., Gao, S., Li, L., Wang, J., Liang, S., & Li, P. (2024). Advances in AI applications in the field of lung cancer. *Frontiers in Oncology*, *14*, 1449068. DOI: 10.3389/fonc.2024.1449068 PMID: 39309740

Yoshimi, J. (2025). *Gaming cancer: How building and playing video games can accelerate scientific discovery*. MIT Press. DOI: 10.7551/mitpress/14967.001.0001

Zhang, G., Lin, L., & Wang, J. (2021). Lung nodule classification in CT images using 3D DenseNet. *Journal of Physics: Conference Series*, *1827*(1), 012155. DOI: 10.1088/1742-6596/1827/1/012155

Zhao, Y., Guo, S., Deng, J., Shen, J., Du, F., Wu, X., Chen, Y., Li, M., Chen, M., Li, X., Li, W., Gu, L., Sun, Y., Wen, Q., Li, J., & Xiao, Z. (2022, May 29). VEGF/VEGFR-targeted therapy and immunotherapy in non-small cell lung cancer: Targeting the tumor microenvironment. *International Journal of Biological Sciences*, *18*(9), 3845–3858. DOI: 10.7150/ijbs.70958 PMID: 35813484

Chapter 10
Therapeutic Approaches in NSCLC:
Navigating Side Effects and Outcomes

Vivek Pazhamalai
https://orcid.org/0000-0003-2088-7545
Department of Bio Engineering, School of Engineering, Vels Institute of Science, Technology, and Advanced Studies, India

Mathumida Rajendran
https://orcid.org/0009-0009-7449-5935
Department of Bio Engineering, School of Engineering, Vels Institute of Science, Technology, and Advanced Studies, India

Manideepa Govindarajan
https://orcid.org/0009-0007-7312-9875
Department of Bio Engineering, School of Engineering, Vels Institute of Science, Technology, and Advanced Studies, India

S. Ivo Romauld
https://orcid.org/0000-0003-0610-0646
Department of Bio Engineering, School of Engineering, Vels Institute of Science, Technology, and Advanced Studies, India

Meenupriya Venkatesan
Department of Bio Engineering, School of Engineering, Vels Institute of Science, Technology, and Advanced Studies, India

S. S. Meenambiga
https://orcid.org/0000-0002-5445-525X
Department of Bio Engineering, School of Engineering, Vels Institute of Science, Technology, and Advanced Studies, India

Jayasri Rajkumar
Department of Bio Engineering, School of Engineering, Vels Institute of Science, Technology, and Advanced Studies, India

DOI: 10.4018/979-8-3373-2096-0.ch010

ABSTRACT

Non-small-cell lung cancer (NSCLC) stands as a predominant and complex malignancy, constituting approximately 85% of all lung cancer diagnoses. The etiology of NSCLC is multifactorial, with tobacco use emerging as the primary risk factor, while air pollution and radon exposure also significantly contribute to its development. The therapeutic landscape for NSCLC has undergone a paradigm shift with the advent of targeted therapies, facilitated by advancements in genetic and biomarker testing. These innovations have enabled the identification of specific mutations, thereby informing personalized treatment strategies tailored to individual patient profiles. This chapter aims to elucidate the current state of NSCLC management, with a particular focus on multimodal treatment approaches for locally advanced disease. It will also explore the role of innovative surgical techniques and contemporary pharmacological interventions in the context of early-stage NSCLC.This chapter aims to provide a nuanced understanding of the current therapeutic options and future directions in NSCLC management.

1. INTRODUCTION

Among the cancers, the deadliest malignancy is lung cancer, which strikes both men and women. Its mortality rate exceeds the sum of the mortality rates of three of the most frequently diagnosed cancers: colon, breast, and pancreatic. More than fifty percent of patients with lung cancer passed away in less than a year of receiving a diagnosis, and the five-year survival rate is approximately 17.8% (Zappa & Mousa, 2016). The lung tumor may spread to nearby tissues or other body regions if treatment is not received. Malignancy that starts in cells of the epithelium accounts for the bulk of lung cancers, commonly known as primary lung malignancies (Akhtar & Bansal, 2017). Around twelve million new instances of lung tumors were reported in 2000, making them one of the most prevalent cancer types worldwide, making up approximately 12 percent of all cancers (Minna et al., 2002). Many behavioral and environmental variables have been linked to lung cancer development. Cigarettes and tobacco usage account for between 85 and 90 percent of cases of lung cancer (Alduais et al., 2023). Lung cancer increased as cigarettes emerged as the main tobacco product produced in the 1900s.The risk of lung cancer varies with the number of periods or packets of cigarettes smoked daily (Zappa & Mousa, 2016). Tobacco usage significantly increases the risk of lung cancer and also genetic ancestry, hazardous chemicals, heavy metals such as asbestos, arsenic, chromium, beryllium, radon gas, and nickel, as well as passive smoking.Furthermore, the carcinogenesis of lung cancer is also caused by alcohol consumption, HIV infection, and pulmonary fibrosis (Alduais et al., 2023).

2. EPIDEMIOLOGY OF LUNG CANCER

According to the International Agency for Research on Cancer's (IARC) most recent estimates, the following are the global cancer statistics by world region for 2022. Nearly 20 million new instances of cancer and 9.7 million cancer-related deaths occurred in 2022. It is estimated that one in five women and men may develop cancer at some point in their life. One in nine men and one in twelve women die from cancer. Lung cancer was the most common cancer diagnosed in 2022. The disease affected 2.5 million new cases, or one in eight malignancies worldwide.

More than 80% of all lung malignancies are NSCLC, which is also one of the leading causes of death worldwide.SCLC is the diagnosis for the twenty percent that is left of patients with lung tumors. For the restricted stage, they often live 12–16 for a period of time, while for the extensive stage, they typically live 7–11 months (Smolarz et al., 2025).

3. CLASSIFICATION OF LUNG CANCER

Histology has traditionally separated lung malignancies into two types.

1. Small-cell lung cancer
2. Non-small-cell lung cancers (NSCLCs).

Squamous cell carcinoma (SCC), adenocarcinoma, and large-cell carcinoma are subtypes of non-small cell lung cancer.Adenocarcinomas account for over 50 percent of all lung cancers. Figure 1 depicts the classification of lung cancer. (Shames & Wistuba, 2014)

Figure 1. Classification of lung cancer

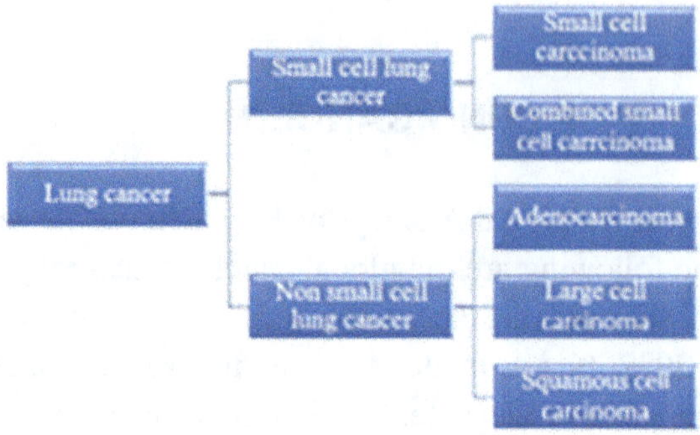

I. **Adenocarcinoma:** The most prevalent histopathological kind of NSCLC is adenocarcinoma. Lung adenocarcinoma typically occurs by cigarette smoking; however, as rates of smoking decline, a substantially higher number of instances arise in never-smokers, who smoke fewer than 100 cigarettes in their lifetime (Cancer Genome Atlas Research Network, 2014).

II. **Large-cell carcinoma:** Having a relatively low prevalence, it has emerged as one of the rarest subtypes of NSCLC. LCC is characterized as "indistinguishable non-small cell carcinoma that exhibits secretory or epithelial differentiation, as well as the morphological and structural attributes" (Rekhtman & Travis, 2019).

III. **Squamous cell carcinoma:** Lung squamous cell carcinoma (SCC) is the most prevalent histologic subtype of non-small cell lung cancer. Thirty percent of NSCLC cases are squamous cell carcinoma (SCC), making it the most common histologic subtype. Although modifications in tobacco use practices are reducing the incidence of lung SCC, SCC remains a serious health concern.

4. TUMOR MICROENVIRONMENT OF NSCLC

Tumor growth, metastasis, and the response to therapeutic interventions are all significantly influenced by the TME, a complex microenvironment. The stromal cells, immune cells, signaling molecules, extracellular matrix, and other cellular and non-cellular components that make up TME interact with one another to control the behavior of tumors. The degree of immune cell infiltration in NSCLC varies according to the stage of the disease, indicating that the lung TME affects carcinogenesis and could be a predictor of outcome. Accordingly, several TME profiles are being researched as possible biomarkers for determining the stage and subtype of the disease, forecasting clinical results, and directing treatment approaches (Edirisinghe et al., 2025).

5. THERAPIES

Chemotherapy, radiation, and surgery are the most often used cancer treatments. Although these techniques are frequently employed in hospitals, their efficacy is constrained by a number of serious issues. For instance, chemotherapy frequently lacks accuracy and has a number of negative consequences. However, surgery and radiation therapy might not always be successful in stopping cancers from growing or coming back. The majority of cancer patients receive treatment with a mix of chemotherapy, radiation, and/or surgery medicines (Schuster et al., 2006).

6. IMMUNOTHERAPY

By strengthening and rebuilding the immune system of the body by managing and eliminating tumor cells, immunotherapy for tumors combats them. The innate capacity of the immune system to combat cancer can be strengthened (active immunity) or given extra support (passive immunity) by this treatment. Immunotherapy in several forms, such as adoptive cell treatment, immune checkpoint inhibitors, and cancer vaccines, has shown encouraging outcomes in the treatment of cancer by influencing distinct immune system components. Further, a number of immunotherapy medications were approved by the U.S. Food and Drug Administration for clinical therapies in cancer treatment (Yuan et al., 2024).

A healthy immune system is essential for preventing the onset and spread of cancer because it recognizes and eliminates tumor antigens. The immune system may use immunoediting to fight against emerging malignancies that have escaped natural tumor suppressors like apoptosis (Forde et al., 2014). One such medication that has impacted lung cancer patients' survival, particularly for those with non-small cell lung cancer, is immunotherapy. Due to the increasing amount of information that is collected regarding the immune mechanisms, driver mutations, neoantigens, and oncogenic pathways involved in non-small cell lung cancer (NSCLC), new immunotherapeutic tools for targetable mutations have been designed with greater understanding of the tumor's microenvironment (TME), mutational load, and heterogeneity (Lahiri et al., 2023).

Immunotherapy is currently widely used to treat NSCLC at various stages (Wang, Li, et al., 2022). Non-Small Cell Lung Cancer (NSCLC) is a very diverse illness with a high mutational burden that codes for numerous potential neoantigens (Malhotra et al., 2017). The adaptive immune response requires two signals between the effector T cells and the antigen-presenting cells (APCs). The first signal is mediated by the major histocompatibility complex classes I or II antigenic peptide and the T-cell receptor. In order to generate the second signal, which is a co-activation signal, the B7 family members on APCs interact with CD28 on the surface of T cells. These signals cause T lymphocytes to become activated and proliferate clonally in response to interleukin-2 (IL-2). Autoimmunity can be avoided by controlling this proliferation. CTLA-4, a homologue of CD28 that was initially identified in 1987 and belongs to the immunoglobulin superfamily, is expressed by T cells after activation (Tomasini et al., 2012). Both single-agent and combination ICI treatments have been studied in numerous cases to dramatically improve clinical efficacy endpoints in patients with extensive-stage small-cell lung carcinoma and locally progressed, metastatic NSCLC patients without mutations in the ALK and EGFR genes (Xiang et al., 2024). According to recent studies, checkpoint inhibitors may particularly reactivate self-antigen-mediated cellular immunity and T cells in healthy tissues, potentially leading to immune-related adverse events (irAE) (Lin et al., 2024).

Different roles in immune regulation are played by PD-1 and CTLA-4. These two checkpoint receptors have been the subject of the most research in the context of clinical cancer immunotherapy (Topalian et al., 2012).

In order to treat patients without a driver mutation, immunotherapy in the form of immune checkpoint inhibitors (ICIs) is a crucial component. One of the prognostic biomarkers that responds to checkpoint inhibitors is programmed cell death ligand-1 (PD-L1). Although PD-L1 expression is the most reliable clinical biomarker, it is not flawless (Mamdani et al., 2022). PD-L1, also known as B7-H1, and PD-L2, also known as B7-DC, are two recognized ligands of the PD-1 receptor. T-cell inhibition and downregulation of the T-cell response arise from PD1 binding to its ligands. On oncogenic cells, both PD-L1 and PD-L2 have been detected. PD-L1 is expressed by tumors on their surface and by cells within the tumor microenvironment; malignancies specifically co-opt this pathway, enabling the tumor to directly suppress anti-tumor cytolytic T-cell activity. In fact, tumor cells' adaptive immune resistance strategy in response to endogenous anti-tumor activity is the activation of the PD1/PD-L1 pathway (Villaruz et al., 2014). CTLA-4, a CD28 homolog, is only expressed by T cells. Through a number of mechanisms, including outcompeting CD28 for the binding of B7 molecules and inhibiting the production of interleukin-2 (IL2), CTLA-4 acts as a negative regulator of T-cell response, causing T-cell responses to be downregulated and stopping cell cycle progression (Malhotra et al., 2017). Through the disruption of inhibitory checkpoints that tumors use to avoid immunological attack, immunotherapy activates the immune system. Monoclonal antibodies in NSCLC target the PD-1/PD-L1 interactions, in which PD-L1 on tumor or antigen-presenting cells binds PD-1 on T cells to suppress cytotoxic activity, rebuilding T-cell proliferation and function. CTLA-4 on T cells also weakens the co-stimulatory signal by competing with CD28 for CD80/CD86 binding; inhibiting CTLA-4 increases early T-cell activation. Checkpoint inhibitors work together to restore anti-tumor T-cell responses and facilitate strong immune-mediated destruction of cancer cells (Stanley et al., 2023). When treating non-small cell lung cancer (NSCLC), immunotherapy mostly consists of immune checkpoint inhibitors like pembrolizumab, nivolumab, atezolizumab, durvalumab, and ipilimumab. These can be administered either alone or in combination with radiation therapy or chemotherapy (Burke & Rashdan, 2021). These substances work by inhibiting the PD-1/PD-L1 or CTLA-4 pathways, which unlocks antitumor immunity. Although usually tolerated, immune-related adverse drug events (irAEs) are often observed; skin and endocrine irAEs are common. These include dermatitis, colitis, hepatitis, thyroid dysfunction, and pneumonitis (Zhou et al., 2022).

Many preclinical studies have demonstrated that blocking the CTLA-4 and PD-1 pathways improves intratumoral immunological responses, and blocking immunological checkpoints has been implemented in the current era of cancer treatment. Fully humanized, ipilimumab is an IgG1 anti-CTLA-4 mAb that inhibits CTLA-4 from binding to its ligand. When ipilimumab was administered after chemotherapy, a randomized phase II clinical study of paclitaxel and carboplatin with or without it in treatment-naïve stage IV NSCLC showed an improvement in immune-related progression-free survival (irPFS) (Anagnostou & Brahmer, 2015). According to preclinical evidence, simultaneous CTLA-4 and PD-1 inhibition markedly boosted tumor-specific immune response (Curran et al., 2010). In melanoma, a phase I trial of nivolumab with ipilimumab showed an ORR of approximately 40% (Wolchok et a., 2013). Immunotherapy has emerged as a viable treatment option for non-small cell lung cancer (NSCLC) after PD-1 and PD-L1 inhibitors were authorized as the current standard of care for the disease's second-line treatment. Pembrolizumab, a PD-1 inhibitor, is also used as a first-line treatment for patients with metastatic non-small cell lung cancer whose tumors express PD-L1.

A total of 191,802 patients were included in this study: 90,807 prior to immunotherapy and 100,995 following it. Overall survival increased and the OS improved dramatically throughout the immunotherapy era (1-year survival, 44.0% vs. 36.8%; 3-year survival, 21.7% vs. 14.4%; 5-year survival, 14.3% vs. 9.0%; median OS, 10 vs. 8 months; $p < .001$ by log-rank test). After taking age, sex, race, wealth, and geographic location into account, multivariate analysis using a Cox proportional hazards model indicated that survival rates were significantly higher during the immunotherapy era (adjusted hazard ratio, 0.830; 95% CI, 0.821–0.840; $p < .001$) (Wang, Kondrat, et al., 2025).

Despite the enormous potential of these medicines, response rates are still low, with the exception of cancers that exhibit high levels of PD-L1 expression (Malhotra et al., 2017). The immune system can be reactivated against oncogenic cells with immunotherapy; however, it also results in a variety of autoimmune side effects, or immune-related adverse events (irAEs), including endocrine dysfunction. One of the most often reported endocrinopathies is pituitary dysfunction, which is significantly more prevalent following anti-CTLA-4 therapy than following other immune-based therapies. The occurrence of hypophysitis due to ipilimumab is above 10% on average. This ipilimumab led to hypophysitis, which is more common in men. Fatigue and headaches are the most common signs of ipilimumab-induced hypophysitis (Cukier et al., 2017).

7. CHEMOTHERAPY

Chemotherapy is a well-known method of treating cancer that uses cytotoxic medications to treat different types of cancer. In order to stop the cancer cell from growing and spreading further, these medications often aim to kill the cancer cell and stop it from reproducing. The majority of chemotherapy medications are either taken orally or intravenously. Numerous chemotherapeutic agents exist, and they are typically categorized into a number of groups, such as plant alkaloids, alkylating agents, anthracycline antibiotics, and antimetabolites. The renowned German chemist Paul Ehrlich began working on the development of drugs to treat infectious diseases in the early 1900s. He was the first to define the term "chemotherapy" as the use of chemicals to treat disease and was the first to document the efficacy of using animal models to screen a number of chemicals for their potential activity against diseases, a feat that had significant implications for the development of cancer drugs (DeVita & Chu, 2008).

In the 1960s, the two cornerstones of cancer treatment were surgery and radiotherapy. When micrometastases and cancer recurrence following surgery and radiation therapy became apparent, combination chemotherapy began to acquire importance (Amjad et al., 2020). Chemotherapy in combination is frequently used to achieve satisfactory results. They seem to encourage cytotoxicity in both resting and dividing cells, which inhibits the formation of resistant clones (Baserga, 1981). The complex cellular processes that either stimulate or inhibit cell division and proliferation involve several genes, receptors, and signal transmissions. The mechanisms of apoptosis, angiogenesis, metastasis, cell signal transmission, differentiation, and growth factor modulation have all been greatly illuminated by research in cancer cell biology (Adjei & Hidalgo, 2005). The role of cytotoxic chemotherapy in treating non-small cell lung cancer is still up for debate, despite the fact that it is frequently used to treat small cell lung cancer. A recent worldwide consensus report came to the conclusion that postoperative chemotherapy should be regarded as experimental because it has not been shown to be beneficial (Non-small Cell Lung Cancer Collaborative Group, 1995). Chemotherapy for non-small cell lung cancer is a remarkable development in cancer treatment. The first chemotherapy drugs were introduced in the 1970s, and their clinical benefits were moderate. In the 1980s and 1990s, treatment was revolutionized with the development of platinum compounds and new-generation agents. A seminal meta-analysis conducted in 1995 showed that, when compared to supportive treatment alone, platinum-based chemotherapy increased survival rates from 5% to 15% at one year. In the treatment of non-small cell lung cancer (NSCLC), chemotherapy is still a vital component that must be used in conjunction with more recent therapeutic modalities. Even with developments in immunotherapy and molecular targeted therapy, chemotherapy is still essential for managing both early-stage and late-stage cancer (Lee, 2019).

8. OUTCOME

The survival rate for advanced non-small cell lung cancer is greatly increased when immunotherapies such as toripalimab are added to conventional platinum-based treatment. A median progression-free survival (PFS) of 8.4 months was achieved with toripalimab plus chemotherapy in the phase III CHOICE-01 study, compared to 5.6 months with chemotherapy alone (HR 0.49; $P < .0001$). Furthermore, the combination showed a hazard ratio of 0.69 ($P = .0099$), indicating an overall survival (OS) benefit. In the toripalimab arm, the median OS was not reached, while in the control group it was almost 17 months (Zhong et al., 2024).

The clinical treatment of lung cancer was dominated by chemotherapy prior to the identification of the gene types of NSCLC. Targeted therapy gradually replaced chemotherapy, but chemotherapy also includes cisplatin combination therapy. Today, chemotherapy for NSCLC primarily consists of cisplatin and carboplatin plus gemcitabine, taxanes, and pemetrexed, along with some targeted therapy medications (Guo et al., 2022). Chemotherapy has a variety of mechanisms, such as cisplatin, carboplatin, and gemcitabine, that may cause DNA damage, interfere with the DNA repair pathway, and cause the cancer cell to undergo apoptosis (Dasari & Tchounwou, 2014; Mini et al., 2006).

9. TYPES OF CHEMOTHERAPY

Chemotherapy for non-small cell lung cancer usually uses platinum-based doublets. Together with pemetrexed (particularly in non-squamous histology), docetaxel, paclitaxel, gemcitabine, or vinorelbine, cisplatin and carboplatin form the backbone of the treatment. According to meta-analyses, pemetrexed-platinum combinations significantly increase overall survival when compared to alternative regimens, especially in non-squamous non-small cell lung cancer (Li et al., 2012). Different medication types and therapeutic modalities, each with unique mechanisms and uses, are included in chemotherapy.

Platinum-based (first-line)

Platinum-based chemotherapy continues to be the most widely used treatment for individuals with non-small cell lung cancer (NSCLC). These days, the platinum compounds employed in NSCLC are carboplatin and cisplatin. Cisplatin should remain the standard reference for treating some patients with non-small cell lung cancer due to several findings showing that third-generation regimens based on cisplatin are slightly more effective than carboplatin-based chemotherapy and have a different safety profile (Rossi & Di Maio, 2016).

In patients with metastatic non-small cell lung cancer (NSCLC), cisplatin-based regimens have demonstrated a slight benefit in extending survival in contrast to the most effective supportive care, but because of its toxicity, cisplatin is still a challenging medication to use. Later, another platinum analogue with fewer adverse effects, carboplatin, was created (Pujol et al., 2006; Rosell et al., 2002). The treatment of solid tumors frequently involves the use of platinum compounds. Platinum medications have transformed the treatment of germ cell cancers, and they are now considered standard therapy because of their remarkable cure rates (Decatris et al., 2004). While researching how electric currents affect microorganisms in 1965, Rosenberg made the coincidental discovery of cisplatin. These have a high frequency of toxicities, namely nephrotoxicity, nausea, and vomiting. First to be used widely in cancer chemotherapy, cisplatin (cis-dichlorodiammineplatinum II) belongs to a new class of powerful anticancer medications called metal coordination complexes. It has been demonstrated that the medication works well either by itself or in combination to treat a wide range of solid tumors in humans (Rosenberg, 1980). An analogue of cisplatin, carboplatin was created in the late 1970s when researchers were actively looking for a substance that had cisplatin's antitumor properties but also showed less toxicity. The initial carboplatin clinical trials were conducted by Calvert and colleagues (de Castria et al., 2013). Tests on a variety of malignancies have demonstrated that carboplatin is just as effective as cisplatin in treating extensive-stage small cell lung cancer (Vasconcellos et al., 2020).

According to extensive clinical studies, oxaliplatin shows promise in treating non-small cell lung cancer (NSCLC) and provides clear benefits for specific patient groups. More effective than conventional platinum-based treatments, with comparable cytotoxic effects while requiring fewer DNA adducts. demonstrates less toxicity and better tolerance than traditional platinum chemical compounds. While stable disease indicates that the tumor did not considerably grow or shrink, partial response shows that the tumor has diminished. exhibits encouraging results in squamous cell NSCLC (Ban et al., 2014).

Non-platinum agents

Expanding on our consideration of platinum-based treatments, a number of non-platinum substances are essential for the treatment of non-small cell lung cancer (NSCLC) due to their varied toxicity profiles and modes of action. Modern chemotherapy regimens require these drugs, especially for certain patient demographics and illness stages.

Pemetrexed

A novel antifolate medication called Pemetrexed has been licensed for advanced non-squamous, non-small cell lung cancer (NSCLC) both in conjunction with cisplatin and as a stand-alone treatment for NSCLC that has relapsed or is chemotherapy-refractory following platinum-containing chemotherapy. It is activated intracellularly by poly-γ-glutamylation, which inhibits important intracellular folate metabolism enzymes. Pemetrexed shows no benefit in squamous-cell histology, while it works well in non-squamous cell non-small cell lung cancer. This makes it possible to treat advanced non-small cell lung cancer with tailored anticancer therapy (Joerger et al., 2010).

Docetaxel

A semisynthetic taxane that was first created to treat breast cancer, docetaxel exhibits considerable activity in lung cancer because of its twice increased binding affinity for beta tubulin. It is the most effective first-line treatment for advanced non-small-cell lung cancer (NSCLC) and the gold standard for second-line therapy (Belani & Eckardt, 2004). Compared to vinorelbine or ifosfamide, docetaxel has shown higher response rates and better 1-year survival rates in individuals who have already undergone treatment. In patients who had never had chemotherapy, docetaxel monotherapy also produced survival rates comparable to the majority of typical combinations involving platinum. The combination of docetaxel with other anticancer medications has also been shown to provide high response rates. Overall, the tolerability profile is acceptable. However, neutropenia is the primary dose-limiting side effect. Docetaxel is more effective at improving survival and patient tolerance than vinorelbine, ifosfamide, or optimal supportive care. Patients with non-small cell lung cancer who received docetaxel 75 or 100 mg/ml as a first-line or second-line monotherapy experienced objective response rates of 20 to 38% and 14 to 25%, respectively, in noncomparative trials (Comer & Goa, 2000).

Paclitaxel

Non-small cell lung cancer (NSCLC) is treated with a platinum compound combination that includes the tubulin-binding drug paclitaxel. Short infusions are more likely to cause neuropathy, and myelosuppression is its dose-limiting hazard. Weekly versus 3-weekly paclitaxel regimens with carboplatin for advanced non-small cell lung cancer are now being compared in a randomized clinical trial. It has been demonstrated that paclitaxel and molecularly targeted medicines interact synergistically (Ramalingam & Belani, 2004). In a research study, patients with stage IV or relapsed non-small-cell lung cancer were evaluated for the toxicity and effectiveness of paclitaxel given by 1-hour infusion. Each dose was given to the patients by 1-hour infusion, and they were either given a single-day or three-day dose. A 3-year actuarial survival rate was observed, with a median survival period of 8 months. Patients receiving 200 mg/m^2 exhibited a higher response rate than those getting 135 mg/m^2. Both dosages and schedules of paclitaxel were well tolerated, and there were no serious hypersensitivity events. The study indicates that patients who have had cisplatin-based regimens in the past may respond to a paclitaxel dose of 200 mg/m^2, which is more effective than 135 mg/m^2 (Hainsworth et al., 1995).

Gemcitabine

The antimetabolite gemcitabine has demonstrated encouraging outcomes in Phase II trials with more than 400 patients, with more than 20% demonstrating response rates. Because of its distinct mode of action and advantageous toxicity profile, it is a perfect fit for combination therapy. With median survival times ranging from 8.4 to 15.4 months, gemcitabine-cisplatin combo response rates vary from 31% to 54%. Several double and triple combinations of gemcitabine with ifosfamide, carboplatin, paclitaxel, docetaxel, and vinorelbine have also been studied, in addition to clinical trials including gemcitabine-cisplatin combinations. (Manegold et al., 2000). Considering that gemcitabine is an active ingredient, its adverse effect profile is rather minimal. Gemcitabine-induced nausea and vomiting are minor and usually manageable with common antiemetics. Gemcitabine does not result in severe baldness, and its hematologic toxicity is mild and unlikely to necessitate hospitalization. For individuals with inoperable non-small cell lung cancer, gemcitabine may be useful as a monotherapy (Abratt et al., 1994).

Vinorelbine

Vinorelbine offers an effective and manageable therapy for both early-stage and advanced non-small cell lung cancer. The most frequent hazard is neutropenia, and patient survival is improved when platinum is administered in combination with other drugs. When used with cisplatin in adjuvant settings, vinorelbine regularly increases survival and is more well-tolerated than other third-generation drugs (Piccirillo et al., 2010). Vinorelbine is known to encourage cancer cells to undergo apoptosis. Numerous specifics remain unclear, and the exact mechanisms underlying this process are intricate. Activation or inactivation of several protein kinases implicated in important signaling pathways, such as p21 WAF1/CIP1 and Ras/Raf, PKC/PKA, and the expression of the tumor suppressor gene p53, are among the impacts of microtubule structural disarray (Wang, Liu, et al., 1999). The phosphorylation and subsequent deactivation of the apoptosis inhibitor Bcl2 are caused by these molecular alterations (Haldar et al., 1995). In non-small cell lung cancer (NSCLC), vinorelbine has been thoroughly investigated in conjunction with cisplatin; cisplatin-navelbine is the most successful combination. A multicenter European trial revealed a higher response rate of 14% for vinorelbine alone and 30% for cisplatin-vindesine. The most successful vinorelbine and cisplatin regimen resulted in significant benefit and cost-effectiveness, according to a pharmaco-economic analysis. Additionally, vinorelbine has been investigated in conjunction with other medications; in advanced non-small cell lung cancer, two-drug combos of cisplatin-vinorelbine have shown promising results (Gregory & Smith, 2000).

10. SIDE EFFECTS AND MANAGEMENT

Chemotherapy is associated with several key toxicities, which can be anticipated and effectively managed with supportive measures.

Hematologic Toxicity

Anemia, thrombocytopenia, and neutropenia are frequent symptoms of myelosuppression. Granulocyte colony-stimulating factor (G-CSF) primary prophylaxis is advised when the risk of febrile neutropenia is ≥20% or 10–20% with other risk factors, including age >65 or comorbidities. In actual use, long-acting G-CSFs have demonstrated a significant decrease in hospitalizations and febrile neutropenia. While platelet transfusions are recommended for severe thrombocytopenia, anemia can be treated palliatively with red blood cell transfusions or erythropoiesis-stimulating drugs (Estcourt et al., 2016).

Gastrointestinal Toxicity

An NK1 receptor antagonist, a 5-HT3 antagonist, dexamethasone, and olanzapine are the four medications needed for antiemetic prophylaxis while using cisplatin and other highly emetogenic regimens. Early loperamide treatment for chemotherapy-induced diarrhea, which is seen with pemetrexed-based combinations, is followed by escalation to octreotide in instances that are not responsive. Oral mucositis is still a common side effect. Preventative measures such as dental care, topical pain relievers, and photobiomodulation treatment are recommended (Venkateswaramurthy, 2024).

Renal and Ototoxicity

Hydration is necessary both before and after therapy since cisplatin is still the most nephrotoxic drug. Supplementing with magnesium has been demonstrated to dramatically lower nephrotoxicity. Baseline audiometry and cumulative dose monitoring are advised since cisplatin can also cause tinnitus and irreversible hearing loss. According to recent studies, sodium thiosulphate has shown promise as an otoprotectant (Lalla et al., 2014; Li et al., 2024).

Neurologic Toxicity

Chemotherapy-induced peripheral neuropathy is often caused by platinum compounds and taxanes (CIPN). For grade ≥2 neuropathy, dosage adjustments and routine screening are necessary. Duloxetine is still the only medication that consistently helps those with painful CIPN (Meijer et al., 2024).

Dermatologic Toxicity

Pemetrexed is linked to redness and other dermatological side effects. Premedication with dexamethasone, vitamin B12, and folic acid is required to reduce this. Extended low-dose dexamethasone successfully lowers the frequency and severity of rash (Desforges et al., 2022).

11. TARGETED THERAPIES

Targeted therapy treats patients with specific mistakes, or abnormalities, in their tumors. If you think of DNA as a book, then errors are like typos in the DNA, and mistakes in the DNA can cause cancer or unchecked cell growth. Targeted therapeutic release at the illness site with minimal off-target adverse effects to healthy tissues is the key to the therapy's effectiveness. It is frequently used with other cancer treatments, such as chemotherapy. Drugs that inhibit the tumor cell proliferation, regulate the cellular cycle, or trigger programmed cell death or autophagy are developed as part of targeted therapy. Toxic compounds are delivered to cancer cells selectively to kill them. Oral tiny medicines or monoclonal antibodies are used in targeted therapy (Gerber, 2008). Targeted therapy works by addressing these "typos," or errors in the DNA, and halting the growth of the cells. For lung cancer tumors exhibiting mistakes or anomalies in the following areas, the FDA presently approves targeted therapies such as EGFR, including exon 20 of EGFR, NTRK, BRAF V600E, ALK, and ROS-1 (Dempke et al., 2010). Targeted therapy has first-line and second-line treatments.

EGFR BLOCKER

EGFR is a promising target in NSCLC because it is frequently overexpressed and because its stimulation results in the downstream activation of important signaling pathways, which increases cell viability, proliferation, blood vessel creation, and metastasis (Barr Kumarakulasinghe et al., 2015). The most significant subcategory of the genetic abnormalities found in lung malignancies is EGFR mutations. The two foremost variations of EGFR are a point replacement in codon 21 (L858R) and an elimination in codon 19 (del E746_A750). Tyrosine-rich cytoplasmic areas are homo/heterodimerized and autophosphorylated by the EGFR tyrosine kinase to auto-activate the receptor after ligand contact (Antonicelli et al., 2013).

Tyrosine kinase (TK) blockers are a group of small chemical drugs that inhibit the tyrosine kinase domain of EGFR. Gefitinib and erlotinib were the first generation of TK blockers to demonstrate therapeutic benefit. These two blockers, which bind to this kinase domain reversibly, are regarded as first generation. In patients with the most prevalent activating EGFR mutations, initially developed EGFR blockers have demonstrated exceptional treatment efficacy (Stewart et al., 2015).

EGFR mutations only show up in mixed adeno-squamous carcinomas; they are not found in pure squamous cell carcinomas (SCCs) (Rekhtman et al., 2012). In response to internal and external stimuli, In many biological processes, such as growth, differentiation, metabolism, and death. They play a crucial role in mediating the signaling cascade as well. It has been demonstrated that a major factor in the pathogenesis of human malignancies is the dysregulation of protein kinase activity. In targeted therapies, one of the first cancer treatments to demonstrate the possibility of such a tailored effect was imatinib. Oral targeted treatment imatinib inhibits tyrosine kinases. Because of its anti-PDGFR action, imatinib has also been shown to include platelet-derived growth factor receptor alpha gene PDGFRA, c-KIT, and BCR-ABL. In addition to its impressive efficacy in CML and GIST, imatinib also helps a number of other cancers brought on by aberrant PDGFR and c-KIT expression. Because it is beneficial in steroid-refractory chronic graft-versus-host disease (Iqbal & Iqbal, 2014).

About 20 years ago, in April 1998, humans were initially given ZD1839, an EGFR-TK blocker that subsequently became gefitinib. The pharmacokinetics, antitumor efficacy, and tolerability of this oral EGFR-TKI were investigated in patients with solid malignant tumors during that phase I investigation. The individuals who were initially selected received fifty milligrams of ZD1839 blocker once a day for 14 days.

They then went another 14 days without taking their prescription. Following the administration of dosages ranging from 300 to 700 milligrams daily, four of sixteen patients with NSCLC were able to demonstrate verifiable partial therapeutic outcomes. Following treatment for advanced non-small cell lung cancer, these results led to 2 dose-finding, randomized clinical studies comparing 250 mg and 500 mg daily in patients (Vansteenkiste & Wauters, 2018; Jänne et al., 2015).

Even with early reactions to EGFR TK blockers (acquired resistance), most of the individuals will experience disease recurrence within 1 to 2 years of beginning treatment. The emergence of a second EGFR variation, EGFR T790M, causes developed resistance in approximately sixty percent of patients (Yun et al., 2008). The T790M mutation accounts for almost half of all resistance to the reversible inhibitors erlotinib and gefitinib. Threonine 790 is referred to as the facilitator domain in EGFR due to its critical location at the entrance to the nonpolar region at the back of the ATP-binding cleft, which influences the blocking selectivity of protein kinases. When this residue in EGFR is swapped out for a big methionine, it was once thought that steric interference with the attachment of TKIs, including gefitinib and erlotinib, causes drug resistance. This allows them to block EGFR kinase activity even when EGFR T790M is present (Jänne et al., 2015; Yun et al., 2008; Engelman et al., 2007).

In patients with EGFR-sensitizing mutations, the second-generation TK blockers dacomitinib and afatinib improved clinical outcomes in comparison to the initial-generation TK blocker and platinum-based chemotherapy. Afatinib also showed promise in treating cancer with uncommon EGFR deletions in a pooled analysis of the LUX-Lung studies; however, patients with exon-20 translocation mutations and de novo T790M saw a diminished therapeutic response (Yang et al., 2015). Under the presence of the T790M variation, fewer EGFR-TK blockers of the first or second generation bind to the nucleotide binding site of EGFR. This may accelerate the course of the disease by lessening the suppression of signaling downstream by EGFR-TKI.

Osimertinib, a third-generation inhibitor, was significantly more successful than platinum treatment with pemetrexed for patients with T790M-positive metastatic

NSCLC (including those with CNS metastases) whose condition worsened after first-line EGFR-targeted therapy (Mok et al., 2017).

NTRK BLOCKER

As a part of the tyrosine receptor kinase family, which also includes NTRK1, NTRK2, and NTRK3, neurotrophic tropomyosin receptor kinase (NTRK) encodes for TRKC, TRKA, and TRKB, respectively. Each of the three NTRKs is essential for the formation of the central nervous system, involving cellular death, division, movement, and growth of cells. The downstream signal pathway and function of NTRK are shown in Figure 2. An internal kinase site, a membrane-spanning site, and external interacting ligand motifs are the typical components of NTRK. NTRK stimulates the subsequent pathway, which supports cellular division and proliferation, when it binds to its ligand. Phospholipase C (PLC), mitogen-activated protein kinase (MAPK), phosphoinositide 3-kinase (PI3K), neurotrophin number four (NT4), neurotrophin nerve growth factor (NGF), and brain-derived neurotrophic factor (BDNF) (Qin & Patel, 2022).

Figure 2. The downstream signal pathway and function of NTRK

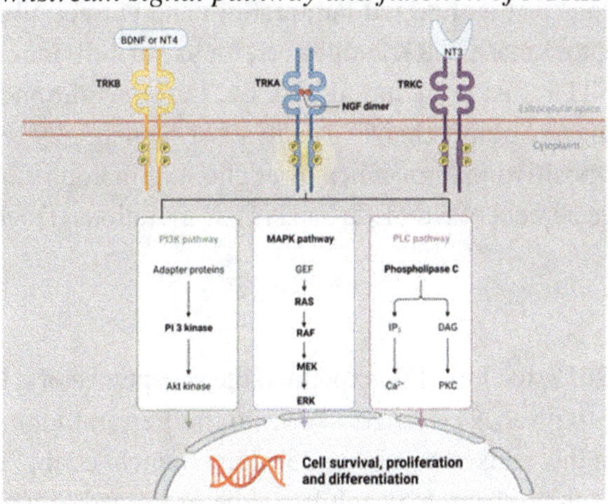

The NTRK1 gene, which is located on chromosomes 1q21–q22, codes for the specific protein TRKA, which interacts with NGF to stimulate the phosphorylation of tyrosine and tyrosine kinase activation. The protein TRKB has a unique interaction with BDNF, and the NTRK2 gene is found on the 9q22.1 allele. Moreover, the 15q5.2 allele contains the NTRK3 gene.

Oncogenic drivers, such as fusion or gene rearrangement involving NTRK1, NTRK2, or NTRK3, are present in a range of tumor forms in both adults and children, including less than one percent of NSCLCs. These gene rearrangements are functionally recognized by a 3′ terminus end that contains an upstream partner gene at the 5′ position and one of the three NTRK genes, which together comprise the whole kinase region (Drilon et al., 2022). Different chromosomal reorganizations can constitutively excite the TRK receptors. This leads to intra-frame gene rearrangement of the NTRK genes' C-terminal TK domain with an N-terminal hybrid target. When the gene rearrangement normally removes the ligand interaction site, cellular receptors dimerize and get phosphorylated without the ligand (Ekman, 2020).

In rare tumors, these fusions might be very common, whereas in more common cancers, they might be far less common (Harada et al., 2021; Hagopian & Nagasaka, 2024). It is undetermined whether gene rearrangement in NTRK returns in NSCLC. Adolescent patients with adenocarcinoma histopathology and little tobacco usage are more likely to have NTRK-mutated NSCLC. In an investigation of 91 lung tumor patients, an NTRK gene fusion was detected in three percent of patients who did not have any other carcinogenic alterations. TPM3-NTRK1, SQSTM1, and ETV6-NTRK3 are frequently detected amalgamation partners in NSCLC with an NTRK mutation (Hagopian & Nagasaka, 2024; Haratake & Seto, 2021).

The US FDA has just authorized larotrectinib and entrectinib, first-generation tropomyosin receptor kinase (TRK) inhibitors, for use in individuals who have solid tumors that have NTRK fusion, including NSCLC. Larotrectinib and entrectinib were approved according to a comprehensive analysis of sequentially registered patients with TRK fusion-positive malignancies throughout numerous clinical trials. Only 0.2 percent to three percent of NSCLCs had NTRK mutations (Doebele et al., 2020).

Larotrectinib

In November 2018, the US FDA expedited the acceptance of it for the therapy of solid malignancies with an NTRK hybrid gene in children and adults who do not have a known mutation that causes resistance (Sartore-Bianchi et al., 2020). The highly efficient pan-Trk inhibitor larotrectinib has been examined in a range of different kinds of tumors in both adult and pediatric patients, and it has shown an ORR of 73% in persons. With a dose reduction of 9% and a cessation of less than 1%, the bulk of the toxicity was grade 1-2. The US, Brazil, and Canada have all authorized larotrectinib. In addition, larotrectinib was recently recommended for approval for solid malignancies with NTRK fusion by the European Medicines Agency (EMA).

Entrectinib

The nucleotide triphosphate-competitive blocker entrectinib is effective and selective; it inhibits ROS1, ALK, TRKB, TRKC, and TRKA in vitro. Tumor cell lines and Ba/f3 cells with changes in the NTRK1 kinase region that made them resistant to another TRK inhibitor, such as the replacement of the key residue F589L and the xDFG motif G667C, were inhibited in their ability to proliferate by entrectinib (Frampton, 2021).

BRAFv600 BLOCKER

Current research has demonstrated that the replacement of a glutamine for a valine at position 600 (V600E) is the most frequent variation in BRAF in a malignant tumor (Khunger et al., 2018; Robinson et al., 2014). Along with ARAF and CRAF, BRAF belongs to the threonine kinase RAF group. The signaling through the MAPK cascade, which regulates the development of cells, growth, and their existence, depends heavily on RAF kinases. It has been found that there are about 300 different BRAF variants in tumor specimens and cancer cell lines from skin cancer, colon, and non-small cell lung cancer (NSCLC) (Tabbò et al., 2022).

BRAFV600 class I mutations show up as monomers that either contain or do not contain activated RAS. When RAS is activated, class II BRAF non-V600 mutations transmit as two molecules of monomers, but class III mutations have increased MAPK pathway signaling but lower kinase activity. This new classification can help anticipate how cancers will respond to targeted treatment (Mazieres et al., 2020). The first BRAF blocker, vemurafenib, was approved for the treatment of advanced BRAF V600E-variant skin cancer. Vemurafenib exhibited a superior progression-free survival (PFS) and a longer overall survival (OS) compared to the PFS and OS of dacarbazine (Khunger et al., 2018).

Initially studied and approved as stand-alone treatments for metastatic melanoma caused by the BRAF V600E mutation, dabrafenib inhibits multiple mutant forms of BRAF, while trametinib is a non-permanently inactivated inhibitor for kinase activity. When compared to dacarbazine, dabrafenib considerably increased PFS for a BRAF V600E or V600K mutation, and when compared to chemotherapy, trametinib significantly increased PFS ("Adverse Event Management in Patients with BRAF V600E-Mutant NSCLC Treated with Dabrafenib plus Trametinib," n.d.).

In line with adenosine triphosphate-competitive blocking, dabrafenib (GSK2118436) is a potent, non-permanently inactivated, and specific antagonist for BRAF V600E kinase activity. The phase I study did not achieve its highest permissible dose. A dose of 150 milligrams oral twice daily was selected depending on the drug kinetics, the impact of dabrafenib on a molecular biological marker target (tumor pERK inhibition), the metabolic processes uptake of FDG-PET, the assessment of the illness as indicated by response according to RECIST criteria at initial restaging, and the safety profile. By day 15, exposure (Cmax and AUC) from 200 milligrams twice daily was no greater than that from 150 mg twice daily (Sánchez-Torres et al., 2013).

According to the National Comprehensive Cancer Network (NCCN) recommendations, individuals suffering from advanced non-squamous NSCLC should be tested for BRAF variants. If the results are positive, dabrafenib plus trametinib should be administered in the first line or later. Trametinib and Dabrafenib together were named a Breakthrough Therapy Designation by the US Food and Drug Administration in 2015 for the treatment of patients with non-small cell lung cancer who had a BRAF V600E alteration and received prior treatment (Anguera & Majem, 2018).

ALK blockers

ALK on the 2p23 allele can express the insulin receptor TK group's anaplastic lymphoma kinase (ALK). The NPM-ALK carcinogenic fusion protein, which is linked to anaplastic large cell lymphoma and is produced by a locational shift between alleles 2 and 5, was first found to contain it (Sullivan & Planchard, 2016). The recurrent deletion and flip of chromosome 2p causes a rare subset of non-small cell lung cancers (NSCLCs) to combine the N-terminus region of the protein expressed by the echinoderm microtubule-associated protein-like 4 (EML4) gene with the signal-regulated section of the ALK receptor TK. Although ALK-related genetic modifications have been found in other tumors, the EML4-ALK recombinant gene seems to be specific to NSCLC. In NSCLCs, a variety of EML4-ALK variants have been found, and they all seem to provide gain-of-function characteristics (Gerber & Minna, 2010).

For advanced NSCLC with ALK rearrangements, the initial choice drug therapy is crizotinib, an oral ALK blocker.

Additionally, more powerful and selective second-generation ALK inhibitors are beginning to be used in clinical settings. Ceritinib (also known as LDK378), the second-generation drug blocker, has shown exceptional efficacy in patients with ALK-driven lung cancer, including those who have developed resistance to crizotinib. The U.S. Food and Drug Administration recently approved crizotinib for use in patients who had previously received crizotinib treatment for advanced ALK-rearranged non-small cell lung cancer. Nevertheless, durability typically manifests within a year, and ALK blocker effectiveness is transient (Wilson et al., 2015).

Most people develop resistance to crizotinib within a year or two of beginning treatment.The ALK blocker resistance is both primary and secondary. Primary resistance occurs when the malignancy is judged unresponsive to the agent at the start of the therapy itself. The primary resistance in ALK+ NSCLC is caused by the many fusion variants of ALK or other partner genes. It has been demonstrated that the ALK variant or fusion gene partner affects the sensitivity to crizotinib. The golden method for detecting ALK mutations in NSCLC at the moment is FISH (Wu et al., 2016).

Developed mechanisms known as secondary resistances emerge following the administration of an ALK antagonist to the malignancy. Secondary resistances are developed responses that emerge after the cancer has been approached with an ALK inhibitor. They can be classified as either ALK-driven or ALK-non-driven. The target ALK gene is mutated in the ALK-driven type, making it impossible to stop the expression of tyrosine kinase (Toyokawa & Seto, 2015).

A multicenter, randomly allocated, stage I/II clinical trial demonstrated that brentinib, another second-generation ALK blocker, can overcome resistance to crizotinib and other first- and second-generation ALK inhibitors in preclinical models, despite the fact that it is not yet approved for use as a first-line treatment (Toyokawa & Seto, 2015). In this study, a dosage of 180 milligrams daily with a 7-day lead-in of 90 milligrams daily produced an excellent outcome for brigatinib with a tolerable safety profile. In evaluable patients with brain metastases, this dose resulted in an overall treatment response rate of 67% (twelve out of eighteen patients) and a total response rate of 54%, including four complete responses. Following the FDA's approval of brigatinib early in the fourth quarter of 2017 for the treatment of crizotinib-resistant, ALK-driven NSCLC, there are now four drugs available to treat ALK-driven NSCLC (Golding et al., 2018).

ROS-1 BLOCKER

ROS1 is an initial oncogene that encodes a tyrosine protein kinase (RTK) receptor that is identical to the Ros sequence of the University of Manchester Tumors virus 2 (UR2) sarcoma virus. Current research is being conducted to identify the virus's ligands. Numerous types of tumors contain ROS1 fusion genes. It functions as an oncoprotein that promotes the growth of cells, stimulation, and progression through the cell cycle by initiating downstream signaling pathways, hence hastening the initiation and spread of non-small cell lung cancer (NSCLC). The first line of treatment for patients with non-small cell lung cancer that is ROS1-positive is ROS1 inhibitors. These tiny molecules provide a reasonable therapeutic option for those who have ROS1 positivity. Sometimes mutations that result in resistance to ROS1 inhibitors inevitably arise, which might cause tumors to develop or reoccur (Yu et al., 2022). The first ROS1 gene fusions were seen in a human glioma cell line (Birchmeier et al., 1987). It was discovered that the 5′ portion of the fused in glioblastoma gene (FIG), also referred to as Golgi-associated PDZ and coiled coil motif including ROS1, was fused to the 3′ area of ROS1 [GOPC] in this cell line through the removal of 240 kilobases on chromosome 6q21, resulting in a constitutively active fusion kinase (Lin & Shaw, 2017). First discovered in 2007, ROS1 rearrangements account for 1-2 percent of NSCLC patients and cause 10,000-15,000 new cases annually worldwide (Rikova et al., 2007). Patients are usually young and either light smokers or non-smokers (D'Angelo et al., 2020). Currently, it is uncertain how ROS1 fusion proteins become constitutively active. For other RTK fusions related to cancer, including ALK, also known as anaplastic lymphoma kinase, the dimerization domain provided by the fusion partner causes constitutive oligomerization, which in turn activates the kinase (Camidge & Doebele, 2012). Whether dimerization plays a role in WT receptor activation for ROS1 is unknown, though. Additionally, it has been revealed that the UR2 avian sarcoma virus's v-ros product and the FIG–ROS1 fusion protein only exist as monomers (Charest et al., 2003). Accordingly, dimerization domains are absent from a large number of the known ROS1 fusion partners (Takeuchi et al., 2012).

12. COMBINATION THERAPIES

The TME's complexity and heterogeneity, the various immune evasion strategies employed by tumor cells, and the drawbacks of mono-immunotherapy provide the justification for combination immunotherapeutic approaches in NSCLC. The goal of combining several immunotherapeutic strategies or other anticancer drugs is to increase the range of antitumor activity, boost antitumor immune responses, and maybe circumvent resistance mechanisms in order to improve treatment results for patients with non-small cell lung cancer. Immune checkpoint inhibitors (ICI) are useful in the treatment of patients with non-small cell lung cancer (NSCLC); nevertheless, because of their limitations when used alone, these medicines are frequently combined with other therapy techniques. Given the limited effectiveness of ICI monotherapy, preclinical studies have shown that neoadjuvant ICIs are more effective than adjuvant ICIs at eradicating distant metastases because they produce a stronger and longer-lasting tumor-specific immune response (Wu et al., 2024). The KEYNOTE-189 study was a double-blind phase III research that assessed the efficacy of pemetrexed in conjunction with platinum-based drugs or a placebo for the treatment of non-squamous metastatic non-small cell lung cancer. The objective response rate (ORR) for the pembrolizumab plus pemetrexed-platinum arm was 48.3%, while the ORR for the placebo plus pemetrexed-platinum arm was only 19.9%. The 5-year overall survival (OS) rate was 19.4% in the pembrolizumab-combination group and 11.3% in the placebo-combination group. The PFS rates for the next five years were 7.5% and 0.6%, respectively (Ma et al., 2025).

13. CONCLUSION

Non-small cell lung cancer (NSCLC) treatment has advanced significantly over the last 20 years, enhancing multimodal therapy and early detection while expanding our knowledge of the illness and the mechanisms behind tumor formation. The use of therapies including immunotherapy, molecularly targeted medications, and chemotherapy, has led to unprecedented increases in survival in some patients. However, overall survival and cure rates for NSCLC remain low, particularly when the disease has progressed. Therefore, additional research into new drugs and combination therapy is required to improve outcomes in NSCLC and increase the clinical benefit to a larger patient group.

REFERENCES

Abratt, R. P., Bezwoda, W. R., Falkson, G., Goedhals, L., Hacking, D., & Rugg, T. A. (1994). Efficacy and safety profile of gemcitabine in non-small-cell lung cancer: A phase II study. *Journal of Clinical Oncology*, *12*(8), 1535–1540. DOI: 10.1200/JCO.1994.12.8.1535 PMID: 8040664

Adjei, A. A., & Hidalgo, M. (2005). Intracellular signal transduction pathway proteins as targets for cancer therapy. *Journal of Clinical Oncology*, *23*(23), 5386–5403. DOI: 10.1200/JCO.2005.23.648 PMID: 15983388

Adverse Event Management in Patients with *BRAF* V600E-Mutant Non-Small Cell Lung Cancer Treated with Dabrafenib plus Trametinib

Akhtar, N., & Bansal, J. G. (2017). Risk factors of Lung Cancer in nonsmoker. *Current Problems in Cancer*, *41*(5), 328–339. DOI: 10.1016/j.currproblcancer.2017.07.002 PMID: 28823540

Alduais, Y., Zhang, H., Fan, F., Chen, J., & Chen, B. (2023). Non-small cell lung cancer (NSCLC): A review of risk factors, diagnosis, and treatment. *Medicine*, *102*(8), e32899. DOI: 10.1097/MD.0000000000032899 PMID: 36827002

Amjad, M. T., Chidharla, A., & Kasi, A. (2020).. . *Cancer & Chemotherapy*.

Anagnostou, V. K., & Brahmer, J. R. (2015). Cancer immunotherapy: A future paradigm shift in the treatment of non–small cell lung cancer. *Clinical Cancer Research*, *21*(5), 976–984. DOI: 10.1158/1078-0432.CCR-14-1187 PMID: 25733707

Anguera, G., & Majem, M. (2018). BRAF inhibitors in metastatic non-small cell lung cancer. *Journal of Thoracic Disease*, *10*(2), 589–592. DOI: 10.21037/jtd.2018.01.129 PMID: 29607117

Antonicelli, A., Cafarotti, S., Indini, A., Galli, A., Russo, A., Cesario, A., Lococo, F. M., Russo, P., Mainini, A. F., Bonifati, L. G., Nosotti, M., Santambrogio, L., Margaritora, S., Granone, P. M., & Dutly, A. E. (2013). EGFR-targeted therapy for non-small cell lung cancer: Focus on EGFR oncogenic mutation. *International Journal of Medical Sciences*, *10*(3), 320–330. DOI: 10.7150/ijms.4609 PMID: 23423768

Ban, H., Kim, K. S., Oh, I. J., Yoon, S. H., Lee, B., Yu, J., Kim, S., Lee, H.-S., Shin, H.-J., Park, C.-K., Kwon, Y.-S., Kim, Y.-I., Lim, S.-C., & Kim, Y. C. (2014). Efficacy and safety of docetaxel plus oxaliplatin as a first-line chemotherapy in patients with advanced or metastatic non-small cell lung cancer. *Thoracic Cancer*, *5*(6), 525–529. DOI: 10.1111/1759-7714.12123 PMID: 26767047

Barr Kumarakulasinghe, N., Zanwijk, N. V., & Soo, R. A. (2015). Molecular targeted therapy in the treatment of advanced stage non-small cell lung cancer (NSCLC). *Respirology (Carlton, Vic.)*, *20*(3), 370–378. DOI: 10.1111/resp.12490 PMID: 25689095

Baserga, R. (1981). The cell cycle. *The New England Journal of Medicine*, *304*(8), 453–459. DOI: 10.1056/NEJM198102193040803 PMID: 6161307

Belani, C. P., & Eckardt, J. (2004). Development of docetaxel inadvanced non-small-cell lung cancer. *Lung Cancer (Amsterdam, Netherlands)*, *46*, S3–S11. DOI: 10.1016/S0169-5002(04)80036-9 PMID: 15698529

Birchmeier, C., Sharma, S., & Wigler, M. (1987). Expression and rearrangement of the ROS1 gene in human glioblastoma cells. *Proceedings of the National Academy of Sciences of the United States of America*, *84*(24), 9270–9274. DOI: 10.1073/pnas.84.24.9270 PMID: 2827175

Burke, M., & Rashdan, S. (2021). Management of Immune-Related Adverse Events in Patients With Non-Small Cell Lung Cancer. *Frontiers in Oncology*, *11*, 720759. DOI: 10.3389/fonc.2021.720759 PMID: 34660286

Camidge, D. R., & Doebele, R. C. (2012). Treating ALK-positive lung cancer—Early successes and future challenges. *Nature Reviews. Clinical Oncology*, *9*(5), 268–277. DOI: 10.1038/nrclinonc.2012.43 PMID: 22473102

Cancer Genome Atlas Research Network. (2014). Comprehensive molecular profiling of lung adenocarcinoma. *Nature*, *511*(7511), 543–550. DOI: 10.1038/nature13385 PMID: 25079552

Charest, A., Kheifets, V., Park, J., Lane, K., McMahon, K., Nutt, C. L., & Housman, D. (2003). Oncogenic targeting of an activated tyrosine kinase to the Golgi apparatus in a glioblastoma. *Proceedings of the National Academy of Sciences of the United States of America*, *100*(3), 916–921. DOI: 10.1073/pnas.242741799 PMID: 12538861

Comer, A. M., & Goa, K. L. (2000). Docetaxel: A review of its use in non-small cell lung cancer. *Drugs & Aging*, *17*(1), 53–80. DOI: 10.2165/00002512-200017010-00004 PMID: 10933515

Cukier, P., Santini, F. C., Scaranti, M., & Hoff, A. O. (2017). Endocrine side effects of cancer immunotherapy. *Endocrine-Related Cancer*, *24*(12), T331–T347. DOI: 10.1530/ERC-17-0358 PMID: 29025857

Curran, M. A., Montalvo, W., Yagita, H., & Allison, J. P. (2010). PD-1 and CTLA-4 combination blockade expands infiltrating T cells and reduces regulatory T and myeloid cells within B16 melanoma tumors. *Proceedings of the National Academy of Sciences of the United States of America*, *107*(9), 4275–4280. DOI: 10.1073/pnas.0915174107 PMID: 20160101

D'Angelo, A., Sobhani, N., Chapman, R., Bagby, S., Bortoletti, C., Traversini, M., Ferrari, K., Voltolini, L., Darlow, J., & Roviello, G. (2020). Focus on ROS1-Positive Non-Small Cell Lung Cancer (NSCLC): Crizotinib, Resistance Mechanisms and the Newer Generation of Targeted Therapies. *Cancers (Basel)*, *12*(11), 3293. DOI: 10.3390/cancers12113293 PMID: 33172113

Dasari, S., & Tchounwou, P. B. (2014). Cisplatin in cancer therapy: Molecular mechanisms of action. *European Journal of Pharmacology*, *740*, 364–378. DOI: 10.1016/j.ejphar.2014.07.025 PMID: 25058905

de Castria, T. B., da Silva, E. M., Gois, A. F., & Riera, R. (2013). Cisplatin versus carboplatin in combination with third-generation drugs for advanced non-small cell lung cancer. *Cochrane Database of Systematic Reviews*, 8. DOI: 10.1002/14651858.CD009256.pub2 PMID: 23949842

Decatris, M. P., Sundar, S., & O'byrne, K. J. (2004). Platinum-based chemotherapy in metastatic breast cancer: Current status. *Cancer Treatment Reviews*, *30*(1), 53–81. DOI: 10.1016/S0305-7372(03)00139-7 PMID: 14766126

Dempke, W. C., Suto, T., & Reck, M. (2010). Targeted therapies for non-small cell lung cancer. *Lung Cancer (Amsterdam, Netherlands)*, *67*(3), 257–274. DOI: 10.1016/j.lungcan.2009.10.012 PMID: 19914732

Desforges, A. D., Hebert, C. M., Spence, A. L., Reid, B., Dhaibar, H. A., Cruz-Topete, D., Cornett, E. M., Kaye, A. D., Urits, I., & Viswanath, O. (2022). Treatment and diagnosis of chemotherapy-induced peripheral neuropathy: An update. *Biomedicine and Pharmacotherapy*, *147*, 112671. DOI: 10.1016/j.biopha.2022.112671 PMID: 35104697

DeVita, V. T.Jr, & Chu, E. (2008). A history of cancer chemotherapy. *Cancer Research*, *68*(21), 8643–8653. DOI: 10.1158/0008-5472.CAN-07-6611 PMID: 18974103

Doebele, R. C., Drilon, A., Paz-Ares, L., Siena, S., Shaw, A. T., Farago, A. F., Blakely, C. M., Seto, T., Cho, B. C., Tosi, D., Besse, B., Chawla, S. P., Bazhenova, L., Krauss, J. C., Chae, Y. K., Barve, M., Garrido-Laguna, I., Liu, S. V., Conkling, P., & Demetri, G. D. (2020). Entrectinib in patients with advanced or metastatic NTRK fusion-positive solid tumours: Integrated analysis of three phase 1–2 trials. *The Lancet. Oncology*, *21*(2), 271–282. DOI: 10.1016/S1470-2045(19)30691-6 PMID: 31838007

Drilon, A., Tan, D. S., Lassen, U. N., Leyvraz, S., Liu, Y., Patel, J. D., Rosen, L., Solomon, B., Norenberg, R., Dima, L., Brega, N., Shen, L., Moreno, V., Kummar, S., & Lin, J. J. (2022). Efficacy and safety of larotrectinib in patients with tropomyosin receptor kinase fusion–positive lung cancers. *JCO Precision Oncology*, *6*(6), e2100418. DOI: 10.1200/PO.21.00418 PMID: 35085007

Edirisinghe, D. T., Kaur, J., Lee, Y. Q., Lim, H. X., Lo, S. W. T., Vishupriyaa, S., Tan, E. W., Wong, R. S. Y., & Goh, B. H. (2025). The role of the tumour microenvironment in lung cancer and its therapeutic implications. *Medical Oncology (Northwood, London, England)*, *42*(6), 219. DOI: 10.1007/s12032-025-02765-7 PMID: 40407951

Ekman, S. (2020). How selecting best therapy for metastatic NTRK fusion-positive non-small cell lung cancer? *Translational Lung Cancer Research*, *9*(6), 2535–2544. DOI: 10.21037/tlcr-20-434 PMID: 33489816

Engelman, J. A., Zejnullahu, K., Gale, C. M., Lifshits, E., Gonzales, A. J., Shimamura, T., Zhao, F., Vincent, P. W., Naumov, G. N., Bradner, J. E., Althaus, I. W., Gandhi, L., Shapiro, G. I., Nelson, J. M., Heymach, J. V., Meyerson, M., Wong, K.-K., & Jänne, P. A. (2007). PF00299804, an irreversible pan-ERBB inhibitor, is effective in lung cancer models with EGFR and ERBB2 mutations that are resistant to gefitinib. *Cancer Research*, *67*(24), 11924–11932. DOI: 10.1158/0008-5472. CAN-07-1885 PMID: 18089823

Estcourt, L., Birchall, J., Allard, S., Bassey, S., Hersey, P., Kerr, J., Mumford, A. D., Stanworth, S. J., & Tinegate, H. (2016). Guidelines for the use of platelet transfusions. *British Journal of Haematology*, *176*(3), 365–394. DOI: 10.1111/bjh.14423 PMID: 28009056

Forde, P. M., Kelly, R. J., & Brahmer, J. R. (2014). New strategies in lung cancer: Translating immunotherapy into clinical practice. *Clinical Cancer Research*, *20*(5), 1067–1073. DOI: 10.1158/1078-0432.CCR-13-0731 PMID: 24470514

Frampton, J. E. (2021). Entrectinib: A review in NTRK+ solid tumours and ROS1+ NSCLC. *Drugs*, *81*(6), 697–708. DOI: 10.1007/s40265-021-01503-3 PMID: 33871816

Gerber, D. E. (2008). Targeted therapies: A new generation of cancer treatments. *American Family Physician*, *77*(3), 311–319. PMID: 18297955

Gerber, D. E., & Minna, J. D. (2010). ALK inhibition for non-small cell lung cancer: From discovery to therapy in record time. *Cancer Cell*, *18*(6), 548–551. DOI: 10.1016/j.ccr.2010.11.033 PMID: 21156280

Golding, B., Luu, A., Jones, R., & Viloria-Petit, A. M. (2018). The function and therapeutic targeting of anaplastic lymphoma kinase (ALK) in non-small cell lung cancer (NSCLC). *Molecular Cancer*, *17*(1), 1–15. DOI: 10.1186/s12943-018-0810-4 PMID: 29455675

Gregory, R. K., & Smith, I. E. (2000). Vinorelbine–a clinical review. *British Journal of Cancer*, *82*(12), 1907–1913. PMID: 10864196

Guo, Q., Liu, L., Chen, Z., Fan, Y., Zhou, Y., Yuan, Z., & Zhang, W. (2022). Current treatments for non-small cell lung cancer. *Frontiers in Oncology*, *12*, 945102. DOI: 10.3389/fonc.2022.945102 PMID: 36033435

Hagopian, G., & Nagasaka, M. (2024). Oncogenic fusions: Targeting NTRK. *Critical Reviews in Oncology/Hematology*, *194*, 104234. DOI: 10.1016/j.critrevonc.2023.104234 PMID: 38122917

Hainsworth, J. D., Thompson, D. S., & Greco, F. A. (1995). Paclitaxel by 1-hour infusion: An active drug in metastatic non-small-cell lung cancer. *Journal of Clinical Oncology*, *13*(7), 1609–1614. DOI: 10.1200/JCO.1995.13.7.1609 PMID: 7602349

Haldar, S., Jena, N., & Croce, C. M. (1995). Inactivation of Bcl-2 by phosphorylation. *Proceedings of the National Academy of Sciences of the United States of America*, *92*(10), 4507–4511. DOI: 10.1073/pnas.92.10.4507 PMID: 7753834

Harada, G., Santini, F. C., Wilhelm, C., & Drilon, A. (2021). NTRK fusions in lung cancer: From biology to therapy. *Lung Cancer (Amsterdam, Netherlands)*, *161*, 108–113. DOI: 10.1016/j.lungcan.2021.09.005 PMID: 34563714

Haratake, N., & Seto, T. (2021). NTRK fusion-positive non–small-cell lung cancer: The diagnosis and targeted therapy. *Clinical Lung Cancer*, *22*(1), 1–5. DOI: 10.1016/j.cllc.2020.10.013 PMID: 33272813

Iqbal, N., & Iqbal, N. (2014). Imatinib: A breakthrough of targeted therapy in cancer. *Chemotherapy Research and Practice*, *2014*(1), 357027. DOI: 10.1155/2014/357027 PMID: 24963404

Jänne, P. A., Yang, J. C. H., Kim, D. W., Planchard, D., Ohe, Y., Ramalingam, S. S., Ahn, M.-J., Kim, S.-W., Su, W.-C., Horn, L., Haggstrom, D., Felip, E., Kim, J.-H., Frewer, P., Cantarini, M., Brown, K. H., Dickinson, P. A., Ghiorghiu, S., & Ranson, M. (2015). AZD9291 in EGFR inhibitor–resistant non–small-cell lung cancer. *The New England Journal of Medicine*, *372*(18), 1689–1699. DOI: 10.1056/NEJMoa1411817 PMID: 25923549

Joerger, M., Omlin, A., Cerny, T., & Fruh, M. (2010). The role of pemetrexed in advanced non small-cell lung cancer: Special focus on pharmacology and mechanism of action. *Current Drug Targets*, *11*(1), 37–47. DOI: 10.2174/138945010790030974 PMID: 19839929

Khunger, A., Khunger, M., & Velcheti, V. (2018). Dabrafenib in combination with trametinib in the treatment of patients with BRAF V600-positive advanced or metastatic non-small cell lung cancer: Clinical evidence and experience. *Therapeutic Advances in Respiratory Disease*, *12*, 1753466618767611. DOI: 10.1177/1753466618767611 PMID: 29595366

Lahiri, A., Maji, A., Potdar, P. D., Singh, N., Parikh, P., Bisht, B., Mukherjee, A., & Paul, M. K. (2023). Lung cancer immunotherapy: Progress, pitfalls, and promises. *Molecular Cancer*, *22*(1), 40. DOI: 10.1186/s12943-023-01740-y PMID: 36810079

Lalla, R. V., Bowen, J., Barasch, A., Elting, L., Epstein, J., Keefe, D. M., McGuire, D. B., Migliorati, C., Nicolatou-Galitis, O., Peterson, D. E., Raber-Durlacher, J. E., Sonis, S. T., & Elad, S. (2014). MASCC/ISOO clinical practice guidelines for the management of mucositis secondary to cancer therapy. *Cancer*, *120*(10), 1453–1461. DOI: 10.1002/cncr.28592 PMID: 24615748

Lee, S. H. (2019). Chemotherapy for lung cancer in the era of personalized medicine. *Tuberculosis and Respiratory Diseases*, *82*(3), 179–189. DOI: 10.4046/trd.2018.0068 PMID: 30841023

Li, J., Wu, Y., Chen, C., Zhang, W., Yue, L., & Liu, T. (2024). A systematic review for prevention of cisplatin-induced nephrotoxicity using different hydration protocols and meta-analysis for magnesium hydrate supplementation. *Clinical and Experimental Nephrology*, *28*(1), 1–12. DOI: 10.1007/s10157-023-02386-2 PMID: 37530867

Li, M., Zhang, Q., Fu, P., Li, P., Peng, A., Zhang, G., Song, X., Tan, M., Li, X., Liu, Y., Wu, Y., Fan, S., & Wang, C. (2012). Pemetrexed plus platinum as the first-line treatment option for advanced non-small cell lung cancer: A meta-analysis of randomized controlled trials. *PLoS One*, *7*(5), e37229. DOI: 10.1371/journal.pone.0037229 PMID: 22615946

Lin, J. J., & Shaw, A. T. (2017). Recent advances in targeting ROS1 in lung cancer. *Journal of Thoracic Oncology*, *12*(11), 1611–1625. DOI: 10.1016/j.jtho.2017.08.002 PMID: 28818606

Lin, X., Xie, M., Yao, J., Ma, X., Qin, L., Zhang, X. M., Song, J., Bao, X., Zhang, X., Zhang, Y., Liu, Y., Han, W., Liang, Y., Jing, Y., & Xue, X. (2024). Immune-related adverse events in non-small cell lung cancer: Occurrence, mechanisms and therapeutic strategies. *Clinical and Translational Medicine*, *14*(3), e1613. DOI: 10.1002/ctm2.1613 PMID: 38451000

Ma, S., Hu, R., Xue, X., Qu, M., & Sun, G. (2025). Novel therapeutic strategies for non-small cell lung cancer: Combination therapies with immune checkpoint inhibitors. *Oncology Letters*, *30*(3), 1–13. DOI: 10.3892/ol.2025.15170 PMID: 40688592

Malhotra, J., Jabbour, S. K., & Aisner, J. (2017). Current state of immunotherapy for non-small cell lung cancer. *Translational Lung Cancer Research*, *6*(2), 196–211. DOI: 10.21037/tlcr.2017.03.01 PMID: 28529902

Malhotra, J., Jabbour, S. K., & Aisner, J. (2017). Current state of immunotherapy for non-small cell lung cancer. *Translational Lung Cancer Research*, *6*(2), 196–211. DOI: 10.21037/tlcr.2017.03.01 PMID: 28529902

Mamdani, H., Matosevic, S., Khalid, A. B., Durm, G., & Jalal, S. I. (2022). Immunotherapy in lung cancer: Current landscape and future directions. *Frontiers in Immunology*, *13*, 823618. DOI: 10.3389/fimmu.2022.823618 PMID: 35222404

Manegold, C., Zatloukal, P., Krejcy, K., & Blatter, J. (2000). Gemcitabine in non-small cell lung cancer (NSCLC). *Investigational New Drugs*, *18*(1), 29–42. DOI: 10.1023/A:1006327729228 PMID: 10830139

Mazieres, J., Cropet, C., Montané, L., Barlesi, F., Souquet, P. J., Quantin, X., Dubos-Arvis, C., Otto, J., Favier, L., Avrillon, V., Cadranel, J., Moro-Sibilot, D., Monnet, I., Westeel, V., Le Treut, J., Brain, E., Trédaniel, J., Jaffro, M., Collot, S., & Blay, J. Y. (2020). Vemurafenib in non-small-cell lung cancer patients with BRAFV600 and BRAFnonV600 mutations. *Annals of Oncology : Official Journal of the European Society for Medical Oncology*, *31*(2), 289–294. DOI: 10.1016/j.annonc.2019.10.022 PMID: 31959346

Meijer, A. J., Diepstraten, F. A., Ansari, M., Bouffet, E., Bleyer, A., Fresneau, B., Geller, J. I., Huitema, A. D. R., Kogner, P., Maibach, R., O'Neill, A. F., Papadakis, V., Rajput, K. M., Veal, G. J., Sullivan, M., van den Heuvel-Eibrink, M. M., & Brock, P. R. (2024). Use of sodium thiosulfate as an otoprotectant in patients with cancer treated with platinum compounds: A review of the literature. *Journal of Clinical Oncology*, *42*(18), 2219–2232. DOI: 10.1200/JCO.23.02353 PMID: 38648563

Mini, E., Nobili, S. F. A. U., Caciagli, B. F. A. U., Landini, I., & Mazzei, T. (2006). Cellular pharmacology of gemcitabine. *Annals of Oncology : Official Journal of the European Society for Medical Oncology*, *17*, v7–v12. DOI: 10.1093/annonc/mdj941 PMID: 16807468

Minna, J. D., Roth, J. A., & Gazdar, A. F. (2002). Focus on lung cancer. *Cancer Cell*, *1*(1), 49–52. DOI: 10.1016/S1535-6108(02)00027-2 PMID: 12086887

Mok, T. S., Wu, Y. L., Ahn, M. J., Garassino, M. C., Kim, H. R., Ramalingam, S. S., Shepherd, F. A., He, Y., Akamatsu, H., Theelen, W. S. M. E., Lee, C. K., Sebastian, M., Templeton, A., Mann, H., Marotti, M., Ghiorghiu, S., & Papadimitrakopoulou, V. A. (2017). Osimertinib or platinum–pemetrexed in EGFR T790M–positive lung cancer. *The New England Journal of Medicine*, *376*(7), 629–640. DOI: 10.1056/NEJMoa1612674 PMID: 27959700

Non-small Cell Lung Cancer Collaborative Group. (1995). Chemotherapy in non-small cell lung cancer: A meta-analysis using updated data on individual patients from 52 randomised clinical trials. *BMJ (Clinical Research Ed.)*, *311*(7010), 899–909. DOI: 10.1136/bmj.311.7010.899 PMID: 7580546

Piccirillo, M. C., Daniele, G., Di Maio, M., Bryce, J., De Feo, G., Del Giudice, A., Perrone, F., & Morabito, A. (2010). Vinorelbine for non-small cell lung cancer. *Expert Opinion on Drug Safety*, *9*(3), 493–510. DOI: 10.1517/14740331003774078 PMID: 20350282

Pujol, J. L., Barlesi, F., & Daurès, J. P. (2006). Should chemotherapy combinations for advanced non-small cell lung cancer be platinum-based? A meta-analysis of phase III randomized trials. *Lung Cancer (Amsterdam, Netherlands)*, *51*(3), 335–345. DOI: 10.1016/j.lungcan.2005.11.001 PMID: 16478643

Qin, H., & Patel, M. R. (2022). The challenge and opportunity of NTRK inhibitors in non-small cell lung cancer. *International Journal of Molecular Sciences*, *23*(6), 2916. DOI: 10.3390/ijms23062916 PMID: 35328336

Ramalingam, S., & Belani, C. P. (2004). Paclitaxel for non-small cell lung cancer. *Expert Opinion on Pharmacotherapy*, *5*(8), 1771–1780. DOI: 10.1517/14656566.5.8.1771 PMID: 15264992

Rekhtman, N., Paik, P. K., Arcila, M. E., Tafe, L. J., Oxnard, G. R., Moreira, A. L., Travis, W. D., Zakowski, M. F., Kris, M. G., & Ladanyi, M. (2012). Clarifying the Spectrum of Driver Oncogene Mutations in Biomarker-Verified Squamous Carcinoma of Lung: Lack of EGFR/KRA S and Presence of PIK3CA/AKT1 Mutations. *Clinical Cancer Research, 18*(4), 1167–1176. DOI: 10.1158/1078-0432.CCR-11-2109 PMID: 22228640

Rekhtman, N., & Travis, W. D. (2019). Large no more: The journey of pulmonary large cell carcinoma from common to rare entity. *Journal of Thoracic Oncology, 14*(7), 1125–1127. DOI: 10.1016/j.jtho.2019.04.014 PMID: 31235033

Rikova, K., Guo, A., Zeng, Q., Possemato, A., Yu, J., Haack, H., Nardone, J., Lee, K., Reeves, C., Li, Y., Hu, Y., Tan, Z., Stokes, M., Sullivan, L., Mitchell, J., Wetzel, R., MacNeill, J., Ren, J. M., Yuan, J., & Comb, M. J. (2007). Global survey of phosphotyrosine signaling identifies oncogenic kinases in lung cancer. *Cell, 131*(6), 1190–1203. DOI: 10.1016/j.cell.2007.11.025 PMID: 18083107

Robinson, S. D., O'Shaughnessy, J. A., Cowey, C. L., & Konduri, K. (2014). BRAF V600E-mutated lung adenocarcinoma with metastases to the brain responding to treatment with vemurafenib. *Lung Cancer (Amsterdam, Netherlands), 85*(2), 326–330. DOI: 10.1016/j.lungcan.2014.05.009 PMID: 24888229

Rosell, R., Gatzemeier, U., Betticher, D. C., Keppler, U., Macha, H. N., Pirker, R., Berthet, P., Breau, J. L., Lianes, P., Nicholson, M., Ardizzoni, A., Chemaissani, A., Bogaerts, J., & Gallant, G. (2002). Phase III randomised trial comparing paclitaxel/carboplatin with paclitaxel/cisplatin in patients with advanced non-small-cell lung cancer: A cooperative multinational trial. *Annals of Oncology : Official Journal of the European Society for Medical Oncology, 13*(10), 1539–1549. DOI: 10.1093/annonc/mdf332 PMID: 12377641

Rosenberg, B. (1980). Cisplatin: Its history and possible mechanisms of action. In *Cisplatin* (pp. 9-20). Academic Press.

Rossi, A., & Di Maio, M. (2016). Platinum-based chemotherapy in advanced non-small-cell lung cancer: Optimal number of treatment cycles. *Expert Review of Anticancer Therapy, 16*(6), 653–660. DOI: 10.1586/14737140.2016.1170596 PMID: 27010977

Sánchez-Torres, J. M., Viteri, S., Molina, M. A., & Rosell, R. (2013). BRAF mutant non-small cell lung cancer and treatment with BRAF inhibitors. *Translational Lung Cancer Research, 2*(3), 244. PMID: 25806238

Sartore-Bianchi, A., Pizzutilo, E. G., Marrapese, G., Tosi, F., Cerea, G., & Siena, S. (2020). Entrectinib for the treatment of metastatic NSCLC: Safety and efficacy. *Expert Review of Anticancer Therapy*, *20*(5), 333–341. DOI: 10.1080/14737140.2020.1747439 PMID: 32223357

Schuster, M., Nechansky, A., & Kircheis, R. (2006). Cancer immunotherapy. *Biotechnology Journal*, *1*(2), 138–147. DOI: 10.1002/biot.200500044 PMID: 16892244

Shames, D. S., & Wistuba, I. I. (2014). The evolving genomic classification of lung cancer. *The Journal of Pathology*, *232*(2), 121–133. DOI: 10.1002/path.4275 PMID: 24114583

Smolarz, B., Łukasiewicz, H., Samulak, D., Piekarska, E., Kołaciński, R., & Romanowicz, H. (2025). Lung Cancer—Epidemiology, Pathogenesis, Treatment and Molecular Aspect (Review of Literature). *International Journal of Molecular Sciences*, *26*(5), 2049. DOI: 10.3390/ijms26052049 PMID: 40076671

Stanley, R., Flanagan, S., Reilly, D. O., Kearney, E., Naidoo, J., & Dowling, C. M. (2023). Immunotherapy through the Lens of Non-Small Cell Lung Cancer. *Cancers (Basel)*, *15*(11), 2996. DOI: 10.3390/cancers15112996 PMID: 37296957

Stewart, E. L., Tan, S. Z., Liu, G., & Tsao, M. S. (2015). Known and putative mechanisms of resistance to EGFR targeted therapies in NSCLC patients with EGFR mutations—A review. *Translational Lung Cancer Research*, *4*(1), 67. PMID: 25806347

Sullivan, I., & Planchard, D. (2016). ALK inhibitors in non-small cell lung cancer: The latest evidence and developments. *Therapeutic Advances in Medical Oncology*, *8*(1), 32–47. DOI: 10.1177/1758834015617355 PMID: 26753004

Tabbò, F., Pisano, C., Mazieres, J., Mezquita, L., Nadal, E., Planchard, D., Pradines, A., Santamaria, D., Swalduz, A., Ambrogio, C., Novello, S., & Ortiz-Cuaran, S.BOLERO Consortium. (2022). How far we have come targeting BRAF-mutant non-small cell lung cancer (NSCLC). *Cancer Treatment Reviews*, *103*, 102335. DOI: 10.1016/j.ctrv.2021.102335 PMID: 35033867

Takeuchi, K., Soda, M., Togashi, Y., Suzuki, R., Sakata, S., Hatano, S., Asaka, R., Hamanaka, W., Ninomiya, H., Uehara, H., Lim Choi, Y., Satoh, Y., Okumura, S., Nakagawa, K., Mano, H., & Ishikawa, Y. (2012). RET, ROS1 and ALK fusions in lung cancer. *Nature Medicine*, *18*(3), 378–381. DOI: 10.1038/nm.2658 PMID: 22327623

Tomasini, P., Khobta, N., Greillier, L., & Barlesi, F. (2012). Ipilimumab: Its potential in non-small cell lung cancer. *Therapeutic Advances in Medical Oncology, 4*(2), 43–50. DOI: 10.1177/1758834011431718 PMID: 22423263

Topalian, S. L., Drake, C. G., & Pardoll, D. M. (2012). Targeting the PD-1/B7-H1(PD-L1) pathway to activate anti-tumor immunity. *Current Opinion in Immunology, 24*(2), 207–212. DOI: 10.1016/j.coi.2011.12.009 PMID: 22236695

Toyokawa, G., & Seto, T. (2015). Updated evidence on the mechanisms of resistance to ALK inhibitors and strategies to overcome such resistance: Clinical and preclinical data. *Oncology Research and Treatment, 38*(6), 291–298. DOI: 10.1159/000430852 PMID: 26045026

Vansteenkiste, J., & Wauters, E. (2018). Tyrosine kinase inhibition of EGFR: A successful history of targeted therapy for NSCLC since 20 years. *Annals of Oncology : Official Journal of the European Society for Medical Oncology, 29*, i1–i2. DOI: 10.1093/annonc/mdx724 PMID: 29462258

Vasconcellos, V. F., Marta, G. N., da Silva, E. M., Gois, A. F., de Castria, T. B., & Riera, R. (2020). Cisplatin versus carboplatin in combination with third-generation drugs for advanced non-small cell lung cancer. *Cochrane Database of Systematic Reviews, 2020*(1), 1. DOI: 10.1002/14651858.CD009256.pub3 PMID: 31930743

Venkateswaramurthy, N., S, A., & P R, E. (2024). Managing Chemotherapy-Induced Diarrhea: Efficacy of Interventions for Cancer Patients. *Biosciences Biotechnology Research Asia, 21*(1), 391–404. DOI: 10.13005/bbra/3233

Villaruz, L. C., Kalyan, A., Zarour, H., & Socinski, M. A. (2014). Immunotherapy in lung cancer. *Translational Lung Cancer Research, 3*(1), 2–14. PMID: 25806276

Wang, L., Liu, X., Kreis, W., & Budman, D. (1999). Activation of MAP kinase during apoptosis mediated by vinorelbine in MCF-7 cells. *Proceedings of the American Association for Cancer Research, 40*, 13.

Wang, Y., Kondrat, K., Adhikari, J., Nguyen, Q., Yu, Q., & Uprety, D. (2025). Survival trends among patients with metastatic non–small cell lung cancer before and after the approval of immunotherapy in the United States: A Surveillance, Epidemiology, and End Results database–based study. *Cancer, 131*(1), e35476. DOI: 10.1002/cncr.35476 PMID: 38985895

Wang, Y., Li, C., Wang, Z., Wang, Z., Wu, R., Wu, Y., Song, Y., & Liu, H. (2022). Comparison between immunotherapy efficacy in early non-small cell lung cancer and advanced non-small cell lung cancer: A systematic review. *BMC Medicine, 20*(1), 426. DOI: 10.1186/s12916-022-02580-1 PMID: 36345004

Wilson, F. H., Johannessen, C. M., Piccioni, F., Tamayo, P., Kim, J. W., Van Allen, E. M., Corsello, S. M., Capelletti, M., Calles, A., Butaney, M., Sharifnia, T., Gabriel, S. B., Mesirov, J. P., Hahn, W. C., Engelman, J. A., Meyerson, M., Root, D. E., Jänne, P. A., & Garraway, L. A. (2015). A functional landscape of resistance to ALK inhibition in lung cancer. *Cancer Cell*, *27*(3), 397–408. DOI: 10.1016/j.ccell.2015.02.005 PMID: 25759024

Wolchok, J. D., Kluger, H., Callahan, M. K., Postow, M. A., Rizvi, N. A., Lesokhin, A. M., Segal, N. H., Ariyan, C. E., Gordon, R.-A., Reed, K., Burke, M. M., Caldwell, A., Kronenberg, S. A., Agunwamba, B. U., Zhang, X., Lowy, I., Inzunza, H. D., Feely, W., Horak, C. E., & Sznol, M. (2013). Nivolumab plus ipilimumab in advanced melanoma. *The New England Journal of Medicine*, *369*(2), 122–133. DOI: 10.1056/NEJMoa1302369 PMID: 23724867

Wu, J., Savooji, J., & Liu, D. (2016). Second-and third-generation ALK inhibitors for non-small cell lung cancer. *Journal of Hematology & Oncology*, *9*(1), 1–7. DOI: 10.1186/s13045-016-0251-8 PMID: 26951079

Wu, Y., Yu, G., Jin, K., & Qian, J. (2024). Advancing non-small cell lung cancer treatment: The power of combination immunotherapies. *Frontiers in Immunology*, *15*, 1349502. DOI: 10.3389/fimmu.2024.1349502 PMID: 39015563

Xiang, Y., Liu, X., Wang, Y., Zheng, D., Meng, Q., Jiang, L., Yang, S., Zhang, S., Zhang, X., Liu, Y., & Wang, B. (2024). Mechanisms of resistance to targeted therapy and immunotherapy in non-small cell lung cancer: Promising strategies to overcoming challenges. *Frontiers in Immunology*, *15*, 1366260. DOI: 10.3389/fimmu.2024.1366260 PMID: 38655260

Yang, J. C., Sequist, L. V., Geater, S. L., Tsai, C. M., Mok, T. S. K., Schuler, M., Yamamoto, N., Yu, C.-J., Ou, S.-H. I., Zhou, C., Massey, D., Zazulina, V., & Wu, Y. L. (2015). Clinical activity of afatinib in patients with advanced non-small-cell lung cancer harbouring uncommon EGFR mutations: A combined post-hoc analysis of LUX-Lung 2, LUX-Lung 3, and LUX-Lung 6. *The Lancet. Oncology*, *16*(7), 830–838. DOI: 10.1016/S1470-2045(15)00026-1 PMID: 26051236

Yu, Z. Q., Wang, M., Zhou, W., Mao, M. X., Chen, Y. Y., Li, N., Peng, X.-C., Cai, J., & Cai, Z. Q. (2022). ROS1-positive non-small cell lung cancer (NSCLC): Biology, diagnostics, therapeutics and resistance. *Journal of Drug Targeting*, *30*(8), 845–857. DOI: 10.1080/1061186X.2022.2085730 PMID: 35658765

Yuan, K., Zhang, C., Pan, X., Hu, B., Zhang, J., & Yang, G. (2024). Immunomodulatory metal-based biomaterials for cancer immunotherapy. *Journal of Controlled Release*, *375*, 249–268. DOI: 10.1016/j.jconrel.2024.09.008 PMID: 39260573

Yun, C. H., Mengwasser, K. E., Toms, A. V., Woo, M. S., Greulich, H., Wong, K. K., Meyerson, M., & Eck, M. J. (2008). The T790M mutation in EGFR kinase causes drug resistance by increasing the affinity for ATP. *Proceedings of the National Academy of Sciences of the United States of America*, *105*(6), 2070–2075. DOI: 10.1073/pnas.0709662105 PMID: 18227510

Zappa, C., & Mousa, S. A. (2016). Non-small cell lung cancer: Current treatment and future advances. *Translational Lung Cancer Research*, *5*(3), 288–300. DOI: 10.21037/tlcr.2016.06.07 PMID: 27413711

Zhong, J., Fei, K., Wu, L., Li, B., Wang, Z., Cheng, Y., Li, X., Wang, X., Han, L., Wu, X., Fan, Y., Yu, Y., Lv, D., Shi, J., Huang, J., Zhou, S., Han, B., Sun, G., Guo, Q., & Wang, J. (2024). Toripalimab plus chemotherapy for first line treatment of advanced non-small cell lung cancer (CHOICE-01): Final OS and biomarker exploration of a randomized, double-blind, phase 3 trial. *Signal Transduction and Targeted Therapy*, *9*(1), 369. DOI: 10.1038/s41392-024-02087-6 PMID: 39715755

Zhou, C., Li, M., Wang, Z., An, D., & Li, B. (2022). Adverse events of immunotherapy in non-small cell lung cancer: A systematic review and network meta-analysis. *International Immunopharmacology*, *102*, 108353. DOI: 10.1016/j.intimp.2021.108353 PMID: 34883352

Chapter 11
Palliative and Supportive Care for Advanced Non-Small Cell Lung Cancer

Mohammad-Salar Hosseini
https://orcid.org/0000-0003-2765-5018
Tabriz University of Medical Sciences, Iran

Yosra Vaez-Gharamaleki
https://orcid.org/0000-0002-2718-321X
Tabriz University of Medical Sciences, Iran

Sarvin Sanaie
https://orcid.org/0000-0003-2325-5631
Tabriz University of Medical Sciences, Iran

Hossein Jabbari Beyrami
https://orcid.org/0000-0002-1749-9915
Iranian Cancer Control Center, Tabriz, Iran

ABSTRACT

The majority of non-small cell lung cancer (NSCLC) patients are diagnosed at advanced stages, where curative treatments may no longer result in optimal outcomes, and the quality of life is limited by disease- or treatment-related adverse events. This chapter explores the principles and practices of palliative and supportive care in NSCLC, emphasizing the importance of early integration into standard oncology care. Core discussed topics include clinical symptom management (including pain, dyspnea, fatigue, cough, nausea/vomiting, anorexia, and cachexia), psychological and psychosocial support (including psychological distress, caregiver burden, financial toxicity, cultural considerations, and spiritual suffering), management of

DOI: 10.4018/979-8-3373-2096-0.ch011

disease- and treatment-related complications (including coagulopathy, malignant pleural effusion, superior vena cava syndrome, spinal cord compression, hypercalcemia, and hematologic, neurological, and dermatologic complications), ethical decision-making, and the role of a multidisciplinary palliative care team.

INTRODUCTION

Non-small cell lung cancer (NSCLC) is a major cause of cancer-related mortality, accounting for almost five out of every six lung cancer cases (Sharma, 2022). Over the past years, the management of NSCLC has undertaken substantial changes, driven by advances in molecular biology, precision diagnostics, and targeted therapies. These developments have not only extended survival but have also reshaped the clinical trajectory, introducing new patterns of symptom burden, treatment-related toxicities, and survivorship challenges. Despite recent advances in molecular diagnostics, targeted therapies, and immuno-oncology, most NSCLC cases are detected at advanced stages, where curative treatments not only no longer result in optimal outcomes but also lead to various life-limiting complications and disease- or treatment-related adverse events. In these cases, the clinical focus primarily shifts from merely curative intent to effective symptom management, maintenance of function, and improvement of quality of life—core principles that define palliative and supportive care. As outcomes improve yet cure remains elusive for the majority, palliative and supportive care assumes an increasingly vital role in optimizing quality of life, tackling complex physical and psychosocial needs, and guiding decision-making process.

Palliative care, as defined by the World Health Organization (WHO), is "an approach that improves the quality of life of patients (adults and children) and their families who are facing problems associated with life-threatening illness" (World Health Organization, 2020). Palliative care relieves suffering through early addressing of the patients' and close carers' physical and psychosocial problems (Dzierżanowski, 2021). In the context of advanced NSCLC, where symptom burden is often severe and multifactorial, palliative care is not only an adjunct to conventional anticancer treatments but a fundamental component of comprehensive cancer management. Clinical conditions, such as dyspnea, cough, pain, and anorexia require precise clinical assessment and often complicated interventions. Moreover, the psychological distress related to the terminal diagnosis, loss of autonomy, and end-of-life uncertainty further highlight the importance of integrated supportive care.

Traditionally, palliative care was perceived as equal to end-of-life care and was often introduced only after active treatment options had been exhausted. However, this paradigm has shifted considerably over the past two decades. Key studies, such as the infamous randomized controlled trial of Temel and colleagues, proved that early implementation of palliative care in metastatic NSCLC improve quality of life and mood, and was also linked with prolonged survival despite reduced use of aggressive end of life care (Temel et al., 2010). This evidence led to a reevaluation of clinical pathways and guidelines, prompting major oncological societies to recommend early referral to palliative care – as early as the first 8 weeks – for patients with advanced or symptomatic NSCLC (Dans et al., 2021; Ferrell et al., 2017).

This chapter aims to provide an inclusive clinical outline of palliative and supportive care in managing advanced NSCLC, exploring evidence-based strategies for symptom management, psychological and psychosocial support, ethical considerations, and integrating palliative care into standard oncology practice.

PRINCIPLES OF PALLIATIVE CARE

Palliative care is a patient- and family-oriented discipline aiming to improve the quality of life in those with life-limiting illnesses. In advanced NSCLC, where optimal curative care is often unreachable, palliative care becomes a central element of treatment rather than a supplementary service. The principles of palliative care are based on patient-centered care, evidence-based practice, and collaborative management.

Patient-Centered and Inclusive Care

A foundational principle of palliative care is its commitment to inclusive care, which acknowledges and addresses the multidimensional nature of management. Patient-centered care should address:

- Physical symptoms, namely pain, dyspnea, and fatigue.
- Psychological distress, anxiety, and depression.
- Social factors, such as the caregiver burden, financial toxicity, and social isolation.
- Spiritual concerns such as the spiritual crisis and preparation for death.

In advanced NSCLC, where symptom burden is often compounded by the progression of disease and treatment-related adverse events, care plans must be individualized. This necessitates a thorough and repeated assessment of patient-reported outcomes, facilitated by validated tools such as the Edmonton Symptom Assessment System (ESAS) or the Functional Assessment of Cancer Therapy – Lung (FACT-L) (Cella et al., 1995; Hui & Bruera, 2017).

Proactive Symptom Management

Palliative care emphasizes the *anticipation* and *prevention* of symptoms, rather than merely responding to crises. In advanced NSCLC, patients frequently experience predictable trajectories of symptom progression due to tumor burden (such as pleural effusion) or the complications of therapy (such as pneumonitis and fatigue) (Rudin et al., 2021). Early intervention, including prophylactic pharmacologic strategies and patient education, can significantly reduce suffering and avoid emergency room visits or hospital admissions (Farbicka & Nowicki, 2013; Yao et al., 2023)

Communication and Shared Decision-Making

Effective, compassionate, and honest communication is a cornerstone of palliative care. This includes not only the delivery of difficult information, such as disease progression, prognosis, and end-of-life expectations, but also the facilitation of shared decision-making (Engel et al., 2023). In advanced NSCLC, patients are often faced with complex choices regarding systemic therapy, radiation, interventional procedures, and hospice enrollment. Palliative care professionals should navigate these conversations with sensitivity and clarity, aligning treatment plans with patient values, priorities, and goals of care (Wilkin et al., 2024). Advance care planning is a key process through which patients are supported in expressing their goals, designating surrogate decision-makers, and documenting their wishes through instruments such as advance directives or Physician Orders for Life-Sustaining Treatment (POLST) (Rosa et al., 2023). In oncology, timely advance care planning is associated with greater satisfaction, reduced decisional regret, and decreased utilization of non-beneficial interventions at the end of life (Starr et al., 2019).

Interdisciplinary and Collaborative Care

Palliative care is an interdisciplinary field relying on a collaborative approach to deliver coordinated and continuous support (Pornrattanakavee et al., 2022). The core team typically includes physicians, nurses, social workers, pharmacists, mental health specialists, rehabilitation specialists, pharmacists, dietitians, and spiritual care specialists. Collaborative care models may be co-managed (parallel care provided by oncology and palliative teams) or integrated (where palliative care is embedded into oncology clinics) (Mathews et al., 2021). Evidence increasingly favors early and integrated models, improving symptom control, caregiver satisfaction, and even survival, particularly in advanced NSCLC cases (Kochovska et al., 2020).

Ethical and Culturally Competent Care

Like every clinical encounter, respect for patient autonomy, beneficence, non-maleficence, and justice must guide palliative care services (Akdeniz et al., 2021). In the setting of advanced NSCLC, where the line between therapeutic benefit and treatment ineffectiveness may become blurred, palliative care teams provide critical guidance in navigating ethically complex scenarios, such as withdrawal from therapy. Cultural sensitivity is also important, and beliefs about illness, suffering, family roles, and death vary widely across populations. Palliative care practice and communications should be culturally sensitive, respectful, and appropriate (Givler et al., 2018).

SYMPTOM MANAGEMENT IN ADVANCED NSCLC

NSCLC patients experience various symptoms, driven by both tumor burden and adverse effects of systemic treatments. Effective symptom management in these patients is fundamental to preserving quality of life, maintaining functional status, and preventing avoidable healthcare utilization.

Pain Management

Pain affects over 75% of patients with advanced NSCLC and may originate from tumor infiltration, treatment sequelae (such as post-thoracotomy pain syndrome and radiation-induced neuropathy), or paraneoplastic syndromes (Nikitas et al., 2024; Simmons et al., 2012). It may be nociceptive, neuropathic, or mixed in nature (Caraceni & Shkodra, 2019). Comprehensive pain assessment involves the characterization of intensity, quality, timing, location, and the exacerbating/relieving factors. Tools such as the Brief Pain Inventory or the Numeric Rating Scale facilitate monitoring (Kumar, 2011).

Mild pain is generally managed with non-opioid analgesics, such as acetaminophen and Non-steroidal anti-inflammatory drugs (NSAIDs). Stepwise escalation per WHO analgesic ladder is recommended, with weak opioids, such as codeine, as initial choices, and more potent opioids, such as morphine and fentanyl, prescribed for moderate-to-severe pain (Anekar et al., 2023). Titration should be guided by pain severity, renal and hepatic function, and prior opioid exposure. Neuropathic pain may require adjuvants, such as gabapentinoids (gabapentin, pregabalin), tricyclic antidepressants, or serotonin-norepinephrine reuptake inhibitors (SNRIs) (Kremer et al., 2016; Mu et al., 2017).

Radiation therapy for localized bone pain or spinal metastases, nerve block or epidural infusions in refractory cases, along with cognitive-behavioral therapy, have been recommended as non-pharmacological approaches (Hamada et al., 2024; Simmons et al., 2012).

Dyspnea

Dyspnea is reported in majority of advanced lung cancer patients, arising from tumor-induced airway obstruction, pleural effusion, lymphangitic spread, anemia, or coexisting cardiopulmonary conditions (Hui et al., 2021). Subjective perception may not always correlate with objective findings; therefore, validated tools such as the Cancer Dyspnea Scale are recommended (Tanaka et al., 2000).

Opioids (such as low-dose morphine) can decrease ventilatory drive and reduce dyspnea perception (Taniguchi et al., 2022). Corticosteroids are indicated in cases of airway compression or lymphangitic carcinomatosis (Hui & Yennurajalingam, 2023). Anti-anxiety medications, including benzodiazepines, should be carefully considered for dyspnea-related anxiety (Simon et al., 2016).

Oxygen supplementation is the first non-pharmacologic choice for hypoxemic patients, although it is not universally beneficial in non-hypoxemic dyspnea (Uronis et al., 2008). Personalized pulmonary rehabilitation has been proven effective in reducing postoperative pulmonary complications in these patients (Zhang et al., 2025). Invasive interventions, such as thoracentesis, endobronchial stenting, or indwelling pleural catheter for malignant pleural effusions, are also indicated in advanced cases (Kastelik, 2013; Saji et al., 2010).

Cough and Hemoptysis

Chronic cough, often refractory, is a distressing symptom in NSCLC. Causes include tumor irritation of the airways, post-obstructive infection, pleural involvement, or therapy-induced pneumonitis (Simoff et al., 2013). Besides, one in every two to five NSCLC patients experiences hemoptysis during their disease course (Razazi et al., 2014).

Minor hemoptysis can be managed conservatively in home care or outpatient settings. However, massive hemoptysis is a medical emergency. It should be noted that massive hemoptysis has diverse definitions across different sources, varying from over 100 mL to over 1000 mL in 24 hours (Gershman et al., 2019). For cough, antitussives, such as hydrocodone or dextromethorphan, could be prescribed based on the cough pattern and patients' co-morbidities (The latest guideline for symptomatic treatment of cough from the CHEST Expert Cough Panel provides clear recommendations regarding the dosage and other details (Molassiotis et al.,

2017)). Nebulized lidocaine, bronchodilators, or corticosteroids are recommended for bronchial hyperreactivity. For hemoptysis of any severity, airway protection and hemodynamic support are the first goals of care (Radchenko et al., 2017). Topical vasoconstrictors and bronchial artery embolization are other practical approaches to control hemoptysis (Han et al., 2019).

Fatigue

Fatigue in advanced NSCLC is multifactorial – rooting in systemic inflammation, anemia, metabolic derangements, treatment side effects, and psychological burden. In fact, fatigue is the most commonly recorded and least successfully treated symptom in this population (Carnio et al., 2016).

Corticosteroids are an appropriate choice for short-term relief. Psychostimulants, such as methylphenidate and modafinil, could also be prescribed in selected cases (Carnio et al., 2016; Spathis et al., 2009). More importantly, personalized nutritional modifications are strongly recommended for addressing fatigue among NSCLC patients (Zhang et al., 2023). Erythropoiesis-stimulating agents are also indicated for anemia-induced fatigue, which should be prescribed cautiously due to thrombotic risk and tumor progression concerns (Heregger & Greil, 2023). Structured physical activity and rehabilitation are effective in NSCLC patients, although the majority of the patients fail to comply with the protocols (Avancini et al., 2020; Temel et al., 2009). Limited evidence supports the role of psychosocial support and energy conservation strategies in managing fatigue in this population (Poort et al., 2017).

Anorexia and Cachexia

Cancer cachexia is described as involuntary weight loss, muscle wasting, and metabolic alterations that are not fully reversed by conventional nutritional support (Ni & Zhang, 2020). Previous studies have suggested an early engagement with dietitians and the inclusion of a nutritionist in the palliative care team to improve outcomes in terms of cachexia (Koshimoto et al., 2023; Roeland & Dunne, 2021). High-calorie, protein-dense supplements and small frequent meals, along with anti-inflammatory agents and omega-3 fatty acids as adjunctive options, are generally recommended in this case; although there are reports of higher prevalence of nausea/vomiting as a complication of these nutritional modifications (de Castro et al., 2021; Ni & Zhang, 2020; van de Worp et al., 2020). Appetite stimulants, such as megestrol acetate and anamorelin, have also been recommended for NSCLC-related anorexia and cachexia in the recent decade (Ruiz Garcia et al., 2013; Wakabayashi et al., 2021; Zhang & Garcia, 2015). GDF15/GFRAL inhibitors, such as ponsegromab, are also under evaluation for lung cancer-related cachexia (Sahebari & Hosseini,

2025). Psychosocial support and addressing family distress related to food refusal and perceived "failure to feed" is also necessary (Hopkinson, 2018).

Nausea and Vomiting

Etiologies include chemotherapy, opioids, gastrointestinal obstruction, brain metastases, or metabolic disturbances (Jovanovic et al., 2024). Current best practices involve the use of combination prophylaxis incorporating a serotonin type 3 receptor antagonist, such as ondansetron or granisetron, a neurokinin-1 receptor antagonist, such as aprepitant, and dexamethasone (He et al., 2021). Etiology-specific treatments are endorsed, with dopamine antagonists, such as metoclopramide and haloperidol, frequently used as first-line agents for many patients (Glare et al., 2011).

PSYCHOLOGICAL AND PSYCHOSOCIAL CARE

Psychological and psychosocial care is an indispensable section of palliative and supportive care in NSCLC. The diagnosis of advanced malignancy frequently triggers profound emotional, existential, and social distress that extends beyond the individual.

Psychological Distress in Advanced NSCLC

Anxiety, depression, demoralization, adjustment disorders, and post-traumatic stress disorder are prevalent among cancer patients, with a higher prevalence among lung cancer (Andersen et al., 2020; Grassi et al., 2023). Depression alone affects one in every three to five NSCLC patients, while clinically significant anxiety is reported in nearly one-third of patients (Arrieta et al., 2013). Psychological distress is often rooted in both disease-related factors (such as functional decline), existential concerns (including fear of death and loss of autonomy), and social or familial disruptions (Vehling & Kissane, 2018).

Early identification of psychological distress is critical, and supportive mental psychosocial care should be integrated into routine clinical assessments (M.-S. Hosseini, 2023). Validated tools such as the National Comprehensive Cancer Network (NCCN) Distress Thermometer and the Hospital Anxiety and Depression Scale (HADS) can be used for this purpose (Michopoulos et al., 2008; National Comprehensive Cancer Network®). Clinicians must maintain a high index of suspicion, particularly in individuals with underreported symptoms or diminished insight due to cultural, cognitive, or emotional barriers. Psychosocial care is strengthened by systematically incorporating patient-reported outcomes (PROs) and lived experiences, which capture symptom burden, emotional distress, functional limitations, and caregiver challenges often missed in routine care. Validated tools such as FACT-L, MDASI-LC, and ESAS, along with patient and caregiver narratives, highlight common themes including uncertainty about prognosis, stigma, role loss, anxiety, anticipatory grief, and financial strain.

Interventions for Psychological Support

Multiple modalities of psychological therapy can be considered for advanced NSCLC patients, including cognitive behavioral and supportive-expressive therapy (Anghel et al., 2025). Mindfulness-based interventions encourage awareness, resilience, and present-focused coping in NSCLC patients (McDonnell et al., 2023; Schellekens et al., 2017; Yu et al., 2025). Access to licensed mental health professionals, psychologists, psychiatrists, and psycho-oncologists, is essential for evidence-based interventions (Mackay et al., 2023).

SSRIs and SNRIs are commonly used for major depressive disorder and generalized anxiety. Anxiolytics such as benzodiazepines may be used for acute symptom relief in these patients, particularly in the context of terminal restlessness, although caution is warranted due to the risk of sedation, dependence, and respiratory depression (O'Donnell et al., 2019; Von Roenn & Brandman, 2004). Close monitoring and collaboration with psychiatric services are advised when initiating or modifying psychotropic medications.

Caregiver Burden and Family Distress

The psychosocial impact of NSCLC extends deeply into the lives of caregivers, who often experience emotional exhaustion, anticipatory grief, and financial strain. Spouses and family members frequently serve as informal care providers, sometimes to the detriment of their own physical and psychological health (Wood et al., 2019). Structured caregiver assessments, including tools like the Zarit Burden Interview or the Caregiver Strain Index, can identify at-risk individuals (Chen & Hu, 2002; Kühnel et al., 2020). Supportive interventions in this regard, may include caregiver counseling and support groups, education on symptom management, respite care, and home care services (Northouse et al., 2010).

Financial Toxicity and Occupational Disruption

Many patients and families face significant economic burdens, especially in systems where out-of-pocket costs for treatment, transportation, or lost wages are substantial (Iragorri et al., 2021). Financial distress has been independently associated with poorer psychological outcomes and diminished treatment adherence (Boulanger et al., 2022). Health policy reforms and insurance frameworks strongly affect access to psychosocial and palliative care, with high-income regions increasingly integrating supportive services while resource-limited settings face financial and structural barriers. Initiatives such as Medicare's coverage for advance care planning in the United States, the National Health Service's integration of palliative services in the United Kingdom, and national cancer strategies in Canada and parts of Europe have sought to embed psychosocial care as a standard component of oncology. Early engagement with social workers and financial navigators can help address these issues through assistance programs, disability claims, or charitable support.

Cultural and Spiritual Considerations

Cultural beliefs and values shape how patients experience illness, express suffering, and seek support. Cultural competence, the ability to respectfully engage with and respond to patients' cultural perspectives, is a critical skill for all palliative care team members (Monette, 2021). Spiritual well-being has been acknowledged as a protective factor against psychological morbidity in lung cancer patients (Clay et al., 2010).

Bereavement Support

Grief is a natural process, but a subset of individuals may experience prolonged grief disorder or complicated bereavement, characterized by persistent longing, functional impairment, and intense sorrow beyond culturally normative expectations. Considering the potential of unfavorable clinical outcomes in advanced NSCLC patients, palliative care teams should be prepared to provide:

- Pre-loss counseling to prepare families emotionally and practically for the anticipated death.
- Post-loss follow-up to identify individuals at risk and offer grief counseling or referrals.
- Community-based bereavement resources, including support groups and memorial services.

Proactive bereavement support improves family outcomes and reflects a compassionate, longitudinal model of care (Cacciatore et al., 2021).

SUPPORTIVE CARE IN NSCLC-RELATED COMPLICATIONS

Malignant Pleural Effusion

Malignant pleural effusion (MPE) occurs in approximately one in every six patients with advanced NSCLC and often signifies pleural dissemination (Yablonskii et al., 2020). MPE is ipsilateral in the majority of cases, and results from lymphatic obstruction and increased capillary permeability due to neoplastic infiltration, leading to fluid accumulation, lung compression, and dyspnea (Lojo-Rodríguez et al., 2024; Yablonskii et al., 2020). Initial work-up includes imaging and diagnostic thoracentesis to confirm malignant cytology. Pleural fluid analysis should include cytopathology, pH, protein, LDH, and microbiologic cultures. A pH of less than 7.30, increased LDH levels, and decreased glucose concentration in the pleural fluid analysis suggest a malignant etiology underlying the fluid accumulation (Pardessus Otero et al., 2024; Sharma & Boster, 2024).

Thoracentesis is the main therapeutic approach that provides symptomatic relief but may be insufficient for recurrent cases. Indwelling pleural catheters, chemical pleurodesis, pleurectomy, and shunt placement may be considered for recurrent effusions unresponsive to less invasive methods (Aydin et al., 2009).

Superior Vena Cava (SVC) Syndrome

SVC syndrome results from external compression or intraluminal obstruction of the SVC, most frequently by right-sided hilar or mediastinal masses (Gupta et al., 2020). It presents with facial edema, dyspnea, cough, and occasionally neurological symptoms due to cerebral edema (Quencer, 2022). Contrast-enhanced chest computed tomography is the imaging modality of choice. Corticosteroids and head elevation may provide transient symptomatic relief. Endovascular stenting is saved for cases with life-threatening obstruction. Radiation therapy and chemotherapy are considered based on tumor histology and treatment responsiveness (Azizi Abdul et al., 2020).

Spinal Cord Compression

Spinal cord compression often results from vertebral metastases that compromise the structural integrity of the spine and exert direct pressure on the spinal cord. Typically presenting with back pain, motor weakness, sensory deficits, and autonomic dysfunction, the related symptoms may progress rapidly, indicating the necessity of a high suspicion index and prompt diagnostic evaluation (Pope et al., 2018). Magnetic resonance imaging (MRI) is the gold standard for confirming the diagnosis (Singleton & Hefner, 2020). Once identified, immediate administration of high-dose corticosteroids is warranted to reduce vasogenic edema and preserve neurologic function. Definitive treatment is determined by patient's neurological status, prognosis, and extent of systemic disease. In case of reasonable life expectancy and focal disease, surgical decompression followed by radiation therapy has been shown to confer functional superiority against radiotherapy alone (Rades et al., 2022).

Thrombosis and Coagulopathy

NSCLC patients are at an elevated venous thromboembolism risk due to hypercoagulability, immobility, systemic inflammation, and treatment exposures, including the anti-angiogenic agents such as bevacizumab (Hansda & Das, 2025). Low molecular weight heparin is preferred for acute treatment, though direct oral anticoagulants, such as apixaban or rivaroxaban, are increasingly used with caution in high-bleeding-risk patients. Extended anticoagulation for a minimum course of 3 to 6 months is typically indicated, especially in patients with ongoing cancer activity or therapy (Chen et al., 2020; Moik et al., 2022). Risk stratification using clinical tools, such as the Khorana risk score, is recommended to guide decisions regarding prophylactic anticoagulation in high-risk ambulatory patients on systemic therapy (Khorana et al., 2008).

Hypercalcemia

Hypercalcemia of malignancy is a frequent metabolic complication, particularly in cases involving extensive skeletal metastases or paraneoplastic secretion of parathyroid hormone-related peptide (PTHrP) (Vakiti et al., 2018). It may manifest acutely or insidiously, often presenting with nonspecific symptoms, including fatigue, anorexia, nausea, constipation, polyuria, polydipsia, altered mental status, and in severe cases, short QTc intervals, cardiac arrhythmias or coma (Vakiti et al., 2018). The pathophysiology typically involves osteolytic activity from bone metastases, increased renal tubular calcium reabsorption, or ectopic hormonal production (Chakhtoura & El-Hajj Fuleihan, 2021). Diagnosis is confirmed through laboratory evaluation showing elevated serum calcium (corrected for albumin), suppressed parathyroid hormone levels, and often elevated PTHrP in the setting of humoral hypercalcemia. Immediate management involves intravenous isotonic hydration in order to correct volume depletion and promote calciuresis. In moderate to severe hypercalcemia, intravenous bisphosphonates such as zoledronic acid are administered to inhibit osteoclastic bone resorption. The monoclonal antibody denosumab is an effective alternative, particularly in patients with renal insufficiency or refractory hypercalcemia (Chakhtoura & El-Hajj Fuleihan, 2021). Adjunctive measures may include loop diuretics (after rehydration) and calcitonin for rapid but transient calcium reduction (Sinha et al., 2020).

Hematologic Complications

Hematologic complications in advanced NSCLC are diverse and clinically significant, often arising as a direct consequence of bone marrow infiltration, nutritional deficiencies, chronic inflammation, or adverse effects of systemic therapy. Anemia is the most prevalent, contributing to fatigue, dyspnea, and reduced performance status, adversely affecting patients' quality of life Kang et al., (2020). Management strategies include transfusion support and, in selected patients with no curative intent, erythropoiesis-stimulating agents (ESAs), although their use requires careful consideration of thromboembolic risks (Bohlius et al., 2019). Thrombocytopenia, though less common, may result from cytotoxic regimens, marrow replacement, or immune-mediated processes, and can predispose patients to bleeding complications. Platelet transfusions may be necessary in severe or symptomatic cases. Neutropenia, particularly when accompanied by fever, is an oncologic emergency (M. S. Hosseini, 2023). Febrile neutropenia mandates immediate initiation of empiric broad-spectrum antibiotics and may require granulocyte colony-stimulating factor (G-CSF) support, especially in high-risk regimens or recurrent episodes. Prophylactic G-CSF may be required in patients with significant treatment-associated myelosuppression.

Central Nervous System Metastases and Neurological Complications

Central nervous system (CNS) metastases are commonly observed among advanced NSCLC patients, as around 20% of CNS metastases are secondary to NSCLC, especially in molecularly defined subtypes such as EGFR-mutated or ALK-rearranged (Lim & Um, 2018). Clinical features include headaches, seizures, cognitive decline, and focal neurologic deficits. The onset of CNS involvement often signals a significant inflection point in disease trajectory and requires urgent palliative and curative intervention. MRI with contrast is the preferred diagnostic modality, and management strategies depend on the extent of CNS disease, systemic disease burden, and overall prognosis. Corticosteroids are commonly used to reduce peritumoral edema. For patients with limited CNS involvement and good performance status, stereotactic radiosurgery offers local control with reduced neurotoxicity compared to whole-brain radiotherapy, which remains an option for patients with multiple or diffuse lesions (De Pietro et al., 2023). In recent years, CNS-penetrant targeted therapies—such as osimertinib for EGFR-mutant NSCLC or alectinib for ALK-positive disease—have transformed the management of brain metastases, offering durable intracranial responses with favorable tolerability (Weller et al., 2024). Seizure management involves the use of antiepileptic agents, though prophylactic use is generally discouraged in asymptomatic patients (Monsour et al., 2020).

Cutaneous and Mucosal Complications

Cutaneous and mucosal complications are relatively prevalent among this group of patients, especially following the emergence of immunotherapies for NSCLC, and significantly affect their quality of life (Yang et al., 2025). In NSCLC patients, the CTCAE grade 1-2 complications are more prevalent than life-threatening adverse events, and may include various clinical manifestations such as simple rash or bullous pemphigoid (Nelson et al., 2022; Vaez-Gharamaleki et al., 2025). However, these adverse events have been associated with a higher treatment response rate among lung cancer patients. Mild cases do not warrant withholding the systemic anticancer therapies, and could be managed through corticosteroids, topical ointments, antihistamines, and gabapentinoids (Vaez-Gharamaleki et al., 2025).

Salivary gland dysfunction secondary to systemic therapy is a common and clinically challenging patient-reported complication, with the management typically involving symptomatic relief with saliva substitutes and stimulants, topical corticosteroids, proper oral hygiene practices, and muscarinic agonists such as pilocarpine (Hosseini et al., 2024). Patient education, regular assessments, and early intervention are essential in addressing the discomfort and preventing secondary oral infections.

INTEGRATING PALLIATIVE CARE EARLY IN THE DISEASE TRAJECTORY

Integrating palliative care early in managing advanced NSCLC prioritizes patient-centered care from the time of diagnosis. Historically conceptualized as end-of-life care, palliative care is now recognized as a concurrent, patient-oriented strategy that enhances the quality of life, optimizes symptom control, facilitates complex decision-making, and improves both patient and caregiver outcomes when introduced alongside disease-modifying treatments. Due to the high symptom burden of NSCLC from both tumor progression and systemic therapies, rapid functional decline and complex psychosocial challenges are prevalent among these patients. They often face uncertainty regarding prognosis, experience distressing symptoms such as discomfort, dyspnea, and depression, and must navigate difficult therapeutic and goals of care decisions. Early palliative care supports these needs through a multidimensional framework that covers physical, psychological, social, and spiritual domains (Yoong et al., 2013).

Core Components and Models of Early Palliative Care

The early palliative care model is best operationalized through interdisciplinary collaboration and routine, structured consultations. Core components include:

- Comprehensive symptom management: Early intervention proactively addresses acute and chronic symptoms, slowing the functional decline and enhancing treatment adherence.
- Prognostic awareness and advance care planning: Skilled communication about disease trajectory and life expectancy enables patients to make informed choices, establish care preferences, and engage in advance directives. It also helps the families to take time and adjust to the upcoming situations.
- Psychosocial and emotional support: Addressing to anxiety, depression, coping mechanisms, caregiver burden, and existential distress improves emotional well-being.
- Facilitation of care coordination: Integration ensures seamless transitions between settings (including hospital, outpatient, home, and hospice) and enhances continuity of care through collaboration with oncology, primary care, and community resources.

Delivery models vary based on resources and infrastructure. Outpatient palliative care clinics embedded within oncology practices are increasingly favored, offering longitudinal support beginning at diagnosis. Inpatient consultation teams are critical during hospital admissions in addressing acute needs, while home-based and telehealth models extend reach to underserved populations.

Timing and Referral

Although early integration is ideal, real-world practice often falls short due to misperceptions that palliative care equates with treatment cessation or impending death (Flieger et al., 2020). As discussed earlier, clinical guidelines from oncology societies recommend routine palliative care consultation within 8–12 weeks of diagnosis for advanced NSCLC, irrespective of ongoing systemic therapy (Dans et al., 2021; Ferrell et al., 2017).

Benefits to Clinical Outcomes

Early palliative care is correlated with several clinically benefits, including improved quality of life, enhanced satisfaction, reduced anxiety and depression, decreased aggressive end-of-life interventions (such as intensive care unit admissions), higher rates of hospice enrollment, and potential improvement in overall survival (Howie & Peppercorn, 2013; Kochovska et al., 2020; Monnery & Droney, 2024).

Barriers to Implementation

Despite strong evidence, integration is often delayed by logistical, educational, and cultural barriers. Key challenges include limited workforce capacity, insufficient training among oncologists and palliative care providers, stigma surrounding palliative care terminology, and variability in healthcare access (Malhotra et al., 2023; Siler et al., 2018). Addressing these requires systemic efforts such as:

- Interdisciplinary collaboration of different services that manage NSCLC patients, including medical oncology, pulmonology, radiation oncology, and surgery
- Developing scalable models using nurse-led or primary palliative care approaches
- Integrating palliative care into undergraduate and graduate training
- Develop digital health and telemedicine initiatives to expand reach
- Promoting public and professional awareness about the significance of supportive care

MULTIDISCIPLINARY TEAM IN PALLIATIVE CARE

Delivering high-quality palliative care in advanced NSCLC requires a coordinated, interdisciplinary approach that integrates the expertise of healthcare professionals. A multidisciplinary team forms the cornerstone of this model, enabling comprehensive, continuous, and patient-centered care that addresses the needs of both patients and their families. As the complexity of care in advanced NSCLC escalates with disease progression and therapeutic advances, the role of the multidisciplinary team becomes increasingly important in ensuring timely symptom management, holistic support, and alignment of care with individual values and goals.

Core Disciplines and Roles

A well-functioning palliative care multidisciplinary team is composed of professionals with distinct but complementary roles. Effective collaboration and communication among these disciplines ensure that no aspect of patient care is overlooked (Ferrell et al., 2011; Ferrell et al., 2015).

Palliative care physicians provide leadership in symptom assessment and management, facilitate prognostic communication and goals-of-care discussions, and oversee complex medical decision-making, where their clinical judgment guides the timing of care transitions and appropriateness of interventions and patient preferences. Medical or clinical oncologists and pulmonologists are also integral to the team and offer insight into disease-specific treatments and progression, as their coordination with palliative care physicians ensures that disease-modifying therapies are integrated with supportive care strategies to maximize benefit and minimize harm. Oncology and palliative care nurses, including nurse practitioners and clinical nurse specialists, provide frontline care through symptom monitoring, patient education, and psychosocial support, and they often detect early changes in status that necessitate intervention before other palliative care team members. Social workers address the psychosocial and practical dimensions of care, including coping strategies, caregiver support, housing, financial needs, and coordination of community resources, and have a pivotal role in family dynamics, counseling, and discharge planning. Mental health professionals, including psychologists and psychiatrists, assess and manage psychological distress, depression, anxiety, and existential concerns that commonly arise in the context of terminal illness. Spiritual care is an essential yet often under-recognized domain of palliative care, and spiritual care specialists provide culturally sensitive spiritual support and offer comfort in times of uncertainty and grief. Their role is particularly critical in end-of-life settings, where questions of meaning, legacy, and reconciliation often surface. Physical and occupational therapists work to preserve independence, manage fatigue, and support adaptive strategies that promote safety and autonomy in daily living, since functional decline is a prominent challenge in advanced NSCLC. Palliative care pharmacists ensure the safe and effective use of complex medication regimens, manage drug interactions, and provide guidance on opioid titration, adjuvant analgesics, and symptom control agents. Finally, as patients with advanced NSCLC often experience weight loss, anorexia, and cachexia, nutritionists tailor dietary plans to address these challenges, provide counseling on nutritional supplements, and support the management of treatment-related gastrointestinal side effects.

ETHICAL CONSIDERATIONS IN PALLIATIVE CARE FOR NSCLC

Ethical considerations are central to the practice of palliative care. As NSCLC progresses and curative intent recedes, ethical dilemmas frequently arise that challenge clinicians, patients, and families (Ullrich et al., 2020). These may include decisions about the appropriateness of continued disease-directed therapy, withdrawal or withholding of life-sustaining interventions, and navigating disagreements regarding care preferences (Lim, 2016). The ethical practice of palliative care is grounded in four cardinal principles, autonomy, beneficence, non-maleficence, and justice, which draw a framework for navigating morally complex situations in a structured and compassionate manner (Akdeniz et al., 2021). Truth-telling, advance care planning, and transparent goals-of-care conversations are essential to maintaining trust, preparing for clinical deterioration, and ensuring that care remains congruent with patient's values (Ghose et al., 2019; Orstad et al., 2023). Moreover, justice demands equitable access to high-quality palliative care across all populations, addressing disparities in availability and ensuring fairness in the distribution of limited resources. Altogether, an ethically grounded approach to palliative care in NSCLC integrates principled decision-making, cultural sensitivity, and clinical compassion to uphold dignity and support patients and families through disease course.

LIMITATIONS AND CHALLENGES

Despite the growing recognition of palliative care as a critical element of comprehensive oncologic management, several limitations and challenges affect the optimal care delivery for NSCLC patients, including:

Delayed Referral and Underutilization of Palliative Services

Despite strong and encouraging evidence of early palliative care integration benefits, most patients are referred only in late stages of life. This delay results from misconceptions among healthcare providers, patients, and their families that palliative care is equal to end-of-life care, leading to reluctance to initiate discussions early in the disease trajectory (Campaña et al., 2025). Additionally, some oncologists may view palliative care as a sign of therapeutic failure or fear that introducing it could undermine hope (Salins et al., 2024).

Workforce Shortages and Resource Constraints

A significant structural obstacle in palliative care access for NSCLC is the widespread shortage of trained specialists. This workforce limitation is particularly observed in rural or resource-limited settings, where generalist providers are often responsible for managing complex symptoms without adequate training or support. Inadequate funding and infrastructure, including insufficient outpatient palliative care clinics or dedicated inpatient consult teams, further constrain service availability

(Zimmermann et al., 2023). These shortages can result in fragmented care, delays in symptom management, and suboptimal coordination across the continuum of care.

Inadequate Symptom Assessment and Management

Effective symptom control is the main goal of palliative care in NSCLC, yet some patients face underrecognition and undertreatment of common symptoms such as pain, dyspnea, fatigue, and psychological distress. Barriers to optimal symptom management include time constraints during clinic visits, lack of standardized assessment tools, and clinician discomfort with opioid prescribing or the use of psychotropic medications (Nwachukwu et al., 2018). Furthermore, cultural differences in the expression of pain and suffering may result in the underreporting of symptoms, especially among minority populations, thereby compromising equitable care. This issue could be addressed by translating and validating common patient assessment palliative care tools and questionnaires.

Communication Challenges

Effective communication between clinicians, patients, and families is important, yet it is frequently suboptimal in practice. Clinicians may lack the training, confidence, or time to initiate and navigate complex conversations around prognosis, goals of care, and end-of-life preferences. These discussions are often delayed or avoided altogether, leading to care that may not align with patient values or priorities (Oliveira & Medeiros Junior, 2020).

Sociocultural and Health Literacy Barriers

Misunderstandings about the purpose of palliative care, differing beliefs about illness and dying, and mistrust of the healthcare system can lead to resistance or disengagement from palliative services. Low health literacy further complicates informed decision-making, especially when patients must interpret complex medical information about prognosis or treatment trade-offs (Golden et al., 2022).

Systemic and Policy-Level Limitations

At a macro level, systemic and policy-level barriers affect the integration and expansion of palliative care services for NSCLC. These include fragmented reimbursement structures incentivizing procedural interventions over time-intensive supportive care, lack of universal coverage for palliative services, and variability in national policies regarding advance care planning and hospice eligibility (Duckett,

2018; Koczywas et al., 2013). Furthermore, the absence of quality metrics specific to palliative care in oncology impedes efforts to evaluate and improve service delivery. Limited investment in research focused on palliative care outcomes in NSCLC populations, particularly in the context of newer treatments such as immunotherapy, further restricts evidence-based innovation in this field.

FUTURE DIRECTIONS

The future of palliative and supportive care for NSCLC patients lies in early integration, personalization, and system-wide reform. As novel therapies extend survival and alter disease trajectories, palliative care must evolve from a late-stage service to a concurrent, proactive component of oncologic care. Precision approaches using predictive analytics, symptom-monitoring tools, and patient-reported outcomes will enable individualized care tailored to evolving needs. Concurrent palliative care models, delivered alongside disease-modifying treatments, are expected to become the standard—particularly in managing unique symptom burdens associated with immunotherapies and targeted agents. Workforce expansion, through training in primary palliative care skills across oncology disciplines, will be critical in addressing existing specialist shortages. Future efforts must also address inequities in access and quality by designing culturally sensitive, community-based interventions and ensuring care is inclusive of historically underserved populations.

CONCLUSION

Palliative and supportive care play a critical role in the comprehensive management of advanced NSCLC, addressing the complex physical, psychological, social, and spiritual challenges faced by patients and their families. As treatment paradigms evolve, the integration of timely, person-centered palliative care alongside disease-directed therapies has become increasingly important to ensuring the quality of life, enhancing symptom control, and supporting informed decision-making throughout the illness trajectory. Despite existing limitations and systemic barriers, ongoing innovations in care delivery, education, technology, and policy hold promise for a more equitable and effective palliative care framework. Workforce expansion, early integration of palliative care, and the development of interdisciplinary palliative care teams can significantly enhance patient outcomes, improve quality of life, and lower the healthcare costs.

REFERENCES

Akdeniz, M., Yardımcı, B., & Kavukcu, E. (2021). Ethical considerations at the end-of-life care. *SAGE Open Medicine*, *9*, 20503121211000918. DOI: 10.1177/20503121211000918 PMID: 33786182

Andersen, B. L., Valentine, T. R., Lo, S. B., Carbone, D. P., Presley, C. J., & Shields, P. G. (2020). Newly diagnosed patients with advanced non-small cell lung cancer: A clinical description of those with moderate to severe depressive symptoms. *Lung Cancer (Amsterdam, Netherlands)*, *145*, 195–204. DOI: 10.1016/j.lungcan.2019.11.015 PMID: 31806360

Anekar, A. A., Hendrix, J. M., & Cascella, M. (2023). WHO analgesic ladder. In *StatPearls* [Internet]. StatPearls Publishing.

Anghel, T., Melania, B. L., Costea, I., Albai, O., Marinca, A., Levai, C. M., & Hogea, L. M. (2025). Review of Psychological Interventions in Oncology: Current Trends and Future Directions. *Medicina, 61*(2), 279. https://www.mdpi.com/1648-9144/61/2/279

Arrieta, Ó., Angulo, L. P., Núñez-Valencia, C., Dorantes-Gallareta, Y., Macedo, E. O., Martínez-López, D., Alvarado, S., Corona-Cruz, J.-F., & Oñate-Ocaña, L. F. (2013). Association of Depression and Anxiety on Quality of Life, Treatment Adherence, and Prognosis in Patients with Advanced Non-small Cell Lung Cancer. *Annals of Surgical Oncology*, *20*(6), 1941–1948. DOI: 10.1245/s10434-012-2793-5 PMID: 23263699

Avancini, A., Sartori, G., Gkountakos, A., Casali, M., Trestini, I., Tregnago, D., Bria, E., Jones, L. W., Milella, M., Lanza, M., & Pilotto, S. (2020). Physical Activity and Exercise in Lung Cancer Care: Will Promises Be Fulfilled? *The Oncologist*, *25*(3), e555–e569. DOI: 10.1634/theoncologist.2019-0463 PMID: 32162811

Aydin, Y., Turkyilmaz, A., Intepe, Y. S., & Eroglu, A. (2009). Malignant pleural effusions: Appropriate treatment approaches. *The Eurasian Journal of Medicine*, *41*(3), 186–193. PMID: 25610100

Azizi Abdul, H., Shafi, I., Shah, N., Rosenfield, K., Schainfeld, R., Sista, A., & Bashir, R. (2020). Superior Vena Cava Syndrome. *JACC: Cardiovascular Interventions*, *13*(24), 2896–2910. DOI: 10.1016/j.jcin.2020.08.038 PMID: 33357528

Bohlius, J., Bohlke, K., Castelli, R., Djulbegovic, B., Lustberg, M. B., Martino, M., Mountzios, G., Peswani, N., Porter, L., Tanaka, T. N., Trifirò, G., Yang, H., & Lazo-Langner, A. (2019). Management of cancer-associated anemia with erythropoiesis-stimulating agents: ASCO/ASH clinical practice guideline update. *Blood Advances*, *3*(8), 1197–1210. DOI: 10.1182/bloodadvances.2018030387 PMID: 30971397

Boulanger, M., Mitchell, C., Zhong, J., & Hsu, M. (2022). Financial toxicity in lung cancer [Review]. *Frontiers in Oncology, Volume 12 - 2022*. https://doi.org/DOI: 10.3389/fonc.2022.1004102

Cacciatore, J., Thieleman, K., Fretts, R., & Jackson, L. B. (2021). What is good grief support? Exploring the actors and actions in social support after traumatic grief. *PLoS One*, *16*(5), e0252324. DOI: 10.1371/journal.pone.0252324 PMID: 34043716

Campaña, C., Cabieses, B., Obach, A., Vezzani, F., Estay, A., & Carrillo, D. (2025). Barriers to accessing formal cancer care from the perspective of informal caregivers: A qualitative study. *Supportive Care in Cancer*, *33*(5), 400. DOI: 10.1007/s00520-025-09426-5 PMID: 40259032

Caraceni, A., & Shkodra, M. (2019). Cancer Pain Assessment and Classification. *Cancers (Basel)*, *11*(4), 510. https://www.mdpi.com/2072-6694/11/4/510. DOI: 10.3390/cancers11040510 PMID: 30974857

Carnio, S., Di Stefano, R. F., & Novello, S. (2016). Fatigue in lung cancer patients: Symptom burden and management of challenges. *Lung Cancer : Targets and Therapy*, •••, 73–82. DOI: 10.2147/LCTT.S85334 PMID: 28210163

Cella, D. F., Bonomi, A. E., Lloyd, S. R., Tulsky, D. S., Kaplan, E., & Bonomi, P. (1995). Reliability and validity of the Functional Assessment of Cancer Therapy-Lung (FACT-L) quality of life instrument. *Lung Cancer (Amsterdam, Netherlands)*, *12*(3), 199–220. DOI: 10.1016/0169-5002(95)00450-F PMID: 7655830

Chakhtoura, M., & El-Hajj Fuleihan, G. (2021). Treatment of Hypercalcemia of Malignancy. *Endocrinology and Metabolism Clinics of North America*, *50*(4), 781–792. DOI: 10.1016/j.ecl.2021.08.002 PMID: 34774248

Chen, A., Stecker, E., & Warden, A., B. (. (2020). Direct Oral Anticoagulant Use: A Practical Guide to Common Clinical Challenges. *Journal of the American Heart Association*, *9*(13), e017559. DOI: 10.1161/JAHA.120.017559 PMID: 32538234

Chen, M.-L., & Hu, L.-C. (2002). The generalizability of Caregiver Strain Index in family caregivers of cancer patients. *International Journal of Nursing Studies*, *39*(8), 823–829. https://doi.org/https://doi.org/10.1016/S0020-7489(02)00021-4. DOI: 10.1016/S0020-7489(02)00021-4 PMID: 12379300

Clay, K. S., Costellia, T., & Young, K. B. (2010). Exploring Spiritual Well-Being Among Survivors of Colorectal and Lung Cancer. *Social Thought*, *29*(1), 14–32. DOI: 10.1080/15426430903479247 PMID: 20625520

Dans, M., Kutner, J. S., Agarwal, R., Baker, J. N., Bauman, J. R., Beck, A. C., & Dalal, S. (2021). NCCN guidelines® insights: palliative care, version 2.2021: featured updates to the NCCN guidelines. *Journal of the National Comprehensive Cancer Network: JNCCN*, *19*(7), 780–788. DOI: 10.6004/jnccn.2021.0033 PMID: 34340208

de Castro, G. S., Andrade, M. F., Pinto, F. C. S., Faiad, J. Z., & Seelaender, M. (2021). Omega-3 Fatty Acid Supplementation and Its Impact on Systemic Inflammation and Body Weight in Patients With Cancer Cachexia-A Systematic Review and Meta-Analysis. *Frontiers in Nutrition*, *8*, 797513. DOI: 10.3389/fnut.2021.797513 PMID: 35174197

De Pietro, R., Zaccaro, L., Marampon, F., Tini, P., De Felice, F., & Minniti, G. (2023). The evolving role of reirradiation in the management of recurrent brain tumors. *Journal of Neuro-Oncology*, *164*(2), 271–286. DOI: 10.1007/s11060-023-04407-2 PMID: 37624529

Duckett, S. (2018). Aligning policy objectives and payment design in palliative care. *BMC Palliative Care*, *17*(1), 42. DOI: 10.1186/s12904-018-0294-4 PMID: 29514639

Dzierżanowski, T. (2021). Definitions of palliative care–narrative review and new proposal. *Medycyna Paliatywna. Medycyna Paliatywna*, *13*(4), 187–200. DOI: 10.5114/pm.2021.114495

Engel, M., Kars, M. C., Teunissen, S., & van der Heide, A. (2023). Effective communication in palliative care from the perspectives of patients and relatives: A systematic review. *Palliative & Supportive Care*, *21*(5), 890–913. DOI: 10.1017/S1478951523001165 PMID: 37646464

Farbicka, P., & Nowicki, A. (2013). Palliative care in patients with lung cancer. *Contemporary Oncology = Współczesna Onkologia*, *17*(3), 238–245. DOI: 10.5114/wo.2013.35033 PMID: 24596508

Ferrell, B., Koczywas, M., Grannis, F., & Harrington, A. (2011). Palliative care in lung cancer. *Surg Clin North Am, 91*(2), 403-417, ix. https://doi.org/DOI: 10.1016/j.suc.2010.12.003

Ferrell, B., Sun, V., Hurria, A., Cristea, M., Raz, D. J., Kim, J. Y., Reckamp, K., Williams, A. C., Borneman, T., Uman, G., & Koczywas, M. (2015). Interdisciplinary Palliative Care for Patients With Lung Cancer. *Journal of Pain and Symptom Management, 50*(6), 758–767. DOI: 10.1016/j.jpainsymman.2015.07.005 PMID: 26296261

Ferrell, B. R., Temel, J. S., Temin, S., & Smith, T. J. (2017). Integration of Palliative Care Into Standard Oncology Care: ASCO Clinical Practice Guideline Update Summary. *Journal of Oncology Practice / American Society of Clinical Oncology, 13*(2), 119–121. DOI: 10.1200/JOP.2016.017897 PMID: 28972832

Flieger, S. P., Chui, K., & Koch-Weser, S. (2020). Lack of Awareness and Common Misconceptions About Palliative Care Among Adults: Insights from a National Survey. *Journal of General Internal Medicine, 35*(7), 2059–2064. DOI: 10.1007/s11606-020-05730-4 PMID: 32157652

Gershman, E., Guthrie, R., Swiatek, K., & Shojaee, S. (2019). Management of hemoptysis in patients with lung cancer. *Annals of Translational Medicine, 7*(15), 358. DOI: 10.21037/atm.2019.04.91 PMID: 31516904

Ghose, S., Radhakrishnan, V., & Bhattacharya, S. (2019). Ethics of cancer care: Beyond biology and medicine. *Ecancermedicalscience, 13*, 911. DOI: 10.3332/ecancer.2019.911 PMID: 31123494

Givler, A., Bhatt, H., & Maani-Fogelman, P. A. (2018). The importance of cultural competence in pain and palliative care.

Glare, P., Miller, J., Nikolova, T., & Tickoo, R. (2011). Treating nausea and vomiting in palliative care: A review. *Clinical Interventions in Aging, 6*, 243–259. DOI: 10.2147/CIA.S13109 PMID: 21966219

Golden, S. E., Disher, N., Dieckmann, N. F., Eden, K. B., Matlock, D., Vranas, K. C., Slatore, C. G., & Sullivan, D. R. (2022). Show me the roads and give me a road map: Development of a patient conversation tool to improve lung cancer treatment decision-making. *PEC Innovation, 1*, 100094. DOI: 10.1016/j.pecinn.2022.100094 PMID: 37213736

Grassi, L., Caruso, R., Riba, M. B., Lloyd-Williams, M., Kissane, D., Rodin, G., McFarland, D., Campos-Ródenas, R., Zachariae, R., Santini, D., & Ripamonti, C. I. (2023). Anxiety and depression in adult cancer patients: ESMO Clinical Practice Guideline†. *ESMO Open, 8*(2), 101155. https://doi.org/https://doi.org/10.1016/j.esmoop.2023.101155. DOI: 10.1016/j.esmoop.2023.101155 PMID: 37087199

Gupta, A., Kim, D. N., Kalva, S., Reznik, S., & Johnson, D. H. (2020). Superior Vena Cava Syndrome. In *Abeloff's Clinical Oncology* (pp. 775-785. e772). Elsevier.

Hamada, T., Ishikawa, H., Rosenzweig, M. Q., Nishimura, N., Sakakibara-Konishi, J., & Itoh, T. (2024). Feasibility of a nurse-initiated brief cognitive behavioral strategy intervention program for symptom clusters experienced by patients with advanced non-small cell lung cancer. *Asia-Pacific Journal of Oncology Nursing*, *11*(11), 100600. https://doi.org/https://doi.org/10.1016/j.apjon.2024.100600. DOI: 10.1016/j.apjon.2024.100600 PMID: 39655228

Han, K., Yoon, K. W., Kim, J. H., & Kim, G. M. (2019). Bronchial Artery Embolization for Hemoptysis in Primary Lung Cancer: A Retrospective Review of 84 Patients. *Journal of Vascular and Interventional Radiology*, *30*(3), 428–434. DOI: 10.1016/j.jvir.2018.08.022 PMID: 30819488

Hansda, S., & Das, H. (2025). Insights into Cancer-Associated Thrombosis Leading Towards Ischemic Stroke. *Biology (Basel)*, *14*(1), 50. Advance online publication. DOI: 10.3390/biology14010050 PMID: 39857281

He, M., Xu, R., Liu, M., Zhang, Y., Yi, F., Wei, Y., Liu, Q., & Zhang, W. (2021). Use of dexamethasone and a 5-HT3 receptor antagonist with or without aprepitant to prevent chemotherapy-induced nausea and vomiting among patients with lung cancer who are treated with platinum-based chemotherapy: A systematic review and meta-analysis of randomized controlled trials. *Annals of Palliative Medicine*, *10*(4), 4308–4319. https://apm.amegroups.org/article/view/67349. DOI: 10.21037/apm-20-2290 PMID: 33894731

Heregger, R., & Greil, R. (2023). Erythropoiesis-stimulating agents—Benefits and harms in the treatment of anemia in cancer patients. *memo -. Magazine of European Medical Oncology*, *16*(4), 259–262. DOI: 10.1007/s12254-023-00902-4

Hopkinson, J. (2018). Psychosocial Support in Cancer Cachexia Syndrome: The Evidence for Supported Self-Management of Eating Problems during Radiotherapy or Chemotherapy Treatment. *Asia-Pacific Journal of Oncology Nursing*, *5*(4), 358–368. https://doi.org/https://doi.org/10.4103/apjon.apjon_12_18. DOI: 10.4103/apjon.apjon_12_18 PMID: 30271817

Hosseini, M.-S. (2023). Exploring the unseen threat: The neglect of suicide risk in people with cancer. *Nature Mental Health*, *1*(6), 375–376. DOI: 10.1038/s44220-023-00074-4

Hosseini, M. S. (2023). Febrile neutropenia: Clinical approach to a controversial presentation of the COVID-19 era. *Journal of the National Cancer Center*, *3*(4), 251–253. DOI: 10.1016/j.jncc.2023.08.005 PMID: 39036663

Hosseini, M.-S., Sanaie, S., Mahmoodpoor, A., Jabbari Beyrami, S., Jabbari Beyrami, H., Fattahi, S., Jahanshahlou, F., Zarei, M., Rahimi Mamaghani, A., & Kuchaki Rafsanjani, M. (2024). Cancer treatment-related xerostomia: Basics, therapeutics, and future perspectives. *European Journal of Medical Research*, *29*(1), 571. DOI: 10.1186/s40001-024-02167-x PMID: 39614391

Howie, L., & Peppercorn, J. (2013). Early palliative care in cancer treatment: Rationale, evidence and clinical implications. *Therapeutic Advances in Medical Oncology*, *5*(6), 318–323. DOI: 10.1177/1758834013500375 PMID: 24179486

Hui, D., Bohlke, K., Bao, T., Campbell, T. C., Coyne, P. J., Currow, D. C., & Nava, S. (2021). Management of dyspnea in advanced cancer: ASCO guideline. *Journal of Clinical Oncology*, *39*(12), 1389–1411. DOI: 10.1200/JCO.20.03465 PMID: 33617290

Hui, D., & Bruera, E. (2017). The Edmonton Symptom Assessment System 25 Years Later: Past, Present, and Future Developments. *Journal of Pain and Symptom Management*, *53*(3), 630–643. DOI: 10.1016/j.jpainsymman.2016.10.370 PMID: 28042071

Hui, D., & Yennurajalingam, S. (2023). The role of corticosteroids in the palliation of dyspnea in cancer patients: An evidence-based review. *Current Opinion in Supportive and Palliative Care*, *17*(4), 270–276. DOI: 10.1097/SPC.0000000000000677 PMID: 37773042

Iragorri, N., de Oliveira, C., Fitzgerald, N., & Essue, B. (2021). The Out-of-Pocket Cost Burden of Cancer Care-A Systematic Literature Review. *Current Oncology (Toronto, Ont.)*, *28*(2), 1216–1248. DOI: 10.3390/curroncol28020117 PMID: 33804288

Jovanovic, D., Ceriman-Krstic, V., Kabalak, P. A., Viola, L., & Papatheodosiou, K. (2024). Palliative care in lung cancer: Tumour- and treatment-related complications in lung cancer and their management. *Breathe (Sheffield, England)*, *20*(3), 230203. DOI: 10.1183/20734735.0203-2023 PMID: 39534495

Kang, H. S., Shin, A. Y., Yeo, C. D., Park, C. K., Kim, J. S., Kim, J. W., Kim, S. J., Lee, S. H., & Kim, S. K. (2020). Clinical significance of anemia as a prognostic factor in non-small cell lung cancer carcinoma with activating epidermal growth factor receptor mutations. *Journal of Thoracic Disease*, *12*(5), 1895–1902. DOI: 10.21037/jtd-19-3932 PMID: 32642093

Kastelik, J. A. (2013). Management of malignant pleural effusion. *Lung*, *191*(2), 165–175. DOI: 10.1007/s00408-012-9445-1 PMID: 23315213

Khorana, A. A., Kuderer, N. M., Culakova, E., Lyman, G. H., & Francis, C. W. (2008). Development and validation of a predictive model for chemotherapy-associated thrombosis. *Blood*, *111*(10), 4902–4907. DOI: 10.1182/blood-2007-10-116327 PMID: 18216292

Kochovska, S., Ferreira, D. H., Luckett, T., Phillips, J. L., & Currow, D. C. (2020). Earlier multidisciplinary palliative care intervention for people with lung cancer: A systematic review and meta-analysis. *Translational Lung Cancer Research*, *9*(4), 1699–1709. DOI: 10.21037/tlcr.2019.12.18 PMID: 32953543

Koczywas, M., Cristea, M., Thomas, J., McCarty, C., Borneman, T., Del Ferraro, C., Sun, V., Uman, G., & Ferrell, B. (2013). Interdisciplinary palliative care intervention in metastatic non-small-cell lung cancer. *Clinical Lung Cancer*, *14*(6), 736–744. DOI: 10.1016/j.cllc.2013.06.008 PMID: 23871439

Koshimoto, S., Amano, K., Mori, N., Oyamada, S., Arakawa, S., Ishiki, H., Satomi, E., Morita, T., & Takeuchi, T. (2023). Perspectives of registered dietitians and factors associated with their personal accomplishment in the management of cancer cachexia. *Supportive Care in Cancer*, *31*(2), 124. DOI: 10.1007/s00520-023-07593-x PMID: 36662333

Kremer, M., Salvat, E., Muller, A., Yalcin, I., & Barrot, M. (2016). Antidepressants and gabapentinoids in neuropathic pain: Mechanistic insights. *Neuroscience*, *338*, 183–206. DOI: 10.1016/j.neuroscience.2016.06.057 PMID: 27401055

Kühnel, M. B., Ramsenthaler, C., Bausewein, C., Fegg, M., & Hodiamont, F. (2020). Validation of two short versions of the Zarit Burden Interview in the palliative care setting: A questionnaire to assess the burden of informal caregivers. *Supportive Care in Cancer*, *28*(11), 5185–5193. DOI: 10.1007/s00520-019-05288-w PMID: 32060707

Kumar, S. P. (2011). Utilization of brief pain inventory as an assessment tool for pain in patients with cancer: A focused review. *Indian Journal of Palliative Care*, *17*(2), 108–115. DOI: 10.4103/0973-1075.84531 PMID: 21976850

Lim, J. H., & Um, S. W. (2018). The risk factors for brain metastases in patients with non-small cell lung cancer. *Annals of Translational Medicine*, *6*(S1, Suppl 1), S66. DOI: 10.21037/atm.2018.10.27 PMID: 30613641

Lim, R. B. (2016). End-of-life care in patients with advanced lung cancer. *Therapeutic Advances in Respiratory Disease*, *10*(5), 455–467. DOI: 10.1177/1753465816660925 PMID: 27585597

Lojo-Rodríguez, I., Botana-Rial, M., González-Montaos, A., Leiro-Fernández, V., González-Piñeiro, A., Ramos-Hernández, C., & Fernández-Villar, A. (2024). Clinical and Molecular Features of Malignant Pleural Effusion in Non-Small Cell Lung Cancer (NSCLC) of a Caucasian Population. *Medicina, 60*(11), 1804. https://www.mdpi.com/1648-9144/60/11/1804

Mackay, S., Ta, V., Dewez, S., & Körner, A. (2023). Evidence-Based Practice in Psychosocial Oncology from the Perspective of Canadian Service Directors. *Current Oncology (Toronto, Ont.), 30*(4), 3998–4020. DOI: 10.3390/curroncol30040303 PMID: 37185416

Malhotra, S., Christopher, M., Chowdry, R. P., Mossman, B., Cooke, A., Deblieux, J., Simmons, C., Fisher, K., Webb, J., & Hoerger, M. (2023). Barriers, blocks, and barricades: Disparities to access of palliative care in cancer care. *Current Problems in Cancer, 47*(5), 101024. https://doi.org/https://doi.org/10.1016/j.currproblcancer.2023.101024. DOI: 10.1016/j.currproblcancer.2023.101024 PMID: 39492069

Mathews, J., Hannon, B., & Zimmermann, C. (2021). Models of Integration of Specialized Palliative Care with Oncology. *Current Treatment Options in Oncology, 22*(5), 44. DOI: 10.1007/s11864-021-00836-1 PMID: 33830352

McDonnell, K. K., Owens, O. L., & Umari, F. (2023). Mindfulness-Based Interventions for Survivors of Lung Cancer and Their Partners: A Systematic Review. *International Journal of Behavioral Medicine, 30*(5), 616–627. DOI: 10.1007/s12529-022-10132-3 PMID: 36224314

Michopoulos, I., Douzenis, A., Kalkavoura, C., Christodoulou, C., Michalopoulou, P., Kalemi, G., Fineti, K., Patapis, P., Protopapas, K., & Lykouras, L. (2008). Hospital Anxiety and Depression Scale (HADS): Validation in a Greek general hospital sample. *Annals of General Psychiatry, 7*(1), 4. DOI: 10.1186/1744-859X-7-4 PMID: 18325093

Moik, F., Colling, M., Mahé, I., Jara-Palomares, L., Pabinger, I., & Ay, C. (2022). Extended anticoagulation treatment for cancer-associated thrombosis-Rates of recurrence and bleeding beyond 6 months: A systematic review. *Journal of Thrombosis and Haemostasis, 20*(3), 619–634. DOI: 10.1111/jth.15599 PMID: 34816583

Molassiotis, A., Smith, J. A., Mazzone, P., Blackhall, F., Irwin, R. S., Adams, T. M., Altman, K. W., Barker, A. F., Birring, S. S., Blackhall, F., Bolser, D. C., Boulet, L.-P., Braman, S. S., Brightling, C., Callahan-Lyon, P., Canning, B. J., Chang, A. B., Cowley, T., Davenport, P., & Weir, K. (2017). Symptomatic Treatment of Cough Among Adult Patients With Lung Cancer: CHEST Guideline and Expert Panel Report. *Chest, 151*(4), 861–874. DOI: 10.1016/j.chest.2016.12.028 PMID: 28108179

Monette, E. M. (2021). Cultural Considerations in Palliative Care Provision: A Scoping Review of Canadian Literature. *Palliative Medicine Reports, 2*(1), 146–156. DOI: 10.1089/pmr.2020.0124 PMID: 34223514

Monnery, D., & Droney, J. (2024). Early palliative care and its impact on end of life care. *Current Opinion in Supportive and Palliative Care, 18*(4), 230–234. DOI: 10.1097/SPC.0000000000000729 PMID: 39351632

Monsour, M. A., Kelly, P. D., & Chambless, L. B. (2020). Antiepileptic Drugs in the Management of Cerebral Metastases. *Neurosurgery Clinics of North America, 31*(4), 589–601. DOI: 10.1016/j.nec.2020.06.008 PMID: 32921354

Mu, A., Weinberg, E., Moulin, D. E., & Clarke, H. (2017). Pharmacologic management of chronic neuropathic pain: Review of the Canadian Pain Society consensus statement. *Canadian Family Physician Médecin de Famille Canadien, 63*(11), 844–852. PMID: 29138154

National Comprehensive Cancer Network®. *NCCN Guidelines Version 1.2025: Distress Management.* Retrieved April 23 from https://www.nccn.org/docs/default-source/patient-resources/nccn_distress_thermometer.pdf

Nelson, C. A., Singer, S., Chen, T., Puleo, A. E., Lian, C. G., Wei, E. X., Giobbie-Hurder, A., Mostaghimi, A., & LeBoeuf, N. R. (2022). Bullous pemphigoid after anti–programmed death-1 therapy: A retrospective case-control study evaluating impact on tumor response and survival outcomes. *Journal of the American Academy of Dermatology, 87*(6), 1400–1402. https://doi.org/https://doi.org/10.1016/j.jaad.2019.12.068. DOI: 10.1016/j.jaad.2019.12.068 PMID: 31931083

Ni, J., & Zhang, L. (2020). Cancer Cachexia: Definition, Staging, and Emerging Treatments. *Cancer Management and Research, 12*, 5597–5605. DOI: 10.2147/CMAR.S261585 PMID: 32753972

Nikitas, J., Yanagawa, J., Sacks, S., Hui, E. K., Lee, A., Deng, J., & Toste, P. (2024). Pathophysiology and Management of Chest Wall Pain after Surgical and Non-Surgical Local Therapies for Lung Cancer. *JTO Clinical and Research Reports, 5*(7), 100690. DOI: 10.1016/j.jtocrr.2024.100690 PMID: 39077624

Northouse, L. L., Katapodi, M. C., Song, L., Zhang, L., & Mood, D. W. (2010). Interventions with family caregivers of cancer patients: Meta-analysis of randomized trials. *CA: a Cancer Journal for Clinicians, 60*(5), 317–339. DOI: 10.3322/caac.20081 PMID: 20709946

Nwachukwu, C. R., Mudasiru, O., Million, L., Sheth, S., Qamoos, H., Onah, J. O., & Banjo, A. A. (2018). Evaluating barriers and opportunities in delivering high-quality oncology care in a resource-limited setting using a comprehensive needs assessment tool. *Journal of Global Oncology*, *4*(4), 1–9. DOI: 10.1200/JGO.18.00125 PMID: 30532992

O'Donnell, S. B., Nicholson, M. K., & Boland, J. W. (2019). The Association Between Benzodiazepines and Survival in Patients With Cancer: A Systematic Review. *Journal of Pain and Symptom Management*, *57*(5), 999–1008.e1011. DOI: 10.1016/j.jpainsymman.2019.01.010 PMID: 30708126

Oliveira, E. P., & Medeiros, P.Junior. (2020). Palliative care in pulmonary medicine. *Jornal Brasileiro de Pneumologia : Publicaçao Oficial da Sociedade Brasileira de Pneumologia e Tisilogia*, *46*(3), e20190280. DOI: 10.36416/1806-3756/e20190280 PMID: 32638839

Orstad, S., Fløtten, Ø., Madebo, T., Gulbrandsen, P., Strand, R., Lindemark, F., Fluge, S., Tilseth, R. H., & Schaufel, M. A. (2023). "The challenge is the complexity" – A qualitative study about decision-making in advanced lung cancer treatment. *Lung Cancer (Amsterdam, Netherlands)*, *183*, 107312. https://doi.org/https://doi.org/10.1016/j.lungcan.2023.107312. DOI: 10.1016/j.lungcan.2023.107312 PMID: 37481888

Pardessus Otero, A., Rafecas-Codern, A., Porcel, J. M., Serra-Mitjà, P., Ferreiro, L., Botana-Rial, M., Ramos-Hernández, C., Brenes, J. M., Canales, L., Camacho, V., Romero-Romero, B., Trujillo, J. C., Martinez, E., Cases, E., Barba, A., Majem, M., Güell, E., & Pajares, V. (2024). Malignant Pleural Effusion: A Multidisciplinary Approach. *Open Respiratory Archives*, *6*(4), 100349. DOI: 10.1016/j.opresp.2024.100349 PMID: 39091982

Poort, H., Peters, M., Bleijenberg, G., Gielissen, M. F., Goedendorp, M. M., Jacobsen, P., Verhagen, S., & Knoop, H. (2017). Psychosocial interventions for fatigue during cancer treatment with palliative intent. *Cochrane Database of Systematic Reviews*, *7*(7), Cd012030. DOI: 10.1002/14651858.CD012030.pub2 PMID: 28708236

Pope, K., Mandel, C., & Tange, D. (2018). Spinal Cord Compression. In MacLeod, R. D., & Van den Block, L. (Eds.), *Textbook of Palliative Care* (pp. 1–22). Springer International Publishing., DOI: 10.1007/978-3-319-31738-0_72-1

Pornrattanakavee, P., Srichan, T., Seetalarom, K., Saichaemchan, S., Oer-areemitr, N., & Prasongsook, N. (2022). Impact of interprofessional collaborative practice in palliative care on outcomes for advanced cancer inpatients in a resource-limited setting. *BMC Palliative Care*, *21*(1), 229. DOI: 10.1186/s12904-022-01121-0 PMID: 36581913

Quencer, K. B. (2022). Superior Vena Cava Syndrome: Etiologies, Manifestations, and Treatments. *Seminars in Interventional Radiology*, *39*(3), 292–303. DOI: 10.1055/s-0042-1753480 PMID: 36062219

Radchenko, C., Alraiyes, A. H., & Shojaee, S. (2017). A systematic approach to the management of massive hemoptysis. *Journal of Thoracic Disease*, *9*(S10, Suppl 10), S1069–s1086. DOI: 10.21037/jtd.2017.06.41 PMID: 29214066

Rades, D., Küchler, J., Graumüller, L., Abusamha, A., Schild, S. E., & Gliemroth, J. (2022). Radiotherapy with or without Decompressive Surgery for Metastatic Spinal Cord Compression: A Retrospective Matched-Pair Study Including Data from Prospectively Evaluated Patients. *Cancers (Basel)*, *14*(5), 1260. https://www.mdpi.com/2072-6694/14/5/1260. DOI: 10.3390/cancers14051260 PMID: 35267568

Razazi, K., Parrot, A., Khalil, A., Djibre, M., Gounant, V., Assouad, J., Carette, M. F., Fartoukh, M., & Cadranel, J. (2014). Severe haemoptysis in patients with nonsmall cell lung carcinoma. *The European Respiratory Journal*, *45*(3), 756–764. DOI: 10.1183/09031936.00010114 PMID: 25359349

Roeland, E. J., & Dunne, R. F. (2021). The Impact of Early Referrals to Dietitians for Patients With Esophagogastric Cancer. *Journal of the National Comprehensive Cancer Network : JNCCN*, *19*(2), 235–238. DOI: 10.6004/jnccn.2021.7006 PMID: 33545687

Rosa, W. E., Izumi, S., Sullivan, D. R., Lakin, J., Rosenberg, A. R., Creutzfeldt, C. J., & Wallace, C. (2023). Advance care planning in serious illness: A narrative review. *Journal of Pain and Symptom Management*, *65*(1), e63–e78. DOI: 10.1016/j.jpainsymman.2022.08.012 PMID: 36028176

Rudin, C. M., Brambilla, E., Faivre-Finn, C., & Sage, J. (2021). Small-cell lung cancer. *Nature Reviews. Disease Primers*, *7*(1), 3. DOI: 10.1038/s41572-020-00235-0 PMID: 33446664

Ruiz Garcia, V., López-Briz, E., Carbonell Sanchis, R., Gonzalvez Perales, J. L., & Bort-Marti, S. (2013). Megestrol acetate for treatment of anorexia-cachexia syndrome. *Cochrane Database of Systematic Reviews*, *2013*(3), Cd004310. DOI: 10.1002/14651858.CD004310.pub3 PMID: 23543530

Sahebari, M., & Hosseini, M.-S. (2025). RET gene and novel pathways: The role of GDF15/GFRAL/RET axis in cancer cachexia. *Journal of the Formosan Medical Association.* https://doi.org/https://doi.org/10.1016/j.jfma.2025.08.015

Saji, H., Furukawa, K., Tsutsui, H., Tsuboi, M., Ichinose, S., Usuda, J., Ohira, T., & Ikeda, N. (2010). Outcomes of airway stenting for advanced lung cancer with central airway obstruction. *Interactive Cardiovascular and Thoracic Surgery, 11*(4), 425–428. DOI: 10.1510/icvts.2010.238196 PMID: 20656802

Salins, N., Hughes, S., & Preston, N. (2024). Oncologists' palliative care referral behaviour: Testing utility of social exchange theory as an explanatory framework. *BMC Palliative Care, 23*(1), 183. DOI: 10.1186/s12904-024-01517-0 PMID: 39048941

Schellekens, M. P. J., van den Hurk, D. G. M., Prins, J. B., Donders, A. R. T., Molema, J., Dekhuijzen, R., van der Drift, M. A., & Speckens, A. E. M. (2017). Mindfulness-based stress reduction added to care as usual for lung cancer patients and/or their partners: A multicentre randomized controlled trial. *Psycho-Oncology, 26*(12), 2118–2126. https://doi.org/https://doi.org/10.1002/pon.4430. DOI: 10.1002/pon.4430 PMID: 28337821

Sharma, R. (2022). Mapping of global, regional and national incidence, mortality and mortality-to-incidence ratio of lung cancer in 2020 and 2050. *International Journal of Clinical Oncology, 27*(4), 665–675. DOI: 10.1007/s10147-021-02108-2 PMID: 35020103

Sharma, S., & Boster, J. (2024). *Malignant pleural effusion.* StatPearls.

Siler, S., Mamier, I., & Winslow, B. (2018). The Perceived Facilitators and Challenges of Translating a Lung Cancer Palliative Care Intervention Into Community-Based Settings. *Journal of Hospice and Palliative Nursing : JHPN : the Official Journal of the Hospice and Palliative Nurses Association, 20*(4), 407–415. DOI: 10.1097/NJH.0000000000000470 PMID: 30063635

Simmons, C. P., Macleod, N., & Laird, B. J. (2012). Clinical management of pain in advanced lung cancer. *Clinical Medicine Insights. Oncology, 6*, 331–346. DOI: 10.4137/CMO.S8360 PMID: 23115483

Simoff, M. J., Lally, B., Slade, M. G., Goldberg, W. G., Lee, P., Michaud, G. C., . . . Chawla, M. (2013). Symptom Management in Patients With Lung Cancer: Diagnosis and Management of Lung Cancer, 3rd ed: American College of Chest Physicians Evidence-Based Clinical Practice Guidelines. *CHEST, 143*(5), e455S-e497S. https://doi.org/DOI: 10.1378/chest.12-2366

Simon, S. T., Higginson, I. J., Booth, S., Harding, R., Weingärtner, V., & Bausewein, C. (2016). Benzodiazepines for the relief of breathlessness in advanced malignant and non-malignant diseases in adults. *Cochrane Database of Systematic Reviews*, *10*(10), Cd007354. DOI: 10.1002/14651858.CD007354.pub3 PMID: 27764523

Singleton, J. M., & Hefner, M. (2020). Spinal cord compression.

Sinha, S., Tham, K., & Seah, D. S. E. (2020). Hypercalcemia of Malignancy. In MacLeod, R. D., & Van den Block, L. (Eds.), *Textbook of Palliative Care* (pp. 1–19). Springer International Publishing., DOI: 10.1007/978-3-319-31738-0_70-2

Spathis, A., Dhillan, R., Booden, D., Forbes, K., Vrotsou, K., & Fife, K. (2009). Modafinil for the treatment of fatigue in lung cancer: A pilot study. *Palliative Medicine*, *23*(4), 325–331. DOI: 10.1177/0269216309102614 PMID: 19270033

Starr, L. T., Ulrich, C. M., Corey, K. L., & Meghani, S. H. (2019). Associations Among End-of-Life Discussions, Health-Care Utilization, and Costs in Persons With Advanced Cancer: A Systematic Review. *The American Journal of Hospice & Palliative Care*, *36*(10), 913–926. DOI: 10.1177/1049909119848148 PMID: 31072109

Tanaka, K., Akechi, T., Okuyama, T., Nishiwaki, Y., & Uchitomi, Y. (2000). Development and validation of the Cancer Dyspnoea Scale: A multidimensional, brief, self-rating scale. *British Journal of Cancer*, *82*(4), 800–805. DOI: 10.1054/bjoc.1999.1002 PMID: 10732749

Taniguchi, Y., Matsuda, Y., Mori, M., Ito, M., Ikari, T., Tokoro, A., Aiki, S., Hoshino, S., Kiuchi, D., Suzuki, K., Igarashi, Y., Odagiri, T., Oya, K., Kubo, E., & Yamaguchi, T. (2022). Effectiveness and safety of opioids for dyspnea in patients with lung cancer: Secondary analysis of multicenter prospective observational study. *Translational Lung Cancer Research*, *11*(12), 2395–2402. DOI: 10.21037/tlcr-22-512 PMID: 36636410

Temel, J. S., Greer, J. A., Goldberg, S., Vogel, P. D., Sullivan, M., Pirl, W. F., Lynch, T. J., Christiani, D. C., & Smith, M. R. (2009). A structured exercise program for patients with advanced non-small cell lung cancer. *Journal of Thoracic Oncology*, *4*(5), 595–601. DOI: 10.1097/JTO.0b013e31819d18e5 PMID: 19276834

Temel, J. S., Greer, J. A., Muzikansky, A., Gallagher, E. R., Admane, S., Jackson, V. A., Dahlin, C. M., Blinderman, C. D., Jacobsen, J., Pirl, W. F., Billings, J. A., & Lynch, T. J. (2010). Early palliative care for patients with metastatic non-small-cell lung cancer. *The New England Journal of Medicine*, *363*(8), 733–742. DOI: 10.1056/NEJMoa1000678 PMID: 20818875

Ullrich, A., Theochari, M., Bergelt, C., Marx, G., Woellert, K., Bokemeyer, C., & Oechsle, K. (2020). Ethical challenges in family caregivers of patients with advanced cancer – a qualitative study. *BMC Palliative Care*, *19*(1), 70. DOI: 10.1186/s12904-020-00573-6 PMID: 32423444

Uronis, H. E., Currow, D. C., McCrory, D. C., Samsa, G. P., & Abernethy, A. P. (2008). Oxygen for relief of dyspnoea in mildly- or non-hypoxaemic patients with cancer: A systematic review and meta-analysis. *British Journal of Cancer*, *98*(2), 294–299. DOI: 10.1038/sj.bjc.6604161 PMID: 18182991

Vaez-Gharamaleki, Y., Akbarzadeh, M. A., Jadidi-Niaragh, F., Mahmoodpoor, A., Sanaie, S., & Hosseini, M.-S. (2025). Dermatologic toxicities related to cancer immunotherapy. *Toxicology Reports*, *14*, 102021. https://doi.org/https://doi.org/10.1016/j.toxrep.2025.102021. DOI: 10.1016/j.toxrep.2025.102021 PMID: 40271531

Vakiti, A., Anastasopoulou, C., & Mewawalla, P. (2018). Malignancy-related hypercalcemia.

van de Worp, W. R. P. H., Schols, A. M. W. J., Theys, J., van Helvoort, A., & Langen, R. C. J. (2020). Nutritional Interventions in Cancer Cachexia: Evidence and Perspectives From Experimental Models [Review]. *Frontiers in Nutrition, Volume 7 - 2020*. https://doi.org/DOI: 10.3389/fnut.2020.601329

Vehling, S., & Kissane, D. W. (2018). Existential distress in cancer: Alleviating suffering from fundamental loss and change. *Psycho-Oncology*, *27*(11), 2525–2530. https://doi.org/https://doi.org/10.1002/pon.4872. DOI: 10.1002/pon.4872 PMID: 30307088

Von Roenn, J. H., & Brandman, J. F. (2004). End-of-Life Care in Patients with Lung Cancer. In J.-P. Sculier & W. A. Fry (Eds.), *Malignant Tumors of the Lung: Evidence-based Management* (pp. 393-402). Springer Berlin Heidelberg. https://doi.org/DOI: 10.1007/978-3-642-18698-1_36

Wakabayashi, H., Arai, H., & Inui, A. (2021). The regulatory approval of anamorelin for treatment of cachexia in patients with non-small cell lung cancer, gastric cancer, pancreatic cancer, and colorectal cancer in Japan: Facts and numbers. *Journal of Cachexia, Sarcopenia and Muscle*, *12*(1), 14–16. DOI: 10.1002/jcsm.12675 PMID: 33382205

Weller, M., Remon, J., Rieken, S., Vollmuth, P., Ahn, M.-J., Minniti, G., Le Rhun, E., Westphal, M., Brastianos, P. K., Soo, R. A., Kirkpatrick, J. P., Goldberg, S. B., Öhrling, K., Hegi-Johnson, F., & Hendriks, L. E. L. (2024). Central nervous system metastases in advanced non-small cell lung cancer: A review of the therapeutic landscape. *Cancer Treatment Reviews, 130,* 102807. https://doi.org/https://doi.org/10.1016/j.ctrv.2024.102807. DOI: 10.1016/j.ctrv.2024.102807 PMID: 39151281

Wilkin, K., Fang, M. L., & Sixsmith, J. (2024). Implementing advance care planning in palliative and end of life care: A scoping review of community nursing perspectives. *BMC Geriatrics*, *24*(1), 294. DOI: 10.1186/s12877-024-04888-4 PMID: 38549045

Wood, R., Taylor-Stokes, G., Smith, F., & Chaib, C. (2019). The humanistic burden of advanced non-small cell lung cancer (NSCLC) in Europe: A real-world survey linking patient clinical factors to patient and caregiver burden. *Quality of Life Research: An International Journal of Quality of Life Aspects of Treatment, Care and Rehabilitation*, *28*(7), 1849–1861. DOI: 10.1007/s11136-019-02152-6 PMID: 30825160

World Health Organization. (2020). *Palliative care*. Retrieved April 23 from https://www.who.int/news-room/fact-sheets/detail/palliative-care

Yablonskii, P., Nefedov, A., Arseniev, A., Kozak, A., Mortada, M., & Patsyuk, A. (2020). Non-small cell lung cancer, pleural effusion and carcinomatosis: Always a criterion of inoperability? *AME Medical Journal*, *5*, 10. https://amj.amegroups.org/article/view/5426. DOI: 10.21037/amj.2020.02.07

Yang, Z., Luo, Y., Lu, R., Liu, X., Liu, H., Liu, S., Huang, C., Tian, J., & Zhang, L. (2025). Incidence Rates of Cutaneous Immune-Related Adverse Events in Patients with Lung Cancer: A Systematic Review and Meta-Analysis. *Current Oncology (Toronto, Ont.)*, *32*(4), 195. https://www.mdpi.com/1718-7729/32/4/195. DOI: 10.3390/curroncol32040195 PMID: 40277752

Yao, J., Novosel, M., Bellampalli, S., Kapo, J., Joseph, J., & Prsic, E. (2023). Lung cancer supportive care and symptom management. *Hematology/Oncology Clinics, 37*(3), 609-622.

Yoong, J., Park, E. R., Greer, J. A., Jackson, V. A., Gallagher, E. R., Pirl, W. F., Back, A. L., & Temel, J. S. (2013). Early Palliative Care in Advanced Lung Cancer: A Qualitative Study. *JAMA Internal Medicine*, *173*(4), 283–290. DOI: 10.1001/jamainternmed.2013.1874 PMID: 23358690

Yu, Y., Liu, E., Zhou, J., Zhao, Q., Deng, R., Li, Q., & Liu, Y. (2025). The effects of mindfulness meditation combined with happiness therapy on the psychological status and survival of patients with middle and advanced non-small cell lung cancer. *Psycho-oncologie*, *19*(2), 3638. DOI: 10.18282/po3638

Zhang, H., & Garcia, J. M. (2015). Anamorelin hydrochloride for the treatment of cancer-anorexia-cachexia in NSCLC. *Expert Opinion on Pharmacotherapy*, *16*(8), 1245–1253. DOI: 10.1517/14656566.2015.1041500 PMID: 25945893

Zhang, J., Wang, Y., Qi, F., & Zhang, T. (2025). Pulmonary rehabilitation in non–small cell lung cancer: A comprehensive review of perioperative strategies and clinical trends. *Journal of Aging and Rehabilitation*, *2*(1), 3–10. https://journals.lww.com/jagr/fulltext/2025/03000/pulmonary_rehabilitation_in_non_small_cell_lung.2.aspx. DOI: 10.1097/jagr.0000000000000023

Zhang, Y., Cui, G., Xiu, Y., & Zhao, M. (2023). The Effect of Nutritional Support Based on the Dietary Anti-Inflammatory Index on Cancer-Related Fatigue in Lung Cancer Patients Undergoing Chemotherapy. *Cancer Nursing*, *46*(5), 394–404. DOI: 10.1097/NCC.0000000000001124 PMID: 37607375

Zimmermann, C., Buss, M. K., Rabow, M. W., Hannon, B., & Hui, D. (2023). Should Outpatient Palliative Care Clinics in Cancer Centers be Stand Alone or Embedded? *Journal of Pain and Symptom Management*, *65*(2), e165–e170. https://doi.org/https://doi.org/10.1016/j.jpainsymman.2022.11.008. DOI: 10.1016/j.jpainsymman.2022.11.008 PMID: 36437178

ADDITIONAL READING

Allende, S., Turcott, J. G., Verástegui, E., Rodríguez-Mayoral, O., Flores-Estrada, D., Pérez Camargo, D. A., Ramos-Ramírez, M., Martínez-Hernández, J.-N., Oñate-Ocaña, L. F., Pina, P. S., Cardona, A. F., & Arrieta, O. (2024). Early Incorporation to Palliative Care (EPC) in Patients With Advanced Non-Small Cell Lung Cancer: The PACO Randomized Clinical Trial. *The Oncologist*, *29*(10), e1373–e1385. DOI: 10.1093/oncolo/oyae050 PMID: 38558247

Ferrell, B., Koczywas, M., Grannis, F., & Harrington, A. (2011). Palliative care in lung cancer. *The Surgical Clinics of North America*, *91*(2), 403–ix. DOI: 10.1016/j.suc.2010.12.003 PMID: 21419260

Ford, D. W., Koch, K. A., Ray, D. E., & Selecky, P. A. (2013). Palliative and end-of-life care in lung cancer: Diagnosis and management of lung cancer, 3rd ed: American College of Chest Physicians evidence-based clinical practice guidelines. Chest, 143(5 Suppl), e498S–e512S. https://doi.org/DOI: 10.1378/chest.12-2367

Hochberg, U., Elgueta, M. F., & Perez, J. (2017). Interventional Analgesic Management of Lung Cancer Pain. *Frontiers in Oncology*, *7*, 17. DOI: 10.3389/fonc.2017.00017 PMID: 28261561

Jordan, K., Aapro, M., Kaasa, S., Ripamonti, C. I., Scotté, F., Strasser, F., Young, A., Bruera, E., Herrstedt, J., Keefe, D., Laird, B., Walsh, D., Douillard, J. Y., & Cervantes, A. (2018). European Society for Medical Oncology (ESMO) position paper on supportive and palliative care. *Annals of Oncology : Official Journal of the European Society for Medical Oncology*, *29*(1), 36–43. DOI: 10.1093/annonc/mdx757 PMID: 29253069

Kaasa, S., Loge, J. H., Aapro, M., Albreht, T., Anderson, R., Bruera, E., Brunelli, C., Caraceni, A., Cervantes, A., Currow, D. C., Deliens, L., Fallon, M., Gómez-Batiste, X., Grotmol, K. S., Hannon, B., Haugen, D. F., Higginson, I. J., Hjermstad, M. J., Hui, D., & Lundeby, T. (2018). Integration of oncology and palliative care: A Lancet Oncology Commission. *The Lancet. Oncology*, *19*(11), e588–e653. DOI: 10.1016/S1470-2045(18)30415-7 PMID: 30344075

Lindell, K. O., & Danoff, S. K. (Eds.). (2021). *Palliative care in lung disease*. Springer Nature., DOI: 10.1007/978-3-030-81788-6

Shinde, A. M., & Dashti, A. (2016). Palliative Care in Lung Cancer. *Cancer Treatment and Research*, *170*, 225–250. DOI: 10.1007/978-3-319-40389-2_11 PMID: 27535397

Temel, J. S., Greer, J. A., Muzikansky, A., Gallagher, E. R., Admane, S., Jackson, V. A., Dahlin, C. M., Blinderman, C. D., Jacobsen, J., Pirl, W. F., Billings, J. A., & Lynch, T. J. (2010). Early palliative care for patients with metastatic non-small-cell lung cancer. *The New England Journal of Medicine*, *363*(8), 733–742. DOI: 10.1056/NEJMoa1000678 PMID: 20818875

Temel, J. S., Petrillo, L. A., & Greer, J. A. (2022). Patient-Centered Palliative Care for Patients With Advanced Lung Cancer. *Journal of Clinical Oncology*, *40*(6), 626–634. DOI: 10.1200/JCO.21.01710 PMID: 34985932

KEY TERMS AND DEFINITIONS

Advance care planning: A process that enables individuals to define and document their goals, values, and preferences regarding future medical care. Advance care planning includes the completion of advance directives and identification of a healthcare proxy, aiming to ensure care aligns with the patient's wishes if they lose decision-making capacity.

Advanced non-small cell lung cancer: A classification of NSCLC that refers to stage IIIB, IIIC, or IV disease, often characterized by unresectable tumors, distant metastases, or both. At this stage, treatment goals slowly shift toward prolonging survival, managing symptoms, and maintaining function and quality of life.

Breakthrough symptoms: Acute exacerbations of a symptom that occur despite baseline symptom control.

Common Terminology Criteria for Adverse Events: CTCAE is a standardized classification and grading system developed by the U.S. National Cancer Institute (NCI) for reporting adverse events in clinical trials and oncology practice.

Financial toxicity: The adverse economic impact of cancer diagnosis and treatment on patients and their families, which may include direct costs (such as medications, transportation, and copayments), indirect costs (such as lost income and caregiver burden), and psychological distress related to financial strain.

Multidisciplinary team: A collaborative group of healthcare professionals from various disciplines, including medicine, nursing, social work, psychology, spiritual care, and rehabilitation, who deliver coordinated and inclusive palliative care based on each patient's needs.

Palliative care: A specialized, interdisciplinary approach to medical care that focuses on improving the quality of life for patients with serious illnesses. In the context of advanced NSCLC, it includes symptom management, psychosocial support, spiritual care, and assistance with complex decision-making, irrespective of prognosis or ongoing disease-modifying treatment.

Patient-centered care: A care approach that respects and responds to individual patient preferences, needs, values, and goals, ensuring that these guide all clinical decisions. In palliative oncology, patient-centered care emphasizes shared decision-making, open communication, and cultural sensitivity, enhancing trust and satisfaction while aligning treatment plans with what matters most to the patient and their family.

Symptom burden: The cumulative impact of multiple physical and psychological symptoms experienced by a patient, often measured using validated tools such as the Edmonton Symptom Assessment System (ESAS). High symptom burden is common in advanced NSCLC and significantly affects quality of life and functional status.

Total pain: A holistic concept introduced by the palliative care pioneer Dame Cicely Saunders that encompasses physical, psychological, social, and spiritual dimensions of pain.

Transitional care: Structured services and supports provided during the transition from hospital to home or hospice. Effective transitional care minimizes readmissions, ensures continuity of care, and facilitates communication across settings.

World Health Organization analgesic ladder: A framework developed by WHO in 1986 for the stepwise management of cancer-related pain. It consists of a three-step ladder: (1) non-opioid analgesics (such as acetaminophen and NSAIDs) for mild pain, (2) weak opioids (such as codeine and tramadol) for moderate pain, and (3) strong opioids (such as morphine and fentanyl) for severe pain.

Chapter 12

Advancements in the Diagnosis and Therapeutics for Non-Small Cell Lung Carcinoma (NSCLC): From Genetic Mutations to Public Health Perspectives

Vivek Pazhamalai
https://orcid.org/0000-0003-2088-7545
Department of Bio Engineering, School of Engineering, Vels Institute of Science, Technology, and Advanced Studies, India

S. Subha Lakshmi
https://orcid.org/0009-0000-2308-185X
Department of Bio Engineering, School of Engineering, Vels Institute of Science, Technology, and Advanced Studies, India

E. Sreeram
https://orcid.org/0009-0001-7797-6824
Department of Bio Engineering, School of Engineering, Vels Institute of Science, Technology, and Advanced Studies, India

S. S. Meenambiga
https://orcid.org/0000-0002-5445-525X
Department of Bio Engineering, School of Engineering, Vels Institute of Science, Technology, and Advanced Studies, India

P. Nimshi
Department of Bio Engineering, School of Engineering, Vels Institute of Science, Technology, and Advanced Studies, India

S. Ivo Romauld
https://orcid.org/0000-0003-0610-0646
Department of Bio Engineering, School of Engineering, Vels Institute of Science, Technology, and Advanced Studies, India

DOI: 10.4018/979-8-3373-2096-0.ch012

R. Chandrasekaran

Department of Bio Engineering, School of Engineering, Vels Institute of Science, Technology, and Advanced Studies, India

ABSTRACT

Lung cancer, particularly non-small cell lung carcinoma (NSCLC), poses significant challenges in oncology. Accounting for approximately 85% of lung cancer-related deaths, NSCLC's aggressive nature demands comprehensive management strategies. Environmental factors like smoking and air pollution, alongside genetic mutations in genes such as EGFR, KRAS, and ALK, contribute to its development. Recent advancements in diagnostic modalities, including low-dose CT scans and molecular profiling, facilitate early detection. Treatment paradigms have evolved to incorporate multimodal approaches, encompassing surgery, radiotherapy, chemotherapy, targeted therapies, and immunotherapy. Collaboration among healthcare professionals is crucial for effective patient care. As research continues to unfold, novel therapeutic strategies and personalized medicine approaches hold promise for improving outcomes in NSCLC patients.

1. INTRODUCTION

Approximately 85% of lung cancer cases globally are attributed to non-small cell lung cancer, or NSCLC for short. And even with new treatments and advances in early detection, it is still a leading cause of cancer death. Hence, it is a very harmful factor for health. Adenocarcinoma, large cell melanoma, and small cell melanoma are the three main types of NSCLC. Their varied reactions lead to the development of different varieties and require an array of treatments. Globally, about 1.8 million NSCLC cases are diagnosed annually. Table 1: Respiratory rates per 1,000 persons by region. Men have the highest rates (33 per 100,000 people) in Asia, while women have the lowest rates. Smoking habits, genetics, environmental toxins, access to healthcare, and other factors influence these differences. In addition, even though the number of smokers has decreased since 2000, the number of cases of NSCLC has increased, indicating how challenging this complaint is to combat (Graph 1). This chapter combines recent research with current medical practices to provide a comprehensive understanding of NSCLC. It investigates the underlying causes of inheritable changes, discovers novel diagnostic techniques, and develops superior treatments to improve patient care and outcomes. The tables and maps' data emphasize the necessity of subtype- and area-specific actions to address this global health issue (Alduais et al., 2023; Ganti et al., 2021; Rodak et al., 2021; Laguna et al., 2024; Lin et al., 2024; Qin et al., 2025; Rakaee et al., 2025).

Figure 1. Types of NSCLC

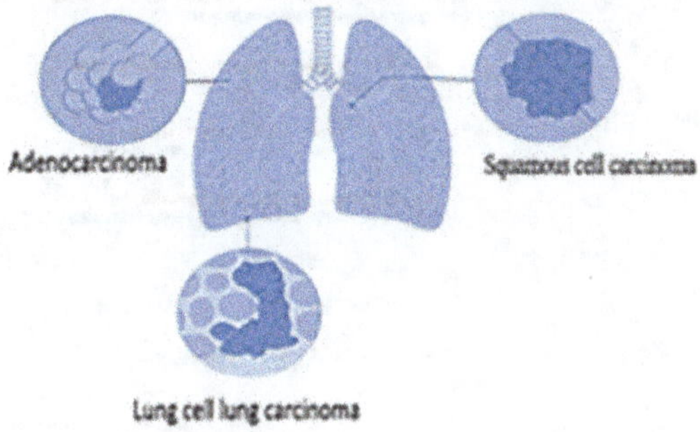

Table 1. NSCLC prevalence rates by region

Region	Prevalence Rate (per 100,000 people)
Asia	33 (Males), 14 (Females)
North America	31.9 (Males), 16.2 (Females)
Europe	28.1 (Males), 22.0 (Females)
South America	14.6 (Males), 11.7 (Females)
Africa	5.8 (Males), 3.2 (Females)
Australia	30.1 (Males), 28.5 (Females)

Figure 2. Smoking rates vs. NSCLC incidence

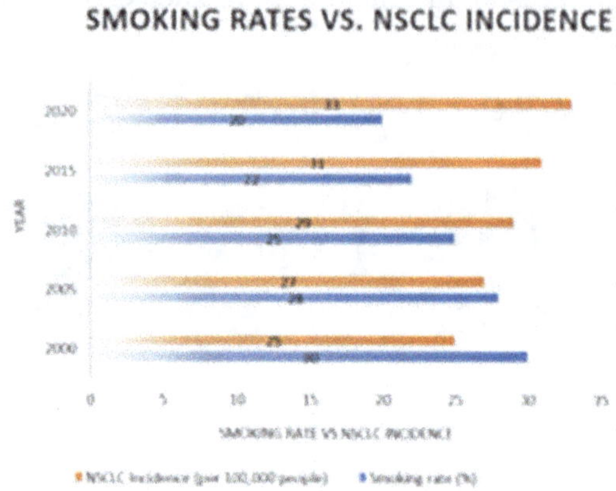

2. TUMOR MICROENVIRONMENT AND IMMUNE EVASION IN NSCLC

2.1 Role of the Tumor Microenvironment (TME)

i. Tumor Microenvironment (TME)

The tumor microenvironment, or TME, consists of numerous elements that support and suppress tumor growth and metastasis. Examples include ECM, signaling molecules (chemokines, growth factors, and cytokines), stroma (fibroblasts and endothelial cells), susceptible cells (T cells, macrophages, dendritic cells, and natural killer (NK) cells), and tumor cells. But behind the unsightly growth, cancer cells that can infiltrate neighbouring tissues and metastasize to distant sites form the ugly core of the excrescence, while stromal cells offer structural and functional support. Cancer can try to kill immune cells or demoralize them to bolster its own growth. Tissues are supported by the extracellular matrix (ECM), and interactions between these factors are facilitated by signaling molecules (Bożyk et al., 2022). The TME is necessary for excrescence growth, irruption, and metastasis because it alters vulnerable responses, alters the gravidity of cancer cells, and creates a protective environment for excrescence cells to thrive in. The stromal cells' influence, the modulation of vulnerable cells, and signaling pathways like those of CD8 T cells, dendritic cells, cancer-associated fibroblasts (CAFs), PD-L1, VEGF, and exosomes are highlighted in Figure 3.

Figure 3. Diagram of the tumor microenvironment

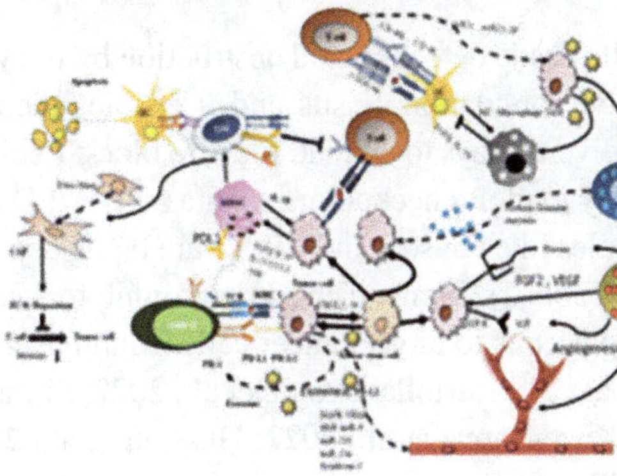

ii. Cellular and Non-Cellular Components of the Tumor Microenvironment

The assemblage of cellular and non-cellular elements that shapes fundamental processes during tumor progression and metastasis is known as the tumor microenvironment (TME). Cellular factors: Cancer-Associated Fibroblasts (CAFs) secrete growth-promoting factors, restructure the extracellular matrix (ECM) and activate angiogenesis, which stimulates cancer cell development, invasion, and spread (Bożyk et al., 2022; Farc et al., 2021; Escobedo-Calvario, A., et al., 2022). CAFs communicate with cancer cells to inject dynamic components to the TME through direct cell-cell contact and through a process called signaling patch stashing. Have either attack cancer — immune T cells, macrophages, dendritic cells, and NK cells — cells can either be reprogrammed to support tumor growth and suppress immune responses that target tumors (Tiwari et al., 2022; Li et al., 2024). The excrescence's growth and metastasis are aided by the formation of new blood vessels by endothelial cells, which grease angiogenesis. MSCs proliferate into different types of cells and modify the extracellular matrix (ECM), as well as sequester factors that promote tumor development and metastasis (Naser et al., 2022; Desai et al., 2025; El-Tanani et al., 2024). In the TME, Extracellular Matrix (ECM), a kind of proteins and glycoproteins, facilitates cell signaling and regulates cell gestation while serving as a structural support. Moreover, cancer cell metabolic reprogramming, characterized by processes such as the Warburg Effect and miscellaneous lipid metabolism, promotes rapid cell division, energy production, and adaptation to stress, and in turn contributes to (Balta et al., 2021; Bagaev et al., 2021; Baghy et al., 2023; Kundu et al., 2024; Li et al., 2023; Dzobo et al., 2023; Xie et al., 2023; Chen et al., 2022; Sadhukhan et al., 2023; Shin et al., 2022; Raju et al., 2022).

2.2 Mechanisms of Immune Evasion

The way cancer cells evade detection and destruction by the vulnerable system loses an immune evasive foundation or sits and it enables them to flourish and spread. And there are several ways to do that. First, to block T cell-mediated attack against cancer cells, they exploit checkpoints such as PD-1/PD-L1 and CTLA-4. New checkpoint molecules like Pause 3 and TIM-3 are being considered for cancer treatment (as shown in Table 2). Immune checkpoint inhibitors can block these relationships, reactivating T cells to target cancer cells.(Malinga et al., 2022; Ziogas et al., 2023; Mimura et al., 2021; Mollavelioglu et al., 2022; Shiravand et al., 2022; Catalano et al., 2022; Kuzevanova et al., 2022; Hussain et al., 2024; El Halabi et al., 2021; Jin et al., 2023).

Table 2. Immune Checkpoints

Checkpoint	Ligand	Function in Immune Evasion	Targeted Therapy (Status)
PD-1	PD-L1/ PD-L2	Inhibits T cell activation, promotes T cell exhaustion	Nivolumab, Pembrolizumab (FDA-approved)
CTLA-4	B7-1/B7-2	Inhibits early T cell priming	Ipilimumab (FDA-approved)
TIM-3	Galectin-9	Suppresses Th1 responses, promotes T cell dysfunction	Clinical trials ongoing
LAG-3	MHC Class II	Limits T cell proliferation and cytokine production	Clinical trials ongoing
TIGIT	CD155	Suppresses NK and T cell cytotoxicity	Clinical trials ongoing

Second, malignant cells store molecules with immune suppression, including cytokines (TGF-β and IL-10, for example) and enzymes (IDO, for example), that inhibit successful cell activity and generate a milieu permissive to evolution (see Table 3). (Abdul-Rahman et al., 2024; Accogli et al., 2021; Lopresti et al., 2024; Khalaf et al., 2021; Soleimani Mamalo et al., 2025).

Table 3. Secretion of Immunosuppressive Molecules

Secretion of Immunosuppressive Molecules	Description
Cytokines (e.g., TGF-β, IL-10)	Suppresses immune cell activity and promotes an immunosuppressive environment.
Enzymes like IDO	IDO depletes tryptophan, which is essential for T cell function, suppressing immune responses.
Prostaglandin E2 (PGE2)	Promotes immune cell suppression, supports regulatory T cell expansion, and enhances angiogenesis.
Adenosine	Accumulates in the TME and binds to A2A receptors on immune cells, leading to suppression of cytotoxic T cell activity.

Third, they slow the elimination of immunosuppressive cells such as regulatory T cells (Tregs), myeloid-derived suppressor cells (MDSCs), and Tumor-associated macrophages (TAMs), that promote excrescence growth and an immune susceptible response (Table 4). (Li et al., 2022; Pietrobon & Marincola, 2021; Qureshi et al., 2021).

Table 4. Immunosuppressive Cells

Immunosuppressive Cells	Function
Regulatory T Cells (Tregs)	suppress killer T cells, creating a calm and restrained immune system.
Myeloid-Derived Suppressor Cells (MDSCs)	Dampen T cell activity and encourage tumor growth with cytokines and enzymes.
Tumor-Associated Macrophages (TAMs)	Encourage the growth of tumors, the formation of new blood vessels (angiogenesis), and immune suppression.

Ultimately, they then mutate major histocompatibility complex (MHC) molecules and downregulate antigen presentation, rendering the already vulnerable system less capable of recognizing and attacking cancer cells. (Dhatchinamoorthy et al., 2021; Yang et al., 2023; Jhunjhunwala et al., 2021; Algarra et al., 2021) Combined, these mechanisms allow cancer cells to avoid the vulnerable system and play a role in the growth of excrescences.

2.3 Implications for Therapy

Targeting the tumor microenvironment (TME) includes creative methods for increasing the efficiency of standard treatments. TME-targeted curatives can be mentioned, such as anti-angiogenic agents (e.g., bevacizumab) and ECM modifiers (e.g., hyaluronidase), which respectively aim to inhibit angiogenesis and ECM formation in the pro-tumorigenic TME in the tumor progression (Huang et al.,

2022). They consist of binding to cancer-associated fibroblasts (CAFs), modifying the extracellular matrix (ECM), and blocking pro-tumorigenic signaling pathways (Ma et al., 2023). Immunotherapy strategies have reinvigorated the cancer-resistant system to a great extent. Immune checkpoint inhibitors activate T cells to attack cancer cells, targeting PD-1, PD-L1, and CTLA-4 checkpoints (Wang et al., 2023). Oncolytic viruses (OV), either in line or reconstituted through lyophilized injection, are designed to infect and kill bacterial cells directly, all the while stimulating a vulnerable response to exosome-specific antigens. (Ghafouri-Fard et al., 2022) Auto T cell therapy involves re-engineering a patient's T cells to express excellent antigen receptors that target specific excrescence antigens, resulting in direct cancer cell elimination (Hou et al., 2022). It is possible to overcome resistance and increase treatment efficacy by combining immunotherapy with conventional therapies like chemotherapy, radiation, and targeted curatives (Sun et al., 2023). These combination curatives work the strengths of different modalities to achieve synergistic goods and address multiple mechanisms of resistance. relating and exercising biomarkers like PD-L1 expression, exome mutational burden (TMB), and other molecular signatures help guide treatment decisions. biomarkers play a crucial role in predicting and covering responses to immunotherapy (Dong et al., 2022). For illustration, PD-L1 expression situations can inform the use of PD-1/PD-L1 inhibitors, while TMB may prognosticate response to vulnerable checkpoint inhibitors (Zhao et al., 2022). Cancer treatment still faces obstacles and limitations, such as treatment resistance, patient response variability, and the need for better biomarkers. Understanding the TME and vulnerable evasion mechanisms shown in Table 5, coming up with new treatments, and solving patient problems with backed drugs are the primary focuses of ongoing research. The objectives of these studies are to address the issues that exist right now, illustrated in Figure 4, and open the way for more efficient cancer treatments in the future (Zhang et al., 2023).

Table 5. Immune Evasion Mechanisms

Immune Evasion Mechanism	Description
Immune Checkpoint Inhibition	Cancer cells upregulate inhibitory molecules like PD-L1 to suppress T-cell activity.
Secretion of Immunosuppressive Cytokines	Tumor cells release factors such as TGF-β and IL-10 to inhibit immune responses.
Tumor-Induced Immune Cell Dysfunction	Tumors can alter the function of immune cells, leading to reduced anti-tumor activity.
Recruitment of Regulatory T Cells (Tregs)	Tumors attract Tregs that suppress the activity of other immune cells.

continued on following page

Table 5. Continued

Immune Evasion Mechanism	Description
Alteration of Antigen Presentation	Tumor cells can downregulate antigen-presenting molecules, making them less recognizable to T cells.
Expression of Immune Checkpoints	Tumor cells express molecules like CTLA-4 to inhibit immune cell activation and proliferation.
Metabolic Competition	Tumor cells consume nutrients and produce waste products, creating an inhospitable environment for immune cells.
Induction of Immune Cell Apoptosis	Tumor cells can induce apoptosis (programmed cell death) in immune cells through various mechanisms.

Figure 4. Immune Response Vs. Tumor Progression

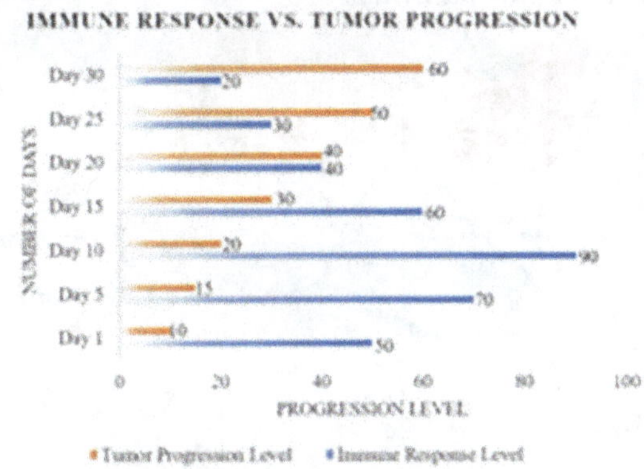

3. GENETIC MUTATIONS AND MOLECULAR SUBTYPES OF NSCLC

3.1 Genetic Mutations in NSCLC

1. Genetic research has changed drastically as a result of inheritable exploration. Treatment of Non-Small Cell Lung Cancer Genes such as EGFR, KRAS, ALK, ROS1, and BRAF drives cancer, illustrated in Figure 5 (NSCLC molecular pathways). Select the appropriate treatment. Take the novel TKI-otinib and its many indications in EGFR-mutated NSCLC. These medicines block dangerous signals to treat cases (Lei et al., 2022). And two ALK inhibitors, crizotinib and alectinib, benefit some patients with ALK mutations (Passaro et al., 2021). This problem was significantly addressed with the introduction of newer KRAS

G12C inhibitors (e.g., Sotorasib) (;;)They treat mutations that were previously difficult to treat. Alternatively, new targeted therapies that target the PD-1/PD-L1 pathways have transformed the medical treatment of the condition, extending some cases to long-term remission (Tan et al., 2022). Improved liquid necropsies that test for ctDNA in the complaint give crooks the ability to monitor the effectiveness of the treatment in real time and provide a more precise diagnosis of the problem (Pop-Bica et al., 2022). Croakers must overcome drug resistance to extend the lives of NSCLC patients. Gene specialists, medical experimenters, and laboratory scientists continue to collaborate in the creation of new medicines and the integration of various treatments (Liu et al., 2025).

Figure 5. NSCLC molecular pathways

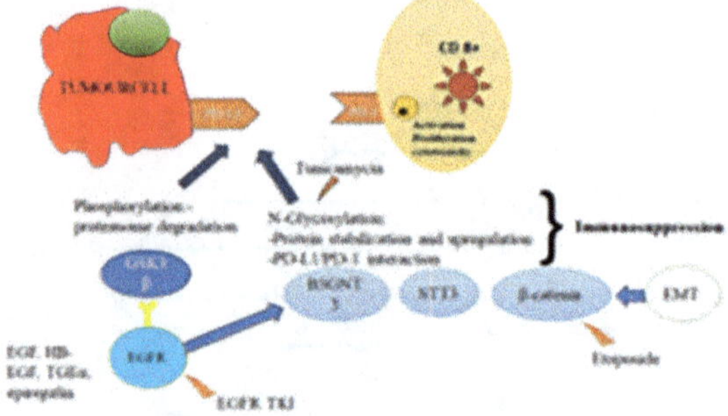

3.2 Clinical Relevance of Genetic Mutations in NSCLC

These tailored approaches have led to the discovery of several targetable mutations in non-small-cell lung cancer (NSCLC), including mutations affecting EGFR, TP53, KRAS, MET, ALK, ROS1, and BRAF.(Koenig et al., 2021; Pruis, 2021) Erlotinib, Gefitinib, and Osimertinib are highly effective for those with EGFR mutations, found in 10–15% of NSCLC patients (eg, adenocarcinoma, especially in Asian women and nonsmokers) (Tada et al., 2022; Tsuboi et al., 2023), but resistance mutations (eg, T790M) will undermine any future combination therapy efforts. (Blaquier et al., 2023). Recent development of treatment options for TP53 mutations, which have an impact on proteins that prevent excretion (Canale et al., 2022). Both of these treatments have negative side effects. Specifics like sotorasib have improved the prognosis for KRAS mutations, which occur in 25 to 30 cases, primarily in smokers; however, the prognosis is still not as good as it is for EGFR or ALK mutations (Koenig et al., 2021). Capmatinib and other inhibitors are being developed to treat cancer and poor health in order to investigate MET mutations that have been linked to aggressive diseases (Koenig et al., 2021). Specific treatments like sotorasib have shown promise for KRAS mutations, which affect approximately 25 to 30 cases, most of which are smokers; however, the prognosis is still not as good as it is for EGFR or ALK mutations (Koenig et al., 2021). Medicines like Crizotinib, Alectinib, and Lorlatinib, which improve survival and quality of life, have seen transformative success with ALK mutations, which are found in 3 to 5 cases (mostly in young, nonsmoking cases) (Fabbri et al., 2023). Capmatinib and other inhibitors are being developed to study MET mutations, which have been linked to aggressive cancers and poor health (Koenig et al., 2021). Besides, targeted curatives such as Dabrafenib and Trametinib are superior in the survival index than conventional chemotherapies for ROS1 mutations, which appear in about one to two cases (predominantly, young nonsmokers) (Dziadziuszko et al., 2021; Fabbri et al., 2023). It's a good disease to have if you have to have one — eventually, crizotinib and entrectinib work well to treat BRAF mutations, seen in one to three cases in smokers and nonsmokers alike (Koenig et al., 2021; Dziadziuszko et al., 2021). The importance of these treatments substantiates the need for ongoing exploration of resistance mechanisms and evidence-based treatment to mitigate the long-term problems posed by NSCLC cases (Yue et al., 2025; Diaz-Jimenez et al., 2024; Oya et al., 2025; Yuan et al., 2024).

3.3 Future Directions and Recent Findings:

Key inheritable mutations EGFR, KRAS, ALK, ROS1, and BRAF that have transformed non-small cell lung cancer (NSCLC) treatment via evidence-based cures have been identified by scientists (Koenig et al., 2021). Tyrosine kinase inhibitors (TKIs) such as Erlotinib, Gefitinib, and Osimertinib specifically target EGFR mutations, thus improving patient outcomes significantly, whereas medications such as Crizotinib and Alectinib have changed the landscape of care for ALK mutations (Herrera-Juárez et al., 2023). The case has been buoyed by the launch of the advanced KRAS G12C asset, Sotorasib, which has offered a new stopgap of sorts in the management of preliminarily recalcitrant cases, and by immunotherapies that target PD-1/PD-L1 pathways still yield durable outcomes (Rodak et al., 2021). Innovations such as liquid autopsies for real-time excrescence shadowing of DNA, oncolytic contagion curatives, and Auto-T cell treatments have an amazing potential to propel cancer treatment (Pezzuto et al., 2023). Continued imaging technologies and the growing cooperation between experimenters, oncologists, and inventors of specifics in medicine enhance the energy evolution that leads to the discovery of new specifics and adjusted curatives based on inheritable biographies (Pan et al., 2021). This heuristic matrix type, which appears in the NSCLC Inherited Mutations Overview table, emphasizes the high influence of targeted treatments aimed at increasing NSCLC patients' quality of life and survival rates (Karagiannakos et al., 2022; Dan et al., 2024; Cognigni et al., 2022; Parvaresh et al., 2024; Gemelli et al., 2024)

Table 6. NSCLC Inheritable Mutations

Mutation	Prevalence (%)	Population	Prognosis	Therapies	References
EGFR	10–15	Non-smokers, Asian women	Improved with TKIs	Erlotinib, Gefitinib, Osimertinib	Koenig et al. (2021); Pezzuto et al. (2023a)
KRAS	25–30	Smokers	Challenging but improving	Sotorasib (KRAS G12C)	Rodak et al. (2021); Pan et al. (2021)
MET	~5	Aggressive cases	Poor prognosis	MET inhibitors in development	Karagiannakos et al. (2022); Dan et al. (2024)
ALK	3–5	Younger, nonsmokers	Favorable with targeted therapies	Crizotinib, Alectinib, Lorlatinib	Cognigni et al. (2022); Parvaresh et al. (2024)
ROS1	1–2	Younger, nonsmokers	Positive with targeted therapies	Crizotinib, Entrectinib	Herrera-Juárez et al. (2023); Rodak et al. (2021)
BRAF	1–3	Smokers, nonsmokers	Improved with BRAF inhibitors	Dabrafenib, Trametinib	Gemelli et al. (2024)

Other mutations:

Infrequently heritable mutations like MET amplifications, RET rearrangements, and HER2 mutations indicate non-small cell lung cancer (NSCLC), paving the way for largely adapted treatments. MET amplifications, for illustration, constantly reduce the efficacy of EGFR inhibitors but can be managed with MET blockers like Capmatinib (Lee et al., 2024; Dagogo-Jack et al., 2023). Also, RET rearrangements, seen in 1 – 2 of NSCLC cases, are effectively treated with targeted antidotes analogous to Selpercatinib and Pralsetinib, offering an expedient for better outcomes (Ali et al., 2022; Syed et al., 2022; Russo et al., 2024; Novello et al., 2023). Advanced treatments like fam-trastuzumab deruxtecan-nxki and ado-trastuzumab emtansine are effective, even though HER2 mutations disrupt cell signaling and proliferation in two to four instances (Olmedo et al., 2022; Lo et al., 2023; Clark et al., 2023). These mutations and their treatments are epitomized in Table 7, Rare heritable Mutations in NSCLC, which highlights their frequency, impact, and the targeted antidotes used (Ghosh et al., 2024; LoPiccolo et al., 2024).

Table 7. Rare Genetic Mutations in NSCLC

Mutation Type	Prevalence in NSCLC	Impact	Targeted Therapy (Examples)	References
MET Amplifications	Associated with resistance to EGFR inhibitors	Continuous activation of the MET pathway	Capmatinib	Lee et al. (2024); Dagogo-Jack et al. (2023)
RET Rearrangements	1–2% of cases	Production of abnormal proteins driving cancer progression	Selpercatinib, Pralsetinib	Ali et al. (2022); Syed (2022); Russo et al. (2024); Novello et al. (2023)
HER2 Mutations	2–4% of cases	Abnormal cell signaling and proliferation	Fam-trastuzumab deruxtecan-nxki, Ado-trastuzumab emtansine	Olmedo et al. (2022); Lo & Lindeman (2023); Clark et al. (2023); Ghosh et al. (2024); LoPiccolo et al. (2024)

3.4 Molecular Subtypes

Treatment plans are heavily influenced by the molecular subtypes of NSCLC, such as adenocarcinoma, gauged cell carcinoma, large cell carcinoma, and mixed-lineage excrescences. Adenocarcinoma, which accounts for roughly 40% of cases, is presently among nonsmokers and responds effectively to targeted therapies, chemotherapy, and immunotherapy (Sen et al., 2024). On the other hand, scaled cell melanoma, explosively linked to smoking and comprising 30% of cases, frequently requires chemotherapy and radiation but generally presents a poorer outlook (Wang et al., 2025). Large cell melanoma, seen in 15 of NSCLC cases, is aggressive and inadequately discerned, challenging individualized approaches that combine targeted and vulnerable curatives (Grilli, 2022; Friedlaender et al., 2024). Incipiently, mixed-lineage excrescences, characterized by features of multiple subtypes, demand acclimatized treatments grounded on their dominant molecular profile (Munteanu et al., 2023; Sulewska et al., 2023). These subtype details are epitomized in Table 8, Molecular Subtypes of NSCLC, which outlines the frequency, characteristics, and treatment strategies for each subtype (Meira, 2023; Wunderlich et al., 2024; Winge et al., 2023; Stanganelli et al., 2022; Sun et al., 2022; Palma et al., 2022; Hyytiäinen et al., 2023; De Jong et al., 2022; Zhu et al., 2024; Koroulakis & Agarwal, 2024).

Table 8. Molecular Subtypes of NSCLC

Subtype	Prevalence (%)	Characteristics	Treatment Strategies	References
Adenocarcinoma	~40	Most common; occurs in both smokers and non-smokers	Targeted therapies, chemotherapy, and immunotherapy	Sen et al. (2024); Friedlaender et al. (2024); Munteanu et al. (2023)
Squamous cell carcinoma	~30	Linked to smoking, it arises in the central airways	Chemotherapy, radiation therapy, and targeted therapies	Wang et al. (2025); Stanganelli et al. (2022); Sun et al. (2022)
Large cell carcinoma	~15	Poorly differentiated; aggressive	Chemotherapy, targeted therapies, and immunotherapy	Sulewska et al. (2023); Palma et al. (2022); De Jong et al. (2022)
Mixed-lineage tumor cells	Varies	Features of multiple subtypes	Treatment based on predominant subtype: chemotherapy, targeted therapies, and immunotherapy	Wunderlich et al. (2024); Winge et al. (2023); Koroulakis & Agarwal (2024)

3.5 Immune Subtypes

Immunological subtypes of non-small cell lung cancer (NSCLC) are separable by molecular entities and infiltration of susceptible cells. Immunotherapy works whenever the lesion has lots of vulnerable cells, when it improves the body's ability to find and count cancer cells (Lei et al., 2022). NOTE: PD-L1 expression and Tumor Mutational Burden (TMB) are both good predictors of treatment efficacy because tumors that have high PD-L1 expression or TMB are typically responsive to susceptible checkpoint inhibitors (Xie et al., 2024; Mamdani et al., 2022; Xing et al., 2022). Table 9 Immunological subtypes of NSCLC, their significance as prognostic factors, and the biomarkers associated with them are presented in Subtypes of NSCLC (Yang et al., 2022; Iglesias-Escudero et al., 2023; Taefehshokr et al., 2022).

Table 9. Immunological Subtypes of NSCLC

Subtype	Definition and Characteristics	Prognostic Significance and Response	Biomarkers	References
Immune Infiltration and Molecular Clustering	Presence of immune cells within the tumor and specific molecular traits	High immune infiltration leads to better immunotherapy responses	PD-L1 expression, Tumor Mutational Burden (TMB)	Lei et al. (2022); Xie et al. (2024); Mamdani et al. (2022)
Prognostic Significance and Response to Immunotherapy	Tumors with high immune infiltration tend to respond better to immunotherapy	Improved outcomes with high immune infiltration	PD-L1 expression, TMB	Xing et al. (2022); Yang et al. (2022); Iglesias-Escudero et al. (2023)
Biomarkers for Predicting Outcomes	Biomarkers such as PD-L1 expression and TMB guide immunotherapy decisions	Better response with high PD-L1 and TMB	PD-L1 expression, TMB	Taefehshokr et al. (2022)

3.6 Prognostic and Predictive Biomarkers

Biomarkers are useful tools for understanding and treating conditions because they give pivotal insight into the progression of complaints and the applicable course of action. Regardless of the treatment, prognostic biomarkers prognosticate the likely course of a condition, such as the likelihood of rushing or overall survival (Tarighati et al., 2023). Predictive biomarkers, on the other hand, help in determining which treatments are most applicable for a given circumstance, ensuring that treatments are acclimatized to the case's condition (Zhang et al., 2023). These natural pointers empower croakers to customize care, relating cases that admit targeted antidotes that meliorate issues, extend survival, and avoid gratuitous or potentially dangerous treatments (Al-Tashi et al., 2023). Personalized medicine is revolutionized by directly relating and using these biomarkers, paving the way for more effective and supported case care (Li et al., 2022; Li et al., 2022; Zhang et al., 2023; Ding et al., 2022; Rosellini et al., 2023; Veyssière et al., 2022; Cao et al., 2022; Su et al., 2023; Győrffy, 2023; Iida et al., 2022).

4 ADVANCED DIAGNOSTIC APPROACHES IN NSCLC

Advanced imaging methods must help in portraying the anatomy of the body organs and their functionality, and also need to detect diseases like non-small cell lung cancer (NSCLC). CT, PET, and MRI are three of the most commonly used imaging modalities; each has its underlying principles, advantages, and drawbacks. CT scans use X-rays to create and generate their slice-by-slice output, the true 3D image of the body. CT scans are a vital part of many medical specialties, including emergency medicine, cardiology, and oncology, as they are very good at early detection of internal bleeding, tumors, and fractures. CT scans are not just fast, mundane, and cheap, but are also going to be a source of radiation exposure for patients and, therefore, are less effective at visualizing soft tissues. Contrast dyes are also uncomfortable for patients with renal disease. PET scans use radioactive tracers, such as fluorodeoxyglucose (FDG), to mark the cellular metabolism of the areas involved. PET is discovered to provide the best optimal outcomes in the diagnosis of brain diseases such as Alzheimer's, cancer diagnosis, tracking cancer growth, and heart disease diagnosis (Nooreldeen et al., 2021; Jin et al., 2023).

Although PET scans may be most useful for cancer detection, they are labor-intensive, difficult to locate, and low in radiation. The heart, brain, joints, and other soft parts of the body are depicted with superior picture quality and detail in MRI scans, which use a strong magnetic field and radio waves. MRIs are needed more for 3D imaging of ligaments and tissues, brain tumors, and scars of multiple sclerosis. MRIs aren't ionizing, but they are much more expensive, take a lot of time, and aren't good for people with heart devices or metal implants, as shown in Table 10, the features of CT, PET, and MRI like imaging modalities (Tan et al., 2025; Pradhan et al., 2023).

Table 10. The features of imaging modalities

Feature	CT (Computed Tomography)	PET (Positron Emission Tomography)	MRI (Magnetic Resonance Imaging)	References
Principle	Separating components based on differential partitioning between stationary and mobile phases, analyzed using computational methods.	Detecting gamma rays from positron annihilation to create detailed images of metabolic activity.	Hydrogen nuclei emit signals when exposed to a strong magnetic field and radiofrequency pulses, producing detailed images.	Rolfo et al. (2021); Abdayem & Planchard (2021); Tomasik et al. (2023)
Best For	Detecting bone fractures, tumors, and internal bleeding.	Assessing metabolic activity, cancer detection, heart disease, and brain disorders.	Imaging soft tissues, brain, spinal cord, and joints.	Qi et al. (2025); Di Capua et al. (2021); Cucchiara et al. (2021)
Radiation	Yes	Yes	No	Smolle et al. (2021); Jin et al. (2023); Nooreldeen & Bach (2021)

continued on following page

Table 10. Continued

Feature	CT (Computed Tomography)	PET (Positron Emission Tomography)	MRI (Magnetic Resonance Imaging)	References
Procedure Time	5-30 minutes	30-60 minutes	15-90 minutes	Malapelle et al. (2021); Ning et al. (2021); Bazhenova et al. (2021)
Contrast Agent	Sometimes required	Required	Sometimes required	Guo et al. (2022); Gandhi et al. (2023); Huang et al. (2023)
Cost	Moderate	High	High	Sharma et al. (2022); Qi et al. (2021); Spira et al. (2021)
Availability	Widely available	Less widely available	Widely available	Pisapia et al. (2022); Liu et al. (2021); Rodrigues et al. (2022)

Advancements in diagnostic technologies have been on the incremental side that resulting in an increase in accuracy over time. The visual representation has been carefully done according to this change, where CT scans have been consistently on the rise, making them the best in anatomical imaging, PET scans have been the first in functional imaging, and MRIs still have the best imaging ability in soft tissue. These methods together are a must for medical professionals to diagnose a situation properly and in the most accurate way that is possible.

Despite having all those imaging technologies, the fact still stands that the new diagnosis of NSCLC was revolutionized by liquid biopsies and molecular profiling. Molecular profiling, which is the analysis of changes in the DNA, RNA, and proteins of cells, is commonly done with methods such as WGS and RNA-Seq. The cross-referencing of the most efficient targetable cancer-causing mutations (for example, EGFR, KRAS, and BRAF) can assist medical professionals in the formulation of a more individualized therapy plan (Spira et al., 2021; Bazhenova et al., 2021). To name one, the identification of cancer cells in blood (CTCs) and circulating tumor DNA (ctDNA) may be carried out through a liquid biopsy, which is a less invasive and more patient-friendly procedure than the conventional body fluid testing, like blood and plasma. The use of ddPCR and NGS, among other methods, can be a potential tool to constantly survey patients and hence have a better chance of providing the necessary treatments while at the same time drastically lowering the number of cancer-causing mutations to the level of sensitivity that is safe for the patients (Rolfo et al., 2021; Tomasik et al., 2023; Qi et al., 2025).

This combination shows that the processes above are an important part of the progress that has been made in NSCLC detection. While, at the same time, they also give us the confidence of more precision, enhanced patient care, and the continued development in the medical field, as shown in Figure 6 (Cucchiara et al., 2021; Malapelle et al., 2021; Liu et al., 2021).

Figure 6. Diagnostic accuracy over time

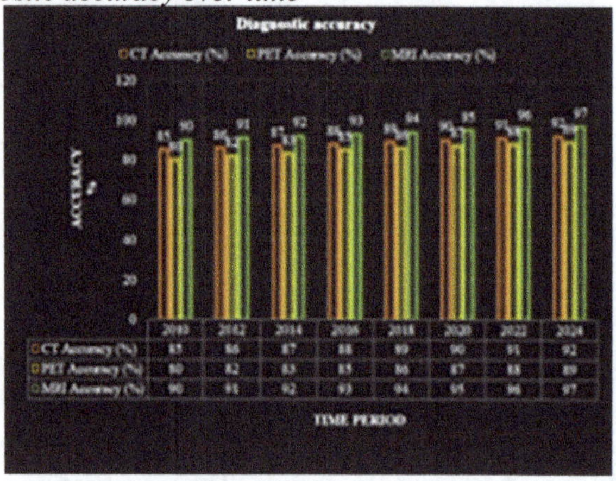

5 SYSTEMIC THERAPIES FOR NSCLC: CHEMOTHERAPY, TARGETED THERAPY, AND IMMUNOTHERAPY

The largest number of cases was set up to be non-small cell lung cancer (NSCLC), which accounts for around 85% of all lung cancers. In late-stage cancers with metastatic diseases, treatment mainly involves the use of drugs falling under the classes of systemic therapy for NSCLC. They can all be taken as immunotherapy, targeted therapy, or cytotoxic chemotherapy. With efficacy and actions being variable, their differences compose each one specific to the specialty of the respective tumor are shown in Table 14& 15 and survival rate variation between therapy is graphically illustrated in Figure 9 (Massafra et al., 2021; Godoy et al., 2023; Lahiri et al., 2023).

5.1 Chemotherapy Mechanisms

Chemotherapy has been used to differentiate some forms of non-small cell lung cancer, or NSCLC. Chemotherapy, on the other hand, causes problems because it affects both cancerous and healthy cells within its range during treatment. This non-selectivity generally results in other side effects, including myelosuppression, nausea, and neuropathy in tumors with particular driver mutations, restricting the overall effect and patient tolerance. As revealed in the following table, the action mechanisms of some reputable chemotherapy agents- Cisplatin, Pemetrexed, Paclitaxel, and Etoposide- are different and attach to cancer cells in their own special way. All these drugs attack specific weaknesses to stop the tumor from growing while killing the cells. The mechanisms of action for the major chemotherapy categories, discussed in Table 11 (Ying et al., 2024; Li et al., 2024; Wang et al., 2024; Xi et al., 2025; Huang et al., 2024; Sito et al., 2024).

i. Platinum-Based Doublet Therapy (Cisplatin)

Chemotherapy places chemical bonds-intrastrand and interstrand cross-links-at DNA-targeted cancer cells. Those bonds cause the deformities in the original structure, which don't let the strands separate in two vital processes for the growth and function of cells-transcription and replication, therefore, don't let the cell develop. The majority of damaged cells trigger a repair process; however, the weight of damage exceeds the capability of these processes and leads to cell cycle arrest and apoptosis (inducement of programmed cell death). The action of cisplatin, which is useful in NSCLC tumors, targets the dividing cells for attack. As shown in the table, this treatment prevents tumor growth through DNA cross-links and the death of cancer cells (Umar et al., 2024; Zou et al., 2024; Lee et al., 2024; Sito et al., 2024; Xi et al., 2025; Wang et al., 2024).

ii. Pemetrexed antimetabolites

Several folate-requiring enzymes involved in the synthesis of DNA and RNA intermediates utilized by the proliferating cancer cells are inhibited by this class of anticancer drugs. In particular, the targets for this drug are thymidylate synthase for the thymidine synthesis, dihydrofolate reductase to sustain folate pool for other generation of DNA precursors, glycinamide ribonucleotide formyl transferase; so upon interference, Pemetrexed could readily stop the S cell cycle, which is utilized for the replication of DNA, leading to cell death. It does a good job of fighting the various subtypes of non-squamous NSCLC, which rely a lot on this kind of metabolic activity to grow faster. Pemetrexed performs one of these interferences in nucleotide synthesis, which will essentially affect tumor survival, as shown in this table (Nardin et al., 2024; Hendriks et al., 2024; Molinaro et al., 2024; Heymach et al., 2025; Nagy et al., 2024).

iii. Taxanes (Paclitaxel)

Paclitaxel involves the cell microtubule structure in the target cells, where the microtubules generate resistance, rigidity, and help in chromosome separation during mitosis (cell division). The mitotic spindles are very effective stabilizers of microtubules because they induce mitotic arrest when paclitaxel is added to the cultures. This causes a metaphase arrest of the cell when paclitaxel stabilizes the microtubules within the spindle. When this checkpoint is prolonged, it results in what is called mitotic catastrophe, which is a cell death mechanism where the divisions go wrong. This artificiality of formation during mitosis uses paclitaxel to kill extensively dividing cancer cells most effectively. - As highlighted in the table, paclitaxel's therapeutic action was ascribed to the stabilization of microtubules and cellular propagation processes within cancer cells (Díaz et al., 2024).

iv. Topoisomerase Inhibitors (Etoposide)

This chemotherapeutic drug works by inhibiting topoisomerase II, an enzyme that resolves DNA supercoiling during transcription and replication. Etoposide stabilizes the intermediate enzyme-DNA complex that prevents DNA strands from religating, causing the cell to accumulate DNA breaks (Jang et al., 2025). The cumulative effect of these breaks affects the replication and transcription processes in the cell. This initiates apoptotic pathways because neither damage repair nor replication can continue (Huang et al., 2024). Etoposide selectively kills cancer cells that are rapidly dividing and that need a functional DNA repair mechanism for survival. In the table, etoposide's therapeutic action involves the disruption of DNA and killing cancer cells by blocking topoisomerase II (Özkaya Gül et al., 2025).

Table 11. Mechanism of action of chemotherapeutic agents

Chemotherapeutic Category	Agents	Mechanism of Action	References
Platinum-Based Doublet Therapy	Cisplatin	Causes DNA cross-links, inducing apoptosis.	Umar et al. (2024); Sito et al. (2024); Zou et al. (2024)
Antimetabolites	Pemetrexed	Inhibits folate-requiring enzymes, disrupting DNA synthesis (effective in non-squamous NSCLC).	Nardin et al. (2024); Hendriks et al. (2024); Molinaro et al. (2024)
Taxanes	Paclitaxel	Stabilizes microtubules, blocking cell division and causing mitotic catastrophe.	Lahiri et al. (2023); Xi et al. (2025); Huang et al. (2024)
Topoisomerase Inhibitors	Etoposide	Inhibits topoisomerase II, preventing DNA repair and replication.	Jang et al. (2025); Huang et al. (2024); Özkaya Gül et al. (2025)

5.2 Targeted Therapy

Targeted therapies are highly specific drug treatments that block one molecular abnormality in cancer cells to promote their growth and spread. This method of treating NSCLC is a refined therapy. The mechanism of targeted therapy is illustrated in Figure 7. Targeted therapy for cancer cells blocks specific signals, whereas chemotherapy is cytotoxic to proliferating cells. As a result, the treatment is expected to have a more specific effect and fewer potentially harmful side effects (Mina et al., 2025). Nearly all of the targeted therapy drugs are oral agents, providing a convenient way for patients to self-treat. Utilizing cancer-targeting medications with minimal off-target toxicity in genetically determined subgroups that the various mutations should reflect within cells is the best way to achieve the best results (Mina et al., 2025). Targeted treatments are, nonetheless, constrained by several limitations such as limited distribution geographically in some areas, treatment costs being prohibitive, occurrence of mutations leading to resistance (Zhao et al., 2024), and overall poor response rate of 20-30% among patients, prompting the necessity for additional research in this area (Mina et al., 2025). The modes of action of major classes of targeted treatment, such as EGFR inhibitors, ALK inhibitors, ROS1 inhibitors, MET inhibitors, and KRAS inhibitors, are described in Table 12.

1. EGFR inhibitors

The inhibition of EGFR with its inhibitors smothers the essential signals needed for the growth of cancer cells and leading to their proliferation. Consequently, these cancer cells ultimately die, and there is no mechanism for them to reproduce any further (Hawash, 2024; Wang et al., 2024). This is the most targeted approach toward types with cancer-potential possessing EGFR mutations (since these mutations are the actual growth inhibitors among the tumor bulk). For instance, if you unplug a light source that doesn't have a cord to plug in, so it doesn't have any energy, just like mutant types' work is likely cut short.

2. ALK Inhibitors

Anaplastic lymphoma kinase (ALK) proteins inhibit the cell-to-cell communication that contributes to the spread of cancer cells. EML4-ALK and other ALK fusion proteins aid in the growth and development of cancer cells. At the same time, ALK inhibitors stop these processes from passing and make it harder for the Interference with the means of communication among the cancer cells greatly stunts their growth, compared to severing the connection of the cancer cells from the network by turning off a Wi-Fi router .

3. ROS1 Inhibitors

The ROS1 inhibitors are designed to disrupt ROS1 gene rearrangement that leads to uncontrollable growth of cancer cells. The cessation of tumor growth by these compounds has prevented or even reversed cancer development (Stanzione et al., 2023; Desilets et al., 2025; Zhao et al., 2024). This approach is aimed at tumors with ROS1 rearrangement, inflicting minimal damage on surrounding normal cells. Picture a road that gets closed to cancer cells, so their passage gets wary and the disease fails to spread.

4. MET Inhibitors

Mutations in the MET gene lead to abnormal, uncontrolled growth of cancer cells, and so-called MET inhibitors aim to address these mutations. By inhibiting MET exon 14 skipping mutations, the drugs bring the equilibrium back to the situation, therefore restraining tumor growth and keeping the cancer in check (Dong et al., 2022; Rosas et al., 2024). It is then that the MET inhibitors directly reverse the aberrant signaling pathways initiated by these mutations and shine. Imagine going and repairing a jammed thermostat: that act prevents the room (or cancer cells) from overheating and getting out of control.

5. KRAS Inhibitors

The mutations in the KRAS gene disrupt normal function, acting like a stuck accelerator that pushes cancer cell growth and tumor formation forward. As a result, KRAS inhibitors slow down this acceleration, effectively stopping the cancer cells' uncontrolled growth (Skoulidis et al., 2021; Singhal et al., 2024). Because it targets only the KRAS G12C mutation, this new class of drugs represents a paradigm shift in how tumors along this pathway have been treated. If one applies the brakes to a speeding car, it would come to a halt. The car won't move, and the cancer cells will die if the brakes work.

Table 12. Targeted Therapy Mechanism

Drug Category	Agents	Target/Mechanism	References
EGFR Inhibitors	Erlotinib, Gefitinib, Osimertinib	Block mutations in EGFR, shutting down growth signals	Hawash, (2024);Wang et al., (2024); Rosas et al. (2024)
ALK Inhibitors	Crizotinib, Alectinib, Lorlatinib	Inhibit ALK fusion proteins (e.g., EML4-ALK)	Tao et al., (2022); Rosas et al. (2024); Mina et al. (2025)
ROS1 Inhibitors	Crizotinib, Entrectinib	Target ROS1 gene rearrangements	Stanzione et al., (2023) ; Desilets et al. (2025); Zhao et al. (2024)
MET Inhibitors	Capmatinib, Tepotinib	Block MET exon 14 skipping mutations	Dong et al., (2022); Rosas et al. (2024); Adamopoulos et al. (2024)
KRAS Inhibitors	Sotorasib	Target KRAS G12C mutation, halting accelerated growth	Skoulidis et al. (2021); Singhal et al. (2024); Wang et al. (2025)

Figure 7. Mechanism of targeted therapy

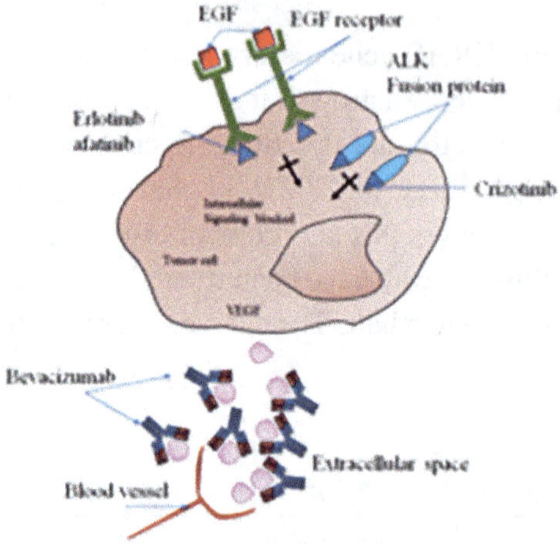

5.3 Immunotherapy

Immunotherapy is the most recent treatment for non-small cell lung cancer, into which the immune-checkpoint stimulators essentially mobilize the quality of the human immune system from delusions, letting it identify and finally engulf the cancer cells. Immunotherapy strikes pathways that are usually exploited by malignant tumors to escape the immune defense—and hence the T-cells, considered to be the warriors of the immune system, aiming to attack the tumors (Cheng et al., 2024). Therefore, in most cases, adjuvant treatments in advanced and early stages of NSCLC treatment are most beneficial to patients with PD-1-positive tumors, with expression greater than 50 percent. The therapy is usually given first alone or in combination with chemotherapy in cases of low-level PD-L1 expression. Some of the advantages include long-standing therapeutic effects, probably being the cause of remissions; comparatively lower systemic toxicity than chemotherapy, and efficacy against most subtypes of NSCLC. However, challenges remain: 20-30 patient efficacy at times shows adverse effects in the form of immune-related toxicities such as colitis, pneumonitis, and endocrinopathies; it is very costly and not widely available (Zhao et al., 2025). Almost all the common immunotherapies are PD-1, PD-L1, and CTLA-4 inhibitors, with their mechanisms of action discussed in Table 13 and illustrated below in Figure 8 (Sharma et al., 2024).

i. PD-1 Inhibitors

The mechanism of action of PD-1 inhibitors is binding to the PD-1 receptor that is expressed by cancer cells to evade immunity. PD-1 serves as a 'shield' and prevents T-cells from the immune system soldiers from recognizing and killing cancer cells. Such drugs act to prevent PD-1, just like taking down that protective shield and exposing the cancer cells to their immunological attackers. The prompt release of this 'shield' will activate the action of T-cells to fight against the cancer cells and restore immunity toward tumor growth. PD-1 inhibitors are highly effective in treating patients with lung cancers that carry marked expression of PD-L1, a related protein (Shen et al., 2024).

ii. PD-L1 Inhibitors

PD-L1 inhibitors intercept a tumor-promoting signaling pathway that is restively expressed by malignant cells-many times. PD-L1 acts as a “disguise” that enables the cancer cells to escape detection from T-cells. These drugs strip the disguise by blocking the activity of PD-L1, allowing the immune system to now view the cancer and destroy it. Once the immune cells identify the cancer, this knowledge broadens and deepens their ability to prosecute the sustained massacre of the tumor (Zabeti Touchaei & Vahidi, 2024). PD-L1 inhibitors work best for patients who have tumors positive for high expression of PD-L1 and represent a powerful arm against cancer evasion mechanisms by bolstering the immune response (Habib, 2024).

iii. CTLA-4 Inhibitors

CTLA-4 blockade releases some brakes on the operation of the immune system. By blocking T-cell activation, CTLA-4 prevents these immune cells from getting overexcited in their reactions. But cancer cells have put a loop in this system, whereby they can manipulate T-cells so that they can no longer become potent against these relentless enemies. Ipilimumab inhibits CTLA-4, making the brakes dysfunctional, thus enabling T-cells to act in full force. Therefore, under these circumstances of optimal strength from T-cells, the latter can unleash an attack against that cancer cell, which ultimately destroys it (Wang, Cheng et al., 2024). CTLA-4 inhibitors are also generally employed together with other therapies, such that victory over NSCLC may ensue with all forces on high gear (Wang, Liu et al., 2024).

Table 13. Common Immunotherapeutic Agents

Inhibitor Type	Agents	Mechanism of Action	References
Programmed Death-1 (PD-1)	Pembrolizumab, Nivolumab	Inhibit PD-1, reactivating T-cell function against cancer cells	Cheng et al. (2024); Zhao et al. (2025); Shen et al. (2024)
Programmed Death-Ligand 1 (PD-L1)	Atezolizumab, Durvalumab	Inhibit PD-L1, preventing tumor immune evasion	Sharma et al. (2024); Zabeti Touchaei & Vahidi (2024); Wang et al. (2024)
CTLA-4 Inhibitors	Ipilimumab	Enhance T-cell priming and activation, boosting the immune response	Habib et al. (2024); Yadav et al. (2024); Ruan et al. (2024)

Figure 8. Mechanism of immunotherapy

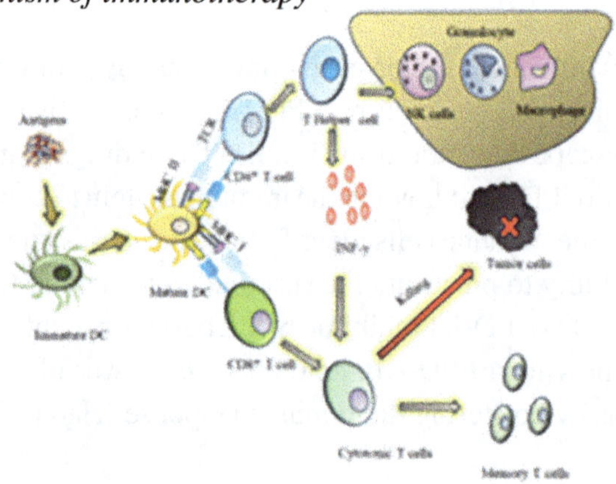

Table 14. outcomes vs therapy types

Treatment Type	Outcomes
Chemotherapy	Effective across various cancer types; significant side effects due to non-selectivity; used as a standard treatment for many cancers.
Targeted Therapy	High specificity for cancer cells; fewer side effects; effectiveness depends on genetic mutations; used for cancers with specific biomarkers.
Immunotherapy	Durable responses with potential long-term remission; less systemic toxicity; effective in certain cancers like melanoma and NSCLC; risk of immune-related toxicities.

Table 15. Survival rates for NSCLC patients

Therapy Type	5-Year Survival Rate	Key Points
Chemotherapy	~25%	Standard treatment; lower survival rates for advanced stages.
Targeted Therapy	~17.4%	Effective for specific genetic mutations; better outcomes for early-stage diagnosis.
Immunotherapy	~18%	Improved survival rates, especially for PD-L1-positive patients.

Figure 9. Patient survival rates by therapy type

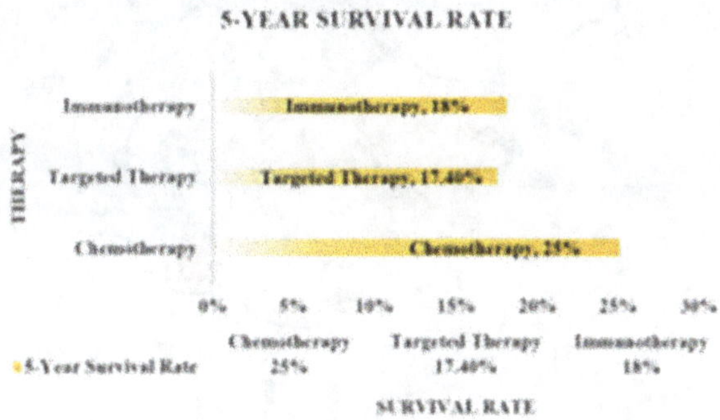

6 EMERGING INNOVATIVE THERAPIES: CAR T CELL THERAPY AND EXPERIMENTAL TREATMENTS

6.1 CAR T Cell Therapy

The overall end of immunotherapy is to use vulnerable checkpoint inhibitors (ICIs) to spark the immune system so that it can attack cancer cells and interfere with the signals that typically inhibit T-cells from being activated (Joy et al., 2024; Gómez-Melero et al., 2025). Ipilimumab, for illustration, enhances T-cell priming and activation by inhibiting CTLA-4 (Yang et al., 2024). In the cancer battle, PD-1 asset pembrolizumab and PD-L1 asset durvalumab both help prevent excrescences from escaping the vulnerable system (Socinski et al., 2021). Immunotherapy typically employs all of these drugs as shown in Figure 10. As a first-line treatment in PD- PD-L1-positive NSCLC (expression of 50 or further), immunotherapy has a part in clinical practice in the form of an adjuvant for advanced NSCLC as well as early NSCLC. In those with low PD-L1 expression, chemotherapy is generally combined with immunotherapy. Immunotherapy can have sustained benefits and grant sustained remission, which is one benefit over chemotherapy. It also has lower systemic toxicity and is effective for most NSCLC subtypes (Nadal et al., 2023). One thing to note, still, is that only 20 to 30 percent of cases will find it salutary. It is also extremely valuable, not always readily available, and it can affect vulnerability-mediated side effects like endocrinopathies, colitis, and pneumonitis described in Table 16, challenges, and proposed solutions (Hu et al., 2024).

Figure 10. CAR -T cell therapy process

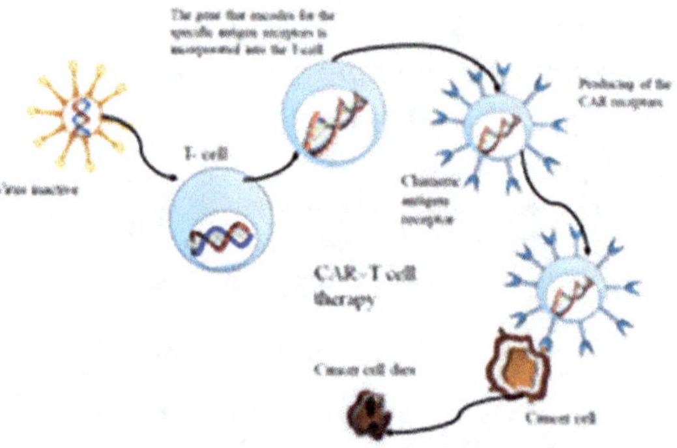

Table 16. Challenges and Proposed Solutions for CAR-T CELL THERAPY

Challenge	Description	Solution	References
Tumor Microenvironment	The immunosuppressive tumor environment can reduce CAR-T cell efficacy.	Combining CAR-T therapy with other immunotherapies or using cytokine support to boost T-cell activity.	Joy et al. (2024); Gómez-Melero et al. (2025); Hu et al. (2024)
On-Target/Off-Tumor Toxicity	CAR-T cells may inadvertently attack healthy cells with low antigen expression.	Developing dual CAR designs or incorporating safety switches to regulate CAR-T cell activity.	Lodka et al. (2024); Huo et al. (2024); Schett et al. (2024)
Neurological Toxicity	Some patients experience severe neurological side effects.	Close monitoring and early intervention with corticosteroids or other supportive care.	Zhang et al. (2023); Chen et al. (2024); Cwynarski et al. (2025)

6.2 Experimental Therapies in NSCLC

New therapies for metastatic or advanced non-small cell lung cancer (NSCLC) are demonstrating true potential in clinical trials (Zhang et al., 2022; Chen et al.,

2024). One of them, DS-1062a, is an experimental drug class known as TROP2 that is often found on cancer cells. Designed as an attack on the cancer without harming healthy tissues, it transmits a potent medicine directly to a tumor. Another exciting approach is measles virotherapy, leveraging a safe, modified measles virus that infects and kills cancer cells and enhances the body's immune response (Li et al., 2022). The drug nivolumab helps immune cells fight the disease by stripping the cancer of its ability to hide. Finally, there's tumor-infiltrating lymphocyte (TIL) therapy, a rarefied treatment in which physicians extract immune cells from the patient's tumor, supercharge them in a lab, and then reinject them into the cancer-killing body (Zhang, Wang & Wang, 2023). These ground-breaking treatments taken together offer patients with advanced NSCLC new hope for improved outcomes, as shown in Figure 11, which illustrates clinical trial results for emerging therapies (Cwynarski et al., 2025).

Figure 11. Clinical trial results for emerging therapies

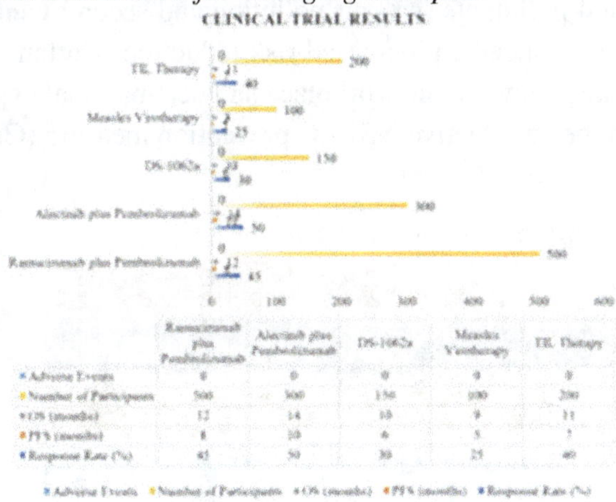

6.3 Future Directions

Researchers are investigating several promising strategies for advancing Auto T cell therapy and innovative treatments to push them forward (Huo, 2024; Lodka et al., 2024). It aims to deliver individualized treatment based on the peculiar genetic and molecular characteristics of a person to maximize efficacy while reducing adverse effects (Zhang & Wang, 2024). Combination therapies seek to bring together several types of therapies to bond into more synergistic properties against more complex problems to solve and enhance outcomes (Li et al., 2022). So-called efforts to defeat treatment resistance are also accelerating, focusing on the ways that cancer escapes therapies (Zhang, Wang & Wang, 2023; Schett et al., 2024). This is an attempt to guarantee long-term effectiveness and sustain consistent patient responses over time, paving the way for cancer care solutions that are more long-lasting and efficient (Ohno & Nakamura, 2024; National Cancer Institute, 2024).

7 PUBLIC HEALTH PERSPECTIVES AND PREVENTION OF NSCLC

Public health initiatives, environmental protections, and smoking cessation programs comprise a large portion of strategies to decrease the burden of non-small cell lung cancer (NSCLC) (Karim et al., 2025). In previous decades, comprehensive tobacco control programs have helped to reduce smoking rates due to lower incidence of NSCLC (Kazerooni et al., 2024). Reducing exposure to tobacco and other environmental pollutants (i.e., air pollution and second-hand smoke) to low or no risk has also produced an increased risk reduction (Cuttano et al., 2024). In addition, maintaining safety in the workplace and occupational exposure to carcinogens continues to be an effective NSCLC prevention measure (Garg et al., 2024).

Figure 12. Diagram of prevention strategies for NSCLC

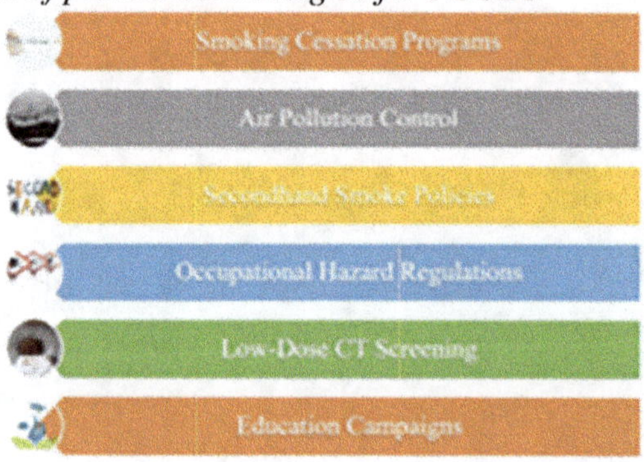

For example, as seen in Figure12, screening programs such as Low-Dose Computed Tomography (LDCT) provide early detection and have been shown to lower the death rate due to NSCLC (Pillay et al., 2024). Public education campaigns also add another layer of protection against lung cancer by inform individuals of the risks involved, discouraging smoking use, and encouraging healthy lifestyle behaviours (Liu et al., 2024).

Policy and regulation have been a particularly important catalyst for prevention. International frameworks (the WHO Framework Convention on Tobacco Control) and national policy approaches (i.e. taxation of tobacco; plain packaging; and restrictions on marketing) have, and will continue to, constrain tobacco consumption by households and populations around the globe.

Further policies to improve the quality of indoor air, provided there is clean energy source and transition to lower exposure to biomass as a fuel source, are also significant risk factors in many low- and middle-income settings.

At the level of individuals and communities, lifestyle and behaviour change are also very important. Eating a range of foods that are balanced in terms of risk, being physically active and reducing alcohol intake all contribute to reducing cancer risk overall. Smoking cessation programs for specific individuals, particularly adolescents or marginalized populations is a special consideration. Technology is increasingly supporting these programs, with mobile health applications and personalized, AI-assisted smoking cessation programs developed to be individually appropriate and broadly available to help support quitting.

Screening and early detection are crucial to saving lives. A recent study of LDCT scans showed that lung cancer could be detected at an earlier stage, but even with evidence for LDCT screening, there are still obstacles, such as false positives, risk of radiation, and whether screening is worth the cost. Research is also exploring various emerging biomarkers including liquid biopsy and circulating tumor DNA, which may one day provide safer, more accurate, non-invasive alternatives. In the meantime, guidelines that identify high-risk populations at the highest risk, and rank populations by risk, also help us to monitor the utilization of LDCT screening resources.

But we also need to work towards equity in prevention. Disparities in access to healthcare often mean that rural areas and low-income populations are usually not privy to either LDCT screening or resources/ supports to successfully quit. Economic barriers, and barriers related to awareness including problem and knowledge of the resources for smoking cessation help keep the divide as wide as it is, particularly for low-income populations and especially indigenous communities. Developing programs that reflect cultural sensitivity and help us begin to reach vulnerable populations & indigenous populations, and work towards equitable prevention strategies.

Looking ahead, we should be excited about what innovation has to offer. The role of electronic cigarettes and vaping devices in tobacco control and as harm reduction products is still controversial and in need of appropriate regulation, but still contribute to the ever-changing tobacco landscape. New developments in genetic risk profiling and artificial intelligence-driven predictive modelling will inevitably bring us to a point of individual prevention strategies. Even public health campaigns are changing, developing new campaigns and using social media and influencer-led initiatives to engage young people to prevent smoking before it starts.

Figure 13. Lung cancer incidence over time with interventions

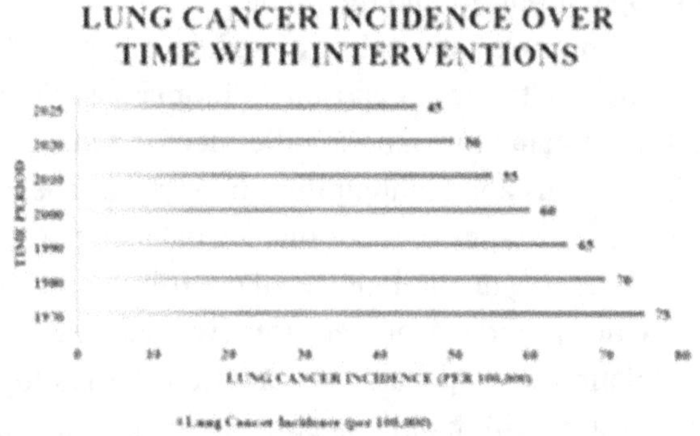

Finally, prevention technologies should be monitored and evaluated at all times. Continuous and longitudinal monitoring of smoking prevalence, air quality indicators, and lung cancer incidence rates is important to evaluate what is working and what should be modified. Japan, Australia and the UK show us that sustained modalities reduce lung cancer incidence. Furthermore, preventative measures—particularly quitting smoking—have considerably bigger health and financial benefits than treatment, according to cost-effectiveness studies. The prevalence of lung cancer has already begun to gradually fall as a result of concerted measures, as seen in Figure 13.

8 CHALLENGES AND FUTURE DIRECTIONS IN NSCLC RESEARCH AND TREATMENT

8.1 Innovations in Research

To address these challenges, exploration is focusing on new strategies including substantiated drugs, immunotherapy, Auto-T cell therapy, oncolytic viruses, and neoadjuvant therapy (Bertolaccini et al., 2024; Li et al., 2025; Tahayneh et al., 2025). Individualized drug leverages inheritable profiling to design acclimatized treatments grounded on specific mutations, while immunotherapy advances aim to enhance excrescence responses through vulnerable checkpoint inhibitors and combination rules. Auto-T cell curatives target NSCLC-specific antigens to ameliorate efficacy and safety. With a high degree of specificity, oncolytic contagions infect and destroy cancer cells in large numbers. Neoadjuvant therapy, involving systemic treatments administered before surgery, helps shrink excrescences and enhances surgical outcomes. These advancements are captured in the Table 17 below.

Table 17. Advancements and their impacts

Future Research Focus	Description	Impact	References
Personalized Medicine	Tailored treatments via genetic profiling.	More effective and less toxic therapies.	Bertolaccini et al., 2024
Immunotherapy	Enhanced immune checkpoint inhibitors and combinations.	Greater tumor response and immune activity.	Li et al., 2025
CAR-T Cell Therapy	Targeting NSCLC-specific antigens.	Increased precision and reduced toxicity.	Tahayneh et al., 2025
Oncolytic Viruses	Viruses are designed to infect and kill cancer cells.	Improved cancer selectivity and potency.	Li et al., 2025; Tahayneh et al., 2025
Neoadjuvant Therapy	Systemic therapy before surgery.	Shrinks tumors and enhances outcomes.	Bertolaccini et al., 2024

8.2 Comprehensive Overview

Non-Small Cell Lung Cancer (NSCLC) exploration and treatment face multiple challenges and opportunities for advancement (Bertolaccini et al., 2024; Li et al., 2025; Tahayneh et al., 2025). Medicine resistance, driven by inheritable mutations, indispensable signaling pathways, and changes in medicine targets, frequently leads to treatment failure and disease progression. Excrescence diversity, encompassing inheritable and phenotypic variations, complicates treatment issues and enables the emergence of resistant subclones. Excretion diversity and the complex progression of cancer make it difficult to identify reliable biomarkers, which are essential for individualized drug development. Additionally, restricted access to advanced curative treatments caused by nonsupervisory, logistical, and financial barriers exacerbates care disparities. The major aspects of these challenges are epitomized in Table 18 below.

Table 18. Challenges in various aspects

Aspect	Description	Impact
Drug Resistance	Genetic mutations, alternative pathways, and changes in drug targets.	Leads to treatment failure and disease progression.
Tumor Heterogeneity	Variations in genetic and cell behaviour and microenvironment interactions.	Causes inconsistent treatment responses and the emergence of resistant clones.
Biomarker Identification	Difficulty in finding sensitive, specific biomarkers due to tumor diversity.	Crucial for improving personalized treatment outcomes.
Access to Treatments	Regulatory and cost-related barriers limit the availability of therapies.	Restricts access to innovative and life-saving treatments.

8.3 Emerging Therapies

Emerging treatment paradigms emphasize the integration of advanced technologies and multidisciplinary collaboration. Precision drug is acclimatizing curatives to individual inheritable biographies, while combination curatives aim to overcome resistance mechanisms. Advanced imaging and biomarker technologies are influenced by prior discovery strategies to identify cancer at earlier, more treatable stages. As demonstrated, global businesses aim to increase the availability of these treatments by reducing costs and improving healthcare structures, as described in Table 19.

Table 19. Emerging therapies

Emerging Paradigm	Description	Impact
Precision Medicine	Treatments tailored to individual genetic profiles.	Enhanced efficacy and reduced side effects.
Combination Therapies	Synergistic use of drugs or modalities.	Overcomes resistance and improves outcomes.
Early Detection	Use of biomarkers and imaging for early diagnosis.	Higher treatment success rates and survival.
Multidisciplinary Care	Collaboration among specialists.	Comprehensive and personalized care.
Global Access	Expanding availability and affordability.	Broader access to innovative treatments.

8.4 Clinical Trials and Future Projections

Active clinical trials are crucial to understanding and perfecting NSCLC treatment approaches. Trials like the ALCHEMIST Trial, targeted radiation studies, and virotherapy exploration are being conducted to identify the most effective strategies for managing NSCLC (Sorin et al., 2024; Hu, 2024; Franceschini et al., 2024; Thomas et al., 2024). A summary of ongoing clinical trials is as follows

Table 20. Clinical trials related to NSCLC

Trial Name	Description	Location	References
ALCHEMIST Trial	Test pembrolizumab with chemotherapy for surgically removed stage IIA-IIIB NSCLC.	1,068 locations worldwide	Sorin et al. (2024)
High Dose, Targeted Radiation Trial	Combines stereotactic body radiation therapy (SBRT) with usual treatment for inoperable NSCLC.	Multiple locations	Hu et al. (2024); Franceschini et al. (2024)
Durvalumab vs Placebo Following SBRT	Evaluates durvalumab's effectiveness post-SBRT in early-stage NSCLC patients.	Rochester, MN	Thomas et al. (2024)
Oraxol and Pembrolizumab	Study oral paclitaxel (Oraxol) with pembrolizumab for advanced solid tumors, including NSCLC.	Scottsdale, AZ; Jacksonville, FL; Rochester, MN	Chen et al. (2025)
Measles Virotherapy with Nivolumab	Phase 1 trial combining measles virus with nivolumab in metastatic NSCLC.	Rochester, MN	Amemiya et al. (2025)
Genome Sequencing for Multifocal Cancers	Assess genome sequencing in treating multifocal lung cancer.	Rochester, MN	Zou et al. (2025)
PT-112 with Avelumab	Studies PT-112 combined with anti-PD-L1 antibody avelumab for advanced solid tumors.	Multiple U.S. locations	Zou et al. (2025)

Projected advancements in treatments like Auto-T remedy, oncolytic contagions, and early discovery methods are anticipated to mainly ameliorate survival rates for NSCLC cases. By 2060, survival rates are projected to increase from 25 in 2025 to 60, driven by inventions in perfect drugs, combination curatives, and a global access enterprise (Chen et al., 2025; Amemiya et al., 2025; Zou et al., 2025). This progress is visually represented in the Graph of Projected Advancements in NSCLC Treatment, pressing a promising future for cases worldwide.

Figure 14. Projected advancements in NSCLC treatment

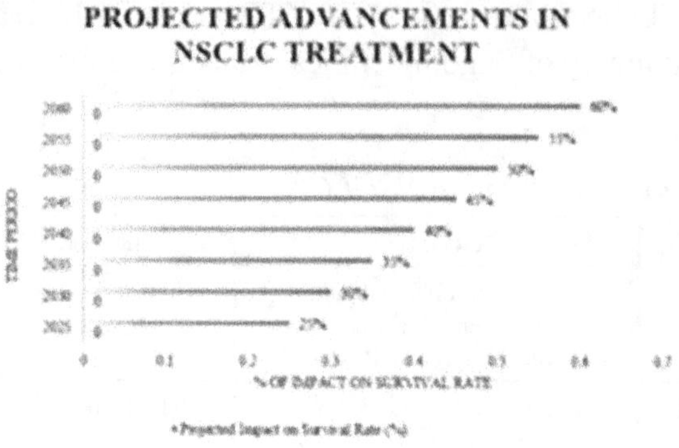

REFERENCES

Abdayem, P., & Planchard, D. (2021). Update on molecular pathology and role of liquid biopsy in nonsmall cell lung cancer. *European Respiratory Review : an Official Journal of the European Respiratory Society*, *30*(161), 200286. DOI: 10.1183/16000617.0294-2020 PMID: 34289984

Abdul-Rahman, T., Ghosh, S., Badar, S. M., Nazir, A., Bamigbade, G. B., Aji, N., Roy, P., Kachani, H., Garg, N., Lawal, L., Bliss, Z. S., Wireko, A. A., Atallah, O., Adebusoye, F. T., Teslyk, T., Sikora, K., & Horbas, V. (2024). The paradoxical role of cytokines and chemokines at the tumor microenvironment: A comprehensive review. *European Journal of Medical Research*, *29*(1), 124. DOI: 10.1186/s40001-024-01711-z PMID: 38360737

Accogli, T., Bruchard, M., & Végran, F. (2021). Modulation of CD4 T cell response according to tumor cytokine microenvironment. *Cancers (Basel)*, *13*(3), 373. DOI: 10.3390/cancers13030373 PMID: 33498483

Al-Tashi, Q., Saad, M. B., Muneer, A., Qureshi, R., Mirjalili, S., Sheshadri, A., Le, X., Vokes, N. I., Zhang, J., & Wu, J. (2023). Machine learning models for the identification of prognostic and predictive cancer biomarkers: A systematic review. *International Journal of Molecular Sciences*, *24*(9), 7781. DOI: 10.3390/ijms24097781 PMID: 37175487

Alduais, Y., Zhang, H., Fan, F., Chen, J., & Chen, B. (2023, February 22). Non-small cell lung cancer (NSCLC): A review of risk factors, diagnosis, and treatment. *Medicine*, *102*(8), e32899. DOI: 10.1097/MD.0000000000032899 PMID: 36827002

Algarra, I., Garrido, F., & Garcia-Lora, A. M. (2021). MHC heterogeneity and response of metastases to immunotherapy. *Cancer and Metastasis Reviews*, *40*(2), 501–517. DOI: 10.1007/s10555-021-09964-4 PMID: 33860434

Ali, F., Neha, K., & Chauhan, G. (2022). Pralsetinib: Chemical and therapeutic development with FDA authorization for the management of RET fusion-positive non-small-cell lung cancers. *Archives of Pharmacal Research*, *45*(5), 309–327. DOI: 10.1007/s12272-022-01385-3 PMID: 35598228

Amemiya, K., Hirotsu, Y., Iimuro, Y., Tajiri, R., Oyama, T., Obi, S., Mochizuki, H., & Omata, M. (2025). Decoding Genomic Diversity to Guide Tumor Lesion-Specific Treatment of Multifocal Hepatocellular Carcinoma. *Cancer Medicine*, *14*(7), e70814. DOI: 10.1002/cam4.70814 PMID: 40145314

Bagaev, A., Kotlov, N., Nomie, K., Svekolkin, V., Gafurov, A., Isaeva, O., Osokin, N., Kozlov, I., Frenkel, F., Gancharova, O., Almog, N., Tsiper, M., Ataullakhanov, R., & Fowler, N. (2021). Conserved pan-cancer microenvironment subtypes predict response to immunotherapy. *Cancer Cell, 39*(6), 845–865. DOI: 10.1016/j.ccell.2021.04.014 PMID: 34019806

Bagaev, A., Kotlov, N., Nomie, K., Svekolkin, V., Gafurov, A., Isaeva, O., Osokin, N., Kozlov, I., Frenkel, F., Gancharova, O., Almog, N., Tsiper, M., Ataullakhanov, R., & Fowler, N. (2021). Conserved pan-cancer microenvironment subtypes predict response to immunotherapy. *Cancer Cell, 39*(6), 845–865. DOI: 10.1016/j.ccell.2021.04.014 PMID: 34019806

Baghy, K., Ladányi, A., Reszegi, A., & Kovalszky, I. (2023). Insights into the tumor microenvironment—Components, functions and therapeutics. *International Journal of Molecular Sciences, 24*(24), 17536. DOI: 10.3390/ijms242417536 PMID: 38139365

Balta, E., Wabnitz, G. H., & Samstag, Y. (2021). Hijacked immune cells in the tumor microenvironment: Molecular mechanisms of immunosuppression and cues to improve T cell-based immunotherapy of solid tumors. *International Journal of Molecular Sciences, 22*(11), 5736. DOI: 10.3390/ijms22115736 PMID: 34072260

Bazhenova, L., Minchom, A., Viteri, S., Bauml, J. M., Ou, S. H. I., Gadgeel, S. M., Trigo, J. M., Backenroth, D., Li, T., Londhe, A., Mahadevia, P., & Girard, N. (2021). Comparative clinical outcomes for patients with advanced NSCLC harboring EGFR exon 20 insertion mutations and common EGFR mutations. *Lung Cancer (Amsterdam, Netherlands), 162*, 154–161. DOI: 10.1016/j.lungcan.2021.10.020 PMID: 34818606

Bertolaccini, L., Casiraghi, M., Uslenghi, C., Maiorca, S., & Spaggiari, L. (2024). Recent advances in lung cancer research: Unravelling the future of treatment. *Updates in Surgery, 76*(6), 2129–2140. DOI: 10.1007/s13304-024-01841-3 PMID: 38581618

Blaquier, J. B., Ortiz-Cuaran, S., Ricciuti, B., Mezquita, L., Cardona, A. F., & Recondo, G. (2023, September 15). Tackling Osimertinib Resistance in EGFR-Mutant Non–Small Cell Lung Cancer. *Clinical Cancer Research, 29*(18), 3579–3591. DOI: 10.1158/1078-0432.CCR-22-1912 PMID: 37093192

Bożyk, A., Wojas-Krawczyk, K., Krawczyk, P., & Milanowski, J. (2022). Tumor microenvironment—A short review of cellular and interaction diversity. *Biology (Basel), 11*(6), 929. DOI: 10.3390/biology11060929 PMID: 35741450

Canale, M., Andrikou, K., Priano, I., Cravero, P., Pasini, L., Urbini, M., Delmonte, A., Crinò, L., Bronte, G., & Ulivi, P. (2022, February 23). The role of TP53 mutations in EGFR-mutated non-small-cell lung cancer: Clinical significance and implications for therapy. *Cancers (Basel)*, *14*(5), 1143. DOI: 10.3390/cancers14051143 PMID: 35267450

Cao, Y., Haring, C. T., Brummel, C., Bhambhani, C., Aryal, M., Lee, C., Heft Neal, M., Bhangale, A., Gu, W., Casper, K., Malloy, K., Sun, Y., Shuman, A., Prince, M. E., Spector, M. E., Chinn, S., Shah, J., Schonewolf, C., McHugh, J. B., & Brenner, J. C. (2022). Early HPV ctDNA kinetics and imaging biomarkers predict therapeutic response in p16+ oropharyngeal squamous cell carcinoma. *Clinical Cancer Research*, *28*(2), 350–359. DOI: 10.1158/1078-0432.CCR-21-2338 PMID: 34702772

Catalano, M., Shabani, S., Venturini, J., Ottanelli, C., Voltolini, L., & Roviello, G. (2022). Lung cancer immunotherapy: Beyond common immune checkpoints inhibitors. *Cancers (Basel)*, *14*(24), 6145. DOI: 10.3390/cancers14246145 PMID: 36551630

Chen, K., Liu, A., Wang, C., Hu, C., Chen, C., Yang, F., Chen, H., Shen, H., Zhang, H., Liu, H., Xiong, J., Wang, J., Zhang, L., Xu, L., Wang, L., Zhao, M., Li, Q., Song, Q., Zhou, Q., & Wang, J. (2025). Multidisciplinary expert consensus on diagnosis and treatment of multiple lung cancers. *Med (New York, N.Y.)*, *6*(4), 100643. DOI: 10.1016/j.medj.2025.100643 PMID: 40220743

Chen, R., Li, Q., Xu, S., Ye, C., Tian, T., Jiang, Q., Shan, J., & Ruan, J. (2022). Modulation of the tumour microenvironment in hepatocellular carcinoma by tyrosine kinase inhibitors: From modulation to combination therapy targeting the microenvironment. *Cancer Cell International*, *22*(1), 73. DOI: 10.1186/s12935-021-02435-4 PMID: 35148789

Chen, T., Wang, M., Chen, Y., & Liu, Y. (2024). Current challenges and therapeutic advances of CAR-T cell therapy for solid tumors. *Cancer Cell International*, *24*(1), 133. DOI: 10.1186/s12935-024-03315-3 PMID: 38622705

Cheng, W., Kang, K., Zhao, A., & Wu, Y. (2024). Dual blockade immunotherapy targeting PD-1/PD-L1 and CTLA-4 in lung cancer. *Journal of Hematology & Oncology*, *17*(1), 54. DOI: 10.1186/s13045-024-01581-2 PMID: 39068460

Clark, L., Fisher, G., Brook, S., Patel, S., & Arkenau, H. T. (2023). Selective RET Inhibitors (SRIs) in Cancer: A Journey from Multi-Kinase Inhibitors to the Next Generation of SRIs. *Cancers (Basel)*, *16*(1), 31. DOI: 10.3390/cancers16010031 PMID: 38201460

Cognigni, V., Pecci, F., Lupi, A., Pinterpe, G., De Filippis, C., Felicetti, C., Cantini, L., & Berardi, R. (2022). The landscape of ALK-rearranged non-small cell lung cancer: A comprehensive review of clinicopathologic, genomic characteristics, and therapeutic perspectives. *Cancers (Basel), 14*(19), 4765. DOI: 10.3390/cancers14194765 PMID: 36230686

Cucchiara, F., Petrini, I., Romei, C., Crucitta, S., Lucchesi, M., Valleggi, S., Scavone, C., Capuano, A., De Liperi, A., Chella, A., Danesi, R., & Del Re, M. (2021). Combining liquid biopsy and radiomics for personalized treatment of lung cancer patients: State of the art and new perspectives. *Pharmacological Research, 169*, 105643. DOI: 10.1016/j.phrs.2021.105643 PMID: 33940185

Cuttano, R., Mazzarelli, F., Afanga, K. M., Bianchi, F., & Dama, E. (2024). MicroRNAs and the Mediterranean diet: A nutri-omics perspective for lung cancer. *Journal of Translational Medicine, 22*(1), 632. DOI: 10.1186/s12967-024-05454-7 PMID: 38972997

Cwynarski, K., Iacoboni, G., Tholouli, E., Menne, T., Irvine, D. A., Balasubramaniam, N., Wood, L., Shang, J., Xue, E., Zhang, Y., Basilico, S., Neves, M., Raymond, M., Scott, I., El-Kholy, M., Jha, R., Dainton-Smith, H., Hussain, R., Day, W., & Pule, M. (2025). TRBC1-CAR T cell therapy in peripheral T cell lymphoma: A phase 1/2 trial. *Nature Medicine, 31*(1), 137–143. DOI: 10.1038/s41591-024-03326-7 PMID: 39528665

Dagogo-Jack, I., Kiedrowski, L. A., Heist, R. S., Lin, J. J., Meador, C. B., Krueger, E. A., Do, A., Peterson, J., Sequist, L. V., Gainor, J. F., Lennerz, J. K., & Digumarthy, S. R. (2023). Efficacy and tolerability of ALK/MET combinations in patients with ALK-rearranged lung cancer with acquired MET amplification: A retrospective analysis. *JTO Clinical and Research Reports, 4*(8), 100534. DOI: 10.1016/j.jtocrr.2023.100534 PMID: 37533439

Dan, A., Burtavel, L. M., Coman, M. C., Focsa, I. O., Duta-Ion, S., Juganaru, I. R., Zaruha, A.-G., Codreanu, P.-C., Strugari, I.-M., Hotinceanu, I.-A., Bohiltea, L.-C., & Radoi, V. E. (2024). Genetic Blueprints in Lung Cancer: Foundations for Targeted Therapies. *Cancers (Basel), 16*(23), 4048. DOI: 10.3390/cancers16234048 PMID: 39682234

De Jong, E., Lammerts, M. U. P. A., Genders, R. E., & Bouwes Bavinck, J. N. (2022). Update of advanced cutaneous squamous cell carcinoma. *Journal of the European Academy of Dermatology and Venereology, 36*(S1), 6–10. DOI: 10.1111/jdv.17728 PMID: 34855246

Desai, S. A., Patel, V. P., Bhosle, K. P., Nagare, S. D., & Thombare, K. C. (2025). The tumor microenvironment: Shaping cancer progression and treatment response. *Journal of Chemotherapy (Florence, Italy)*, *37*(1), 15–44. DOI: 10.1080/1120009X.2023.2300224 PMID: 38179655

Desilets, A., Repetto, M., Yang, S. R., & Drilon, A. (2025). Targeting ROS1 rearrangements in non–small cell lung cancer: Current insights and future directions. *Cancer*, *131*(S1), e35784. DOI: 10.1002/cncr.35784 PMID: 40171848

Dhatchinamoorthy, K., Colbert, J. D., & Rock, K. L. (2021). Cancer immune evasion through loss of MHC class I antigen presentation. *Frontiers in Immunology*, *12*, 636568. DOI: 10.3389/fimmu.2021.636568 PMID: 33767702

Di Capua, D., Bracken-Clarke, D., Ronan, K., Baird, A. M., & Finn, S. (2021). The liquid biopsy for lung cancer: State of the art, limitations and future developments. *Cancers (Basel)*, *13*(16), 3923. DOI: 10.3390/cancers13163923 PMID: 34439082

Díaz, M. A., Fusco, M., Benítez, C. A., Gayet, F., García, L., Victoria, L., Jaramillo, S., Bayo, J., Zubieta, M. R., Rizzo, M. M., Piccioni, F., & Malvicini, M. (2024). Targeting hyaluronan metabolism-related molecules associated with resistant tumor-initiating cells potentiates chemotherapy efficacy in lung cancer. *Scientific Reports*, *14*(1), 16803. DOI: 10.1038/s41598-024-66914-0 PMID: 39039104

Diaz-Jimenez, A., Shuldiner, E. G., Somogyi, K., Gonzalez, O., Akkas, F., Murray, C. W., ... EML4-ALK variant-specific genetic interactions shape lung tumorigenesis. bioRxiv. 2024 Aug 27:2024-08.

Ding, L., Gosh, A., Lee, D. J., Emri, G., Huss, W. J., Bogner, P. N., & Paragh, G. (2022). Prognostic biomarkers of cutaneous melanoma. *Photodermatology, Photoimmunology & Photomedicine*, *38*(5), 418–434. DOI: 10.1111/phpp.12770 PMID: 34981569

Dong, Y., Xu, J., Sun, B., Wang, J., & Wang, Z. (2022). MET-targeted therapies and clinical outcomes: A systematic literature review. *Molecular Diagnosis & Therapy*, *26*(2), 203–227. DOI: 10.1007/s40291-021-00568-w PMID: 35266116

Dziadziuszko, R., Krebs, M. G., De Braud, F., Siena, S., Drilon, A., Doebele, R. C., Patel, M. R., Cho, B. C., Liu, S. V., Ahn, M.-J., Chiu, C.-H., Farago, A. F., Lin, C.-C., Karapetis, C. S., Li, Y.-C., Day, B., Chen, D., Wilson, T. R., & Barlesi, F. (2021, April 10). Updated integrated analysis of the efficacy and safety of entrectinib in locally advanced or metastatic ROS1 fusion–positive non–small-cell lung cancer. *Journal of Clinical Oncology*, *39*(11), 1253–1263. DOI: 10.1200/JCO.20.03025 PMID: 33646820

Dzobo, K., Senthebane, D. A., & Dandara, C. (2023). The tumor microenvironment in tumorigenesis and therapy resistance revisited. *Cancers (Basel)*, *15*(2), 376. DOI: 10.3390/cancers15020376 PMID: 36672326

El Halabi, L., Adam, J., Gravelle, P., Marty, V., Danu, A., Lazarovici, J., Ribrag, V., Bosq, J., Camara-Clayette, V., Laurent, C., & Ghez, D. (2021). Expression of the immune checkpoint regulators LAG-3 and TIM-3 in classical Hodgkin lymphoma. *Clinical Lymphoma, Myeloma & Leukemia*, *21*(4), 257–266. DOI: 10.1016/j.clml.2020.11.009 PMID: 33277223

El-Tanani, M., Rabbani, S. A., Babiker, R., Rangraze, I., Kapre, S., Palakurthi, S. S., Alnuqaydan, A. M., Aljabali, A. A., Rizzo, M., El-Tanani, Y., & Tambuwala, M. M. (2024, April 16). Unraveling the tumor microenvironment: Insights into cancer metastasis and therapeutic strategies. *Cancer Letters*, *591*, 216894. DOI: 10.1016/j.canlet.2024.216894 PMID: 38626856

Escobedo-Calvario, A., Chávez-Rodríguez, L., Simoni-Nieves, A., Souza-Arroyo, V., Miranda-Labra, R. U., Gomez-Quiroz, L. E., & Gutiérrez-Ruíz, M. C. (2022). Tumor immune microenvironment modulation by cholesterol in hepatocellular carcinoma. *Exploration of Digestive Diseases*, *1*, 21–39. DOI: 10.37349/edd.2022.00003

Fabbri, L., Di Federico, A., Astore, M., Marchiori, V., Rejtano, A., Seminerio, R., Gelsomino, F., & De Giglio, A. (2023, December 25). From development to place in therapy of Lorlatinib for the treatment of ALK and ROS1 rearranged non-small cell lung cancer (NSCLC). *Diagnostics (Basel)*, *14*(1), 48. DOI: 10.3390/diagnostics14010048 PMID: 38201357

Farc, O., & Cristea, V. (2021). An overview of the tumor microenvironment, from cells to complex networks. *Experimental and Therapeutic Medicine*, *21*(1), 96. DOI: 10.3892/etm.2020.9528 PMID: 33363607

Franceschini, D., Franzese, C., Comito, T., Ilieva, M. B., Spoto, R., Marzo, A. M., Dominici, L., Massaro, M., Bellu, L., Badalamenti, M., Mancosu, P., & Scorsetti, M. (2024). Definitive results of a prospective non-randomized phase 2 study on stereotactic body radiation therapy (SBRT) for medically inoperable lung and liver oligometastases from breast cancer. *Radiotherapy and Oncology : Journal of the European Society for Therapeutic Radiology and Oncology*, *195*, 110240. DOI: 10.1016/j.radonc.2024.110240 PMID: 38522597

Friedlaender, A., Perol, M., Banna, G. L., Parikh, K., & Addeo, A. (2024). Oncogenic alterations in advanced NSCLC: A molecular super-highway. *Biomarker Research*, *12*(1), 24. DOI: 10.1186/s40364-024-00566-0 PMID: 38347643

Gandhi, Z., Gurram, P., Amgai, B., Lekkala, S. P., Lokhandwala, A., Manne, S., Mohammed, A., Koshiya, H., Dewaswala, N., Desai, R., Bhopalwala, H., Ganti, S., & Surani, S. (2023). Artificial intelligence and lung cancer: Impact on improving patient outcomes. *Cancers (Basel)*, *15*(21), 5236. DOI: 10.3390/cancers15215236 PMID: 37958411

Ganti, A. K., Klein, A. B., Cotarla, I., Seal, B., & Chou, E. (2021, December 1). Update of incidence, prevalence, survival, and initial treatment in patients with non–small cell lung cancer in the US. *JAMA Oncology*, *7*(12), 1824–1832. DOI: 10.1001/jamaoncol.2021.4932 PMID: 34673888

Garg, P., Singhal, S., Kulkarni, P., Horne, D., Malhotra, J., Salgia, R., & Singhal, S. S. (2024). Advances in non-small cell lung cancer: Current insights and future directions. *Journal of Clinical Medicine*, *13*(14), 4189. DOI: 10.3390/jcm13144189 PMID: 39064229

Gemelli, M., Albini, A., Catalano, G., Incarbone, M., Cannone, M., Balladore, E., Ricotta, R., & Pelosi, G. (2024). Navigating resistance to ALK inhibitors in the lorlatinib era: A comprehensive perspective on NSCLC. *Expert Review of Anticancer Therapy*, *24*(6), 347–361. DOI: 10.1080/14737140.2024.2344648 PMID: 38630549

Ghosh, D. D., McDonald, H., Dutta, R., Krishnan, K., Thilakan, J., Paul, M. K., Arya, N., Rao, M., & Rangnekar, V. M. (2024). Prognostic Indicators for Precision Treatment of Non-Small Cell Lung Carcinoma. *Cells*, *13*(21), 1785. DOI: 10.3390/cells13211785 PMID: 39513892

Godoy, L. A., Chen, J., Ma, W., Lally, J., Toomey, K. A., Rajappa, P., Sheridan, R., Mahajan, S., Stollenwerk, N., Phan, C. T., Cheng, D., Knebel, R. J., & Li, T. (2023). Emerging precision neoadjuvant systemic therapy for patients with resectable non-small cell lung cancer: Current status and perspectives. *Biomarker Research*, *11*(1), 7. DOI: 10.1186/s40364-022-00444-7 PMID: 36650586

Gómez-Melero, S., Hassouneh, F., Vallejo-Bermúdez, I. M., Agüera-Morales, E., Solana, R., & Caballero-Villarraso, J. (2025). Tandem CAR-T cell therapy: Recent advances and current challenges. *Frontiers in Immunology*, *16*, 1546172. DOI: 10.3389/fimmu.2025.1546172 PMID: 40092990

. Grilli, G. (2022). Molecular target therapy and immunotherapy of rare lung tumors.

Guo, Q., Liu, L., Chen, Z., Fan, Y., Zhou, Y., Yuan, Z., & Zhang, W. (2022). Current treatments for non-small cell lung cancer. *Frontiers in Oncology*, *12*, 945102. DOI: 10.3389/fonc.2022.945102 PMID: 36033435

Győrffy, B. (2023). Discovery and ranking of the most robust prognostic biomarkers in serous ovarian cancer. *GeroScience*, *45*(3), 1889–1898. DOI: 10.1007/s11357-023-00742-4 PMID: 36856946

. Habib, P. (2024). Review of immunotherapy in non-small cell lung cancer: mechanisms, clinical applications, and future prospects.

Hawash, M. (2024). Advances in cancer therapy: A comprehensive review of CDK and EGFR inhibitors. *Cells*, *13*(19), 1656. DOI: 10.3390/cells13191656 PMID: 39404419

Hendriks, L. E., Remon, J., Faivre-Finn, C., Garassino, M. C., Heymach, J. V., Kerr, K. M., Tan, D. S. W., Veronesi, G., & Reck, M. (2024). Non-small-cell lung cancer. *Nature Reviews. Disease Primers*, *10*(1), 71. DOI: 10.1038/s41572-024-00551-9 PMID: 39327441

Herrera-Juárez, M., Serrano-Gómez, C., Bote-de-Cabo, H., & Paz-Ares, L. (2023). Targeted therapy for lung cancer: Beyond EGFR and ALK. *Cancer*, *129*(12), 1803–1820. DOI: 10.1002/cncr.34757 PMID: 37073562

Heymach, J. V., Yu, H. A., Besse, B., Cheng, Y., Tan, D. S., Wei, L., Wacheck, V., & Nishio, M. (2025). REZILIENT3: Randomized phase III study of first-line zipalertinib plus chemotherapy in patients with EGFR exon 20 insertion-mutated NSCLC. *Future Oncology (London, England)*, *21*(5), 549–556. DOI: 10.1080/14796694.2025.2457294 PMID: 39957151

Hu, C. (2024). Stereotactic Body Radiotherapy for Medically Inoperable Early-Stage Non–Small Cell Lung Cancer. *JAMA Oncology*, *10*(11), 1576–1577. DOI: 10.1001/jamaoncol.2024.2905 PMID: 39298175

Hu, D., Yang, R., Wang, G., Li, H., Fan, X., & Liang, G. (2024). Emerging strategies to overcome current CAR-T therapy dilemmas—Exosomes derived from CAR-T cells. *International Journal of Nanomedicine*, *19*, 2773–2791. DOI: 10.2147/IJN.S445101 PMID: 38525009

Huang, J., Zhang, J., Sun, C., Yang, R., Sheng, M., Hu, J., Kai, G., & Han, B. (2024). Adjuvant role of Salvia miltiorrhiza bunge in cancer chemotherapy: A review of its bioactive components, health-promotion effect and mechanisms. *Journal of Ethnopharmacology*, *318*, 117022. DOI: 10.1016/j.jep.2023.117022 PMID: 37572929

Huang, R., Chen, H., Pi, D., He, X., Yu, C., & Yu, C. (2024). Preparation of etoposide liposomes for enhancing antitumor efficacy on small cell lung cancer and reducing hematotoxicity of drugs. *European Journal of Pharmaceutics and Biopharmaceutics*, *198*, 114239. DOI: 10.1016/j.ejpb.2024.114239 PMID: 38452907

Huang, S., Yang, J., Shen, N., Xu, Q., & Zhao, Q. (2023, February). Artificial intelligence in lung cancer diagnosis and prognosis: Current application and future perspective. *Seminars in Cancer Biology*, *89*, 30–37. DOI: 10.1016/j.semcancer.2023.01.006 PMID: 36682439

Huo, T. (2024). Next-gen CAR-T therapy: Innovations, challenges and future directions. BioTechniques. Retrieved from https://www.biotechniques.com/cancer-research/next-gen-car-t-therapy-innovations-challenges-and-future-directions/

Hussain, F. H., & Raza, A. (2024). Immune checkpoint inhibitors in cancer immunotherapy. In *Critical Developments in Cancer Immunotherapy* (pp. 123–156). IGI Global., DOI: 10.4018/979-8-3693-3976-3.ch004

Hyytiäinen, A., Mroueh, R., Peltonen, J., Wennerstrand, P., Mäkitie, A., Al-Samadi, A., Ventelä, S., & Salo, T. (2023). Prognostic histological markers in oral tongue squamous cell carcinoma patients treated with (chemo) radiotherapy. *APMIS*, *131*(4), 142–151. DOI: 10.1111/apm.13298 PMID: 36695633

Iglesias-Escudero, M., Arias-González, N., & Martínez-Cáceres, E. (2023). Regulatory cells and the effect of cancer immunotherapy. *Molecular Cancer*, *22*(1), 26. DOI: 10.1186/s12943-023-01714-0 PMID: 36739406

Iida, H., Tani, M., Komeda, K., Nomi, T., Matsushima, H., Tanaka, S., Ueno, M., Nakai, T., Maehira, H., Mori, H., Matsui, K., Hirokawa, F., Kaibori, M., & Kubo, S. (2022). Superiority of CRP-albumin-lymphocyte index (CALLY index) as a non-invasive prognostic biomarker after hepatectomy for hepatocellular carcinoma. *HPB : The Official Journal of the International Hepato Pancreato Biliary Association*, *24*(1), 101–115. DOI: 10.1016/j.hpb.2021.06.414 PMID: 34244053

Jang, J. Y., Kim, D., Im, E., & Kim, N. D. (2025). Etoposide as a key therapeutic agent in lung cancer: Mechanisms, efficacy, and emerging strategies. *International Journal of Molecular Sciences*, *26*(2), 796. DOI: 10.3390/ijms26020796 PMID: 39859509

Jhunjhunwala, S., Hammer, C., & Delamarre, L. (2021). Antigen presentation in cancer: Insights into tumour immunogenicity and immune evasion. *Nature Reviews. Cancer*, *21*(5), 298–312. DOI: 10.1038/s41568-021-00339-z PMID: 33750922

Jin, S., Shang, Z., Wang, W., Gu, C., Wei, Y., Zhu, Y., Yang, C., Zhang, T., Zhu, Y., Zhu, Y., Wu, J., & Ye, D. (2023). Immune co-inhibitory receptors CTLA-4, PD-1, TIGIT, LAG-3, and TIM-3 in upper tract urothelial carcinomas: A large cohort study. *Journal of Immunotherapy*, *46*(4), 154–159. DOI: 10.1097/CJI.0000000000000466 PMID: 37017991

Jin, Y., Yang, F., & Chen, K. (2023). An overview of current development and barriers on liquid biopsy in patients with early-stage non-small-cell lung cancer. *Holistic Integrative Oncology.*, *2*(1), 43–49. DOI: 10.1007/s44178-023-00066-5

Joy, R., Phair, K., O'Hara, R., & Brady, D. (2024). Recent advances and current challenges in CAR-T cell therapy. *Biotechnology Letters*, *46*(1), 115–126. DOI: 10.1007/s10529-023-03461-0 PMID: 38150098

Karagiannakos, A., Adamaki, M., Tsintarakis, A., Vojtesek, B., Fåhraeus, R., Zoumpourlis, V., & Karakostis, K. (2022). Targeting oncogenic pathways in the era of personalized oncology: A systemic analysis reveals highly mutated signaling pathways in cancer patients and potential therapeutic targets. *Cancers (Basel)*, *14*(3), 664. DOI: 10.3390/cancers14030664 PMID: 35158934

Karim, N. A., Rabea, A. M., Mack, P. C., Subramanian, J., Khalil, E., Sherif, M., Marawan, R., Gaafar, T., Shash, L., Suzuki, K., Ahluwalia, M., Wahba, H., Aboelela, S., Al Ahmadi, A., Al Husaini, H., Mohsen, N., Khaled, R., Kassem, N., Khaled, H., & Sen, T. (2025). State of Lung Cancer in Egypt: Moving Towards Improved Guidelines for Prevention, Screening, Treatment, and Clinical Care Programs. *JTO Clinical and Research Reports*, *6*(1), 100776. DOI: 10.1016/j.jtocrr.2024.100776 PMID: 39790369

Kazerooni, E. A., Wood, D. E., Rosenthal, L. S., & Smith, R. A. (2024). The American Cancer Society National Lung Cancer Roundtable strategic plan: Introduction. *Cancer*, *130*(23), 3948–3960. DOI: 10.1002/cncr.35385 PMID: 39302215

Khalaf, K., Hana, D., Chou, J. T., Singh, C., Mackiewicz, A., & Kaczmarek, M. (2021). Aspects of the tumor microenvironment involved in immune resistance and drug resistance. *Frontiers in Immunology*, *12*, 656364. DOI: 10.3389/fimmu.2021.656364 PMID: 34122412

Koenig, D., Savic Prince, S., & Rothschild, S. I. (2021, February 15). Targeted therapy in advanced and metastatic non-small cell lung cancer. An update on treatment of the most important actionable oncogenic driver alterations. *Cancers (Basel)*, *13*(4), 804. DOI: 10.3390/cancers13040804 PMID: 33671873

Koroulakis, A., & Agarwal, M. (2024). Laryngeal cancer. In *StatPearls* [Internet]. StatPearls Publishing.

Kundu, M., Butti, R., Panda, V. K., Malhotra, D., Das, S., Mitra, T., Kapse, P., Gosavi, S. W., & Kundu, G. C. (2024). Modulation of the tumor microenvironment and mechanism of immunotherapy-based drug resistance in breast cancer. *Molecular Cancer*, *23*(1), 92. DOI: 10.1186/s12943-024-01990-4 PMID: 38715072

Kuzevanova, A., Apanovich, N., Mansorunov, D., Korotaeva, A., & Karpukhin, A. (2022). The features of checkpoint receptor–ligand interaction in cancer and the therapeutic effectiveness of their inhibition. *Biomedicines*, *10*(9), 2081. DOI: 10.3390/biomedicines10092081 PMID: 36140182

Laguna, J. C., Tagliamento, M., Lambertini, M., Hiznay, J., & Mezquita, L. (2024, June). Tackling non–small cell lung cancer in young adults: From risk factors and genetic susceptibility to lung cancer profile and outcomes. *American Society of Clinical Oncology Educational Book*, *44*(3), e432488. DOI: 10.1200/EDBK_432488 PMID: 38788188

Lahiri, A., Maji, A., Potdar, P. D., Singh, N., Parikh, P., Bisht, B., Mukherjee, A., & Paul, M. K. (2023). Lung cancer immunotherapy: Progress, pitfalls, and promises. *Molecular Cancer*, *22*(1), 40. DOI: 10.1186/s12943-023-01740-y PMID: 36810079

Lee, J. Y., Bhandare, R. R., Boddu, S. H., Shaik, A. B., Saktivel, L. P., Gupta, G., Negi, P., Barakat, M., Singh, S. K., Dua, K., & Chellappan, D. K. (2024). Molecular mechanisms underlying the regulation of tumour suppressor genes in lung cancer. *Biomedicine and Pharmacotherapy*, *173*, 116275. DOI: 10.1016/j.biopha.2024.116275 PMID: 38394846

Lei, Y., Wang, K., Liu, Y., Wang, X., Xiang, X., Ning, X., Ding, W., Duan, J., Li, D., Zhao, W., Li, Y., Zhang, F., Luo, X., Shi, Y., Wang, Y., Huang, D., Bai, Y., & Zhang, H. (2022). Various subtypes of EGFR mutations in patients with NSCLC define genetic, immunologic diversity and possess different prognostic biomarkers. *Frontiers in Immunology*, *13*, 811601. DOI: 10.3389/fimmu.2022.811601 PMID: 35265073

Li, C. L., Yuan, X., & Yi, P. (2025). The role of immunotherapy in lung cancer treatment: Current strategies, future directions, and insights into metastasis and immune microenvironment. *Current Gene Therapy*, *25*(4), 453–466. DOI: 10.2174/0115665232340926241105064739 PMID: 39779552

Li, Q., Guo, C., Cao, B., Zhou, F., Wang, J., Ren, H., Li, Y., Wang, M., Liu, Y., Zhang, H., & Ma, L. (2024). Safety and efficacy evaluation of personalized exercise prescription during chemotherapy for lung cancer patients. *Thoracic Cancer*, *15*(11), 906–918. DOI: 10.1111/1759-7714.15272 PMID: 38462754

Li, W., Li, T., Sun, C., Du, Y., Chen, L., Du, C., Shi, J., & Wang, W. (2022). Identification and prognostic analysis of biomarkers to predict the progression of pancreatic cancer patients. *Molecular Medicine (Cambridge, Mass.)*, *28*(1), 43. DOI: 10.1186/s10020-022-00467-8 PMID: 35428170

Li, X., Gulati, M., Larson, A. C., Solheim, J. C., Jain, M., Kumar, S., & Batra, S. K. (2022). Immune checkpoint blockade in pancreatic cancer: Trudging through the immune desert. In *Seminars in Cancer Biology* (Vol. 86, pp. 14–27). Academic Press., DOI: 10.1016/j.semcancer.2022.08.009

Li, X. Y., Zhao, Z. J., Wang, J. B., Shao, Y. H., You, J. X., & Yang, X. T. (2022). m7G methylation-related genes as biomarkers for predicting overall survival outcomes for hepatocellular carcinoma. *Frontiers in Bioengineering and Biotechnology*, *10*, 849756. DOI: 10.3389/fbioe.2022.849756 PMID: 35620469

Li, Y., Liu, X., & Wang, Y. (2022). CAR-T cell combination therapy: The next revolution in cancer treatment. *Cancer Cell International*, *22*(1), 1–15. DOI: 10.1186/s12935-022-02778-6 PMID: 34980127

Li, Y. R., Fang, Y., Lyu, Z., Zhu, Y., & Yang, L. (2023). Exploring the dynamic interplay between cancer stem cells and the tumor microenvironment: Implications for novel therapeutic strategies. *Journal of Translational Medicine*, *21*(1), 686. DOI: 10.1186/s12967-023-04575-9 PMID: 37784157

Li, Z., Li, J., Bai, X., Huang, X., & Wang, Q. (2024, September 28). Tumor microenvironment as a complex milieu driving cancer progression: A mini review. *Clinical & Translational Oncology*, *27*(5), 1–0. DOI: 10.1007/s12094-024-03697-w PMID: 39342061

Lin, H. L., Lin, Q. Y., Feng, J. N., Zheng, W. E., Yang, C., & Yuan, S. F. (2024, September 18). Plasma fatty acid levels and risk of non-small cell lung cancer: A large-scale prospective cohort study. *Frontiers in Nutrition*, *11*, 1462300. DOI: 10.3389/fnut.2024.1462300 PMID: 39376792

Liu, J., Wang, H., Aggarwal, A., Ortiz-Ruiz, M. J., Zapatero-Solana, E., Lallena, M. J., Peregrina, S., del Hoyo, G. M., Velasco, S., Ebert, P. J., Gong, X., Hossain, A. M., & Estrem, S. T. (2025). Survival benefit from abemaciclib in non–small cell lung cancer by Kirsten rat sarcoma–mutation gene expression subtype: Retrospective analysis from the JUNIPER Trial. *Frontiers in Oncology*, *15*, 1461530. DOI: 10.3389/fonc.2025.1461530 PMID: 40231258

Liu, L., Bai, H., Wang, C., Seery, S., Wang, Z., Duan, J., Li, S., Xue, P., Wang, G., Sun, Y., Du, X., Zhang, X., Ma, Z., & Wang, J. (2021). Efficacy and safety of first-line immunotherapy combinations for advanced NSCLC: A systematic review and network meta-analysis. *Journal of Thoracic Oncology*, *16*(7), 1099–1117. DOI: 10.1016/j.jtho.2021.03.016 PMID: 33839365

Liu, M., Liu, L., Lv, Z., Mao, Y., & Liu, Y. (2024). Investigating the determinants of fear of cancer recurrence in patients with early-stage non-small cell lung cancer: Insights from a restricted cubic spline model. *Cancer Medicine*, *13*(12), e7406. DOI: 10.1002/cam4.7406

Lo, Y. C., & Lindeman, N. I. (2023). Molecular Pathology of Lung Tumors. In *Molecular Surgical Pathology* (pp. 231–245). Springer International Publishing. DOI: 10.1007/978-3-031-35118-1_9

Lodka, D., Zschummel, M., Bunse, M., Rousselle, A., Sonnemann, J., Kettritz, R., Höpken, U. E., & Schreiber, A. (2024). CD19-targeting CAR T cells protect from ANCA-induced acute kidney injury. *Annals of the Rheumatic Diseases*, *83*(4), 499–507. DOI: 10.1136/ard-2023-224875 PMID: 38182404

LoPiccolo, J., Gusev, A., Christiani, D. C., & Jänne, P. A. (2024). Lung cancer in patients who have never smoked—An emerging disease. *Nature Reviews. Clinical Oncology*, *21*(2), 121–146. DOI: 10.1038/s41571-023-00844-0 PMID: 38195910

Lopresti, L., Tatangelo, V., Baldari, C. T., & Patrussi, L. (2024). Rewiring the T cell-suppressive cytokine landscape of the tumor microenvironment: A new frontier for precision anti-cancer therapy. *Frontiers in Immunology*, *15*, 1418527. DOI: 10.3389/fimmu.2024.1418527 PMID: 39281678

Malapelle, U., Leprieur, E. G., Kamga, P. T., Chiasseu, M. T., & Rolfo, C. (2021). Emerging biomarkers for NSCLC: Recent advances in diagnosis and therapy. *Frontiers in Oncology*, *11*, 694578. DOI: 10.3389/fonc.2021.694578 PMID: 34055656

Malinga, N. Z., Siwele, S. C., Steel, H. C., Kwofie, L. L., Meyer, P. W., Smit, T., Anderson, R., Rapoport, B. L., & Kgokolo, M. C. (2022). Systemic levels of the soluble co-inhibitory immune checkpoints, CTLA-4, LAG-3, PD-1/PD-L1 and TIM-3 are markedly increased in basal cell carcinoma. *Translational Oncology*, *19*, 101384. DOI: 10.1016/j.tranon.2022.101384 PMID: 35255355

Mamdani, H., Matosevic, S., Khalid, A. B., Durm, G., & Jalal, S. I. (2022). Immunotherapy in lung cancer: Current landscape and future directions. *Frontiers in Immunology*, *13*, 823618. DOI: 10.3389/fimmu.2022.823618 PMID: 35222404

Massafra, M., Passalacqua, M. I., Gebbia, V., Macrì, P., Lazzari, C., Gregorc, V., & Santarpia, M. (2021). Immunotherapeutic advances for NSCLC. *Biologics*, •••, 399–417. PMID: 34675481

Meira, D. D. (2023). de Castro e Caetano. *Lung Cancer (Amsterdam, Netherlands)*, *24*, 26.

Mimura, K., Kua, L. F., Xiao, J. F., Asuncion, B. R., Nakayama, Y., Syn, N., Fazreen, Z., Soong, R., Kono, K., & Yong, W. P. (2021). Combined inhibition of PD-1/PD-L1, LAG-3, and TIM-3 axes augments antitumor immunity in gastric cancer–T cell coculture models. *Gastric Cancer*, *24*(3), 611–623. DOI: 10.1007/s10120-020-01151-8 PMID: 33611641

Mina, S. A., Shanshal, M., Leventakos, K., & Parikh, K. (2025). Emerging Targeted Therapies in Non-Small-Cell Lung Cancer (NSCLC). *Cancers (Basel)*, *17*(3), 353. DOI: 10.3390/cancers17030353 PMID: 39941723

Molinaro, M., Skrodzki, D., & Pan, D. (2024). Chemoradiotherapy and nanomedicine: Drug mechanisms and delivery systems. *Wiley Interdisciplinary Reviews. Nanomedicine and Nanobiotechnology*, *16*(4), e1984. DOI: 10.1002/wnan.1984 PMID: 39109509

Mollavelioglu, B., Cetin Aktas, E., Cabioglu, N., Abbasov, A., Onder, S., Emiroglu, S., Tükenmez, M., Muslumanoglu, M., Igci, A., Deniz, G., & Ozmen, V. (2022). High co-expression of immune checkpoint receptors PD-1, CTLA-4, LAG-3, TIM-3, and TIGIT on tumor-infiltrating lymphocytes in early-stage breast cancer. *World Journal of Surgical Oncology*, *20*(1), 349. DOI: 10.1186/s12957-022-02810-z PMID: 36271406

Munteanu, R., Tomuleasa, C., Iuga, C. A., Gulei, D., & Ciuleanu, T. E. (2023). Exploring therapeutic avenues in lung cancer: The epigenetic perspective. *Cancers (Basel)*, *15*(22), 5394. DOI: 10.3390/cancers15225394 PMID: 38001653

Nadal, E., Saleh, M., Ponce Aix, S., Ochoa-de-Olza, M., Patel, S. P., Antonia, S., Zhao, Y., Gueorguieva, I., Man, M., Estrem, S. T., Liu, J., Avsar, E., Lin, W. H., Benhadji, K. A., Gandhi, L., Guba, S. C., & Ales Diaz, I. (2023). A phase Ib/II study of galunisertib in combination with nivolumab in solid tumors and non-small cell lung cancer. *BMC Cancer*, *23*(1), 11153. Advance online publication. DOI: 10.1186/s12885-023-11153-1 PMID: 37507657

Nagy, A., Börzsei, D., Hoffmann, A., Török, S., Veszelka, M., Almási, N., Varga, C., & Szabó, R. (2024). A comprehensive overview on chemotherapy-induced cardiotoxicity: Insights into the underlying inflammatory and oxidative mechanisms. *Cardiovascular Drugs and Therapy*, •••, 1–15. DOI: 10.1007/s10557-024-07574-0 PMID: 38492161

Nardin, S., Sacco, G., Lagodin D'Amato, A., Barcellini, L., Rovere, M., Santamaria, S., Marconi, S., Coco, S., & Genova, C. (2024). Updates in pharmacotherapy for non-small cell lung cancer: A focus on emerging tubulin inhibitors. *Expert Opinion on Pharmacotherapy*, *25*(8), 1051–1069. DOI: 10.1080/14656566.2024.2369196 PMID: 38935538

Naser, R., Fakhoury, I., El-Fouani, A., Abi-Habib, R., & El-Sibai, M. (2022). Role of the tumor microenvironment in cancer hallmarks and targeted therapy. *International Journal of Oncology*, *62*(2), 23. DOI: 10.3892/ijo.2022.5471 PMID: 36579669

National Cancer Institute. (2024). CAR T cells: Engineering patients' immune cells to treat their cancers. Retrieved from https://www.cancer.gov/about-cancer/treatment/research/car-t-cells

Ning, J., Ge, T., Jiang, M., Jia, K., Wang, L., Li, W., Chen, B., Liu, Y., Wang, H., Zhao, S., & He, Y. (2021). Early diagnosis of lung cancer: Which is the optimal choice? *Aging (Albany NY)*, *13*(4), 6214–6229. DOI: 10.18632/aging.202504 PMID: 33591942

Nooreldeen, R., & Bach, H. (2021). Current and future development in lung cancer diagnosis. *International Journal of Molecular Sciences*, *22*(16), 8661. DOI: 10.3390/ijms22168661 PMID: 34445366

Novello, S., Califano, R., Reinmuth, N., Tamma, A., & Puri, T. (2023). RET fusion-positive non small cell lung cancer: The evolving treatment landscape. *The Oncologist*, *28*(5), 402–413. DOI: 10.1093/oncolo/oyac264 PMID: 36821595

Ohno, R., & Nakamura, A. (2024, May). Advancing autoimmune rheumatic disease treatment: CAR-T Cell Therapies—Evidence, safety, and future directions. In *Seminars in Arthritis and Rheumatism* (p. 152479). WB Saunders. DOI: 10.1016/j.semarthrit.2024.152479

Olmedo, M. E., Cervera, R., Cabezon-Gutierrez, L., Lage, Y., de la Fuente, E. C., Rueda, A. G., & Couñago, F. (2022). New horizons for uncommon mutations in non-small cell lung cancer: BRAF, KRAS, RET, MET, NTRK, HER2. *World Journal of Clinical Oncology*, *13*(4), 276–286. DOI: 10.5306/wjco.v13.i4.276 PMID: 35582653

Oya, Y., Tanaka, I., & Soo, R. A. (2025, April 8). Integration of Liquid Biopsy for Optimal Management of NSCLC. *Tuberculosis and Respiratory Diseases*. Advance online publication. DOI: 10.4046/trd.2024.0146

Özkaya Gül, S., Şimşek, B., Yıldız, F., & Aydemir, E. (2025). Cytotoxic effect of escitalopram/etoposide combination on etoposide-resistant lung cancer. *Pharmaceuticals (Basel, Switzerland)*, *18*(4), 531. DOI: 10.3390/ph18040531 PMID: 40283966

Palma, D. A., Prisman, E., Berthelet, E., Tran, E., Hamilton, S., Wu, J., Eskander, A., Higgins, K., Karam, I., Poon, I., Husain, Z., Enepekides, D., Hier, M., Sultanem, K., Richardson, K., Mlynarek, A., Johnson-Obaseki, S., Odell, M., Bayley, A., & Nichols, A. C. (2022). Assessment of toxic effects and survival in treatment deescalation with radiotherapy vs transoral surgery for HPV-associated oropharyngeal squamous cell carcinoma: The ORATOR2 phase 2 randomized clinical trial. *JAMA Oncology*, *8*(6), 845–851. DOI: 10.1001/jamaoncol.2022.0615 PMID: 35482348

Pan, D., Hu, A. Y., Antonia, S. J., & Li, C. Y. (2021). A gene mutation signature predicting immunotherapy benefits in patients with NSCLC. *Journal of Thoracic Oncology*, *16*(3), 419–427. DOI: 10.1016/j.jtho.2020.11.021 PMID: 33307194

Parvaresh, H., Roozitalab, G., Golandam, F., Behzadi, P., & Jabbarzadeh Kaboli, P. (2024). Unraveling the potential of ALK-targeted therapies in non-small cell lung cancer: Comprehensive insights and future directions. *Biomedicines*, *12*(2), 297. DOI: 10.3390/biomedicines12020297 PMID: 38397899

Passaro, A., Attili, I., Rappa, A., Vacirca, D., Ranghiero, A., Fumagalli, C., Guarize, J., Spaggiari, L., de Marinis, F., Barberis, M., & Guerini-Rocco, E. (2021). Genomic characterization of concurrent alterations in Non-Small Cell Lung Cancer (NSCLC) harboring actionable mutations. *Cancers (Basel)*, *13*(9), 2172. DOI: 10.3390/cancers13092172 PMID: 33946519

Pezzuto, F., Hofman, V., Bontoux, C., Fortarezza, F., Lunardi, F., Calabrese, F., & Hofman, P. (2023a). The significance of co-mutations in EGFR-mutated non-small cell lung cancer: Optimizing the efficacy of targeted therapies? *Lung Cancer (Amsterdam, Netherlands)*, *181*, 107249. DOI: 10.1016/j.lungcan.2023.107249 PMID: 37244040

Pietrobon, V., & Marincola, F. M. (2021). Hypoxia and the phenomenon of immune exclusion. *Journal of Translational Medicine*, *19*(1), 9. DOI: 10.1186/s12967-020-02667-4 PMID: 33407613

Pillay, J., Rahman, S., Klarenbach, S., Reynolds, D. L., Tessier, L. A., Thériault, G., Persaud, N., Finley, C., Leighl, N., McInnes, M. D. F., Garritty, C., Traversy, G., Tan, M., & Hartling, L. (2024). Screening for lung cancer with computed tomography: Protocol for systematic reviews for the Canadian Task Force on Preventive Health Care. *Systematic Reviews*, *13*(1), 88. DOI: 10.1186/s13643-024-02506-3 PMID: 38493159

Pisapia, P., Pepe, F., Baggi, A., Barberis, M., Galvano, A., Gristina, V., Mastrilli, F., Novello, S., Pagni, F., Pasini, S., Perrone, G., Righi, D., Russo, A., Troncone, G., & Malapelle, U. (2022). Next generation diagnostic algorithm in non-small cell lung cancer predictive molecular pathology: The KWAY Italian multicenter cost evaluation study. *Critical Reviews in Oncology/Hematology*, *169*, 103525. DOI: 10.1016/j.critrevonc.2021.103525 PMID: 34813925

Pop-Bica, C., Ciocan, C. A., Braicu, C., Harangu , A., Simon, M., Nutu, A., Pop, L. A., Slaby, O., Atanasov, A. G., Pirlog, R., Al Hajjar, N., & Berindan-Neagoe, I. (2022). Next-generation sequencing in lung cancer patients: A comparative approach in NSCLC and SCLC mutational landscapes. *Journal of Personalized Medicine*, *12*(3), 453. DOI: 10.3390/jpm12030453 PMID: 35330454

Pradhan, K. S., Chawla, P., & Tiwari, R. (2023). HRDEL: High ranking deep ensemble learning-based lung cancer diagnosis model. *Expert Systems with Applications*, *213*, 118956. DOI: 10.1016/j.eswa.2022.118956

. Pruis M. Genotype-guided anti-cancer therapy: development, associated diagnostics and clinical applications: From mutation to patient.

Qi, S. A., Wu, Q., Chen, Z., Zhang, W., Zhou, Y., Mao, K., Li, J., Li, Y., Chen, J., Huang, Y., & Huang, Y. (2021). High-resolution metabolomic biomarkers for lung cancer diagnosis and prognosis. *Scientific Reports*, *11*(1), 11805. DOI: 10.1038/s41598-021-91276-2 PMID: 34083687

Qi, W., Tian, L., Xu, J., Li, Z., & Wang, T. (2025). Multimodal framework in lung cancer management: Integrating liquid biopsy with traditional diagnostic techniques. *Cancer Management and Research*, *17*, 461–481. DOI: 10.2147/CMAR.S506630 PMID: 40060704

Qin, Y., Mo, Y., Li, P., Liang, X., Yu, J., & Chen, D. (2025, April 16). Concurrent immunotherapy improves progression-free survival but increases toxicity in unresectable stage III NSCLC. *Lung Cancer (Amsterdam, Netherlands)*, *203*, 108544. DOI: 10.1016/j.lungcan.2025.108544 PMID: 40253944

Qureshi, M., Afridi, H. I., & Unar, A. (n.d.). [-dioxygenase in primary biliary cholangitis: A comprehensive review of its role, clinical applications, and regulatory mechanisms.]. *Indoleamine*, *2*, 3.

Raju, G. S., Pavitra, E., Varaprasad, G. L., Bandaru, S. S., Nagaraju, G. P., Farran, B., Huh, Y. S., & Han, Y.-K. (2022). Nanoparticles mediated tumor microenvironment modulation: Current advances and applications. *Journal of Nanobiotechnology*, *20*(1), 274. DOI: 10.1186/s12951-022-01476-9 PMID: 35701781

Raju, G. S., Pavitra, E., Varaprasad, G. L., Bandaru, S. S., Nagaraju, G. P., Farran, B., Huh, Y. S., & Han, Y.-K. (2022). Nanoparticles mediated tumor microenvironment modulation: Current advances and applications. *Journal of Nanobiotechnology*, *20*(1), 274. DOI: 10.1186/s12951-022-01476-9 PMID: 35701781

Rakaee, M., Tafavvoghi, M., Ricciuti, B., Alessi, J. V., Cortellini, A., Citarella, F., Nibid, L., Perrone, G., Adib, E., Fulgenzi, C. A., Hidalgo Filho, C. M., Di Federico, A., Jabar, F., Hashemi, S., Houda, I., Richardsen, E., Rasmussen Busund, L.-T., Donnem, T., Bahce, I., & Kwiatkowski, D. J. (2025, February 1). Deep Learning Model for Predicting Immunotherapy Response in Advanced Non– Small Cell Lung Cancer. *JAMA Oncology*, *11*(2), 109–118. DOI: 10.1001/jamaoncol.2024.5356 PMID: 39724105

Rodak, O., Peris-Díaz, M. D., Olbromski, M., Podhorska-Okołów, M., & Dzięgiel, P. (2021, September 20). Current landscape of non-small cell lung cancer: Epidemiology, histological classification, targeted therapies, and immunotherapy. *Cancers (Basel)*, *13*(18), 4705. DOI: 10.3390/cancers13184705 PMID: 34572931

Rodrigues, A., Chauhan, J., Sagkriotis, A., Aasaithambi, S., & Montrone, M. (2022). Understanding the lived experience of lung cancer: A European social media listening study. *BMC Cancer*, *22*(1), 475. DOI: 10.1186/s12885-022-09505-4 PMID: 35490223

Rolfo, C., Mack, P., Scagliotti, G. V., Aggarwal, C., Arcila, M. E., Barlesi, F., Bivona, T., Diehn, M., Dive, C., Dziadziuszko, R., Leighl, N., Malapelle, U., Mok, T., Peled, N., Raez, L. E., Sequist, L., Sholl, L., Swanton, C., Abbosh, C., & Gandara, D. (2021). Liquid biopsy for advanced NSCLC: A consensus statement from the International Association for the Study of Lung Cancer. *Journal of Thoracic Oncology*, *16*(10), 1647–1662. DOI: 10.1016/j.jtho.2021.06.017 PMID: 34246791

Rosas, D., Jones, C., Akinbobuyi, O., Yee Theik, N. W., & Alvarez-Pinzon, A. (2024). Molecular Targeting in Non-Small Cell Lung Cancer: Advances in EGFR, ROS1, ALK, and MET Pathways. *Journal of Oncology Research and Therapy*, *9*, 10214.

Rosellini, M., Marchetti, A., Mollica, V., Rizzo, A., Santoni, M., & Massari, F. (2023). Prognostic and predictive biomarkers for immunotherapy in advanced renal cell carcinoma. *Nature Reviews. Urology*, *20*(3), 133–157. DOI: 10.1038/s41585-022-00676-0 PMID: 36414800

Russo, G. L., Bironzo, P., Bennati, C., Bonanno, L., Catino, A., Metro, G., Petrini, I., Russano, M., & Passaro, A. (2024). Clinical evidence and adverse event management update of patients with RET-rearranged advanced non-small-cell lung cancer (NSCLC) treated with pralsetinib. *Critical Reviews in Oncology/Hematology*, *194*, 104243. DOI: 10.1016/j.critrevonc.2023.104243 PMID: 38135019

Sadhukhan, P., & Seiwert, T. Y. (2023). The role of macrophages in the tumor microenvironment and tumor metabolism. *Seminars in Immunopathology*, *45*(2), 187–201. DOI: 10.1007/s00281-023-00988-2 PMID: 37002376

Scheffler, M., Ihle, M. A., Hein, R., Merkelbach-Bruse, S., Scheel, A. H., Siemanowski, J., Brägelmann, J., Kron, A., Abedpour, N., Ueckeroth, F., Schüller, M., Koleczko, S., Michels, S., Fassunke, J., Pasternack, H., Heydt, C., Serke, M., Fischer, R., Schulte, W., & Wolf, J. (2019). K-ras mutation subtypes in NSCLC and associated co-occurring mutations in other oncogenic pathways. *Journal of Thoracic Oncology*, *14*(4), 606–616. DOI: 10.1016/j.jtho.2018.12.013 PMID: 30605727

Schett, G., Müller, F., Taubmann, J., Mackensen, A., Wang, W., Furie, R. A., Gold, R., Haghikia, A., Merkel, P. A., Caricchio, R., D'Agostino, M.-A., Locatelli, F., June, C. H., & Mougiakakos, D. (2024). Advancements and challenges in CAR T cell therapy in autoimmune diseases. *Nature Reviews. Rheumatology*, *20*(9), 531–544. DOI: 10.1038/s41584-024-01139-z PMID: 39107407

Sen, T., Takahashi, N., Chakraborty, S., Takebe, N., Nassar, A. H., Karim, N. A., Puri, S., & Naqash, A. R. (2024). Emerging advances in defining the molecular and therapeutic landscape of small-cell lung cancer. *Nature Reviews. Clinical Oncology*, *21*(8), 610–627. DOI: 10.1038/s41571-024-00914-x PMID: 38965396

Sharma, A., Shambhwani, D., Pandey, S., Singh, J., Lalhlenmawia, H., Kumarasamy, M., Singh, S. K., Chellappan, D. K., Gupta, G., Prasher, P., Dua, K., & Kumar, D. (2022). Advances in lung cancer treatment using nanomedicines. *ACS Omega*, *8*(1), 10–41. DOI: 10.1021/acsomega.2c04078 PMID: 36643475

Sharma, K., Saini, K., Chimaniya, P., Sahu, S., Gantayat, D., Sharma, R., & Shilpi, S. (2024). Lung Cancer Therapy: Synergistic Potential of PD-1/PD-L1 and CTLA-4 Inhibitors. In *Immunotherapy Against Lung Cancer: Emerging Opportunities and Challenges* (pp. 297–316). Springer Nature Singapore. DOI: 10.1007/978-981-99-7141-1_15

Shen, S., Hong, Y., Huang, J., Qu, X., Sooranna, S. R., Lu, S., Li, T., & Niu, B. (2024). Targeting PD-1/PD-L1 in tumor immunotherapy: Mechanisms and interactions with host growth regulatory pathways. *Cytokine & Growth Factor Reviews*, *79*, 16–28. DOI: 10.1016/j.cytogfr.2024.08.001 PMID: 39179486

Shin, S.. (2022, April 1). Tumor microenvironment modulating functional nanoparticles for effective cancer treatments. *Tissue Engineering and Regenerative Medicine*, •••, 1–5. PMID: 34674182

Shiravand, Y., Khodadadi, F., Kashani, S. M., Hosseini-Fard, S. R., Hosseini, S., Sadeghirad, H., Ladwa, R., O'Byrne, K., & Kulasinghe, A. (2022). Immune checkpoint inhibitors in cancer therapy. *Current Oncology (Toronto, Ont.)*, *29*(5), 3044–3060. DOI: 10.3390/curroncol29050247 PMID: 35621637

Shiravand, Y., Khodadadi, F., Kashani, S. M. A., Hosseini-Fard, S. R., Hosseini, S., Sadeghirad, H., Ladwa, R., O'Byrne, K., & Kulasinghe, A. (2022). Immune checkpoint inhibitors in cancer therapy. *Current Oncology (Toronto, Ont.)*, *29*(5), 3044–3060. DOI: 10.3390/curroncol29050247 PMID: 35621637

Singhal, A., Li, B. T., & O'Reilly, E. M. (2024). Targeting KRAS in cancer. *Nature Medicine*, *30*(4), 969–983. DOI: 10.1038/s41591-024-02903-0 PMID: 38637634

Sito, H., Sharzehan, M. A. K., Islam, M. A., & Tan, S. C. (2024). Genetic variants associated with response to platinum-based chemotherapy in non-small cell lung cancer patients: A field synopsis and meta-analysis. *British Journal of Biomedical Science*, *81*, 11835. DOI: 10.3389/bjbs.2024.11835 PMID: 38450253

Sito, H., & Tan, S. C. (2024). Genetic polymorphisms as potential pharmacogenetic biomarkers for platinum-based chemotherapy in non-small cell lung cancer. *Molecular Biology Reports*, *51*(1), 102. DOI: 10.1007/s11033-023-08915-2 PMID: 38217759

Skoulidis, F., Li, B. T., Dy, G. K., Price, T. J., Falchook, G. S., Wolf, J., & Riely, G. J. (2021). Sotorasib for lung cancers with KRAS p.G12C mutation. *The New England Journal of Medicine*, *384*(25), 2371–2381. DOI: 10.1056/NEJMoa2103695 PMID: 34096690

Smolle, E., Taucher, V., Lindenmann, J., Pichler, M., & Smolle-Juettner, F. M. (2021). Liquid biopsy in non-small cell lung cancer—Current status and future outlook: A narrative review. *Translational Lung Cancer Research*, *10*(5), 2237–2252. DOI: 10.21037/tlcr-21-3 PMID: 34164273

Socinski, M. A., Özgüroğlu, M., Villegas, A., Daniel, D., Vicente, D., Murakami, S., Hui, R., Gray, J. E., Park, K., Vincent, M., Mann, H., Newton, M., Dennis, P. A., & Antonia, S. J. (2021, November 1). Durvalumab after concurrent chemoradiotherapy in elderly patients with unresectable stage III non–small–cell lung cancer (PACIFIC). *Clinical Lung Cancer*, *22*(6), 549–561. DOI: 10.1016/j.cllc.2021.05.009 PMID: 34294595

Soleimani Mamalo, A., Pashaei, M., Valilo, M., & Ojarudi, M. (2025). Cytokine-mediated regulation of immune cell metabolic pathways in the tumor microenvironment. *Naunyn-Schmiedeberg's Archives of Pharmacology*, *398*(9), 1–9. DOI: 10.1007/s00210-025-04133-8 PMID: 40220026

Sorin, M., Prosty, C., Ghaleb, L., Nie, K., Katergi, K., Shahzad, M. H., Dubé, L.-R., Atallah, A., Swaby, A., Dankner, M., Crump, T., Walsh, L. A., Fiset, P. O., Sepesi, B., Forde, P. M., Cascone, T., Provencio, M., & Spicer, J. D. (2024). Neoadjuvant chemoimmunotherapy for NSCLC: A systematic review and meta-analysis. *JAMA Oncology*, *10*(5), 621–633. DOI: 10.1001/jamaoncol.2024.0057 PMID: 38512301

Spira, A. I., Tu, H., Aggarwal, S., Hsu, H., Carrigan, G., Wang, X., Ngarmchamnanrith, G., Chia, V., & Gray, J. E. (2021). A retrospective observational study of the natural history of advanced non–small-cell lung cancer in patients with KRAS p. G12C mutated or wild-type disease. *Lung Cancer (Amsterdam, Netherlands)*, *159*, 1–9. DOI: 10.1016/j.lungcan.2021.05.026 PMID: 34293517

Stanganelli, I., Spagnolo, F., Argenziano, G., Ascierto, P. A., Bassetto, F., Bossi, P., Donato, V., Massi, D., Massone, C., Patuzzo, R., Pellacani, G., Quaglino, P., Queirolo, P., Zalaudek, I., & Palmieri, G. (2022). The multidisciplinary management of cutaneous squamous cell carcinoma: A comprehensive review and clinical recommendations by a panel of experts. *Cancers (Basel)*, *14*(2), 377. DOI: 10.3390/cancers14020377 PMID: 35053539

Stanzione, B., Del Conte, A., Bertoli, E., De Carlo, E., Revelant, A., Spina, M., & Bearz, A. (2023). Therapeutical options in ROS1-rearranged advanced non-small cell lung cancer. *International Journal of Molecular Sciences*, *24*(14), 11495. DOI: 10.3390/ijms241411495 PMID: 37511255

Su, K., Huang, W., Li, X., Xu, K., Gu, T., Liu, Y., Song, J., Qian, K., Xu, Y., Zeng, H., Yang, Y., Guo, L., & Han, Y. (2023). Evaluation of lactate dehydrogenase and alkaline phosphatase as predictive biomarkers in the prognosis of hepatocellular carcinoma and development of a new nomogram. *Journal of Hepatocellular Carcinoma*, *10*, 69–79. DOI: 10.2147/JHC.S398632 PMID: 36685113

Sulewska, A., Pilz, L., Manegold, C., Ramlau, R., Charkiewicz, R., & Niklinski, J. (2023). A systematic review of progress toward unlocking the power of epigenetics in NSCLC: Latest updates and perspectives. *Cells*, *12*(6), 905. DOI: 10.3390/cells12060905 PMID: 36980246

Sun, Z., Sun, X., Chen, Z., Du, J., & Wu, Y. (2022). Head and neck squamous cell carcinoma: Risk factors, molecular alterations, immunology and peptide vaccines. *International Journal of Peptide Research and Therapeutics*, *28*(1), 1–18. DOI: 10.1007/s10989-021-10334-5 PMID: 34903958

Syed, Y. Y. (2022). Pralsetinib: A review in advanced RET fusion-positive NSCLC. *Drugs*, *82*(7), 811–816. DOI: 10.1007/s40265-022-01720-4 PMID: 35587858

Tada, H., Mitsudomi, T., Misumi, T., Sugio, K., Tsuboi, M., Okamoto, I., Iwamoto, Y., Sakakura, N., Sugawara, S., Atagi, S., Takahashi, T., Hayashi, H., Okada, M., Inokawa, H., Yoshioka, H., Takahashi, K., Higashiyama, M., Yoshino, I., & Nakagawa, K. (2022, January 20). Randomized phase III study of gefitinib versus cisplatin plus vinorelbine for patients with resected stage II-IIIA non–small-cell lung cancer with EGFR mutation (IMPACT). *Journal of Clinical Oncology*, *40*(3), 231–241. DOI: 10.1200/JCO.21.01729 PMID: 34726958

Taefehshokr, S., Parhizkar, A., Hayati, S., Mousapour, M., Mahmoudpour, A., Eleid, L., Rahmanpour, D., Fattahi, S., Shabani, H., & Taefehshokr, N. (2022). Cancer immunotherapy: Challenges and limitations. *Pathology, Research and Practice*, *229*, 153723. DOI: 10.1016/j.prp.2021.153723 PMID: 34952426

Tahayneh, K., Idkedek, M., & Abu Akar, F. (2025). NSCLC: Current evidence on its pathogenesis, integrated treatment, and future perspectives. *Journal of Clinical Medicine*, *14*(3), 1025. DOI: 10.3390/jcm14031025 PMID: 39941694

Tan, A. C., Saw, S. P., Chen, J., Lai, G. G., Oo, H. N., Takano, A., Lau, D. P. X., Yeong, J. P. S., Tan, G. S., Lim, K. H., Skanderup, A. J., Chan, J. W. K., Teh, Y. L., Rajasekaran, T., Jain, A., Tan, W. L., Ng, Q. S., Kanesvaran, R., Lim, W.-T., & Tan, D. S. W. (2022). Clinical and genomic features of HER2 exon 20 insertion mutations and characterization of HER2 expression by immunohistochemistry in east Asian non–small-cell lung cancer. *JCO Precision Oncology*, *6*(6), e2200278. DOI: 10.1200/PO.22.00278 PMID: 36240473

Tan, S. L., Selvachandran, G., Paramesran, R., & Ding, W. (2025). Lung cancer detection systems applied to medical images: A state-of-the-art survey. *Archives of Computational Methods in Engineering*, *32*(1), 343–380. DOI: 10.1007/s11831-024-10141-3

Tao, Y., Zhou, Y., Tang, L., Chen, H., Feng, Y., & Shi, Y. (2022). Toxicity profile of anaplastic lymphoma kinase tyrosine kinase inhibitors for patients with non-small cell lung cancer: A systematic review and meta-analysis. *Investigational New Drugs*, *40*(4), 831–840. DOI: 10.1007/s10637-022-01242-6 PMID: 35435628

Tarighati, E., Keivan, H., & Mahani, H. (2023). A review of prognostic and predictive biomarkers in breast cancer. *Clinical and Experimental Medicine*, *23*(1), 1–16. PMID: 35031885

Thomas, Q. D., Chaabouni, M., Al Herk, A., Lefevbre, C., Cavaillon, S., Sinoquet, L., Pouderoux, S., Viala, M., Roca, L., & Quantin, X. (2024). Exploring the Efficacy of Pembrolizumab in Combination with Carboplatin and Weekly Paclitaxel for Frail Patients with Advanced Non-Small-Cell Lung Cancer: A Key Investigative Study. *Cancers (Basel)*, *16*(5), 992. DOI: 10.3390/cancers16050992 PMID: 38473356

Tiwari, A., Trivedi, R., & Lin, S. Y. (2022). Tumor microenvironment: Barrier or opportunity towards effective cancer therapy. *Journal of Biomedical Science*, *29*(1), 83. DOI: 10.1186/s12929-022-00866-3 PMID: 36253762

Tomasik, B., Skrzypski, M., Bieńkowski, M., Dziadziuszko, R., & Jassem, J. (2023). Current and future applications of liquid biopsy in non-small-cell lung cancer—A narrative review. *Translational Lung Cancer Research*, *12*(3), 594–608. DOI: 10.21037/tlcr-22-742 PMID: 37057121

Tsuboi, M., Herbst, R. S., John, T., Kato, T., Majem, M., Grohé, C., Wang, J., Goldman, J. W., Lu, S., Su, W.-C., de Marinis, F., Shepherd, F. A., Lee, K. H., Le, N. T., Dechaphunkul, A., Kowalski, D., Poole, L., Bolanos, A., Rukazenkov, Y., & Wu, Y.-L. (2023, July 13). Overall survival with osimertinib in resected EGFR-mutated NSCLC. *The New England Journal of Medicine*, *389*(2), 137–147. DOI: 10.1056/NEJMoa2304594 PMID: 37272535

Umar, H., Wahab, H. A., Attiq, A., Amjad, M. W., Bukhari, S. N. A., & Ahmad, W. (2024). Platinum-based targeted chemotherapies and reversal of cisplatin resistance in non-small cell lung cancer (NSCLC). *Mutation Research. Fundamental and Molecular Mechanisms of Mutagenesis*, *828*, 111856. DOI: 10.1016/j.mrfmmm.2024.111856 PMID: 38520879

Veyssière, H., Bidet, Y., Penault-Llorca, F., Radosevic-Robin, N., & Durando, X. (2022). Circulating proteins as predictive and prognostic biomarkers in breast cancer. *Clinical Proteomics*, *19*(1), 25. DOI: 10.1186/s12014-022-09362-0 PMID: 35818030

Wang, B., Shen, C., Liu, D., Dong, Z., Lin, X., & Liao, H. (2025). A Comprehensive Review of Advances in Molecular Mechanisms and Targeted Therapies for the Specific Type of Cystic Lung Cancer. *OncoTargets and Therapy*, *18*, 211–224. DOI: 10.2147/OTT.S495018 PMID: 39959914

Wang, H., Cheng, X., Yang, F., Chen, L., Zhang, A., Zhong, L., Long, H., Zhu, B., & Wang, Z. (2024). Subsequent strategies and underlying mechanism of acquired resistance to PD-1 axis inhibitors in advanced non-small cell lung cancer. *Chinese Medical Journal*, *137*(7), 880–882. DOI: 10.1097/CM9.0000000000003015 PMID: 38494340

Wang, Q., Li, H., Wu, T., Yu, B., Cong, H., & Shen, Y. (2024). Nanodrugs based on co-delivery strategies to combat cisplatin resistance. *Journal of Controlled Release, 370*, 14–42. DOI: 10.1016/j.jconrel.2024.04.020 PMID: 38615892

Wang, S., Liu, C., Yang, C., Jin, Y., Cui, Q., Wang, D., Ge, T., He, G., Li, W., Zhang, G., Liu, A., Xia, Y., Liu, Y., & Yu, J. (2024). PI3K/AKT/mTOR and PD-1/CTLA-4/CD28 pathways as key targets of cancer immunotherapy. *Oncology Letters, 28*(6), 567. DOI: 10.3892/ol.2024.14700 PMID: 39390982

Wang, Y., Hu, J., Fleishman, J. S., Li, Y., Ren, Z., Wang, J., Feng, Y., Chen, J., & Wang, H. (2024). Inducing ferroptosis by traditional medicines: A novel approach to reverse chemoresistance in lung cancer. *Frontiers in Pharmacology, 15*, 1290183. DOI: 10.3389/fphar.2024.1290183 PMID: 38855750

Wang, Y. T., Yang, P. C., Zhang, J. Y., & Sun, J. F. (2024). Synthetic routes and clinical application of representative small-molecule EGFR inhibitors for cancer therapy. *Molecules (Basel, Switzerland), 29*(7), 1448. DOI: 10.3390/molecules29071448 PMID: 38611728

Winge, M. C., Kellman, L. N., Guo, K., Tang, J. Y., Swetter, S. M., Aasi, S. Z., Sarin, K. Y., Chang, A. L. S., & Khavari, P. A. (2023). Advances in cutaneous squamous cell carcinoma. *Nature Reviews. Cancer, 23*(7), 430–449. DOI: 10.1038/s41568-023-00583-5 PMID: 37286893

Wunderlich, K., Suppa, M., Gandini, S., Lipski, J., White, J. M., & Del Marmol, V. (2024). Risk factors and innovations in risk assessment for melanoma, basal cell carcinoma, and squamous cell carcinoma. *Cancers (Basel), 16*(5), 1016. DOI: 10.3390/cancers16051016 PMID: 38473375

Xi, Z., Dai, R., Ze, Y., Jiang, X., Liu, M., & Xu, H. (2025). Traditional Chinese medicine in lung cancer treatment. *Molecular Cancer, 24*(1), 57. DOI: 10.1186/s12943-025-02245-6 PMID: 40001110

Xie, M., Vuko, M., Rodriguez-Canales, J., Zimmermann, J., Schick, M., O'Brien, C., Paz-Ares, L., Goldman, J. W., Garassino, M. C., Gay, C. M., Heymach, J. V., Jiang, H., Barrett, J. C., Stewart, R. A., Lai, Z., Byers, L. A., Rudin, C. M., & Shrestha, Y. (2024). Molecular classification and biomarkers of outcome with immunotherapy in extensive-stage small-cell lung cancer: Analyses of the CASPIAN phase 3 study. *Molecular Cancer, 23*(1), 115. DOI: 10.1186/s12943-024-02014-x PMID: 38811992

Xie, Z., Zhou, Z., Yang, S., Zhang, S., & Shao, B. (2023). Epigenetic regulation and therapeutic targets in the tumor microenvironment. *Molecular Biomedicine, 4*(1), 17. DOI: 10.1186/s43556-023-00126-2 PMID: 37273004

Xie, Z., Zhou, Z., Yang, S., Zhang, S., & Shao, B. (2023). Epigenetic regulation and therapeutic targets in the tumor microenvironment. *Molecular Biomedicine*, *4*(1), 17. DOI: 10.1186/s43556-023-00126-2 PMID: 37273004

Xing, S., Hu, K., & Wang, Y. (2022). Tumor immune microenvironment and immunotherapy in non-small cell lung cancer: Update and new challenges. *Aging and Disease*, *13*(6), 1615. DOI: 10.14336/AD.2022.0407 PMID: 36465180

Yang, K., Halima, A., & Chan, T. A. (2023). Antigen presentation in cancer—Mechanisms and clinical implications for immunotherapy. *Nature Reviews. Clinical Oncology*, *20*(9), 604–623. DOI: 10.1038/s41571-023-00789-4 PMID: 37328642

Yang, M., Cao, H., Wang, C., Yu, C., & Sun, P. (2024). Incidence of thromboembolic events in non-small cell lung cancer patients treated with immune checkpoint inhibitors: A systematic review and meta-analysis. *Journal of Cancer Research and Therapeutics*, *20*(2), 509–521. DOI: 10.4103/jcrt.jcrt_1031_23 PMID: 38687920

Yang, T., Xiong, Y., Zeng, Y., Wang, Y., Zeng, J., Liu, J., Xu, S., & Li, L. S. (2022). Current status of immunotherapy for non-small cell lung cancer. *Frontiers in Pharmacology*, *13*, 989461. DOI: 10.3389/fphar.2022.989461 PMID: 36313314

Ying, Q., Fan, R., Shen, Y., Chen, B., Zhang, J., Li, Q., & Shi, X. (2024). Small cell lung cancer—An update on chemotherapy resistance. *Current Treatment Options in Oncology*, *25*(8), 1112–1123. DOI: 10.1007/s11864-024-01245-w PMID: 39066852

Yuan, W., Shi, X., & Lee, L. T. (2024, April 24). RNA therapeutics in targeting G protein-coupled receptors: Recent advances and challenges. *Molecular Therapy. Nucleic Acids*, *35*(2), 102195. DOI: 10.1016/j.omtn.2024.102195 PMID: 38741614

Zabeti Touchaei, A., & Vahidi, S. (2024). MicroRNAs as regulators of immune checkpoints in cancer immunotherapy: Targeting PD-1/PD-L1 and CTLA-4 pathways. *Cancer Cell International*, *24*(1), 102. DOI: 10.1186/s12935-024-03293-6 PMID: 38462628

Zhang, C., Wang, Y., & Wang, Y. (2023). Antigen escape in CAR-T cell therapy: Mechanisms and overcoming strategies. *European Journal of Cancer*, *180*, 1–10. DOI: 10.1016/j.ejca.2023.10.001

Zhang, L., Feng, J., Kuang, T., Chai, D., Qiu, Z., Deng, W., Dong, K., Zhao, K., & Wang, W. (2023). Blood biomarkers predict outcomes in patients with hepatocellular carcinoma treated with immune checkpoint inhibitors: A pooled analysis of 44 retrospective studies. *International Immunopharmacology*, *118*, 110019. DOI: 10.1016/j.intimp.2023.110019 PMID: 36933492

Zhang, L., Ma, W., Qiu, Z., Kuang, T., Wang, K., Hu, B., & Wang, W. (2023). Prognostic nutritional index as a prognostic biomarker for gastrointestinal cancer patients treated with immune checkpoint inhibitors. *Frontiers in Immunology, 14*, 1219929. DOI: 10.3389/fimmu.2023.1219929 PMID: 37545502

Zhang, Y., & Wang, Y. (2024). Advancements and future directions of dual-target chimeric antigen receptor T-cell therapy. *Journal of Immunology Research*. PMID: 39844819

Zhang, Z., Wang, T., Wang, X., Zhang, Y., Song, S., & Ma, C. (2022). Improving the ability of CAR-T cells to hit solid tumors: Challenges and strategies. *Pharmacological Research, 175*, 106003. DOI: 10.1016/j.phrs.2021.106036 PMID: 34920118

Zhao, H., Huang, S., Wu, J., Lu, Y., Zou, Y., Zeng, H., Li, C., Wang, J., Zhang, X., Duan, S., & Liang, W. (2025). Efficacy and safety of first-line PD-1/PD-L1 inhibitor in combination with CTLA-4 inhibitor in the treatment of patients with advanced non-small cell lung cancer: A systemic review and meta-analysis. *Frontiers in Immunology, 16*, 1515027. DOI: 10.3389/fimmu.2025.1515027 PMID: 39981238

Zhao, X., Zhang, X., Chen, H., Bao, H., Wu, X., Wang, H., Bao, H., Pang, J., Wang, S., & Wang, J. (2024). Mechanisms of resistance to tyrosine kinase inhibitors in ROS1 fusion-positive nonsmall cell lung cancer. *Clinical Chemistry, 70*(4), 629–641. DOI: 10.1093/clinchem/hvae008 PMID: 38416709

Zhu, J., Lu, H., Wang, K., Liu, B., & Yan, J. (2024). Tertiary lymphoid structures in head and neck squamous cell carcinoma. *Translational Oncology, 44*, 101949. DOI: 10.1016/j.tranon.2024.101949 PMID: 38583352

Ziogas, D. C., Theocharopoulos, C., Lialios, P. P., Foteinou, D., Koumprentziotis, I. A., Xynos, G., & Gogas, H. (2023). Beyond CTLA-4 and PD-1 inhibition: Novel immune checkpoint molecules for melanoma treatment. *Cancers (Basel), 15*(10), 2718. DOI: 10.3390/cancers15102718 PMID: 37345056

Ziogas, D. C., Theocharopoulos, C., Lialios, P.-P., Foteinou, D., Koumprentziotis, I.-A., Xynos, G., & Gogas, H. (2023). Beyond CTLA-4 and PD-1 inhibition: Novel immune checkpoint molecules for melanoma treatment. *Cancers (Basel), 15*(10), 2718. DOI: 10.3390/cancers15102718 PMID: 37345056

Zou, J. X., Chang, M. R., Kuznetsov, N. A., Kee, J. X., Babak, M. V., & Ang, W. H. (2025). Metal-based immunogenic cell death inducers for cancer immunotherapy. *Chemical Science (Cambridge), 16*(15), 6160–6187. DOI: 10.1039/D4SC08495K PMID: 40160356

Zou, T., Liu, J. Y., Liu, Z. Q., Xiao, D., & Chen, J. (2024). The role of ADCY1 in regulating the sensitivity of platinum-based chemotherapy in NSCLC. *Pharmaceuticals (Basel, Switzerland)*, *17*(9), 1118. DOI: 10.3390/ph17091118 PMID: 39338283

Chapter 13
Future Trends in NSCLC and Care

Reyhane Alidousti Shahraki
https://orcid.org/0009-0007-0269-1844
Tarbiat Modares University, Iran

ABSTRACT

Several treatment methods have been proposed for lung cancer, each exhibiting different success rates. Efforts in this field aim to enhance the effectiveness of these treatments while reducing their side effects. New technologies are being utilized to improve treatment methods and facilitate early diagnosis, ultimately increasing patients' survival rates and life expectancy. Although current methods face challenges, ongoing advancements are being made to address these issues. In this chapter, we will first review the current approaches to treating NSCLC and the challenges associated with them. We will then introduce emerging fields and technologies in these treatment methods that are expected to experience significant growth in the near future, along with the concerns and limitations that accompany their use. Additionally, we will specifically discuss the importance of artificial intelligence in the treatment process and outline essential tools for managing the disease, as well as the palliative and supportive care options available for patients and their families.

INTRODUCTION

Present Challenges of NSCL and Care

In this chapter, we will survey the current challenges associated with non-small cell lung cancer (NSCLC) and its care. This topic is extremely important because the incidence rate of lung cancer is rising due to various risk factors. The most

DOI: 10.4018/979-8-3373-2096-0.ch013

significant risk factor is smoking, and the increasing rate of smoking among young people is heightening the risk of developing this cancer. Additionally, air pollution and industrial gas emissions are critical environmental factors contributing to this issue. Recent statistics indicate there are approximately 2.2 million new cases of lung cancer and 1.8 million deaths each year. One prediction study suggests that these numbers will rise to 4.62 million new cases and 3.55 million deaths in the future. Alarming trends underscore the urgent need for further research into effective early detection and treatment strategies (Zhou et al., 2024).

Non-small cell lung cancer accounts for approximately 80% of lung cancer cases (Padinharayil et al., 2023). In this type of cancer, lung cells grow uncontrollably to form tumors that are less aggressive than those of small cell lung cancer (SCLC). This cancer is divided into three groups based on histological characteristics. Adenocarcinoma, which accounts for approximately 40% of cases, is the most common type of this cancer. The second group is squamous cell carcinoma, which accounts for 25-30% of cases. Large cell carcinoma, which is relatively rare and accounts for approximately 5-10%, exhibits relatively aggressive characteristics. Different clinical and therapeutic approaches are considered for the aforementioned subgroups based on their molecular characteristics (Travis et al., 2015).

The development of early detection methods and high-quality treatment options has become increasingly important, as it provides the best chance for effective outcomes, reduces therapy costs, and improves survival rates (Kenaan et al., 2024).

Less than 20 percent of people with NSCLC are diagnosed in the early stages, when the tumor is still localized, while about 47 percent of patients are diagnosed in stages III or IV. At these stages, the tumor has metastasized to lymph nodes or distant organs. In fact, late detection is one of the main challenges in managing NSCLC, as many of these symptoms often appear only in the later stages of the disease (Kumar & Sarkar, 2022). The 5-year relative survival rate for patients diagnosed in the advanced stages is approximately 6 percent, compared with about 61 percent for patients diagnosed in the early stages (Šutić et al., 2021).

Critical challenges significantly impact patient survival and contribute to over 1.5 million deaths from non-small cell lung cancer (NSCLC) worldwide. Common clinical symptoms of NSCLC include chest, neck, and head pain, difficulty breathing, and coughing up blood. The other current challenge in the treatment of non-small cell lung cancer (NSCLC) is that cytotoxic chemotherapy remains the standard approach for advanced stages. While this method can extend survival and enhance the quality of life for patients, it has the significant drawback of lacking durable clinical benefits. Recent advancements in technology and research have led to the development of innovative methods, including targeted therapy. However, targeted therapy presents its own set of unique challenges, including primary and acquired resistance, limitations in accessibility, and both "on-target" and "off-target" effects of the therapeutic agents. These challenges can result in toxicity. Additionally, factors such as age, central nervous system (CNS) toxicity, drug-drug interactions, and the impact of food on drug bioavailability are crucial in determining toxicity levels. Therefore, it is essential to identify appropriate targets for targeted therapy, understand oncogenic pathways, and develop strategies to address tumor heterogeneity. These considerations are vital for advancing new therapies for NSCLC (Ali, 2024).

Personalized Medicine

Analyzing genomic profiles through personalized medicine for various diseases, including non-small cell lung cancer (NSCLC), can lead to targeted treatments and improved outcomes. For instance, mutation-targeting therapies can facilitate the design of drugs tailored to specific mutations.

Personalized medical care can optimize drug efficacy and reduce toxicity through pharmacogenetics, an essential step in treating NSCLC (Rivera-Concepcion et al., 2022). For example, Osimertinib, a third-generation inhibitor, exhibits better efficacy against the mutant form of EGFR (T790M mutation) (Fu et al., 2022). Since the AURA3 clinical trial showed that patients with this mutation experienced a longer progression-free survival (PFS) (median 10.1 months), a higher percentage of objective response to treatment (ORR) of about 71%, and a longer median overall survival (OS), and these results made osemitinib a major breakthrough in the treatment of this disease depending on the existing mutations (Hizal et al., 2022).

Additionally, treatment plans based on genetic profiles can involve the production of monoclonal antibodies. This approach enables the determination of optimal drug dosages based on the target genes (W. Jiang et al., 2018).

Another advanced method for personalized medicine detection is the development of sequencing approaches. Techniques such as multiplex genotyping, next-generation sequencing, transcriptome analysis, and epigenome analysis offer high-throughput platforms for diagnosis, significantly improving speed and sensitivity. By identifying mutational profiles and oncogenic drivers, such as EGFR, KRAS, and ALK, in a single reaction, these methods can enhance patient survival rates by providing comprehensive and cost-effective data (Vadakara & Borghaei, 2012; Gadgeel, 2016; Okimoto & Bivona, 2014).

New Trends and Growing Technologies

While previous methods are still being developed, more innovative approaches for diagnosing and treating non-small cell lung cancer are emerging, promising a brighter future for those affected by this disease. These research efforts aim to minimize side effects, enhance detection accuracy, improve patient outcomes, increase survival rates, and enhance the quality of life for patients. Currently, cutting-edge techniques being explored in NSCLC research include studies on epigenetic changes such as histone modifications and DNA methylation, investigations into therapeutic strategies based on the tumor microenvironment, CAR-T cell therapy, oncolytic viruses, and combination immunotherapies. Additionally, advancements in high-resolution imaging technologies, molecular biomarker studies, robotic-assisted surgery, and video-assisted thoracoscopic surgery (VATS) are at the forefront of NSCLC research(Garg et al., 2024).

Role of AI in The Present and Future of NSCLC

With the advent of AI, methods for diagnosing and prognosing NSCLC, evaluating treatment responses, and predicting outcomes based on histological, pathological features, and mutations have all significantly improved. The perspective of AI-based methods can enhance patient outcomes (Lococo et al., 2024).

Combination Therapy and Systemic Treatment

Systemic therapy and combination therapy are being developed to improve therapeutic effectiveness. Targeted therapy is often integrated with immunotherapy, chemotherapy, or precision medicine based on genomic profiles. This innovative approach aims to enhance treatment outcomes by managing toxicity and overcoming resistance mechanisms. As a result, these strategies can lead to increased survival and improved response rates(Garg et al., 2024).

Concern Management, Limitations, and Global Disparities

Despite advances in the diagnosis and treatment of non-small cell lung cancer (NSCLC), there are still significant challenges in its management, including financial limitations, ethical issues, and patient accessibility. Individuals from low-income backgrounds, particularly those living in underprivileged areas, often struggle to access advanced treatments and healthcare facilities. As a result, patients may experience delays in diagnosis, misdiagnoses, or incomplete treatments. To address these barriers, authorities should implement policies that promote equitable access to healthcare and improve infrastructure. Additionally, financial constraints can lead patients to opt for less effective treatment options. Policymakers need to prioritize a balance between treatment methods and patient outcomes, regardless of socioeconomic status, as financial limitations can significantly influence treatment choices and decision-making. Furthermore, establishing ethical frameworks to protect patients' privacy and genetic information is crucial. Ensuring that patients provide informed consent before any treatment is essential for maintaining trust and upholding ethical standards in healthcare(Garg et al., 2024).

The treatment process can be influenced by various economic and environmental factors, leading to inequalities in access to treatment, which can impact the mortality, diagnosis, and quality of life of individuals. In high-income countries, despite access to more advanced treatments, due to the high prevalence of smoking and longer life expectancy, people have a higher mortality rate from lung cancer. Low and middle-income countries have an increasing rate of lung cancer due to air pollution, tobacco use, and limitations in diagnostic and treatment infrastructure. Studies have shown that the geographical distance from treatment centers can be a significant factor in the survival of non-small cell lung cancer (NSCLC) patients.

In patients residing in rural areas, the 12-month survival rate is lower than that of patients in urban areas. In fact, the difference in survival and access to treatment between urban and rural NSCLC patients emphasizes the role of geographical and economic inequalities in lung cancer health. Additionally, genetic burden and differences in the type of population mutations can impact the response to treatment in various climates (Laguna et al., 2024; Paakkola et al., 2024; Sharma, 2022).

Challenges and Post-Treatment Measures

One important topic regarding future trends in non-small cell lung cancer (NSCLC) is the duration of patient follow-up, which is determined by clinicopathologic characteristics and patterns of recurrence. Key factors influencing this duration include the patient's sex, smoking history, TNM stage at the time of first recurrence, age, type of treatment received, and tumor size. Establishing an appropriate follow-up duration is crucial for enhancing long-term survival and for the potential implementation of future diagnostic tests. Additionally, developing online tools can help patients and healthcare specialists alleviate potential psychological and economic burdens in the future (M. Zhang et al., 2025).

Additionally, adopting a personalized lifestyle that includes a healthy diet, regular physical exercise, maintaining a healthy body weight, getting vaccinations, and limiting alcohol and processed foods after cancer treatment can decrease the likelihood of recurrence (Murphy et al., 2023; Ko et al., 2023).

Survival-related needs are crucial in the treatment process for lung cancer. Improving the survival rates of patients with non-small cell lung cancer (NSCLC) requires increased awareness among both the lung cancer community and the general public, including family and friends who support these patients. Survivors' needs can be categorized into different domains: physical, financial, spiritual, and social. Addressing these needs as an essential part of the treatment process is vital for enhancing personalized survivorship care and improving the overall quality of life for lung cancer patients(Luszczynska et al., 2013; Curran Jr et al., 2008).

Future trends for NSCLC and care are summarized in Figure 1 and will be explained in detail in the following sections.

Figure 1. Future trend of NSCLC and care

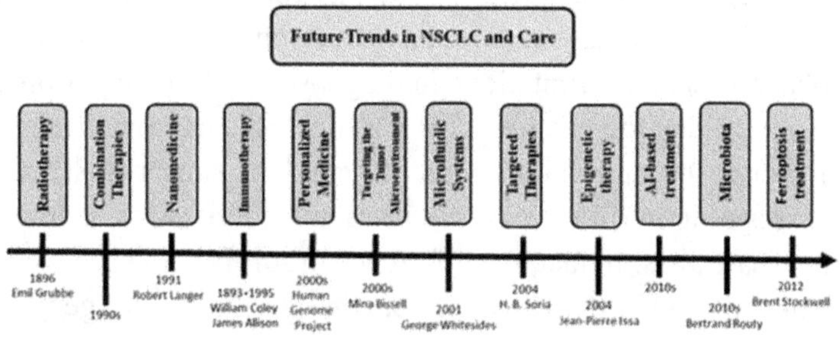

Present approaches, challenges, and growing methods

As mentioned in the introduction, Lung adenocarcinoma (LUAD), with a prevalence of 40%, lung cancer small cell (LUSC), with a prevalence of 30%, and large cell carcinoma (LCC), with 10 -15% are the three most common subtypes of NSCLC and other/mixed types which are being less common are about (3%–5%). Adenocarcinoma originates from the epithelial parenchyma of the lung, LUSC originates from the basal cells of the airways in the lung, and large cell carcinoma is less differentiated. New studies from JMDB and Advances in Precision Medicine suggest specific treatment approaches for each subtype, as specific driver genes in each subtype may influence prognosis and response to targeted therapies (Das & Tisch, 2017).

In the diagnosis of adenocarcinoma (LUAD), biopsy is a challenging process due to the often small tumor environment. Also, the diagnosis process is difficult due to the high tumor heterogeneity. Therefore, the need for accurate identification of molecular mutations is necessary to select a targeted therapy. Squamous cell carcinoma (LUSC) also presents challenges in the differential diagnosis process compared to other squamous cell cancers caused by inflammatory diseases or chronic injuries. Large cell carcinoma (LCC) also presents difficulties in morphological diagnosis due to the low differentiation of the cells. Additionally, the lack of specific markers and high genetic and biological heterogeneity make it challenging to distinguish different subtypes from one another. Therefore, the use of advanced molecular and genomic methods for more accurate diagnosis can be very helpful (Petersen, 2011).

Mutations in the EGFR (10%-15%), ALK (5%), and KRAS (20%-30%) genes are the most common types of mutations in Adenocarcinoma, while ROS1, MET, BRAF, RET, and HER2 are other less common mutations. In squamous cell carcinoma FGFR1(20%), DDR2(3%), and PIK3CA (12%) are most common mutations and, TP53, NOTCH1, CDKN2A, and PTEN are other less common mutations in population. Large cell carcinoma, as a combination of the other two groups, shows mutations in TP53, KRAS, and EGFR (Shen et al., 2025).

Accurate classification is crucial for determining the timing of treatment and identifying diagnostic molecular markers, which are based on genetic differences and response to treatment. Adenocarcinoma is further divided into several subgroups based on growth pattern, namely pre-invasive lesions, including minimally invasive adenocarcinoma (MIA), and invasive adenocarcinomas (Petersen, 2011).

The treatment methods for NSCLC, discussed in detail in the following sections, include surgery, chemotherapy, radiotherapy, targeted therapy, and immunotherapy. However, the effectiveness of these methods varies depending on the subtype. For example, in adenocarcinoma (LUAD), targeted therapies based on EGFR and ALK mutations are more important.

In squamous cell carcinoma (LUSC), targeted therapy has shown less success, while immunotherapy has shown more progress. In large cell carcinoma (LCC), surgery and chemotherapy have also shown better results. However, in general, the combination of immunotherapy with chemotherapy is the first choice of treatment in many cases for NSCLC due to better results (Guo et al., 2022).

In the following parts, we will examine diagnostic methods in detail.

1. THERAPEUTIC STRATEGIES WITH LIQUID BIOPSY

Various cancer screening programs for non-small cell lung cancer (NSCLC) aim to enhance early detection and prevent cancer-related deaths. Currently, most of these programs target high-risk populations due to their increased likelihood of developing cancer. Biomarkers are fundamental in screening, making the establishment of effective policies for practical biomarker research essential. These biomarkers serve as indicators for cytological and molecular diagnostics, prognostics, and assessments of treatment response. They have transformed cancer detection methods, moving beyond traditional techniques. Traditional methods often depend on tissue biopsies and surgical specimens, which can be uncomfortable for patients and may lead to incomplete data due to tumor heterogeneity, resulting in the need for multiple samples. Conversely, body fluids such as sputum, blood, saliva, and urine present attractive alternatives for cancer detection. In the case of NSCLC, the anatomical location of tumors often complicates biopsy sampling. Body fluids not only allow for resampling and sequencing but also minimize invasiveness, provide insights into tumor heterogeneity, enhance early detection, and facilitate real-time monitoring. The most common biomarkers in NSCLC include mRNA, microRNAs (miRNAs), circular RNA (circRNA), serum proteins, circulating DNA (ctDNA), and circulating tumor cells (CTCs). For instance, analyzing the expression levels of specific genes, such as EGFR, KRAS, and PIK3CA, in isolated CTCs, or detecting mutations with digital droplet PCR (ddPCR), can help predict cancer progression. Combining biomarkers with other diagnostic methods can improve accuracy and ensure precise detection. For example, potential miRNAs could serve as biomarkers in conjunction with CT imaging, particularly when definitive diagnostic signs are absent. Moreover, research into exosomes and their components, including exosomal DNA, proteins, RNA, and miRNAs, as potential biomarkers is progressing, alongside growing studies on other types of extracellular bodies. Identifying new, high-performance biomarkers is an ongoing endeavor. New methodologies and research areas related to liquid biopsies and body fluid biomarkers are emerging from the integration of diverse cancer research fields, including multi-omics studies. The advent of artificial intelligence and machine learning-based computational methods is expediting biomarker identification, making them increasingly feasible for routine clinical use. Epigenetic studies and methylation modifications can yield insights into mutations and changes. Methylation studies can detect markers in cell-free DNA (cfDNA) and circulating tumor DNA (ctDNA). Additionally, methylation panels, methylation fragments, and plasma DNA methylation represent other promising avenues for future studies in liquid biopsy and biomarker research. Circulating antibodies, such as autoantibodies targeting tumor-associated antigens (TAAs), are also detectable biomarkers in liquid biopsies, with immunoenzymatic assays enabling the detection and monitoring of these stable proteins. P53 antibodies and their mutations could serve as potential candidates for biomarkers. Furthermore, ongoing metabolite research is contributing to the discovery of biomarkers, such as plasma metabolites. Plasma cell-free RNA (cfRNA) and tumor-educated platelets are potential biomarkers likely to become more prevalent in future liquid biopsy studies and approaches. Despite the heightened focus on identifying new biomarkers, many remain in the preclinical phase due to challenges associated with their routine clinical application, including issues with specificity and sensitivity, the absence of established standards and reliable cutoffs, high costs, and the necessity for extensive clinical trials for final validation(Casagrande et al., 2023; Tomasik et al., 2023; Frullanti & Serrano, 2023).

In Figure 2, developing biomarkers are summarized in body fluids that are being developed to determine treatment strategies, particularly in the early stages.

Figure 2. Present and future key biomarkers

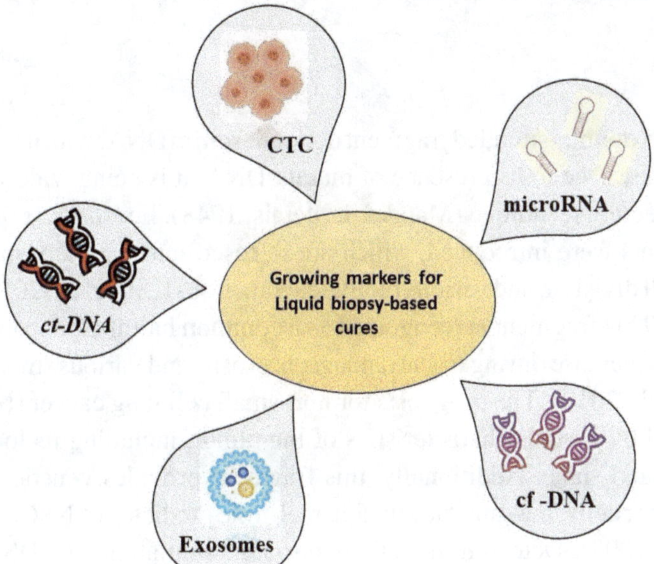

1.1 CTCs

Another emerging marker for the detection of NSCLC is CTCs, which were first introduced by Dr. Ashworth in 1869 (Apostolou et al., 2017). Circulating tumor cells (CTCs) can serve as markers for early detection in plasma samples because they can spread from the primary tumor and travel through the bloodstream (Wirtz et al., 2011). Based on research, higher numbers of CTCs can be related to the rate of progression, metastasis, and advanced stage of NSCLC, shorter OS, and guiding treatment decisions (Heidrich et al., 2023; Cristofanilli et al., 2004; Cohen et al., 2006; Krebs et al., 2011; Tanaka et al., 2009).

1.2 microRNAs

Micrornas (miRNAs) are well-known biomarkers for diagnosing and predicting outcomes in NSCLC because they are significantly influenced by gene expression and cellular signaling pathways. Recently, cell-derived exosomal miRNAs have emerged as promising predictors for early cancer detection and the metastatic process (Tai et al., 2018) (Q. Liu et al., 2016). These markers may enable future detection methods, including personalized medicine and targeted therapy (Iliescu et al., 2019) Reclusa et al., 2017; Araújo, 2016).

1.3 cf DNA

cfDNA is a double-stranded fragment derived from cfDNA, with a length of 150-200 nucleotides. Due to its presence of mutant DNA, it is being widely adopted as a reliable detection technique (Mandel & Metais, 1948). For the first time in 1948, these fragments were introduced, which are released into the bloodstream during apoptosis, cell division, and various biological functions (Liao et al., 2011) Mouliere et al., 2018). This fragment is recognized as a common hallmark of cancer because cfDNA levels increase during tissue damage, necrosis, and various stress conditions (Catarino et al., 2012). The prognosis for non-small cell lung cancer (NSCLC) can be influenced by various characteristics of the tumor, including its location, size, progression, and stage. Additionally, this fragment provides genetic information about the tumor cells, making it a valuable real-time predictor of NSCLC prognosis (Diehl et al., 2008). Detecting mutations through circulating free DNA (cfDNA) is important because it creates opportunities for targeted therapy (Ou et al., 2018). Digital PCR, BEAMing, NGS, ARMS, and next-generation sequencing (NGS) can identify gene rearrangements, copy number alterations, and single-nucleotide variants in NSCLC candidate genes, such as ALK and EGFR (Dono et al., 2019; Vanni et al., 2015; Herbreteau et al., 2019).

1.4 ct DNA

Circulating tumor DNA (ctDNA) is developing more and more as a prognostic and predictive marker for screening populations in order to reduce deaths related to non-small cell lung cancer (NSCLC) due to its noninvasive nature. However, further research is necessary to improve its negative predictive value (NPV) and sensitivity. Currently, using ctDNA as a follow-up tool or for early detection is not feasible because of the high rate of false negative results (Marinello et al., 2024) Waldeck et al., 2022; Zografos et al., 2022; J.-T. Zhang et al., 2022). In fact, due to the low secretion of DNA from cancer cells into the blood, the accuracy of diagnosis can be affected and creating a challenging process. However, the development of new methods, such as sequencing, is helping to address this challenge. However, other limitations, such as the need for a large volume of plasma to obtain sufficient amounts of ctDNA, detecting ctDNA mutations in the background noise, and the lack of clinical approvals, have made the use of ctDNA require further research and studies, and prevent its routine use as a diagnostic marker. On the other hand, some advantages, such as non-invasiveness and the possibility of continuous monitoring, are two important factors, despite the existing weaknesses (Dang & Park, 2022; S.-C. Liu, 2024).

Moreover, cost (Ezeife et al., 2022; (Marino et al., 2018), diagnostic accuracy, and invasiveness are common disadvantages, whereas invasiveness is a key advantage in diagnostic investigations that provide both qualitative and quantitative information (Zaman et al., 2023) Malapelle et al., 2021). Two advantages of tumor heterogeneity analysis include its ability to detect sub-clonal cell populations. Additionally, circulating tumor DNA (ctDNA) profiling can reveal the diverse mechanisms of resistance to EGFR inhibitors in patients with lung cancer. The integration of ctDNA data with radiomics represents a new and intriguing field in artificial intelligence that is still under development. Researchers worldwide are utilizing machine learning models and clustering algorithms to identify specific prognostic and predictive phenotypes for monitoring patients (Costa et al., 2024).

1.5 Extracellular Vesicles and Exosomes

Extracellular vesicles (EVs) are bilayer vesicles classified into three groups based on their size: exomers (<30 nm), small exosomes (30 nm–90 nm), and large exosomes (90 nm–150 nm). They can be purified from whole blood and other body fluids, such as saliva and urine, through various filtration and centrifugation methods. EVs play a significant role in cancer detection and treatment as they reflect the characteristics of their source tissue and cells. These vesicles contain active molecules, including proteins, nucleic acids, and lipids. Because these molecules can serve as biomarkers, EVs are recognized as carriers of biomarkers in different cancers, including non-small cell lung cancer (NSCLC). Several EV markers for NSCLC have already been identified. For instance:

1. Exosomal miRNAs: The profile of miRNAs found in exosomes closely resembles that of primary cells and is equally important. These exosomal miRNAs are associated with gene mutations in NSCLC, making their expression profiles a critical area of research in cancer studies.
2. Exosomal proteins: Certain proteins present in exosomes, such as EGFR, KRAS, claudins, and the RAB family, can serve as diagnostic biomarkers since they are involved in the main pathways associated with NSCLC tumorigenicity. Furthermore, studies suggest that specific exosomal proteins, such as CD171 and CD151, may be associated with lung cancer.
3. Exosomal DNA: The use of exosomal dsDNA as a biomarker is limited to NSCLC cell lines. While these biomarkers are invaluable due to their physical isolation, further research is needed to enhance their effectiveness

Apart from their diagnostic roles, exosomes have several other identified functions. They are often more favorable than liposomes and nanoparticles due to certain disadvantages associated with those alternatives. For instance, exosomes exhibit lower immunogenicity and toxicity, facilitate distribution in body fluids, can cross the blood-brain barrier, and effectively target specific sites through their surface markers. Exosomes are being used as drug delivery vectors because they can transport biomolecules, including drugs. Their significant role in clinical applications is largely due to their emerging function in nanomedicine, particularly in delivering peptides as therapeutic agents. Additionally, they contribute significantly to targeted therapies. Their potential as immunotherapeutic agents could further enhance their role in immune-targeting treatments. For example, exosomes play a role in producing vaccines, delivering genes, and facilitating antigen delivery, as seen in Chimeric Antigen Receptor T (CAR-T) therapies, which enhance the targeting of cancer cells in immunotherapy. Although research on exosomes is rapidly advancing, with numerous papers published in recent years, several limitations remain that need to be addressed. One major challenge is distinguishing normal extracellular vesicles (EVs) from tumor-derived EVs. Additionally, detecting EV surface markers for clinical applications can be expensive, time-consuming, and may require specialized equipment that is not readily available in many clinics. Furthermore, identifying EVs as viable markers necessitates a complex study involving transcriptomics, proteomics, and metabolomics to establish valid EV markers. Many studies have shortcomings in these areas, which represent key limitations in the use of exosomes. However, innovations such as microfluidic systems and organoids, classified as New Approach Methodologies, could accelerate the clinical application of exosomes and lead to exciting new discoveries in this field(Vetsika et al., 2021) Hasan et al., 2022; (Zheng et al., 2018)(Masaoutis et al., 2018) Mullen & Movia, 2023; J. Wu & Chen, 2024).

1.6 Liquid biopsy, challenges and concerns

While the use of liquid biopsies has many advantages, it has also created disadvantages and challenges. Lower sensitivity in early stages of cancer or in cancers with small tumor volumes can lead to false-negative results. Access to advanced equipment and skilled personnel to perform laboratory procedures, and the need for training and patient acceptance for repeated tests and molecular data analysis in underserved areas can be challenging. Additionally, the high cost of implementing the relevant techniques can exacerbate accessibility issues. The universal adoption of liquid biopsies necessitates the standardization of methods and compensation for the current lack of clinical studies. The absence of established standards hinders the full acceptance of liquid biopsy as a standard method in medical centers. Ethical concerns related to protecting patient privacy and data security are also consistently a challenge (Garg et al., 2024).

2. NEXT-GENERATION TARGETED THERAPIES

Next-generation sequencing (NGS) for treating patients with non-small cell lung cancer (NSCLC) is an advanced approach that offers personalized treatment based on targeted panels. These panels identify specific tumor molecular profiles, which are essential for effectively managing patient care. NGS provides targeted therapy by focusing on gene alterations involved in various pathways. Currently, companies like Illumina and Thermo Fisher Scientific offer targeted panels specifically designed for NGS. These panels enable high-resolution analysis of mutations in selected candidate genes. The most commonly targeted genes in NSCLC panels include EGFR, KRAS, ALK, and ROS1. NGS-based methods are continuously evolving to deliver quick, cost-effective, and comprehensive profiling with high sensitivity and specificity. They are also improving in their ability to detect alterations in genes at low densities, particularly in heterogeneous tumors with low mutation rates. These platforms analyze the genome, exome, and transcriptome to identify chromosomal rearrangements and changes in gene copy number. New platforms are being developed for chromatin immunoprecipitation (ChIP) assays, which provide complementary data for validation purposes. Additionally, NGS platforms are advancing to help prevent drug resistance in NSCLC treatments caused by gene alterations. Current advancements in this field can predict genetic resistance before it leads to further medical challenges, facilitating more effective treatment strategies. Identifying driver genes and improving early diagnosis are other anticipated applications of NGS platforms in the near future. Liquid biopsies, which contain circulating tumor DNA (ctDNA), circulating tumor cells, and circulating RNA (ctRNA), can be utilized to create early detection methods based on NGS. These biomarkers offer minimally invasive ways to monitor tumor heterogeneity and point mutations, including deletions, insertions, and epigenetic modifications in NSCLC genes like EGFR and ALK(Ferreira et al., 2021)Tsoulos et al., 2017; (Lu & Lu, 2017).

2.1 Multi-omics integration

In omics analyses, genomic, transcriptomic, and physiogenetic data, as well as single-cell sequencing, are examined to investigate gene mutation patterns, gene expression, and cellular interactions. Examples of combining these data to understand the complexity of NSCLC have been carried out so far, which have led to the identification of mutations that are effective in disease recurrence. Advanced deep learning models, such as the MOLUNGN model, utilize these data and distinguish different subtypes of this cancer by establishing distinct networks and correlation relationships. Pathways of progression and key axes within these pathways are identified to select genes effective in growth and survival, as well as therapeutic and drug targets. Studies are also being conducted on the use of medical images (D. Zhang et al., 2025).

Multi-omics analyses are one of the newest methods in the field of biological data analysis, combining genomic, transcriptomic, epigenetic, metabolomic, immunological, and liquid biopsies with single-cell sequencing data to investigate gene mutation patterns, gene expression, and cellular interactions. Examples of combining these data to understand the complexity of NSCLC have been carried out so far, which have led to the identification of effective mutations and biomarkers such as IL-6 and IL-8 in disease recurrence. Advanced deep learning models, such as the MOLUNGN model, also utilize these data and distinguish the subtypes of this cancer by establishing different networks and correlation relationships. They identify the progression pathways and key axes within these pathways to select genes effective in growth and survival, including biomarkers and the best therapeutic and drug targets. The results of these studies include various commercialized tests. For example, the Pervenio Lung RS utilizes 14 selected genes, including KRAS, BRAF, EGFR, HER2, ALK, and p53, to identify patients with early-stage non-squamous non-small cell lung cancer (NSCLC). The test is being introduced by Pinpoint Genomics or Life Technologies (Kratz et al., 2012; Kratz, Mann, et al., 2013; Kratz, Tham, et al., 2013).

MyPlan Lung Cancer, offered by Myriad Genetics, also uses cell cycle gene expression data, with microarray analysis. The test provides specialists with quantitative and scored indicators to guide treatment decisions (Bueno et al., 2015; Wistuba et al., 2013).

MicroRNA tests, such as MSC (MicroRNA Signature Classifier, plasma microRNA signature) and miR-Test (serum microRNA signature), are another common test derived from omics data analysis. Molecular data and detailed bioinformatics analyses that use microRNA markers in patients' blood or plasma for prognosis and diagnosis. These tests are very useful for screening and reducing unnecessary biopsies (F. Bianchi et al., 2011; Boeri et al., 2011; Montani et al., 2015; Sozzi et al., 2014).

3. IMMUNOTHERAPY

One of the most effective therapeutic approaches for non-small cell lung cancer (NSCLC) is immunotherapy, which encompasses several methods. While this approach has its limitations and not all patients respond positively, the development of new antibodies combined with innovative techniques has proven effective in minimizing side effects and enhancing the overall efficacy of treatment methods(Krzyżanowska et al., 2022).

3.1 CAR-T Cell Therapy

Chimeric antigen receptors (CARs) provide engineered specificity for T cells by utilizing fusion proteins. To date, five generations of CAR T cells have been developed, each aimed at enhancing the efficacy of the therapy through various designs and modifications of intracellular and extracellular domains. This innovative treatment approach has revolutionized the management of hematologic malignancies, particularly when used in combination therapy to enhance treatment outcomes. Regarding NSCLC, common antigens targeted in CAR T cell therapy include epidermal growth factor receptor (EGFR), mesothelin (MSLN), prostate stem cell antigen (PSCA), and mucin 1 (MUC1). These antigens are considered attractive targets because they are overexpressed in NSCLC. Additionally, researchers are investigating new antigens such as erythropoietin-producing hepatocellular carcinoma A2 (EphA2), tissue factor (TF), and protein tyrosine kinase 7 (PTK7) as potential targets for CAR T cell therapy (H. Y. Ma et al., 2023).

The most common challenges regarding this treatment are:

1. Poor T-cell filtration into the microenvironment and T-cell exhaustion. In non-small cell lung cancer (NSCLC), T-cell infiltration into the tumor microenvironment is often inadequate, resulting in T-cell exhaustion. To enhance treatment efficiency, synchronizing gene editing methods like CRISPR-Cas9 with CAR T cell therapy can be beneficial by knocking out genes responsible for this exhaustion.
2. Heterogeneous tumor antigens in NSCC. To address heterogeneity in non-small cell carcinoma (NSCC), multi-targeting CARs, including dual, bicistronic, tandem, and inhibitory CARs, are being developed and tested in animal models and clinical trials.

3.CAR T cell manufacturing is costly and time-consuming. However, using automated manufacturing systems and closed bioreactor systems can help lower costs, reduce production time, and minimize contamination rates. Additionally, optimizing growth media can enhance the functionality of the cells. Technologies such as AI, machine learning, and neural networks can further optimize the production process, assist in the design of CARs, and provide predictions about patient outcomes, ultimately reducing expenses (Alaa Ali & DiPersio, 2024).

4.The tumor microenvironment is immunosuppressive. Binding CAR-T cells to checkpoint inhibitors can effectively reduce immunosuppression in the tumor microenvironment. Checkpoint inhibitor immunotherapy, a novel approach to counteracting the immunosuppressive tumor environment, can enhance the efficacy of immune responses, such as those mediated by PD-1/PD-L1 inhibitors (H. Y. Ma et al., 2023). The second generation of strategies based on CAR T cell therapy utilizes multitargeted CARs, enhancing T cell specificity while reducing toxicities and on-target/off-tumor effects (Qu et al., 2021).

Current studies have focused on enhancing the efficacy of CAR T cell therapy, particularly in the context of metastatic cancers. This approach enhances drug bioavailability in targeted areas, particularly where barriers such as the blood-brain barrier can limit its effectiveness. In metastatic NSCLC, the co-expression of certain receptors, such as CCL2 or CCR2b, alongside CAR T cells has been shown to improve treatment efficacy. Another strategy involves using microwave ablation (MWA) to remodel the tumor microenvironment (TME). This technique enhances tumor suppression by specifically targeting receptors. However, tracking CAR T cells in NSCLC to fully understand their mechanism of action can be challenging. Molecular imaging provides valuable assessment tools for various cancers, utilizing radionuclides through positron emission tomography (PET) or other methods, such as single-photon emission computed tomography (SPECT). For instance, 18-F-fluorodeoxyglucose (F-FDG) with PET/CT is a recognized method for staging and monitoring treatment response in NSCLC. To address the tracking challenges, two preclinical imaging techniques are employed: direct and indirect labeling using reporter genes, including antibodies, enzymes, and symporters. Additionally, small and nano molecules facilitate in vivo tracking of cell migration. However, these methods are not without limitations. For example, direct labeling may be hindered by potentially toxic effects from small tracker molecules or their short half-lives. Further research is essential for effectively monitoring CAR T therapy in solid tumors, such as NSCLC, to advance its development and clinical application (H. Y. Ma et al., 2023).

3.2 Immune Checkpoint Inhibitors

Immune checkpoint inhibitors are an emerging approach in immunotherapy that focuses on enhancing the immune system's ability to combat cancer rather than directly killing cancer cells. These pharmacologic agents work by targeting specific checkpoints, inhibiting ligand/receptor interactions, and preventing immune escape. This process can restore the activity of cytotoxic T-cells as well as improve their activation, proliferation, and differentiation. Common checkpoint inhibitors used to treat non-small cell lung cancer (NSCLC) include the anti-PD-1 monoclonal antibodies nivolumab and pembrolizumab, the anti-PD-L1 monoclonal antibodies atezolizumab and nivolumab, and the anti-CTLA-4 monoclonal antibodies ipilimumab and tremelimumab. Despite benefits, there are some potential adverse effects associated with checkpoint inhibitor therapy. These can include immune reactions and toxicity in various organ systems, such as gastrointestinal, endocrine, dermatologic, neurological, cardiovascular, and pulmonary systems. Additionally, patients may experience infusion reactions, which can manifest as allergic reactions, rashes, or dizziness (H. Y. Ma et al., 2023; Tang et al., 2022).

3.3 Cancer Vaccines

One of the most effective strategies for cancer treatment is the development of vaccines. Vaccines, a form of immunotherapy, play a significant role in treating and preventing tumor progression. Their production has notably increased following the COVID-19 pandemic. Most cancer vaccines are either DNA or peptide-based, and the advancements in mRNA-based vaccines for COVID-19 have also spurred growth in cancer vaccine development. Despite progress, the vaccines developed thus far still face several challenges. Common issues include the risk of non-specific immune reactions, the necessity for effective gene delivery methods (such as electroporation), the requirement for adjuvants (which act as immune boosters), and limitations related to patients' specific HLA types (which is important for genetic compatibility). The most common vaccines in development for the treatment of NSCLC are:

Peptide/Protein with Dendritic Cell:

These vaccines are made from peptides derived from tumor antigens that the immune system targets. They can be administered intravenously, intradermally, or intramuscularly. One promising protein-peptide vaccine is CIMAvax-EGF, which is produced from epidermal growth factor (EGF) and binds to EGF receptors. This vaccine was developed in the United States and has shown increased effectiveness when used in combination with immunotherapy drugs, such as Nivolumab. Other antigen vaccines currently undergoing clinical trials for the treatment of NSCLC include MAGE-A3, NY-ESO-1, and L-BLP25 (Tecemotide)(Flores Banda et al., 2025).

DNA Vaccines:

These vaccines are currently in development and have not yet reached the clinical phase. However, they seem to be more effective than peptide vaccines because they stimulate multiple components of the immune system simultaneously. Additionally, they tend to be less expensive and more stable (Lopes et al., 2019).

Vector Vaccines

These vaccines include modified viruses that carry genes coding for antigens, which trigger the immune system's response. They are currently in clinical trials, and two common side effects include inflammation and allergic reactions (Sasso et al., 2020). The combination vaccine MG1-MAGEA3 + Ad-MAGEA3 is currently undergoing clinical trials (Pol et al., 2019).

Dendritic Cell (DC) Vaccines

A type of advanced immunotherapy vaccine uses dendritic cells to activate the immune system. These vaccines are currently undergoing clinical trials; however, they are not expected to be widely available due to their high cost and complexity. Alongside these vaccines, drugs like pembrolizumab are considered powerful treatment options (Murphy et al., 2023)Y.-L. Wu et al., 2011).

Allogenic Vaccines

These vaccines are currently in the research and clinical trial stages, aiming to provide stronger immunity to recipients by utilizing tumor antigens derived from infected donors. Because they are administered subcutaneously, these vaccines tend to have few side effects. Additionally, they are less expensive to produce and more readily available compared to other methods. However, since their primary targets are tumor cells, there is a potential risk of inducing immune system-suppressing responses (Satoh et al., 1997; Klopp et al., 2007).

Messenger RNA (mRNA) Vaccines

The success of Moderna and Pfizer's COVID-19 vaccines has opened new avenues for cancer treatment. Unlike traditional vaccines that inject proteins, these mRNA vaccines use messenger RNA to deliver genetic instructions for creating the antigen. Currently, BNT116 and V940 are two mRNA-based vaccines undergoing clinical trials, with BNT116 currently in the trial phase across seven countries (Teo, 2022; Lorentzen et al., 2022; Flores Banda et al., 2025).

Neoantigens Vaccines

Neoantigens are unique short peptides found in tumor cells that may address resistance to current treatments. However, they have only been tested in a limited number of patients, necessitating larger studies (Su et al., 2023).

3.4 Immunotherapy, concerns and challenges

Despite significant advances in immunotherapy, several problems and challenges persist that hinder the full success of this new technology. Serious side effects, such as immune-related adverse events (irAEs), cause hyperactive immune reactions that require special care for patients. Additionally, inflammation and damage to healthy tissues, as well as the difficulty in controlling and predicting side effects, create limitations in the use of this method. In addition, the high cost of immunotherapy drugs, including CAR-T cells and immune checkpoint inhibitors, as well as the need for specialized infrastructure, creates accessibility issues for some patients. In some patients, tumor resistance to some immunotherapies and the patient's diverse responses to treatment create challenges in the treatment process. Moreover, ethical considerations in the use of genetic and clinical data from patients in new treatments are a persistent concern related to the use of new technologies, which require more extensive studies to ensure safety and efficacy in the clinic (Sui et al., 2024).

4. TARGETING THE TUMOR MICROENVIRONMENT

Recent studies have shown that the environment surrounding a tumor plays a crucial role in understanding cancer cells and applying effective treatment methods. This environment consists of various components, including immune cells, fibroblasts, the extracellular matrix, and stem cells. A promising area of research in the study of the tumor microenvironment is targeting these components as part of cancer treatment strategies(Lopes et al., 2019).

Different therapeutic approaches are being developed to investigate the tumor microenvironment, and we will discuss these separately. Examining the microenvironment can serve as a biomarker to assess the severity of cancer. It offers insights into gene expression patterns within this environment, which can be predictive of tumor progression and can be analyzed alongside other biomarkers(Qu et al., 2021).

Changes in T-cell numbers within this environment improved therapeutic strategies and predicted treatment effectiveness and response rates (Bremnes et al., 2016).

4.1 Targeted Therapy and TME

Research indicates that targeting components of the tumor microenvironment in personalized therapy can enhance the effectiveness of existing treatments. Ongoing studies focus on cancer-associated fibroblasts (CAFs), vascular growth factors, immune cells, hypoxia, and other elements within this environment to improve therapeutic methods and treatment responses (L. Chen et al., 2022).

4.2 Immunotherapy and TME

One of the emerging fields in microenvironment studies is the use of immunotherapy methods. For instance, bispecific antibodies can stimulate a more active immune response in tumor cells by targeting these cells and recruiting additional immune cells to the area (L. Wang et al., 2023).

4.3 Microbiome and TME

One of the emerging topics in the field of microenvironments is the study of the tumor microbiome and its surrounding environment. Each tumor has a unique microbiome that can influence the onset of cancer, the rate of its progression, and the tumor's response to treatment (Wong-Rolle et al., 2021). Research indicates that tumor-associated microbes activate cancer pathways, including the PI3K pathway, in non-small cell lung cancer (Gustafson et al., 2010). Modulating the microbiome and its composition through the use of inhaled antibiotics or probiotics could lead to new treatment options (Le Noci et al., 2018).

4.4 Liquid Biopsy and TME

Liquid biopsies have been introduced as a noninvasive method for diagnosis. When obtained from the peritumoral area, these biopsies can reveal dynamic changes in the tumor microenvironment (TME). This area contains compounds secreted by the tumor, which can provide important diagnostic markers, inflammatory factors, indicators of treatment response, and even prognostic information (She et al., 2024).

4.5 Omics Analysis and TME

Omics studies provide detailed insights into the tumor microenvironment, enabling personalized and targeted treatment approaches that ultimately improve treatment responses. For instance, analyzing gene expression data, protein expression levels, and signaling pathways can help predict a patient's response to immunotherapy. This information allows doctors to make wiser decisions regarding drug prescriptions and treatment plans (Z. Huang et al., 2021).

4.6 Nanoparticle-Based Delivery and TME

In addition to investigating the tumor microenvironment, nanoparticles have emerged as a promising approach in targeted therapeutic methods. The macroenvironment can contribute to resistance against immunotherapy. However, nanoparticles have the ability to cross biological barriers and accumulate in tumor areas, which enhances drug delivery. This advancement has the potential to lead to more effective treatments (P. Wu et al., 2022).

4.7 Organoids and TME

To understand the significance of macroenvironment components, researchers are developing organoid and three-dimensional culture models. These models are designed to investigate the effects of various therapeutic methods, including immunotherapy, targeted therapy, treatment responses, and the interactions between the components of the macroenvironment (Neal et al., 2018; Xia et al., 2021).

5. MICROFLUIDIC SYSTEMS

Microfluidic platforms represent a cutting-edge technology in cancer research. Developing Precision Oncology has led to the creation of high-precision sampling techniques based on molecular abnormalities. Circulating Tumor Cells (CTCs) have the potential to be diagnostic markers, particularly in the early stages of cancer. A microfluidic chip can efficiently capture and isolate CTCs for the analysis of genetic mutations. For example, in NSCLC patients, mutations such as EGFR, KRAS, and BRAF can be detected on a chip, which may not be identifiable through standard cell searches. Although this innovative technology has significant applications for cancer detection, further research is necessary to enhance detection sensitivity (Ogidi et al., 2024; Watanabe et al., 2018; S.-Q. Wang et al., 2020).

6. COMBINATION THERAPIES

One of the advanced treatments for non-small cell lung cancer (NSCLC) is combination therapy. This approach can enhance patients' survival rates, as using multiple treatments can lead to more effective results. Combination therapy typically involves a mix of immunotherapy with chemotherapy, radiotherapy, dual immunotherapy, and targeted therapy. The low objective response rate (ORR) of immunotherapy prompts oncologists to combine it with traditional and newer treatments to improve effectiveness. Combination therapy is crucial for managing metastatic non-small cell lung cancer and can lead to improved patient outcomes (Tang et al., 2022).

7. MICROBIOTA AND HOST FACTORS

One of the emerging areas in cancer research is the study of the microbiome. Recent investigations have revealed the impact of the lung microbiome on the development of lung cancer and the response to treatment. There is a growing interest in exploring this relationship using various methods, including meta-transcriptomics (RNA sequencing), metabolomics (small-molecule analysis), bioinformatics, and software tools such as QIIME2 (Quantitative Insights into Microbial Ecology), PICRUSt2 (Phylogenetic Investigation of Communities by Reconstruction of Unobserved States), and MaAsLin2 (Microbiome Multivariable Association with Linear Models)(Caporaso et al., 2010; Bolyen et al., 2019; Langille et al., 2013; Douglas et al., 2020).

Investigating entire microbial communities can yield significant insights into cancer research. Sputum and bronchoalveolar lavage (BAL) fluid are commonly used samples for these studies (Whiteside et al., 2021). In addition to age and sex, the lung microbiome can be influenced by smoking and certain medications. Specific bacteria, such as Acidovorax, Capnocytophaga, and Veillonella, are strongly associated with lung cancer. (Yan et al., 2015; García-Pachón & Padilla-Navas, 2020; Maldonado et al., 2023).

The importance of the lung microbiome profile in relation to lung cancer risk, including both malignant and benign forms, as well as its role in classification, early detection, and metastasis, is a significant topic in this field (Ji et al., 2023; Wang et al., 2023; Xue et al., 2023).

In addition to the tumor microbiome, the intratumor microbiome is an interesting and emerging field of study in cancer treatment (Giraldo et al., 2019; Xue et al., 2023). It is a significant component of the tumor microenvironment, and any changes in its composition or the metabolites encoded by intratumor bacteria can affect cancer, tumorigenesis, cancer progression, and drug resistance(M. Wang et al., 2023; Dejea et al., 2018; Nejman et al., 2020). The study of the microbiome has several limitations that require further investigation. For example, concerns regarding accuracy, low-biomass microbial populations, and complex computational challenges for microbiome analysis are common challenges to address (Souza et al., 2023). The study of the microbiome has limitations that require further investigation. For instance, issues related to accuracy, low-biomass microbial populations, and the complex computational challenges in microbiome analysis are common obstacles to overcome (J. Liu & Zhang, 2022; Bharti & Grimm, 2021).

Recent research has revealed the impact of microbiomes on the effectiveness of immunotherapy methods. Studies indicate that altering microbiome composition through diet, probiotics, or inhaled microbial therapies can improve treatment outcomes. These modifications enhance immune responses, reduce immune suppression, and offer personalized immunotherapy strategies. For example, the gut microbiome can increase the efficacy of immune checkpoint inhibitors, while the lung microbiome can help decrease lung metastasis (Shaikh et al., 2019; Sivan et al., 2015; Vétizou et al., 2015; Le Noci et al., 2018).

Future combination therapies that incorporate immunotherapy and microbiome modulation are expected to be among the emerging methods in cancer treatment. Additionally, understanding the specific combinations of microbiomes is crucial because the occurrence of cancer can be influenced by chemical substances produced by bacteria, such as Clostridium cholephorum, as well as genomic instability(Cuevas-Ramos et al., 2010; He et al., 2019; Attene-Ramos et al., 2006; Carbonero et al., 2012), Damage to a host's DNA caused by bacteria, alteration of gene expression by bacterial toxins, and integration of bacterial DNA into the host's genome (Greathouse et al., 2018; Tsay et al., 2018).

As mentioned, modifying the composition of the microbiome is an emerging strategy aligned with personalized treatment for non-small cell lung cancer (NSCLC). Preclinical models are utilized in clinical trials to enhance our understanding of how the microbiome impacts cancer treatment. Some personalized approaches to cancer therapy include dietary management, as research has shown that high-fiber diets, fasting, long-term calorie restrictions, and ketogenic diets can influence the structure of the gut microbiome. These dietary changes can lead to improved immune responses and enhance anticancer immunosurveillance (Park et al., 2022; Costa et al., 2024; Dai et al., 2021).

The developing field of NSCLC therapy includes fecal microbiota transplantation (FMT). Eiseman first introduced this concept in 1958, and subsequent researchers have continued to explore it as a modern treatment approach (D. Chen et al., 2019; Shaikh et al., 2019).

The objective of microbiome studies is to identify non-invasive and reliable biomarkers for detection and diagnosis. Researchers aim to pinpoint therapeutic targets based on microbiome communities and to manage tumor growth by using antibiotics, probiotics, or microbial metabolites that influence tumor cell proliferation. Additionally, these studies seek to establish the microbiome as a supplementary diagnostic tool. This area of research can be considered a subset of precision oncology and personalized therapy (Dong et al., 2021). Diversity in microbiome communities among individuals, regions, and ethnic groups presents challenges for researchers (Lee et al., 2024).

8. EPIGENETIC THERAPY APPROACH

Research has concentrated on combining epigenetic agents with standard cancer treatments. Epigenetic drugs may be suitable for patients who cannot undergo aggressive chemotherapy and for those with high-risk NSCLC (Sandoval et al., 2013). Epigenetic therapy involves the silencing or activation of specific genes, targeting only cancer cells and resulting in fewer side effects. These therapies are often used in combination with other treatments. Clinical trials have demonstrated that combining epigenetic drugs with other methods can produce a priming effect. This means that epigenetic drugs enhance the responsiveness of tumor cells to other types of treatments. Two common examples of epigenetic drugs are DNMT inhibitors (DNMTi) and histone deacetylase inhibitors (HDACi), which are often used in combination with chemotherapy, monoclonal antibodies, or tyrosine kinase inhibitors (Schiffmann et al., 2016). In addition to epigenetic therapies, several epigenetic biomarkers are emerging for the detection of NSCLC and for guiding therapeutic options. Common epigenetic changes include DNA cytosine methylation, alterations in microRNA expression, and modifications to histone proteins. However, further investigations are needed for clinical application (Ansari et al., 2016; Balgkouranidou et al., 2013; Van Den Broeck et al., 2008; Miyanaga et al., 2008; Xi et al., 2013; Ansari et al., 2016). Investigations are ongoing, revealing significant opportunities for these drugs in the treatment of NSCLC.

9. NANOMEDICINE AND NSCLC

The development of nanotechnology is very promising due to the use of small, biocompatible particles in the process of cancer diagnosis and treatment. The use of nanotechnology is developing in various areas of diagnosis and treatment, which we will discuss below (Chaturvedi et al., 2019).

9.1 Nanoparticles for the treatment and diagnosis of NSCLC

Nanoparticles are increasingly being utilized in the treatment of NSCLC because nano-based approaches can effectively reach cancer cells and penetrate tissues, improving bioavailability (Siddique & Chow, 2022). This technology has helped address the problem of drug resistance, reduce toxicity, enhance early detection pathways, facilitate precise treatment management, increase survival, and improve the quality of life for patients. Various common nanoparticles, including gold nanoparticles, carbon nanotubes, aptamer-based nanoparticles, liposomes, micelles, polymeric nanoparticles, and solid lipid nanoparticles, are currently being researched (Sibuyi et al., 2021; Cai et al., 2023). Studies show that, so far, polylactic acid-glycolic acid (PLGA) nanoparticle modified with chitosan and RGD peptide have been used for targeted drug delivery of paclitaxel-cyclic doxorubicin based on RGD peptide - various types of advanced organic and inorganic nanoparticles have been used (Carrasco-Esteban et al., 2021; J. Wang et al., 2021)

9.2 Bio-conjugated nanoparticles and molecular targeting in NSCLC

The attachment of biological ligands, such as antibodies, aptamers, peptides, or small molecules, to nanoparticles enables them to specifically bind to cancer cells. In this way, most nanoparticles can be more effective and less toxic. However, the possibility of immune recognition and elimination remains; to overcome this challenge, biomimetic methods are used to coat nanoparticles, achieving more precise drug delivery. The attachment of these particles to diagnostic and therapeutic markers for non-small cell lung cancer (NSCLC), such as EGFR, RET, KRAS, ALK, ROS1, and NTRK1, is an emerging area of development. This process leads to the creation of bioconjugated drugs and revolutionizes treatment options(J. Wang et al., 2021).

9.3 Nanoimaging and early diagnosis of NSCLC

One of the newest applications of nanotechnology in the imaging and early diagnosis of NSCLC is the use of multimodal MRI, gadolinium-iron oxide nanoparticles, and extracorporeal optical coherence tomography (EOCT). These methods are highly accurate and precise, allowing for non-invasive and reproducible performance. These methods utilize nanoparticles carrying targeted drugs to the tumor area, thereby reducing drug toxicity while increasing the accuracy of drug dosing and diagnosis. Iron oxide and gadolinium nanoparticles with their superparamagnetic and special properties as contrast agents in MRI increase the sensitivity and accuracy of NSCLC tumor diagnosis. These nanoparticles have the ability to bind to tumor cells, enabling high-resolution and non-invasive imaging. Additionally, using the inhalation route to deliver these nanoparticles, compared to intravenous injection, leads to higher sensitivity and contrast-to-noise ratio (CNR) and lower toxicity (A. Bianchi et al., 2014).

9.4 Nanocarriers and targeted drug delivery for NSCLC

Precision nanomedicine has emerged from the integration of innovative therapeutic strategies, including targeted therapy and drug delivery. For these approaches, liposomal nanoparticles are used as drug carriers in the treatment of NSCLC. The use of nanocarriers offers greater efficacy due to reduced toxicity and targeted drug release, thereby reducing drug side effects on healthy tissues (Jin et al., 2018; D. Liu et al., 2011). These carriers utilize lapatinib-perfluorocarbon nanoparticles coated with PEG for enhanced stability in the bloodstream and increased solubility, as well as specific peptides incorporated into the structure of these particles to facilitate deeper tissue penetration (Majumder & Minko, 2021; Y. Sun et al., 2022).

9.5 Nanomedicine and targeted therapies and immunotherapy

Nanomedicine is a targeted therapy that delivers drug carriers precisely to cancer cells with the aid of immunotherapy, thereby increasing the effective dose of the drug and enhancing its effectiveness while reducing systemic toxicity. The use of immune checkpoint inhibitors (such as PD-1/PD-L1 and CTLA-4) and nano-immune systems that precisely and simultaneously deliver chemotherapeutic drugs, targeted antibodies, and multiple immunological factors to the tumor and its microenvironment leads to targeting of cancer-related biological pathways and remodeling of the immune response, increasing the effectiveness of treatment, reducing side effects, reducing tumor resistance, and improving the immune response. For example, studies have shown that ARAC nanoparticles, a combination of a PLK1 inhibitor and an anti-PD-L1 antibody, have led to a reduction in drug doses and an improved therapeutic response in animal models of lung cancer, resulting in fewer drug side effects (Doroudian et al., 2023).

9.6 Clinical problems and challenges of nanomedicines

In addition to the advantages mentioned for nanomedicine, there are also challenges and limitations for this technology. Among them, we can mention the high cost of nanomedicines, which limits access for low-income patients. Additionally, the technological complexity of this technology necessitates advanced infrastructure and the presence of specialized personnel, which limits its accessibility in various locations. Concerns about the safety and toxicity of nanoparticles in long-term use and the development of drug resistance also reduce the effectiveness of drugs(Doroudian et al., 2023).

10. ORGANOIDS & PATIENT-DERIVED XENOGRAFTS

One of the current models used to study non-small cell lung cancer (NSCLC) is the patient-derived xenograft (PDX) model. These platforms are designed to display the histopathological and therapeutic characteristics of primary tumor cells, as well as tumor heterogeneities, gene expression, and mutations. PDX models are commonly utilized for preclinical screening, drug testing, biomarker discovery, and translational research(X. Chen et al., 2021).

11. PERSONALIZED MEDICINE, BIOMARKER-DRIVEN THERAPY

Until now, standard care for non-small cell lung cancer (NSCLC) has been based on the tumor's primary location and the patient's histology. However, the advent of precision medicine in the early 2000s initiated a revolution in cancer treatment. Recent advancements in this field present potentially effective strategies. In precision oncology, treatment plans are tailored based on specific biomarkers, aiming for maximum effectiveness, suggesting targeted therapies, and minimizing drug toxicity. Currently, personalized medicine approaches in cancer treatment are interdisciplinary and focus on the following:

* Tumor histology
* molecular profile of tumor cells
* Immune profile of patients
* patient's microbiota

Histological types, such as adenocarcinoma, large cell carcinoma, squamous cell carcinoma, and NSCLC, play a significant role in determining appropriate medications and drug combinations. In terms of molecular profiling, mutations in genes such as BRAF, EGFR, HER2, ROS1, as well as ALK rearrangements, RET fusions, and MET amplification are crucial for guiding targeted therapy. Multiplex and next-generation sequencing (NGS) panels are becoming increasingly common due to their affordability, which surpasses that of single-gene analyses. These methods are also more affordable and help save time and reduce the need for tissue samples. Regarding immune profiling, research has led to the development of immunotherapy drugs. Anti-cancer vaccines exemplify treatment approaches based on immune profiles, as they harness adaptive immunity mechanisms, immune checkpoint inhibitors (ICIs), and signals that modulate immune responses (Mascaux et al., 2017). Research indicates that gut microbiota can influence anti-cancer responses. Precision medicine now integrates pharmacogenomics with microbial organisms and their specific metabolites to enhance therapeutic outcomes (Roy & Trinchieri, 2017).

12. RADIOTHERAPY

One method for managing the treatment of non-small cell lung cancer (NSCLC) is radiotherapy, which has seen significant improvements and advancements in recent years. Radiotherapy serves as an effective monotherapy for advanced stages of NSCLC or in combination with other methods, such as chemotherapy, to enhance its effectiveness. One of the major challenges in radiotherapy is precisely targeting the tumor site. Recent developments in this field include three-dimensional conformal techniques (3D-CRT), designed to minimize damage to healthy tissues surrounding the tumor. In contrast, conventional two-dimensional (2-D) techniques are limited by their low accuracy in distinguishing tumor boundaries, particularly due to the movement of lung tissue (Koka et al., 2022). This treatment method has notable side effects such as fatigue, nausea, and vomiting. New methods have been developed in radiotherapy, including several that are emerging in this field:

12.1 XPDT / EBRT

One of the emerging trends in radiotherapy is Combinatorial Radiotherapy, which includes X-ray-induced Photodynamic Therapy (X-PDT). This innovative approach utilizes radiation to both kill cancer cells and activate therapeutic drugs. X-PDT is particularly useful for treating deep tumors that cannot be addressed with traditional Photodynamic Therapy (PDT). By generating free radicals, this method damages the DNA of cancer cells, allowing for targeted treatment. The development of advanced technologies, such as smart nanodevices like IRaGAZ, exemplifies the progress being made in this field(Tetzlaff et al., 2006)H. Liu et al., 2020). Drugs such as ALA, MAL, HAL, Photofrin, Curcumin, and Anthraquinones are among the photosensitizing medications that are being utilized and have received the necessary approvals for this method (Wilson, 2002; Ormond & Freeman, 2013).

12.2 FLASH Radiotherapy (FLASH-RT)

This is one of the newest and most promising treatment methods for non-small cell lung cancer (NSCLC), although it has not yet been widely adopted in clinical practice. In this approach, a high dose of radiation is delivered rapidly to the tumor area, significantly minimizing damage to surrounding healthy tissues. So far, this method has primarily utilized electrons, which are effective for superficial or shallow tumors, but research is also being conducted on protons, photons, and ionic flashes. Because individual responses to treatment can vary based on the biological characteristics of the cells and the tumor environment, this method must be tailored to each patient and cannot be applied uniformly to everyone(Matuszak et al., 2022).

The integration of artificial intelligence into radiotherapy techniques has led to advancements that enable specialists to pinpoint the precise location for radiation exposure, create treatment plans, and analyze the structure and size of tumors for effective radiotherapy. One notable device that incorporates AI is the MR-Linac. Below, we provide a table comparing the advantages and disadvantages of the latest and emerging radiotherapy methods for non-small cell lung cancer (NSCLC) (Saadeddin, 2012).

Table 1. Advantages and disadvantages of growing radiotherapy methods

Methods	Advantages	Disadvantages
IGRT (Image-Guided Radiotherapy)	High precision during treatment - suitable for moving organs such as the lungs	The time-consuming process of taking photos
SBRT (Stereotactic Body Radiation Therapy)	Suitable for small tumors or inoperable patients	High possible side effects
Particle Therapy	Extremely high accuracy and drastically reduced side effects	Very expensive and complicated
XPDT	For deep tumors - minimal damage to adjacent tissues	Not yet usable

12.3 Radiation Therapy Innovations

Particle Therapy

One of the newest types of radiation therapy utilizes heavy particles, including protons, neutrons, and carbon ions. However, this method is currently only available in a limited number of centers worldwide and is very expensive. Despite these challenges, it is considered one of the most promising treatment options. The use of proton particles also prevents damage to surrounding healthy tissues, such as the heart and esophagus, because their radiation is highly focused on the tumor area and passes through healthy tissues without causing the side effects associated with radiation therapy. For this reason, this method is particularly suitable for tumors located in central and vital areas due to the controlled radiation (Bayasgalan et al., 2021). FALBA (Fractionated Ablative Radio-Boron Neutron Capture Therapy) is recommended for advanced stages of non-small cell lung cancer (NSCLC) and requires specialized equipment and facilities. Three specific methods that fall under this category include Proton Beam Therapy, Boron Neutron Capture Therapy, and Carbon Ion Radiotherapy(Dell'Oro et al., 2020; G.-L. Jiang, 2012; Kinashi et al., 2017).

stereotactic body radiotherapy (SBRT)

SBRT is one of the newest radiotherapy methods used in the early stages of non-small cell lung cancer or inoperable cancers. In this method, high-precision radiation is directed at the tumor from multiple directions without damaging healthy tissue. Due to its effectiveness, the duration of treatment with this method is 3 to 5 sessions per week. This short period is a significant advantage of this treatment method, as it reduces side effects for the patient (Zhu et al., 2023).

12.4 Radiotherapy, challenges and concerns

The use of radiotherapy and imaging techniques, due to the need for advanced devices and technologies, consistently faces the challenge of financial constraints in providing equipment and the need for skilled professionals to operate these devices safely and prevent harm to patients. These challenges create limitations in access to medical centers for patients in remote geographical areas.

13. NSCLC THERAPY BASED ON FERROPTOSIS

One of the newest therapeutic approaches for non-small cell lung cancer (NSCLC) and overcoming drug resistance in this condition is the induction of ferroptosis. Ferroptosis is an iron-dependent mechanism that triggers cell death through a chemical process known as the Fenton reaction. This process results in lipid peroxidation and the accumulation of toxic reactive oxygen species (ROS) within the cell, ultimately leading to apoptosis. The Fenton reaction occurs between divalent iron (Fe^{2+}) and hydrogen peroxide (H_2O_2), producing highly toxic hydroxyl radicals (•OH). Various strategies, including gene therapy, small-molecule drugs, and nanoparticles, are being explored to induce ferroptosis. Iron nanoparticles can take different forms, such as amorphous particles, those combined with drugs, or Iron–Organic Frameworks (MONs). The use of nanoparticles and combination drug engineering plays a significant role in developing promising strategies for inducing ferroptosis in NSCLC(Zou et al., 2021).

The use of iron oxide nanoparticles (IO NPs), such as Ferumoxytol—which the FDA has approved for the treatment of anemia—takes advantage of their ability to accumulate in tumor tissue. These nanoparticles can produce divalent (Fe^{2+}) and trivalent (Fe^{3+}) iron ions, which react with hydrogen peroxide found in the tumor microenvironment. This reaction generates toxic hydroxyl radicals (•OH) that severely damage DNA, proteins, and membrane lipids. Ultimately, this process leads to ferroptosis and the death of cancer cells(P. Ma et al., 2017).

The combination of iron nanoparticles with fatty peroxides, such as LAHP, in the tumor's acidic environment leads to the release of singlet oxygen ($^1O_2$) and reactive oxygen species (ROS), thereby inducing ferroptosis (Z. Zhou et al., 2017). Amorphous iron nanoparticles (AFeNPs) have a disordered structure, making them highly reactive in acidic environments. This reactivity leads to rapid production of reactive oxygen species (ROS) and induces cell death (C. Zhang et al., 2016; P. Zhang et al., 2016).

Metal-organic frameworks (MOFs) are crystalline structures with high porosity that can induce both apoptosis and ferroptosis pathways in cancer cells by carrying genes such as p53, thereby inhibiting tumor growth (Z. Liu et al., 2022). In addition to iron nanoparticles, non-iron nanoparticles can also play a significant role in targeting cancer cells while minimizing harm to healthy cells. This approach is known as Indirect Iron-Based Nanomaterials. It utilizes α-MSH-PEG-C′ dot nanoparticles, which are composed of a fluorescent core (Cy5), a polyethylene glycol (PEG) coating, and α-MSH, a hormone with high receptor presence in certain cancers. These nanoparticles are injected into cancer cells under starvation conditions, leading to the induction of apoptosis (Shen et al., 2018).

In genetic engineering, apoptosis is often induced as part of the process. Two well-known mechanisms for this are gene transfection and gene knockdown. Apoptosis can be induced through the action of certain genes, such as p53 and ACSL4, while the knockdown of genes like NRF2 and p62, as well as the proteins CISD1, HSF1, and HSPB1, can also play a role in this process (Doll et al., 2017; S.-J. Wang et al., 2016; Kamp et al., 2016; H. Yuan et al., 2016b; Xiaofang Sun et al., 2016; H. Yuan et al., 2016a; X Sun et al., 2015).

Research has explored the effects of both natural and extracted drugs, as well as chemical and synthetic drugs, on the regulation of apoptosis induction. Notable examples of effective natural and herbal medicines include Artemisinin and its derivatives (ART and DHA), Huaier extract, Zinc, Curcumin, and Ginkgetin. Additionally, several chemical compounds have been studied, including Ammonium

Ferric Citrate (AFC), Erastin, XAV939, Levobupivacaine, and Auranofin (AF) (Zou et al., 2021).

Since this therapeutic pathway is new, ongoing research aims to uncover its effective functions. Bioinformatics studies and advanced statistical methods are identifying the genes involved in this pathway. Researchers are also focusing on understanding the relationships between miRNA, lncRNA, and drug interactions. For instance, non-coding RNAs—particularly miRNA and lncRNA—play a role in regulating cell death and ferroptosis by interfering with the reactive oxygen species (ROS) GPX4 pathways and cystine/glutamate transporters. As a result, these non-coding RNAs can serve as potential targets for targeted therapies aimed at modulating these pathways and cell death processes. Among the non-coding RNAs that have been studied and investigated in this pathway:

- miR-302a-3p
- miR-4443
- lncRNA NEAT1
- lncRNA MT1DP
- lncRNA LINC00336

Ferroptosis is being investigated as a way to tackle and manage treatment resistance problems in non-small cell lung cancer, particularly when chemotherapy, radiotherapy, and targeted therapies prove ineffective, such as in cases of drug resistance associated with Lapatinib and Cisplatin. An example of this approach involves Cisplatin-loaded iron nanoparticles, which deliver the anticancer drug cisplatin directly to tumor cells while simultaneously increasing reactive oxygen species (ROS) production upon drug release. This multifunctional system not only enhances the antitumor effect of the drug but also helps to reduce drug resistance (P. Ma et al., 2017).

Overall, the benefits of gene therapy include long-lasting effects, precise genetic modifications, and consistent induction. Nevertheless, ethical, legal, and safety concerns have hindered its widespread use in clinical settings (Zou et al., 2021).

Therapeutic small molecules that can serve as drugs are essential in cancer treatment due to their long half-lives, rapid metabolism, and low toxicity. However, they also have notable drawbacks, including side effects on healthy tissues, a lack of specificity for tumors, quick clearance from the bloodstream, and low accumulation in tumor sites. On the other hand, ferroptosis-inducing nanoparticles offer advantages in this context due to their precise targeting of tumors and the durability of ligand binding for active targeting. Nonetheless, these nanoparticles also have limitations, such as a shorter shelf life and potential long-term toxicity(Shen et al., 2018).

14. TUMOR-EDUCATED PLATELETS (TEPS) AS BIOMARKERS

One of the most recent diagnostic biomarkers for determining treatment options is tumor-derived platelets (TEPs), which contain tumor-related RNAs. TEPs can aid in the early detection of cancer, the localization of tumors, and the monitoring of treatment responses. Indicators for cancer diagnosis and treatment monitoring using TEPs include a high platelet count, platelet factor PF4, the platelet-to-lymphocyte ratio, and platelet infiltration into the tumor(Pucci et al., 2016; Rachidi et al., 2017; Best et al., 2018).

Analysis of RNA expression patterns in tumor endothelial cells (TEPs) and the application of machine learning algorithms for detecting RNA splicing patterns have led to the development of the thromboSeq platform, which is used for tumor subtype detection (Best et al., 2015). Another algorithm, known as Swarm Intelligence, utilizes RNAs as biomarkers for diagnosing non-small cell lung cancer(Best et al., 2017).

15. ARTIFICIAL INTELLIGENCE AND DIGITAL HEALTH

With the emergence of AI and machine learning-based medical platforms, a range of new AI tools has been developed to support oncologists, radiologists, patients, pharmacists, and healthcare professionals. Regarding NSCLC, these AI-based platforms could significantly contribute to cancer screening and diagnosis, differentiation of histological subtypes, treatment planning, and patient follow-up. The most common applications of AI in medicine and oncology include digital pathology, biomarker development, early diagnosis, cancer image classification, and outcome prediction (Senthil Kumar et al., 2023; Ladbury et al., 2023).

Deep learning, a key technology in machine learning (ML), involves the processing of multilayer or multistage nonlinear models. Several network learning models, such as Convolutional Neural Networks (CNNs), are commonly used for classifying input data. Artificial Neural Networks (ANN) are another example of these classifiers. Deep learning primarily employs two methods for data processing: supervised learning and unsupervised learning. In these methods, information is classified based on specific labels or similarities. Currently, the main areas of focus in artificial intelligence (AI) include genomics, transcriptomics, proteomics, metabolomics, immunomics, and microbiomics. In the field of genomics, AI-based tools are utilized to assess mutations, variations, and genomic instability, as well as to analyze gene amplification, chromosome numbers, and chromosomal structural variations (Y. Liu, 2020).

15.1 AI's role in screening and diagnosis

Integrated AI and clinical oncology diagnostic tools are being developed to enhance the treatment and medical management of patients. For instance, in the imaging process, AI can significantly assist radiologists by improving the accuracy of image readings. This not only leads to more precise detection but also reduces the time required for diagnosis. Regarding NSCLC, AI-based platforms can identify small nodules with high sensitivity, decreasing the likelihood of missed diagnoses, especially at early stages. Additionally, deep learning algorithms can help characterize these nodules more effectively(Y. Liu, 2020).

15.2 Radiomics and AI-driven imaging

AI's increased sensitivity and specificity, particularly in detecting smaller nodules, can enhance its performance as a secondary reader in cancer-related chest imaging, including CT and PET scans. However, further research is needed to improve AI's efficacy and conduct cost-effectiveness analyses (Megat Ramli et al., 2025).

In predicting early-stage metastasis, radiomics enhanced with AI shows promise. The combination of AI and PET/CT imaging can identify lymph node metastasis through radiomic ML markers and responses to immunotherapy (Rabbani et al., 2018; Zhong et al., 2023). In the genomic classification of various subtypes of non-small cell lung cancer (NSCLC), machine learning (ML) algorithms and classifiers can enhance the accurate characterization of tumors based on genomic data. While ML methods in clinical pathology are not yet widely adopted, they show promise for personalized therapy. Decision trees are used in marker detection. Moreover, support vector machines (SVMs), as another machine learning technique, are combined with immunohistochemistry (IHC) panels to achieve the highest detection accuracy (Rabbani et al., 2018).

AI is being developed to produce point-of-care biosensors for the detection of lung cancer. Research focuses on developing user-friendly tools that reduce labor intensity and provide minimally invasive applications. These biosensors typically utilize body fluids such as blood, serum, saliva, and urine to analyze a comprehensive array of protein and nucleic acid data, allowing for the differentiation between lung cancer patients and healthy individuals. The goal is to predict the risk of cancer metastasis, with sensitivity and selectivity being critical factors for these biosensors. However, challenges remain regarding the clinical use of these tools due to the lack of standardization in valid cut-off values, the number of biomarkers used, and the types of biomarkers present. The ongoing evolution of AI-assisted biosensors aims to enhance their performance and accuracy for detection, as well as create monitoring systems and recurrence surveillance, which can include wireless connectivity features

(Ng et al., 2025). I3LUNG is an AI decision-support tool that combines images, pathological data, genomic and transcriptomic data, and electronic health records (EHRs) to predict individual treatment responses, therapeutic recommendations, and survival rates (Senthil Kumar et al., 2023).

15.3 AI in treatment

AI can accelerate and improve the drug discovery process. Bringing new drugs to market can be both expensive and time-consuming, but AI has the potential to accelerate this process. Machine learning algorithms and AI-based simulations play a crucial role in identifying various compounds that interact with biological targets. Understanding protein folding and protein structures is essential for effective drug design. This understanding is facilitated by high-performance AI platforms, such as DeepMind's AlphaFold. This technology has the potential to advance the development of personalized medications (Lei, 2024).

Radiation oncology is a promising field for development using machine learning tools. Radiotherapy systems offer detailed information about patients, with high-quality digital records that track treatment history, including treatment volumes, durations, and dose rates. AI tools can analyze this raw data to create integrative predictive models, leading to improved clinical decisions, safer and more personalized radiation treatments, and a reduction in complications (Rabbani et al., 2018).

15.4 ML Models for Prognosis Prediction

Serial CTRS is an AI model developed by Onc.AI to predict treatment outcomes in patients with non-small cell lung cancer (NSCLC). This model is trained using CT scan data to forecast overall survival rates. A significant advancement in device designation from the FDA, supported by researchers from The James Cancer Center at Ohio State University (Sako et al., 2024).

15.5 Remote Patient Monitoring

During the Monitoring and Follow-Up phase, AI diagnostic tools can collect accurate data on nodule size, mass, and density over time. This information can inform potential treatments based on the behavior of nodules or help avoid unnecessary treatment for indolent nodules(Y. Liu, 2020).

15.6 Wearable devices

One of the non-invasive medical tools used in cancer treatment is wearable devices. According to Medical Device News Network, a notable example is Optune, developed by Novocure, which has been approved by the U.S. FDA for the treatment of metastatic non-small cell lung cancer (NSCLC). This device is placed on the skin over the lungs and uses alternating electric fields to disrupt electrically charged structures within tumor cells. This disruption interferes with cell division and growth, ultimately leading to cell death. Additionally, the device stimulates immune responses, influences cell mobility, and regulates gene expression, which can help prevent cell proliferation and metastasis. Optune Lua is intended for use in combination with immune therapy and chemotherapy to enhance effectiveness. The JAMA Network reported that the second type of wearable technology is home-based monitoring devices, which are used during the recovery phase. It's crucial to monitor patients after surgery, and one popular option is the Fitbit. This wearable device helps track and improve patients' physical activity to alleviate symptoms and enhance rehabilitation. Fitbit monitors daily steps, the intensity of physical activity, heart rate, sleep quality, and exercise duration. With this information, patients can receive instant feedback and make real-time adjustments to their activity levels. These personalized cancer care devices are emerging as valuable modern tools to support patients in their recovery.

About AI implications

There is ongoing investment in the actual clinical application of AI, particularly in clinical oncology. However, doctors and assistants face several challenges, including infrastructure issues, data validation, legal and ethical implications, as well as regulatory and economic considerations. Additionally, patient privacy and data protection against potential cyberattacks are significant concerns, making privacy policies crucial. In the near future, establishing a standardized, world-class database and promoting regulatory frameworks and audit systems will be essential for advancing AI in medicine and oncology, enabling more accurate and personalized therapies (Lei, 2024).

16. High-Impact Clinical Trial

Recent clinical trials report the results of the FLAURA2 study on the treatment of patients with NSCLC with EGFR mutations. The study was conducted by Professor Pasi A. Jänne of the Dana-Farber Cancer Institute on 550 patients in 21 countries worldwide. This study examined the effect of concomitant osimertinib (a third-generation tyrosine kinase inhibitor for EGFR) with chemotherapy and showed that this combination can increase progression-free survival (PFS) from 16.7 to 25.5 months. This result occurs despite an increase in the response rate among patients, and this combination has received FDA approval as a first-line treatment. The LAURA study on stage III NSCLC patients with EGFR mutations also showed that this drug, as an adjuvant treatment, leads to a significant improvement in patient survival, and the results of this study confirmed the FDA approval of this drug to improve the quality and length of life of patients(Garg et al., 2024; Planchard et al., 2025).

17. POST-TREATMENT MEASURES AND SURVIVORSHIP CARE PLAN

The survivorship care program should begin at the time of diagnosis and continue throughout the treatment process. These programs, along with post-treatment care, include various aspects of medical, psychological, social, and economic support, which we will discuss below. This care is carried out in 4 key areas, including relapse prevention, relapse monitoring - side effect management, and coordination of various specialists to manage the treatment process. Since surgery does not mean a definitive cure or no recurrence of the disease, regular follow-up after treatment is essential to prevent relapse and timely diagnosis if necessary, and helps increase the number of survivors. It is recommended that surveillance programs, including clinical examination and CT scan, be performed regularly at intervals of 6 to 12 months in the first 2 years(Vijayvergia et al., 2015).

17.1 Quality of Life Management

The survivorship care program should begin at the time of diagnosis and continue throughout the treatment process. These programs, along with post-treatment care, include various aspects of medical, psychological, social, and economic support, which we will discuss below. This care is carried out in 4 key areas, including relapse prevention, relapse monitoring, side effect management, and coordination of various specialists to manage the treatment process. Since surgery does not mean a definitive cure or no relapse of the disease, and a population study shows a 27% relapse rate of this disease, regular follow-up after treatment is essential to prevent relapse and timely diagnosis if necessary, and helps increase the number of survivors. It is recommended that surveillance programs, including clinical examination and CT scan, be performed regularly at intervals of 6 to 12 months in the first 2 years, and smoking cessation is also strongly emphasized in order to prevent relapse and the occurrence of secondary tumors. We will discuss the types of post-treatment care in detail below(Martini et al., 1995; Matsuda et al., 2012).

16.2 Palliative and Supportive Care

With the advent of cutting-edge technology and modern personalized medicine approaches, palliative care is no longer limited to the end of life. It has evolved into an innovative and specialized field of paramount importance that encompasses the entire journey from diagnosis to survivorship and end-of-life care. Today, palliative care not only reduces symptoms and improves quality of life but is also involved in early cancer detection through the use of advanced diagnostic methods. Furthermore, the expansion of psychotherapy has highlighted the significance of emotional support and psychological assistance for patients. Supportive care has also broadened to include managing side effects, providing nutritional counseling, and aiding in decision-making to select the most effective oncologic treatments. It is advisable for individuals experiencing clinical, physical, psychosocial, spiritual, and caregiver distress to consult a specialist in palliative care. A comprehensive and personalized care plan should be established, incorporating screening, assessment, diagnosis, treatment, and the post-treatment phase. Despite advancements in this field, a need remains for further research and replication of previous studies to enhance and develop palliative care frameworks from the moment of diagnosis through the entire disease process. Additionally, establishing a foundation for the involvement of specialists in both medical and legal aspects will facilitate quicker decision-making and ensure that patients and their families receive the most appropriate treatment together. As the severity of symptoms tends to escalate with disease progression, it is crucial to develop effective methods for controlling and monitoring symptoms. Two strategies that could be implemented in this regard are the provision of reliable tools for managing symptoms and ensuring access to a specialized support team that accompanies the patient throughout their journey (Chandrasekar et al., 2016).

16.2 Exercise, Nutrition, and Pain Management

This section highlights the most significant changes and emerging areas in palliative care. One of the most common symptoms experienced by patients with non-small cell lung cancer (NSCLC) is fatigue. These patients are also more likely to suffer from depression, leading to a decreased interest in socializing and exercising. These issues often become more pronounced during treatment due to physical weakness. Recent findings emphasize the importance of exercise interventions both before and after treatment, as patients who engage in physical activity tend to recover mentally and physically more quickly. As a result, there is a growing need to refer patients to rehabilitation centers that offer targeted exercise programs (Catherine L. Granger et al., 2014; Payne et al., 2013; Kuehr et al., 2014; C. L. Granger et al., 2011).

One common symptom in patients with MS is weight loss and a decreased appetite, which often begins at the time of diagnosis and may persist during various treatment methods. This is significant because patients require strong physical and mental capabilities to manage their condition effectively. Having a nutritionist to provide suitable nutritional supplements and a strengthening diet is essential. Additionally, regularly assessing the patient's physical condition during treatment and monitoring the impact of nutritional interventions are important considerations in this area (Fearon et al., 2006; Ross et al., 2004; van der Meij et al., 2012).

One of the most important issues in this field is pain management. During treatment, they often experience increased levels of pain. Effectively managing this pain requires collaboration among various specialists, including oncologists, pain specialists, psychiatrists, and nursing professionals. In addition to pain caused by the disease itself, patients may also encounter varying degrees of discomfort due to the metabolic effects of medications and their individual psychological tolerance. Consequently, the integration of complementary methods into the treatment process is becoming increasingly common. For example, patient treatment plans may now include education on meditation and mindfulness, as well as recommendations for therapies such as massage or acupuncture (Cassileth et al., 2007; C.-S. Yuan, 2007; Chute et al., 1985).

The treatment plan for the patient includes interventional methods such as radiofrequency ablation and radiotherapy, alongside the WHO Analgesic Ladder for effective pain management and analgesic prescriptions (Organization, 1996; Cassileth et al., 2007).

16.3 Respiratory support

In lung cancer, one important issue to address, alongside the different stages of the disease, is the dyspnea (difficulty breathing) that some patients experience. Providing education on necessary preventive measures as well as emotional and psychological support is crucial in palliative care for these patients. In addition to common medication prescriptions, recommended interventions include proper breathing training, lifestyle modifications, and the provision of portable oxygen devices(Cheville et al., 2011; Abernethy et al., 2010).

16.4 Psychological Support

Managing a patient's psychological stress is one of the most important aspects of palliative care. Stress and depression can worsen the disease and hinder the recovery process. Many patients experience depression during their treatment, and neglecting both the physiological and psychological aspects of care in the context of advanced treatment methods can reduce the effects of the treatment (Fujisawa et al., 2015).

Tools like the Distress Thermometer have become essential in palliative care for evaluating the psychological stress experienced by patients and their coping strategies regarding their illness. Specialists should consider the patient's family relationships, financial concerns, and emotional well-being, and they are expected to refer patients to the appropriate specialists as needed(Graves et al., 2007).

Additionally, based on the mentioned cases, the Patient Support Associations Foundation is an advanced solution to enhance the role of spirituality in patients' health and address mental health concerns. These associations provide a platform for patients to express their challenges and concerns after treatment, as well as to follow up and monitor their condition to help prevent relapse (V. Sun et al., 2016).

An important aspect of palliative care is setting the proper time for hospice care. This decision is crucial as it allows the patient to experience less pain and suffering and provides the family with the opportunity to say goodbye and process their grief. Typically, this decision is made when the patient's life expectancy is estimated to be less than six months. Taking the necessary measures and planning effectively for this stage is essential(Lövgren et al., 2008; von Plessen et al., 2006; Greer et al., 2012).

Supporting and educating the patient's family is crucial, as concerns about losing a loved one, financial difficulties, and shifting responsibilities can lead to anxiety and depression among family members. This education should begin early in the patient's treatment process (Hendriksen et al., 2015; Porter et al., 2011).

18. GLOBAL DISPARITIES AND CARE ACCESS

Studies in the field of treatment inequalities reveal that economic, social, and racial factors are among the most significant factors influencing patient treatment outcomes. Low-income areas and deprived communities, due to lack of access to advanced treatments - modern drugs - early diagnostic methods - and lack of appropriate insurance coverage to cover treatment costs, show lower survival rates and more treatment complications. In addition to the factors mentioned, racial differences can also influence responses to treatment. For example, studies show that blacks have a higher rate of lung cancer than whites, and that socio-economic factors and access to diagnostic and therapeutic services are among the factors affecting this issue. Addressing this problem and ensuring justice in the care and treatment process, as well as increasing the quality and quantity of patient treatment, requires increased measures for medical infrastructure, including facilitating access to medical services, training specialist personnel, and cooperation between various bodies to provide medicine and financial support. In addition, taking specific measures for cultural education to raise awareness among individuals, providing medical services that are appropriate to the culture and social conditions of individuals, improving patient-doctor relationships to increase health literacy in society, risk assessment and population screening measures in high-risk groups, and using electronic patient monitoring programs and guiding individuals towards treatment paths with the help of digital technologies can provide more equitable access in society and improve treatment outcomes in deprived areas(Harrison et al., 2022; Ohta & Sano, 2024; Shehata et al., 2025)

Ethical Concerns

Like other cancers, treatment considerations for non-small cell lung cancer (NSCLC) involve various complex issues. Decision-making in cancer treatment is particularly challenging. Alongside scientific methods, it is essential to consider patient values, beliefs, desires, costs, and potential side effects. Before starting treatment, doctors must evaluate not only whether it is effective for the patient but also their financial limitations. Striking a balance between ethics, economics, and treatment effectiveness is crucial, as these factors significantly influence the development of future treatment methods. Additionally, new treatment methods give rise to new ethical dilemmas. Key issues include fair access to innovative and effective treatments for different patients, the high costs associated with these new methods, their actual effectiveness, and the risk of implementing unnecessary and profit-driven treatments. These considerations illustrate that ethical issues serve as a guiding principle in the advancement of future treatment options. Therefore, ethical considerations should always be prioritized in the development of new therapies. (Brescia, 2001).

The development and application of new technologies, along with the benefits they bring, also raise concerns and ethical issues. For this reason, regulatory organizations such as the FDA (USA) and the EMA (Europe) are responsible for monitoring the development and acceptance of these technologies. Clinical data of patients - the process of conducting clinical trials and the quality of data generation must be monitored to ensure patient safety. Especially in the use of technologies such as artificial intelligence, determining regulatory frameworks to protect patient privacy, ensuring transparency in the use of various algorithms, and defining legal responsibilities in the event of errors are necessary to protect patient rights, which are monitored by the FDA. The use of emerging technologies, such as CAR-T cell therapy, also requires long-term follow-up after treatment due to potential serious side effects, for which the necessary rules and regulations must be established. For this purpose, the FDA has provided the Biological Evaluation Bureaus (CBER) along with the INTERACT program to help researchers and developers of these clinical methods. The EMA has also developed guidelines for modern therapeutic methods, overseeing Advanced Therapy Medicinal Products (ATMPs) and CAR-T cell-based therapies. In addition to clinical trials, ethical considerations must also be taken into account in the process of using these new methods to treat patients, and patient consent must be obtained after informing them of the risks and possible complications and ensuring the confidentiality of patient data(Coppola et al., 2025; D. Huang et al., 2024; S S et al., 2024; Yang et al., 2023).

CONCLUSION AND FUTURE PERSPECTIVES

Today, we are observing the integration of various scientific disciplines and the rise of interdisciplinary technologies. Recent advancements in different fields have significantly improved medicine and treatment. The rapid pace of technological growth suggests a promising future for cancer treatments, including non-small cell lung cancer (NSCLC). Future trends will focus on enhancing treatment efficacy while minimizing side effects. These innovations aim to increase life expectancy and improve recovery for patients with NSCLC, ensuring that cancer doesn't dictate the course of their lives.

REFERENCES

Abernethy, A. P., McDonald, C. F., Frith, P. A., Clark, K., Herndon, J. E.II, Marcello, J., Young, I. H., Bull, J., Wilcock, A., Booth, S., Wheeler, J. L., Tulsky, J. A., Crockett, A. J., & Currow, D. C. (2010). Effect of palliative oxygen versus room air in relief of breathlessness in patients with refractory dyspnoea: A double-blind, randomised controlled trial. *Lancet*, *376*(9743), 784–793. DOI: 10.1016/S0140-6736(10)61115-4 PMID: 20816546

Ali, A. (2024). Advances in Non-Small Cell Lung Cancer (NSCLC) Treatment—A Paradigm Shift in Oncology. In *Pharmaceuticals* (Vol. 17, Issue 2, p. 246). MDPI. https://doi.org/https://doi.org/10.3390/ph17020246

Ali, A., & DiPersio, J. F. (2024). ReCARving the future: Bridging CAR T-cell therapy gaps with synthetic biology, engineering, and economic insights. *Frontiers in Immunology*, *15*, 1432799. DOI: 10.3389/fimmu.2024.1432799

Ansari, J., Shackelford, R. E., & El-Osta, H. (2016). Epigenetics in non-small cell lung cancer: From basics to therapeutics. *Translational Lung Cancer Research*, *5*(2), 155–171. DOI: 10.3978/j.issn.2218-6751.2016.02.07

Apostolou, P., Papadimitriou, M., & Papasotiriou, I. (2017). Stemness gene profiles of circulating tumor cells. *Journal of Cancer Therapy*, *8*(2), 155–167. https://www.scirp.org/journal/paperinformation?paperid=74104. DOI: 10.4236/jct.2017.82013

Araújo, A. (2016). *Exosomes isolation and characterization in serum is feasible in non-small cell lung cancer patients: critical analysis of evidence and potential role in clinical practice.* https://pubmed.ncbi.nlm.nih.gov/26919248/

Attene-Ramos, M. S., Wagner, E. D., Plewa, M. J., & Gaskins, H. R. (2006). Evidence that hydrogen sulfide is a genotoxic agent. *Molecular Cancer Research*, *4*(1), 9–14. DOI: 10.1158/1541-7786.MCR-05-0126 PMID: 16446402

Balgkouranidou, I., & Liloglou, T. (2013). Lung cancer epigenetics: Emerging biomarkers. *Biomarkers in Medicine*, *7*(5), 771–782. DOI: 10.2217/bmm.12.111

Bayasgalan, U., Moon, S. H., Kim, T. H., Kim, T. Y., Lee, S. H., & Suh, Y.-G. (2021). Dosimetric Comparisons between Proton Beam Therapy and Modern Photon Radiation Techniques for Stage I Non-Small Cell Lung Cancer According to Tumor Location. *Cancers (Basel)*, *13*(24), 6356. Advance online publication. DOI: 10.3390/cancers13246356 PMID: 34944976

Best, M. G., & Sol, N. In 't Veld, S. G. J. G., Vancura, A., Muller, M., Niemeijer, A. L. N., … Wurdinger, T. (2017). Swarm intelligence-enhanced detection of non-small-cell lung cancer using tumor-educated platelets. Cancer Cell, 32(2), 238-252. e9. DOI: 10.1016/j.ccell.2017.07.004

Bharti, R., & Grimm, D. G. (2021). Current challenges and best-practice protocols for microbiome analysis. *Briefings in Bioinformatics*, *22*(1), 178–193. DOI: 10.1093/bib/bbz155 PMID: 31848574

Bianchi, A., Dufort, S., Lux, F., Fortin, P.-Y., Tassali, N., Tillement, O., Coll, J.-L., & Crémillieux, Y. (2014). Targeting and in vivo imaging of non-small-cell lung cancer using nebulized multimodal contrast agents. *Proceedings of the National Academy of Sciences of the United States of America*, *111*(25), 9247–9252. DOI: 10.1073/pnas.1402196111 PMID: 24927562

Bianchi, F., Nicassio, F., Marzi, M., Belloni, E., Dall'olio, V., Bernard, L., Pelosi, G., Maisonneuve, P., Veronesi, G., & Di Fiore, P. P. (2011). A serum circulating miRNA diagnostic test to identify asymptomatic high-risk individuals with early stage lung cancer. *EMBO Molecular Medicine*, *3*(8), 495–503. DOI: 10.1002/emmm.201100154 PMID: 21744498

Boeri, M., Verri, C., Conte, D., Roz, L., Modena, P., Facchinetti, F., Calabrò, E., Croce, C. M., Pastorino, U., & Sozzi, G. (2011). MicroRNA signatures in tissues and plasma predict development and prognosis of computed tomography detected lung cancer. *Proceedings of the National Academy of Sciences of the United States of America*, *108*(9), 3713–3718. DOI: 10.1073/pnas.1100048108 PMID: 21300873

Bolyen, E., Rideout, J. R., Dillon, M. R., Bokulich, N. A., Abnet, C. C., Al-Ghalith, G. A., Alexander, H., Alm, E. J., Arumugam, M., Asnicar, F., Bai, Y., Bisanz, J. E., Bittinger, K., Brejnrod, A., Brislawn, C. J., Brown, C. T., Callahan, B. J., Caraballo-Rodríguez, A. M., Chase, J., . . . Caporaso, J. G. (2019). Reproducible, interactive, scalable and extensible microbiome data science using QIIME 2. In *Nature biotechnology* (Vol. 37, Issue 8, pp. 852–857). DOI: 10.1038/s41587-019-0209-9

Bremnes, R. M., Busund, L.-T., Kilvær, T. L., Andersen, S., Richardsen, E., Paulsen, E. E., Hald, S., Khanehkenari, M. R., Cooper, W. A., Kao, S. C., & Dønnem, T. (2016). The Role of Tumor-Infiltrating Lymphocytes in Development, Progression, and Prognosis of Non-Small Cell Lung Cancer. *Journal of Thoracic Oncology*, *11*(6), 789–800. DOI: 10.1016/j.jtho.2016.01.015 PMID: 26845192

Brescia, F. J. (2001). Lung cancer—A philosophical, ethical, and personal perspective. *Critical Reviews in Oncology/Hematology*, *40*(2), 139–148. DOI: 10.1016/S1040-8428(01)00140-8

Bueno, R., Hughes, E., Wagner, S., Gutin, A. S., Lanchbury, J. S., Zheng, Y., Archer, M. A., Gustafson, C., Jones, J. T., Rushton, K., Saam, J., Kim, E., Barberis, M., Wistuba, I., Wenstrup, R. J., Wallace, W. A., Hartman, A.-R., & Harrison, D. J. (2015). Validation of a molecular and pathological model for five-year mortality risk in patients with early stage lung adenocarcinoma. *Journal of Thoracic Oncology*, *10*(1), 67–73. DOI: 10.1097/JTO.0000000000000365 PMID: 25396679

Cai, K., Pi, W., Qin, J., Peng, C., Wang, D., Gu, Y., & Mei, Y. (2023). Detection of CYFRA 21-1 in human serum by an electrochemical immunosensor based on UiO -66-NH_2@CMWCNTs and CS@AuNPs. *Colloids and Surfaces. B, Biointerfaces*, *230*, 113517. DOI: 10.1016/j.colsurfb.2023.113517

Caporaso, J. G., Kuczynski, J., Stombaugh, J., Bittinger, K., Bushman, F. D., Costello, E. K., Fierer, N., Peña, A. G., Goodrich, J. K., Gordon, J. I., Huttley, G. A., Kelley, S. T., Knights, D., Koenig, J. E., Ley, R. E., Lozupone, C. A., McDonald, D., Muegge, B. D., Pirrung, M., . . . Knight, R. (2010). QIIME allows analysis of high-throughput community sequencing data. In *Nature methods* (Vol. 7, Issue 5, pp. 335–336). DOI: 10.1038/nmeth.f.303

Carbonero, F., Benefiel, A. C., Alizadeh-Ghamsari, A. H., & Gaskins, H. R. (2012). Microbial pathways in colonic sulfur metabolism and links with health and disease. *Frontiers in Physiology*, *3*, 448. DOI: 10.3389/fphys.2012.00448 PMID: 23226130

Carrasco-Esteban, E., Domínguez-Rullán, J. A., Barrionuevo-Castillo, P., Pelari-Mici, L., Leaman, O., Sastre-Gallego, S., & López-Campos, F. (2021). Current role of nanoparticles in the treatment of lung cancer. *Journal of Clinical and Translational Research*, *7*(2), 140–155. https://pubmed.ncbi.nlm.nih.gov/34104817/ PMID: 34104817

Casagrande, G. M. S., Silva, M. de O., Reis, R. M., & Leal, L. F. (2023). Liquid biopsy for lung cancer: Up-to-date and perspectives for screening programs. *International Journal of Molecular Sciences*, *24*(3), 2505. https://pubmed.ncbi.nlm.nih.gov/36768828/. DOI: 10.3390/ijms24032505 PMID: 36768828

Cassileth, B. R., Deng, G. E., Gomez, J. E., Johnstone, P. A. S., Kumar, N., & Vickers, A. J. (2007). Complementary therapies and integrative oncology in lung cancer: ACCP evidence-based clinical practice guidelines (2nd edition). Chest, 132(3 Suppl.), 340S-354S. DOI: 10.1378/chest.07-1389

Catarino, R., Coelho, A., Araújo, A., Gomes, M., Nogueira, A., Lopes, C., & Medeiros, R. (2012). Circulating DNA: Diagnostic tool and predictive marker for overall survival of NSCLC patients. *PLoS One*, *7*(6), e38559. https://pubmed.ncbi.nlm.nih.gov/22701665/. DOI: 10.1371/journal.pone.0038559 PMID: 22701665

Chandrasekar, D., Tribett, E., & Ramchandran, K. (2016). Integrated Palliative Care and Oncologic Care in Non-Small-Cell Lung Cancer. *Current Treatment Options in Oncology, 17*(5), 23. DOI: 10.1007/s11864-016-0397-1 PMID: 27032645

Chaturvedi, V. K., Singh, A., Singh, V. K., & Singh, M. P. (2019). Cancer Nanotechnology: A New Revolution for Cancer Diagnosis and Therapy. *Current Drug Metabolism, 20*(6), 416–429. DOI: 10.2174/1389200219666180918111528 PMID: 30227814

Chen, D., Wu, J., Jin, D., Wang, B., & Cao, H. (2019). Fecal microbiota transplantation in cancer management: Current status and perspectives. *International Journal of Cancer, 145*(8), 2021–2031. DOI: 10.1002/ijc.32003 PMID: 30458058

Chen, L., Chen, F., Li, J., Pu, Y., Yang, C., Wang, Y., Lei, Y., & Huang, Y. (2022). CAR-T cell therapy for lung cancer: Potential and perspective. *Thoracic Cancer, 13*(7), 889–899. DOI: 10.1111/1759-7714.14375 PMID: 35289077

Chen, X., Shen, C., Wei, Z., Zhang, R., Wang, Y., Jiang, L., Chen, K., Qiu, S., Zhang, Y., Zhang, T., Chen, B., Xu, Y., Feng, Q., Huang, J., Zhong, Z., Li, H., Che, G., & Xiao, K. (2021). Patient-derived non-small cell lung cancer xenograft mirrors complex tumor heterogeneity. *Cancer Biology & Medicine, 18*(1), 184–198. DOI: 10.20892/j.issn.2095-3941.2020.0012 PMID: 33628593

Cheville, A. L., Novotny, P. J., Sloan, J. A., Basford, J. R., Wampfler, J. A., Garces, Y. I., Jatoi, A., & Yang, P. (2011). The value of a symptom cluster of fatigue, dyspnea, and cough in predicting clinical outcomes in lung cancer survivors. *Journal of Pain and Symptom Management, 42*(2), 213–221. DOI: 10.1016/j.jpainsymman.2010.11.005 PMID: 21398089

Chute, C. G., Greenberg, E. R., Baron, J., Korson, R., Baker, J., & Yates, J. (1985). Presenting conditions of 1539 population-based lung cancer patients by cell type and stage in New Hampshire and Vermont. *Cancer, 56*(8), 2107–2111. DOI: 10.1002/1097-0142(19851015)56:8<2107:AID-CNCR2820560837>3.0.CO;2-T

Cohen, S. J., Alpaugh, R. K., Gross, S., O'Hara, S. M., Smirnov, D. A., Terstappen, L. W. M. M., Allard, W. J., Bilbee, M., Cheng, J. D., Hoffman, J. P., Lewis, N. L., Pellegrino, A., Rogatko, A., Sigurdson, E., Wang, H., Watson, J. C., Weiner, L. M., & Meropol, N. J. (2006). Isolation and characterization of circulating tumor cells in patients with metastatic colorectal cancer. *Clinical Colorectal Cancer, 6*(2), 125–132. https://pubmed.ncbi.nlm.nih.gov/16945168/. DOI: 10.3816/CCC.2006.n.029 PMID: 16945168

Coppola, C. A., De Summa, S., Matera, G., Pilato, B., Traversa, D., & Tommasi, S. (2025). Liquid Biopsy: The Challenges of a Revolutionary Approach in Oncology. *International Journal of Molecular Sciences*, *26*(11), 5013. Advance online publication. DOI: 10.3390/ijms26115013 PMID: 40507825

Costa, J., Membrino, A., Zanchetta, C., Rizzato, S., Cortiula, F., Rossetto, C., Pelizzari, G., Aprile, G., & Macerelli, M. (2024). The Role of ctDNA in the Management of Non-Small-Cell Lung Cancer in the AI and NGS Era. *International Journal of Molecular Sciences*, *25*(24), 13669. Advance online publication. DOI: 10.3390/ijms252413669 PMID: 39769431

Cristofanilli, M., Budd, G. T., Ellis, M. J., Stopeck, A., Matera, J., Miller, M. C., Reuben, J. M., Doyle, G. V., Allard, W. J., Terstappen, L. W. M. M., & Hayes, D. F. (2004). Circulating tumor cells, disease progression, and survival in metastatic breast cancer. *The New England Journal of Medicine*, *351*(8), 781–791. https://pubmed.ncbi.nlm.nih.gov/15317891/. DOI: 10.1056/NEJMoa040766 PMID: 15317891

Cuevas-Ramos, G., Petit, C. R., Marcq, I., Boury, M., Oswald, E., & Nougayrède, J.-P. (2010). Escherichia coli induces DNA damage in vivo and triggers genomic instability in mammalian cells. *Proceedings of the National Academy of Sciences of the United States of America*, *107*(25), 11537–11542. DOI: 10.1073/pnas.1001261107 PMID: 20534522

Curran, W. J., Jr., Schiller, J. H., Wolkin, A. C., Comis, R. L., & Groups, S. L. C. in L. C. of the C. of C. C. (2008). Addressing the current challenges of non–small-cell lung cancer clinical trial accrual. *Clinical Lung Cancer,* *9*(4), 222–226. https://pubmed.ncbi.nlm.nih.gov/18650170/

Dai, X., Bu, X., Gao, Y., Guo, J., Hu, J., Jiang, C., Zhang, Z., Xu, K., Duan, J., He, S., Zhang, J., Wan, L., Liu, T., Zhou, X., Hung, M.-C., Freeman, G. J., & Wei, W. (2021). Energy status dictates PD-L1 protein abundance and anti-tumor immunity to enable checkpoint blockade. *Molecular Cell*, *81*(11), 2317–2331.e6. DOI: 10.1016/j.molcel.2021.03.037 PMID: 33909988

Dang, D. K., & Park, B. H. (2022). Circulating tumor DNA: Current challenges for clinical utility. *The Journal of Clinical Investigation*, *132*(12), e154941. Advance online publication. DOI: 10.1172/JCI154941 PMID: 35703177

Das, M., & Tisch, A. H. (2017). Diagnosis and Treatment of Adenocarcinomas and Squamous Cell Carcinomas of the Lung. *Journal of the Advanced Practitioner in Oncology*, *8*(3), 267–272. https://pubmed.ncbi.nlm.nih.gov/29928550/ PMID: 29928550

Dejea, C. M., Fathi, P., Craig, J. M., Boleij, A., Taddese, R., Geis, A. L., Wu, X., DeStefano Shields, C. E., Hechenbleikner, E. M., Huso, D. L., Anders, R. A., Giardiello, F. M., Wick, E. C., Wang, H., Wu, S., Pardoll, D. M., Housseau, F., & Sears, C. L. (2018). Patients with familial adenomatous polyposis harbor colonic biofilms containing tumorigenic bacteria. *Science*, *359*(6375), 592–597. DOI: 10.1126/science.aah3648 PMID: 29420293

Dell'Oro, M., Short, M., Wilson, P., & Bezak, E. (2020). Clinical Limitations of Photon, Proton and Carbon Ion Therapy for Pancreatic Cancer. *Cancers (Basel)*, *12*(1), 163. Advance online publication. DOI: 10.3390/cancers12010163 PMID: 31936565

Diehl, F., Schmidt, K., Choti, M. A., Romans, K., Goodman, S., Li, M., Thornton, K., Agrawal, N., Sokoll, L., Szabo, S. A., Kinzler, K. W., Vogelstein, B., & Diaz, L. A.Jr. (2008). Circulating mutant DNA to assess tumor dynamics. *Nature Medicine*, *14*(9), 985–990. https://pubmed.ncbi.nlm.nih.gov/18670422/. DOI: 10.1038/nm.1789 PMID: 18670422

Doll, S., Proneth, B., Tyurina, Y. Y., Panzilius, E., Kobayashi, S., Ingold, I., Irmler, M., Beckers, J., Aichler, M., Walch, A., Prozorovski, T., Stark, G., Wurst, W., & Conrad, M. (2017). ACSL4 dictates ferroptosis sensitivity by shaping cellular lipid composition. *Nature Chemical Biology*, *13*(1), 91–98. DOI: 10.1038/nchembio.2239

Dong, Q., Chen, E. S., Zhao, C., & Jin, C. (2021). Host-Microbiome Interaction in Lung Cancer. *Frontiers in Immunology*, *12*, 679829. DOI: 10.3389/fimmu.2021.679829 PMID: 34108973

Dono, M., De Luca, G., Lastraioli, S., Anselmi, G., Dal Bello, M. G., Coco, S., Vanni, I., Grossi, F., Vigani, A., Genova, C., Ferrarini, M., Ravetti, J. L., & Zupo, S. (2019). Tag-based next generation sequencing: A feasible and reliable assay for EGFR T790M mutation detection in circulating tumor DNA of non small cell lung cancer patients. *Molecular Medicine (Cambridge, Mass.)*, *25*(1), 1–13. https://pubmed.ncbi.nlm.nih.gov/31029076/. DOI: 10.1186/s10020-019-0082-5 PMID: 31029076

Doroudian, M., Zanganeh, S., Abbasgholinejad, E., & Donnelly, S. C. (2023). Nanomedicine in Lung Cancer Immunotherapy. *Frontiers in Bioengineering and Biotechnology*, *11*, 1144653. DOI: 10.3389/fbioe.2023.1144653 PMID: 37008041

Douglas, G. M., Maffei, V. J., Zaneveld, J. R., Yurgel, S. N., Brown, J. R., Taylor, C. M., Huttenhower, C., & Langille, M. G. I. (2020). PICRUSt2 for prediction of metagenome functions. In *Nature biotechnology* (Vol. 38, Issue 6, pp. 685–688). DOI: 10.1038/s41587-020-0548-6

Ezeife, D. A., Spackman, E., Juergens, R. A., Laskin, J. J., Agulnik, J. S., Hao, D., Laurie, S. A., Law, J. H., Le, L. W., Kiedrowski, L. A., Melosky, B., Shepherd, F. A., Cohen, V., Wheatley-Price, P., Vandermeer, R., Li, J. J., Fernandes, R., Shokoohi, A., Lanman, R. B., & Leighl, N. B. (2022). The economic value of liquid biopsy for genomic profiling in advanced non-small cell lung cancer. *Therapeutic Advances in Medical Oncology*, *14*, 17588359221112696. DOI: 10.1177/17588359221112696 PMID: 35923926

Fearon, K. C. H., Voss, A. C., & Hustead, D. S. (2006). Definition of cancer cachexia: Effect of weight loss, reduced food intake, and systemic inflammation on functional status and prognosis. *The American Journal of Clinical Nutrition*, *83*(6), 1345–1350. DOI: 10.1093/ajcn/83.6.1345

Ferreira, D., Miranda, J., Martins-Lopes, P., Adega, F., & Chaves, R. (2021). Future Perspectives in Detecting EGFR and ALK Gene Alterations in Liquid Biopsies of Patients with NSCLC. *International Journal of Molecular Sciences*, *22*(8), 3815. Advance online publication. DOI: 10.3390/ijms22083815 PMID: 33916986

Flores Banda, J. S., Gangane, S., Raza, F., & Massarelli, E. (2025). Current Development of Therapeutic Vaccines in Lung Cancer. *Vaccines*, *13*(2), 185. Advance online publication. DOI: 10.3390/vaccines13020185 PMID: 40006732

Frullanti, E., & Serrano, M. J. (2023). Current trends and future perspectives about liquid biopsy. In *Frontiers in Genetics* (Vol. 14, p. 1345876). Frontiers Media SA. https://www.frontiersin.org/journals/genetics/articles/10.3389/fgene.2023.1345876/full

Fu, K., Xie, F., Wang, F., & Fu, L. (2022). Therapeutic strategies for EGFR-mutated non-small cell lung cancer patients with osimertinib resistance. *Journal of Hematology & Oncology*, *15*(1), 173. DOI: 10.1186/s13045-022-01391-4 PMID: 36482474

Fujisawa, D., Temel, J. S., Traeger, L., Greer, J. A., Lennes, I. T., Mimura, M., & Pirl, W. F. (2015). Psychological factors at early stage of treatment as predictors of receiving chemotherapy at the end of life. *Psycho-Oncology*, *24*(12), 1731–1737. DOI: 10.1002/pon.3840

Gadgeel, S. M. (2016). Personalized therapy of non-small cell lung cancer (NSCLC). *Lung Cancer and Personalized Medicine: Novel Therapies and Clinical Management*, 203–222. https://pubmed.ncbi.nlm.nih.gov/26703806/

García-Pachón, E., & Padilla-Navas, I. (2020). Microbioma de la vía aérea inferior y cáncer de pulmón. *Arch. Bronconeumol.(Ed. Impr.)*, 410. https://www.archbronconeumol.org/en-microbioma-via-aerea-inferior-cancer-articulo-S0300289620300521

Garg, P., Singhal, S., Kulkarni, P., Horne, D., Malhotra, J., Salgia, R., & Singhal, S. S. (2024). Advances in non-small cell lung cancer: Current insights and future directions. *Journal of Clinical Medicine*, *13*(14), 4189. https://pubmed.ncbi.nlm.nih.gov/39064229/. DOI: 10.3390/jcm13144189 PMID: 39064229

Giraldo, N. A., Sanchez-Salas, R., Peske, J. D., Vano, Y., Becht, E., Petitprez, F., Validire, P., Ingels, A., Cathelineau, X., Fridman, W. H., & Sautès-Fridman, C. (2019). The clinical role of the TME in solid cancer. *British Journal of Cancer*, *120*(1), 45–53. DOI: 10.1038/s41416-018-0327-z PMID: 30413828

Granger, C. L., Denehy, L., McDonald, C. F., Irving, L., & Clark, R. A. (2014). Physical activity measured using global positioning system tracking in non-small cell lung cancer: An observational study. *Integrative Cancer Therapies*, *13*(6), 482–492. DOI: 10.1177/1534735414542484

Granger, C. L., McDonald, C. F., Berney, S., Chao, C., & Denehy, L. (2011). Exercise intervention to improve exercise capacity and health related quality of life for patients with Non-small cell lung cancer: A systematic review. *Lung Cancer (Amsterdam, Netherlands)*, *72*(2), 139–153. DOI: 10.1016/j.lungcan.2011.01.006

Graves, K. D., Arnold, S. M., Love, C. L., Kirsh, K. L., Moore, P. G., & Passik, S. D. (2007). Distress screening in a multidisciplinary lung cancer clinic: Prevalence and predictors of clinically significant distress. *Lung Cancer (Amsterdam, Netherlands)*, *55*(2), 215–224. DOI: 10.1016/j.lungcan.2006.10.001

Greathouse, K. L., White, J. R., Vargas, A. J., Bliskovsky, V. V., Beck, J. A., von Muhlinen, N., Polley, E. C., Bowman, E. D., Khan, M. A., Robles, A. I., Cooks, T., Ryan, B. M., Padgett, N., Dzutsev, A. H., Trinchieri, G., Pineda, M. A., Bilke, S., Meltzer, P. S., Hokenstad, A. N., & Harris, C. C. (2018). Interaction between the microbiome and TP53 in human lung cancer. *Genome Biology*, *19*(1), 123. DOI: 10.1186/s13059-018-1501-6 PMID: 30143034

Greer, J. A., Pirl, W. F., Jackson, V. A., Muzikansky, A., Lennes, I. T., Heist, R. S., Gallagher, E. R., & Temel, J. S. (2012). Effect of early palliative care on chemotherapy use and end-of-life care in patients with metastatic non-small-cell lung cancer. *Journal of Clinical Oncology*, *30*(4), 394–400. DOI: 10.1200/JCO.2011.35.7996

Guo, Q., Liu, L., Chen, Z., Fan, Y., Zhou, Y., Yuan, Z., & Zhang, W. (2022). Current treatments for non-small cell lung cancer. *Frontiers in Oncology*, *12*, 945102. DOI: 10.3389/fonc.2022.945102 PMID: 36033435

Gustafson, A. M., Soldi, R., Anderlind, C., Scholand, M. B., Qian, J., Zhang, X., Cooper, K., Walker, D., McWilliams, A., Liu, G., Szabo, E., Brody, J., Massion, P. P., Lenburg, M. E., Lam, S., Bild, A. H., & Spira, A. (2010). Airway PI3K pathway activation is an early and reversible event in lung cancer development. *Science Translational Medicine*, *2*(26), 26ra25. Advance online publication. DOI: 10.1126/scitranslmed.3000251 PMID: 20375364

Harrison, S., Judd, J., Chin, S., & Ragin, C. (2022). Disparities in Lung Cancer Treatment. *Current Oncology Reports*, *24*(2), 241–248. DOI: 10.1007/s11912-022-01193-4 PMID: 35080738

Hasan, H., Sohal, I. S., Soto-Vargas, Z., Byappanahalli, A. M., Humphrey, S. E., Kubo, H., Kitdumrongthum, S., Copeland, S., Tian, F., Chairoungdua, A., & Kasinski, A. L. (2022). Extracellular vesicles released by non-small cell lung cancer cells drive invasion and permeability in non-tumorigenic lung epithelial cells. *Scientific Reports*, *12*(1), 972. DOI: 10.1038/s41598-022-04940-6 PMID: 35046472

He, Z., Gharaibeh, R. Z., Newsome, R. C., Pope, J. L., Dougherty, M. W., Tomkovich, S., Pons, B., Mirey, G., Vignard, J., Hendrixson, D. R., & Jobin, C. (2019). Campylobacter jejuni promotes colorectal tumorigenesis through the action of cytolethal distending toxin. *Gut*, *68*(2), 289–300. DOI: 10.1136/gutjnl-2018-317200 PMID: 30377189

Heidrich, I., Deitert, B., Werner, S., & Pantel, K. (2023). Liquid biopsy for monitoring of tumor dormancy and early detection of disease recurrence in solid tumors. *Cancer and Metastasis Reviews*, *42*(1), 161–182. https://pubmed.ncbi.nlm.nih.gov/36607507/. DOI: 10.1007/s10555-022-10075-x PMID: 36607507

Hendriksen, E., Williams, E., Sporn, N., Greer, J., DeGrange, A., & Koopman, C. (2015). Worried together: A qualitative study of shared anxiety in patients with metastatic non-small cell lung cancer and their family caregivers. *Supportive Care in Cancer*, *23*(4), 1035–1041. DOI: 10.1007/s00520-014-2431-9

Herbreteau, G., Vallée, A., Charpentier, S., Normanno, N., Hofman, P., & Denis, M. G. (2019). Circulating free tumor DNA in non-small cell lung cancer (NSCLC): Clinical application and future perspectives. *Journal of Thoracic Disease*, *11*(S1, Suppl 1), S113–S126. DOI: 10.21037/jtd.2018.12.18 PMID: 30775034

Hizal, M., Bilgin, B., Paksoy, N., Açıkgöz, Ö., Sezer, A., Gürbüz, M., Ak, N., Yücel, Ş., Ayhan, M., Erol, C., Demirkıran, A., Mandel, N. M., Shbair, A., Gökmen, İ., Başoğlu, T., Paydaş, S., Demiray, A. G., İriağaç, Y., Şakalar, T., & Şendur, M. A. N. (2022). The real-life efficacy and safety of osimertinib in pretreated advanced non-small cell lung cancer patients with T790M mutation: A Turkish Oncology Group Study. *Journal of Cancer Research and Clinical Oncology*, *148*(6), 1501–1508. DOI: 10.1007/s00432-021-03748-7 PMID: 34331582

Huang, D., Li, Z., Jiang, T., Yang, C., & Li, N. (2024). Artificial intelligence in lung cancer: Current applications, future perspectives, and challenges. *Frontiers in Oncology*, *14*, 1486310. DOI: 10.3389/fonc.2024.1486310 PMID: 39763611

Huang, Z., Li, B., Guo, Y., Wu, L., Kou, F., & Yang, L. (2021). Signatures of Multi-Omics Reveal Distinct Tumor Immune Microenvironment Contributing to Immunotherapy in Lung Adenocarcinoma. *Frontiers in Immunology*, *12*, 723172. DOI: 10.3389/fimmu.2021.723172 PMID: 34539658

Iliescu, F. S., Vrtačnik, D., Neuzil, P., & Iliescu, C. (2019). Microfluidic technology for clinical applications of exosomes. *Micromachines*, *10*(6), 392. https://pmc.ncbi.nlm.nih.gov/articles/PMC6631586/. DOI: 10.3390/mi10060392 PMID: 31212754

Ji, H., Jiang, Z., Wei, C., Ma, Y., Zhao, J., Wang, F., Zhao, B., Wang, D., & Tang, D. (2023). Intratumoural microbiota: From theory to clinical application. *Cell Communication and Signaling : CCS*, *21*(1), 164. DOI: 10.1186/s12964-023-01134-z PMID: 37381018

Jiang, G.-L. (2012). Particle therapy for cancers: A new weapon in radiation therapy. *Frontiers of Medicine*, *6*(2), 165–172. DOI: 10.1007/s11684-012-0196-4 PMID: 22573221

Jiang, W., Cai, G., Hu, P. C., & Wang, Y. (2018). Personalized medicine in non-small cell lung cancer: A review from a pharmacogenomics perspective. *Acta Pharmaceutica Sinica. B*, *8*(4), 530–538. https://pubmed.ncbi.nlm.nih.gov/30109178/. DOI: 10.1016/j.apsb.2018.04.005 PMID: 30109178

Jin, X., Zhou, J., Zhang, Z. & Lv, H. (2018). The combined administration of parthenolide and ginsenoside CK in long circulation liposomes with targeted tLyp-1 ligand induce mitochondria-mediated lung cancer apoptosis. *Artificial Cells, Nanomedicine, and Biotechnology, 46*(sup3), S931–S942. DOI: 10.1080/21691401.2018.1518913

Kamp, W. M., Wang, P., & Hwang, P. M. (2016). TP53 mutation, mitochondria and cancer. *Current Opinion in Genetics & Development*, *38*, 16–22. DOI: 10.1016/j.gde.2016.02.007

Kenaan, N., Hanna, G., Sardini, M., Iyoun, M. O., Layka, K., Hannouneh, Z. A., & Alshehabi, Z. (2024). Advances in early detection of non-small cell lung cancer: A comprehensive review. *Cancer Medicine*, *13*(18), e70156. https://pubmed.ncbi.nlm.nih.gov/39300939/. DOI: 10.1002/cam4.70156 PMID: 39300939

Kinashi, Y., Yokomizo, N., & Takahashi, S. (2017). DNA Double-strand Breaks Induced byFractionated Neutron Beam Irradiation for Boron Neutron Capture Therapy. *Anticancer Research*, *37*(4), 1681–1685. DOI: 10.21873/anticanres.11499 PMID: 28373429

Klopp, A. H., Spaeth, E. L., Dembinski, J. L., Woodward, W. A., Munshi, A., Meyn, R. E., Cox, J. D., Andreeff, M., & Marini, F. C. (2007). Tumor irradiation increases the recruitment of circulating mesenchymal stem cells into the tumor microenvironment. *Cancer Research*, *67*(24), 11687–11695. DOI: 10.1158/0008-5472.CAN-07-1406 PMID: 18089798

Ko, J. J., Banerji, S., Blais, N., Brade, A., Clelland, C., Schellenberg, D., Snow, S., Wheatley-Price, P., Yuan, R., & Melosky, B. (2023). Follow-Up Imaging Guidelines for Patients with Stage III Unresectable NSCLC: Recommendations Based on the PACIFIC Trial. *Current Oncology (Toronto, Ont.)*, *30*(4), 3817–3828. DOI: 10.3390/curroncol30040289 PMID: 37185402

Koka, K., Verma, A., Dwarakanath, B. S., & Papineni, R. V. L. (2022). Technological advancements in external beam radiation therapy (EBRT): An indispensable tool for cancer treatment. *Cancer Management and Research*, *14*, 1421–1429. DOI: 10.2147/CMAR.S351744

Kratz, J. R., He, J., Van Den Eeden, S. K., Zhu, Z.-H., Gao, W., Pham, P. T., Mulvihill, M. S., Ziaei, F., Zhang, H., Su, B., Zhi, X., Quesenberry, C. P., Habel, L. A., Deng, Q., Wang, Z., Zhou, J., Li, H., Huang, M.-C., Yeh, C.-C., & Jablons, D. M. (2012). A practical molecular assay to predict survival in resected non-squamous, non-small-cell lung cancer: Development and international validation studies. *Lancet*, *379*(9818), 823–832. DOI: 10.1016/S0140-6736(11)61941-7 PMID: 22285053

Kratz, J. R., Mann, M. J., & Jablons, D. M. (2013). International trial of adjuvant therapy in high risk stage I non-squamous cell carcinoma identified by a 14-gene prognostic signature. *Translational Lung Cancer Research*, *2*(3), 222–225. DOI: 10.3978/j.issn.2218-6751.2013.05.01 PMID: 25806235

Kratz, J. R., Tham, P. T., Mulvihill, M. S., Ziaei, F., Ray, M. R., Hurst, J. W., Segal, M. R., Berryman, D. M., Chu, W., He, B., Jablons, D. M., & Mann, M. J. (2013). Analytical validation of a practical molecular assay prognostic of survival in nonsquamous non-small cell lung cancer. *Diagnostic Molecular Pathology : The American Journal of Surgical Pathology. Diagnostic Molecular Pathology*, *22*(2), 65–69. DOI: 10.1097/PDM.0b013e318273fb61 PMID: 23628816

Krebs, M. G., Sloane, R., Priest, L., Lancashire, L., Hou, J.-M., Greystoke, A., Ward, T. H., Ferraldeschi, R., Hughes, A., Clack, G., Ranson, M., Dive, C., & Blackhall, F. H. (2011). Evaluation and prognostic significance of circulating tumor cells in patients with non–small-cell lung cancer. *Journal of Clinical Oncology*, *29*(12), 1556–1563. https://pubmed.ncbi.nlm.nih.gov/21422424/. DOI: 10.1200/JCO.2010.28.7045 PMID: 21422424

Krzyżanowska, N., Wojas-Krawczyk, K., Milanowski, J., & Krawczyk, P. (2022). Future prospects of immunotherapy in non-small-cell lung cancer patients: Is there hope in other immune checkpoints targeting molecules? *International Journal of Molecular Sciences*, *23*(6), 3087. DOI: 10.3390/ijms23063087

Kuehr, L., Micke, O., & Fischbach, R. (2014). Exercise in patients with non-small cell lung cancer: Feasibility and effects of an eight-week combined resistance and endurance exercise program. *Medicine and Science in Sports and Exercise*, *46*(11), 2011–2018. DOI: 10.1249/MSS.0000000000000158

Kumar, K. S., Somani, C., Sheth, K., Mathavan, N., Lim, D. T., Khor, L.-Y., & Ng, I. (2023). Artificial intelligence in clinical oncology: From data to digital pathology and treatment. *ASCO Educational Book*, *43*, e390084. DOI: 10.1200/EDBK_390084

Kumar, M., & Sarkar, A. (2022). Current therapeutic strategies and challenges in NSCLC treatment: A comprehensive review. *Experimental Oncology*, *44*(1), 7–16. https://pubmed.ncbi.nlm.nih.gov/35548961/. DOI: 10.32471/exp-oncology.2312-8852.vol-44-no-1.17411 PMID: 35548961

Ladbury, C., Amini, A., Govindarajan, A., Mambetsariev, I., Raz, D. J., Massarelli, E., Williams, T., Rodin, A., & Salgia, R. (2023). Integration of artificial intelligence in lung cancer: Rise of the machine. *Cell Reports Medicine*, *4*(4), 100933. DOI: 10.1016/j.xcrm.2023.100933

Laguna, J. C., García-Pardo, M., Alessi, J., Barrios, C., Singh, N., Al-Shamsi, H. O., Loong, H., Ferriol, M., Recondo, G., & Mezquita, L. (2024). Geographic differences in lung cancer: Focus on carcinogens, genetic predisposition, and molecular epidemiology. *Therapeutic Advances in Medical Oncology*, *16*, 17588359241231260. DOI: 10.1177/17588359241231260 PMID: 38455708

Langille, M. G. I., Zaneveld, J., Caporaso, J. G., McDonald, D., Knights, D., Reyes, J. A., Clemente, J. C., Burkepile, D. E., Vega Thurber, R. L., Knight, R., Beiko, R. G., & Huttenhower, C. (2013). Predictive functional profiling of microbial communities using 16S rRNA marker gene sequences. *Nature Biotechnology*, *31*(9), 814–821. DOI: 10.1038/nbt.2676 PMID: 23975157

Le Noci, V., Guglielmetti, S., Arioli, S., Camisaschi, C., Bianchi, F., Sommariva, M., Storti, C., Triulzi, T., Castelli, C., Balsari, A., Tagliabue, E., & Sfondrini, L. (2018). Modulation of Pulmonary Microbiota by Antibiotic or Probiotic Aerosol Therapy: A Strategy to Promote Immunosurveillance against Lung Metastases. *Cell Reports*, *24*(13), 3528–3538. DOI: 10.1016/j.celrep.2018.08.090 PMID: 30257213

Lee, J. B., Huang, Y., Oya, Y., Nutzinger, J., Ang, Y. L. E., Sooi, K., Cho, B. C., & Soo, R. A. (2024). Modulating the gut microbiome in non-small cell lung cancer: Challenges and opportunities. *Lung Cancer (Amsterdam, Netherlands)*, *107862*, •••. https://pubmed.ncbi.nlm.nih.gov/38959670/

Lei, F. (2024). The Application of Artificial Intelligence in Lung Cancer Research. *Cancer Control : Journal of the Moffitt Cancer Center*, *31*, 10732748241297372. DOI: 10.1177/10732748241297373 PMID: 39460384

Liao, G. J. W., Lun, F. M. F., Zheng, Y. W. L., Chan, K. C. A., Leung, T. Y., Lau, T. K., Chiu, R. W. K., & Lo, Y. M. D. (2011). Targeted massively parallel sequencing of maternal plasma DNA permits efficient and unbiased detection of fetal alleles. *Clinical Chemistry*, *57*(1), 92–101. https://pubmed.ncbi.nlm.nih.gov/21078840/. DOI: 10.1373/clinchem.2010.154336 PMID: 21078840

Liu, D., Liu, F., Liu, Z., Wang, L., & Zhang, N. (2011). Tumor specific delivery and therapy by double-targeted nanostructured lipid carriers with anti-VEGFR-2 antibody. *Molecular Pharmaceutics*, *8*(6), 2291–2301. DOI: 10.1021/mp200402e PMID: 21923159

Liu, H., Laan, A. C., Plomp, J., Parnell, S. R., Men, Y., Dalgliesh, R. M., Eelkema, R., & Denkova, A. G. (2020). Ionizing Radiation-Induced Release from Poly (ε-caprolactone-b-ethylene glycol) Micelles. *ACS Applied Polymer Materials*, *3*(2), 968–975. https://repository.tudelft.nl/record/uuid:aa6e2f08-436d-43cd-a928-74461628d66d. DOI: 10.1021/acsapm.0c01258

Liu, J., & Zhang, Y. (2022). Intratumor microbiome in cancer progression: Current developments, challenges and future trends. *Biomarker Research*, *10*(1), 37. DOI: 10.1186/s40364-022-00381-5 PMID: 35642013

Liu, Q., Yu, Z., Yuan, S., Xie, W., Li, C., Hu, Z., Xiang, Y., Wu, N., Wu, L., Bai, L., & Li, Y. (2016). Circulating exosomal microRNAs as prognostic biomarkers for non-small-cell lung cancer. *Oncotarget*, *8*(8), 13048–13058. https://pubmed.ncbi.nlm.nih.gov/28055956/. DOI: 10.18632/oncotarget.14369 PMID: 28055956

Liu, S.-C. (2024). Circulating tumor DNA in liquid biopsy: Current diagnostic limitation. In *World journal of gastroenterology* (Vol. 30, Issue 15, pp. 2175–2178). DOI: 10.3748/wjg.v30.i15.2175

Liu, Y. (2020). Application of artificial intelligence in clinical non-small cell lung cancer. *Artificial Intelligence in Cancer, 1*(1), 19–30. https://pmc.ncbi.nlm.nih.gov/articles/PMC8946647/

Liu, Z., Li, T., Li, N., Wang, Y., Chen, L., Tang, X., Wan, M., & Mao, C. (2022). GSH-induced chemotaxis nanomotors for cancer treatment by ferroptosis strategy. *Science China. Chemistry*, *65*(5), 989–1002. DOI: 10.1007/s11426-021-1208-6

Lococo, F., Ghaly, G., Flamini, S., Campanella, A., Chiappetta, M., Bria, E., Vita, E., Tortora, G., Evangelista, J., Sassorossi, C., Congedo, M. T., Valentini, V., Sala, E., Cesario, A., Margaritora, S., Boldrini, L., & Mohammed, A. (2024). Artificial intelligence applications in personalizing lung cancer management: State of the art and future perspectives. *Journal of Thoracic Disease*, *16*(10), 7096–7110. https://pubmed.ncbi.nlm.nih.gov/39552872/. DOI: 10.21037/jtd-24-244 PMID: 39552872

Lopes, A., Vandermeulen, G., & Préat, V. (2019). Cancer DNA vaccines: Current preclinical and clinical developments and future perspectives. *Journal of Experimental & Clinical Cancer Research : CR*, *38*(1), 146. DOI: 10.1186/s13046-019-1154-7 PMID: 30953535

Lorentzen, C. L., Haanen, J. B., Met, Ö., & Svane, I. M. (2022). Clinical advances and ongoing trials on mRNA vaccines for cancer treatment. *The Lancet. Oncology*, *23*(10), e450–e458. DOI: 10.1016/S1470-2045(22)00372-2 PMID: 36174631

Lövgren, M., Tishelman, C., Sprangers, M., Koyi, H., & Hamberg, K. (2008). Symptoms and problems with functioning among women and men with inoperable lung cancer—a longitudinal study. *Lung Cancer (Amsterdam, Netherlands)*, *60*(1), 113–124. DOI: 10.1016/j.lungcan.2007.09.015

Lu, Y.-Q., & Lu, K.-H. (2017). Advancements in next-generation sequencing for diagnosis and treatment of non-small-cell lung cancer. In *Chronic diseases and translational medicine* (Vol. 3, Issue 1, pp. 1–7). DOI: 10.1016/j.cdtm.2017.02.009

Luszczynska, A., Pawlowska, I., Cieslak, R., Knoll, N., & Scholz, U. (2013). Social support and quality of life among lung cancer patients: A systematic review. *Psycho-Oncology*, *22*(10), 2160–2168. https://pubmed.ncbi.nlm.nih.gov/23097417/. DOI: 10.1002/pon.3218 PMID: 23097417

Ma, H. Y., Das, J., Prendergast, C., De Jong, D., Braumuller, B., Paily, J., Huang, S., Liou, C., Giarratana, A., Hosseini, M., Yeh, R., & Capaccione, K. M. (2023). Advances in CAR T cell therapy for non-small cell lung cancer. *Current Issues in Molecular Biology*, *45*(11), 9019–9038. DOI: 10.3390/cimb45110566

Ma, P., Xiao, H., Yu, C., Liu, J., Cheng, Z., Song, H., Zhang, X., Li, C., Wang, J., Gu, Z., & Lin, J. (2017). Enhanced cisplatin chemotherapy by iron oxide nanocarrier-mediated generation of highly toxic reactive oxygen species. *Nano Letters*, *17*(2), 928–937. DOI: 10.1021/acs.nanolett.6b04269

Majumder, J., & Minko, T. (2021). Multifunctional lipid-based nanoparticles for codelivery of anticancer drugs and siRNA for treatment of non-small cell lung cancer with different level of resistance and EGFR mutations. *Pharmaceutics*, *13*(7), 1063. DOI: 10.3390/pharmaceutics13071063

Malapelle, U., Tiseo, M., Vivancos, A., Kapp, J., Serrano, M. J., & Tiemann, M. (2021). Liquid biopsy for biomarker testing in non-small cell lung cancer: A European perspective. *Journal of Molecular Pathology*, *2*(3), 255–273. https://www.mdpi.com/2673-5261/2/3/22. DOI: 10.3390/jmp2030022

Maldonado, J., Czarnecka, B., Harmon, D. E., & Ruiz, C. (2023). The multidrug efflux pump regulator AcrR directly represses motility in Escherichia coli. *MSphere*, *8*(5), e0043023. DOI: 10.1128/msphere.00430-23 PMID: 37787551

Mandel, P. & Metais, P. (1948). [Nuclear Acids In Human Blood Plasma]. *Comptes rendus des seances de la Societe de biologie et de ses filiales, 142*(3–4), 241–243. https://pubmed.ncbi.nlm.nih.gov/18875018/

Marinello, A., Tagliamento, M., Pagliaro, A., Conci, N., Cella, E., Vasseur, D., Remon, J., Levy, A., Dall'Olio, F. G., & Besse, B. (2024). Circulating tumor DNA to guide diagnosis and treatment of localized and locally advanced non-small cell lung cancer. *Cancer Treatment Reviews*, *129*, 102791. DOI: 10.1016/j.ctrv.2024.102791 PMID: 38963991

Marino, P., Touzani, R., Perrier, L., Rouleau, E., Kossi, D. S., Zhaomin, Z., Charrier, N., Goardon, N., Preudhomme, C., Durand-Zaleski, I., Borget, I., & Baffert, S. (2018). Cost of cancer diagnosis using next-generation sequencing targeted gene panels in routine practice: A nationwide French study. *European Journal of Human Genetics : EJHG*, *26*(3), 314–323. DOI: 10.1038/s41431-017-0081-3 PMID: 29367707

Martini, N., Bains, M. S., Burt, M. E., Zakowski, M. F., McCormack, P., Rusch, V. W., & Ginsberg, R. J. (1995). Incidence of local recurrence and second primary tumors in resected stage I lung cancer. *The Journal of Thoracic and Cardiovascular Surgery*, *109*(1), 120–129. DOI: 10.1016/S0022-5223(95)70427-2 PMID: 7815787

Masaoutis, C., Mihailidou, C., Tsourouflis, G., & Theocharis, S. (2018). Exosomes in lung cancer diagnosis and treatment. From the translating research into future clinical practice. *Biochimie*, *151*, 27–36. DOI: 10.1016/j.biochi.2018.05.014 PMID: 29857182

Mascaux, C. (2017). Personalised medicine for nonsmall cell lung cancer. *European Respiratory Review : an Official Journal of the European Respiratory Society*, *26*(146), 170066. DOI: 10.1183/16000617.0066-2017

Matsuda, A., Yamaoka, K., & Tango, T. (2012). Quality of life in advanced non-small cell lung cancer patients receiving palliative chemotherapy: A meta-analysis of randomized controlled trials. *Experimental and Therapeutic Medicine*, *3*(1), 134–140. DOI: 10.3892/etm.2011.368 PMID: 22969858

Matuszak, N., Suchorska, W. M., Milecki, P., Kruszyna-Mochalska, M., Misiarz, A., Pracz, J., & Malicki, J. (2022). FLASH radiotherapy: An emerging approach in radiation therapy. *Reports of Practical Oncology and Radiotherapy : Journal of Greatpoland Cancer Center in Poznan and Polish Society of Radiation Oncology*, *27*(2), 344–351. DOI: 10.5603/RPOR.a2022.0038 PMID: 36299375

Miyanaga, A., Gemma, A., Noro, R., Kataoka, K., Matsuda, K., Nara, M., & Jin, Y. (2008). Antitumor activity of histone deacetylase inhibitors in non-small cell lung cancer cells: Development of a molecular predictive model. *Molecular Cancer Therapeutics*, *7*(7), 1923–1930. DOI: 10.1158/1535-7163.MCT-07-2140

Montani, F., Marzi, M. J., Dezi, F., Dama, E., Carletti, R. M., Bonizzi, G., Bertolotti, R., Bellomi, M., Rampinelli, C., Maisonneuve, P., Spaggiari, L., Veronesi, G., Nicassio, F., Di Fiore, P. P., & Bianchi, F. (2015). miR-Test: A blood test for lung cancer early detection. *Journal of the National Cancer Institute*, *107*(6), djv063. Advance online publication. DOI: 10.1093/jnci/djv063 PMID: 25794889

Mouliere, F., Chandrananda, D., Piskorz, A. M., Moore, E. K., Morris, J., Ahlborn, L. B., Mair, R., Goranova, T., Marass, F., Heider, K., Wan, J. C. M., Supernat, A., Hudecova, I., Gounaris, I., Ros, S., Jimenez-Linan, M., Garcia-Corbacho, J., Patel, K., Østrup, O., & Rosenfeld, N. (2018). Enhanced detection of circulating tumor DNA by fragment size analysis. *Science Translational Medicine*, *10*(466), eaat4921. https://pubmed.ncbi.nlm.nih.gov/30404863/. DOI: 10.1126/scitranslmed.aat4921 PMID: 30404863

Mullen, S., & Movia, D. (2023). The role of extracellular vesicles in non-small-cell lung cancer, the unknowns, and how new approach methodologies can support new knowledge generation in the field. *European Journal of Pharmaceutical Sciences*, *188*, 106516. DOI: 10.1016/j.ejps.2023.106516 PMID: 37406971

Murphy, D. J., Mayoral, M., Larici, A. R., Ginsberg, M. S., Cicchetti, G., Fintelmann, F. J., Marom, E. M., Truong, M. T., & Gill, R. R. (2023). Imaging Follow-Up of Nonsurgical Therapies for Lung Cancer: AJR Expert Panel Narrative Review. *AJR. American Journal of Roentgenology*, *221*(4), 409–424. DOI: 10.2214/AJR.23.29104 PMID: 37095669

Neal, J. T., Li, X., Zhu, J., Giangarra, V., Grzeskowiak, C. L., Ju, J., Liu, I. H., Chiou, S.-H., Salahudeen, A. A., Smith, A. R., Deutsch, B. C., Liao, L., Zemek, A. J., Zhao, F., Karlsson, K., Schultz, L. M., Metzner, T. J., Nadauld, L. D., Tseng, Y.-Y., & Kuo, C. J. (2018). Organoid Modeling of the Tumor Immune Microenvironment. *Cell*, *175*(7), 1972–1988.e16. DOI: 10.1016/j.cell.2018.11.021 PMID: 30550791

Nejman, D., Livyatan, I., Fuks, G., Gavert, N., Zwang, Y., Geller, L. T., Rotter-Maskowitz, A., Weiser, R., Mallel, G., Gigi, E., Meltser, A., Douglas, G. M., Kamer, I., Gopalakrishnan, V., Dadosh, T., Levin-Zaidman, S., Avnet, S., Atlan, T., Cooper, Z. A., & Straussman, R. (2020). The human tumor microbiome is composed of tumor type-specific intracellular bacteria. *Science*, *368*(6494), 973–980. DOI: 10.1126/science.aay9189 PMID: 32467386

Ng, X. J. K., Mohd Khairuddin, A. S., Liu, H. C., Loh, T. C., Tan, J. L., Khor, S. M., & Leo, B. F. (2025). Artificial intelligence-assisted point-of-care devices for lung cancer. *Clinica Chimica Acta*, *570*, 120191. DOI: 10.1016/j.cca.2025.120191

Ogidi, N. O., Lind, M. J., & Greenman, J. (2024). A new immunomagnetic microfluidic device for characterizing EGFR mutations in circulating tumor cells from patients with non-small cell lung cancer. *Tumor Discovery*, *3*(4), 3987. Advance online publication. DOI: 10.36922/td.3987

Ohta, R., & Sano, C. (2024). Disparity of the Treatment of Unresectable Non-small Cell Lung Cancer Regarding Chemotherapy: A Systematic Review and Meta-Analysis. *Cureus*, *16*(5), e60635. DOI: 10.7759/cureus.60635 PMID: 38899245

Okimoto, R. A., & Bivona, T. G. (2014). Recent advances in personalized lung cancer medicine. *Personalized Medicine*, *11*(3), 309–321. https://pubmed.ncbi.nlm.nih.gov/25506379/. DOI: 10.2217/pme.14.19 PMID: 25506379

Ormond, A. B., & Freeman, H. S. (2013). Dye Sensitizers for Photodynamic Therapy. *Materials (Basel)*, *6*(3), 817–840. DOI: 10.3390/ma6030817 PMID: 28809342

Ou, S.-H. I., Nagasaka, M., & Zhu, V. W. (2018). Liquid biopsy to identify actionable genomic alterations. *American Society of Clinical Oncology Educational Book. American Society of Clinical Oncology. Annual Meeting, 38*, 978. https://pubmed.ncbi.nlm.nih.gov/30231331/

Paakkola, N.-M., Jekunen, A., Sihvo, E., Johansson, M., & Andersén, H. (2024). Area-based disparities in non-small-cell lung cancer survival. *Acta Oncologica (Stockholm, Sweden), 63*, 146–153. DOI: 10.2340/1651-226X.2024.27507 PMID: 38591350

Padinharayil, H., Varghese, J., John, M. C., Rajanikant, G. K., Wilson, C. M., Al-Yozbaki, M., Renu, K., Dewanjee, S., Sanyal, R., Dey, A., Mukherjee, A. G., Wanjari, U. R., Gopalakrishnan, A. V., & George, A. (2023). Non-small cell lung carcinoma (NSCLC): Implications on molecular pathology and advances in early diagnostics and therapeutics. *Genes & Diseases, 10*(3), 960–989. DOI: 10.1016/j.gendis.2022.07.023 PMID: 37396553

Park, E. M., Chelvanambi, M., Bhutiani, N., Kroemer, G., Zitvogel, L., & Wargo, J. A. (2022). Targeting the gut and tumor microbiota in cancer. *Nature Medicine, 28*(4), 690–703. DOI: 10.1038/s41591-022-01779-2 PMID: 35440726

Payne, C., Larkin, P. J., McIlfatrick, S., Dunwoody, L., & Gracey, J. H. (2013). Exercise and nutrition interventions in advanced lung cancer: A systematic review. *Current Oncology (Toronto, Ont.), 20*(4), e321–e337. DOI: 10.3747/co.20.1431

Petersen, I. (2011). The morphological and molecular diagnosis of lung cancer. *Deutsches Ärzteblatt International, 108*(31–32), 525–531. DOI: 10.3238/arztebl.2011.0525 PMID: 21886665

Planchard, D., Jänne, P. A., Cheng, Y., Yang, J. C.-H., Yanagitani, N., Kim, S.-W., Sugawara, S., Yu, Y., Fan, Y., Geater, S. L., Laktionov, K., Lee, C. K., Valdiviezo, N., Ahmed, S., Maurel, J.-M., Andrasina, I., Goldman, J., Ghiorghiu, D., Rukazenkov, Y., & Kobayashi, K. (2025). A plain language summary of results from the FLAURA2 study: Initial (first-line) osimertinib treatment with or without chemotherapy in patients with untreated EGFR-mutated advanced NSCLC. *Future Oncology (London, England), 21*(8), 903–915. DOI: 10.1080/14796694.2025.2463880 PMID: 39995095

Pol, J. G., Acuna, S. A., Yadollahi, B., Tang, N., Stephenson, K. B., Atherton, M. J., Hanwell, D., El-Warrak, A., Goldstein, A., Moloo, B., Turner, P. V., Lopez, R., LaFrance, S., Evelegh, C., Denisova, G., Parsons, R., Millar, J., Stoll, G., Martin, C. G., & McCart, J. A. (2019). Preclinical evaluation of a MAGE-A3 vaccination utilizing the oncolytic Maraba virus currently in first-in-human trials. *OncoImmunology, 8*(1), e1512329. DOI: 10.1080/2162402X.2018.1512329 PMID: 30546947

Porter, L. S., Keefe, F. J., Garst, J., Baucom, D. H., McBride, C. M., McKee, D. C., Sutton, L., Carson, K., Knowles, V., Rumble, M., & Scipio, C. (2011). Caregiver-assisted coping skills training for lung cancer: Results of a randomized clinical trial. *Journal of Pain and Symptom Management*, *41*(1), 1–13. DOI: 10.1016/j.jpainsymman.2010.04.014

Pucci, F., Rickelt, S., Newton, A. P., Garris, C., Nunes, E., Evavold, C., Pfirschke, C., Engblom, C., Mino-Kenudson, M., Hynes, R. O., Weissleder, R., & Pittet, M. J. (2016). PF4 promotes platelet production and lung cancer growth. *Cell Reports*, *17*(7), 1764–1772. DOI: 10.1016/j.celrep.2016.10.031

Puteri Norliza Megat Ramli, P. N., Aizuddin, A. N., Ahmad, N., Abdul Hamid, Z., & Ismail, K. I. (2025). A systematic review: The role of artificial intelligence in lung cancer screening in detecting lung nodules on chest X-rays. *Diagnostics (Basel)*, *15*(3), 246. DOI: 10.3390/diagnostics15030246

Qu, J., Mei, Q., Chen, L., & Zhou, J. (2021). Chimeric antigen receptor (CAR)-T-cell therapy in non-small-cell lung cancer (NSCLC): Current status and future perspectives. *Cancer Immunology, Immunotherapy : CII*, *70*(3), 619–631. DOI: 10.1007/s00262-020-02735-0 PMID: 33025047

Rabbani, M., O'Sullivan, J., Gnanasekaran, S., & Kalapara, A. (2018). Role of artificial intelligence in the care of patients with non-small cell lung cancer. *European Journal of Cancer Care*, *27*(1), e12901. DOI: 10.1111/ecc.12901

Rachidi, S., Metelli, A., Riesenberg, B., Wu, B. X., Nelson, M. H., Wallace, C., Paulos, C. M., Rubinstein, M. P., Garrett-Mayer, E., Hennig, M., Bearden, D. W., Yang, Y., Liu, B., & Li, Z. (2017). Platelets subvert T cell immunity against cancer via GARP-TGFβ axis. *Science Immunology*, *2*(11), eaai7911. Advance online publication. DOI: 10.1126/sciimmunol.aai7911

Reclusa, P., Taverna, S., Pucci, M., Durendez, E., Calabuig, S., Manca, P., Serrano, M. J., Sober, L., Pauwels, P., Russo, A., & Rolfo, C. (2017). Exosomes as diagnostic and predictive biomarkers in lung cancer. *Journal of Thoracic Disease*, *9*(S13, Suppl 13), S1373–S1382. https://pubmed.ncbi.nlm.nih.gov/29184676/. DOI: 10.21037/jtd.2017.10.67 PMID: 29184676

Rivera-Concepcion, J., Uprety, D., & Adjei, A. A. (2022). Challenges in the use of targeted therapies in non-small cell lung cancer. *Cancer Research and Treatment*, *54*(2), 315–329. https://pubmed.ncbi.nlm.nih.gov/35209703/. DOI: 10.4143/crt.2022.078 PMID: 35209703

Ross, P. J., Ashley, S., Norton, A., Priest, K., Waters, J. S., Eisen, T., Smith, I. E., & O'Brien, M. E. R. (2004). Do patients with weight loss have a worse outcome when undergoing chemotherapy for lung cancers? *British Journal of Cancer*, *90*(10), 1905–1911. DOI: 10.1038/sj.bjc.6601781

Roy, S., & Trinchieri, G. (2017). Microbiota: A key orchestrator of cancer therapy. *Nature Reviews. Cancer*, *17*(3), 271–285. DOI: 10.1038/nrc.2017.13

S S, K. D., Joga, R., Srivastava, S., Nagpal, K., Dhamija, I., Grover, P. & Kumar, S. (2024). Regulatory landscape and challenges in CAR-T cell therapy development in the US, EU, Japan, and India. *European Journal of Pharmaceutics and Biopharmaceutics : Official Journal of Arbeitsgemeinschaft Fur Pharmazeutische Verfahrenstechnik e.V*, *201*, 114361. DOI: 10.1016/j.ejpb.2024.114361

Saadeddin, A. (2012). Radiotherapy for NSCLC: Review of conventional and new treatment techniques. *Journal of Infection and Public Health*, *5*(Suppl 1), S45–S49. DOI: 10.1016/j.jiph.2012.09.002 PMID: 23244188

Sako, C., Schmidt, T. G., Patel, A. A., Owen, D. H., Amini, A., Curti, B. D., Kelly, R. J., Page, R. D., Swalduz, A., Beregi, J.-P., Chrusciel, J., Sanchez, S., Rosenberg, R., Snyder, E., Weiss, J., Wentland, A. L., Kirpalani, A., Liu, A., Gevaert, O., & Jordan, P. (2024). Deep learning serial CT response score predicts overall survival in advanced non-small cell lung cancer treated with PD-(L)1 immune checkpoint inhibitors. *Journal for Immunotherapy of Cancer*, *12*(Suppl 2), A1381. DOI: 10.1136/jitc-2024-SITC2024.1237

Sandoval, J., Mendez-Gonzalez, J., Nadal, E., Chen, G., Carmona, F. J., Sayols, S., Moran, S., Heyn, H., Vizoso, M., Gomez, A., Sanchez-Cespedes, M., Assenov, Y., Müller, F., Bock, C., Taron, M., Mora, J., Muscarella, L. A., Liloglou, T., Davies, M., & Esteller, M. (2013). A prognostic DNA methylation signature for stage I non-small-cell lung cancer. *Journal of Clinical Oncology*, *31*(32), 4140–4147. DOI: 10.1200/JCO.2012.48.5516

Sasso, E., D'Alise, A. M., Zambrano, N., Scarselli, E., Folgori, A., & Nicosia, A. (2020). New viral vectors for infectious diseases and cancer. *Seminars in Immunology*, *50*, 101430. DOI: 10.1016/j.smim.2020.101430 PMID: 33262065

Satoh, E., Naganuma, H., Sasaki, A., Nagasaka, M., Ogata, H., & Nukui, H. (1997). Effect of irradiation on transforming growth factor-beta secretion by malignant glioma cells. *Journal of Neuro-Oncology*, *33*(3), 195–200. DOI: 10.1023/A:1005791621265 PMID: 9195490

Schiffmann, I., Greve, G., Jung, M., & Lübbert, M. (2016). Epigenetic therapy approaches in non-small cell lung cancer: Update and perspectives. *Epigenetics, 11*(12), 858–870. DOI: 10.1080/15592294.2016.1237345

Shaikh, F. Y., Gills, J. J., & Sears, C. L. (2019). Impact of the microbiome on checkpoint inhibitor treatment in patients with non-small cell lung cancer and melanoma. *EBioMedicine, 48*, 642–647. DOI: 10.1016/j.ebiom.2019.08.076 PMID: 31597596

Sharma, R. (2022). Mapping of global, regional and national incidence, mortality and mortality-to-incidence ratio of lung cancer in 2020 and 2050. *International Journal of Clinical Oncology, 27*(4), 665–675. DOI: 10.1007/s10147-021-02108-2 PMID: 35020103

She, W., Garitaonaindia, Y., & Lin, Y. (2024). The latest advances in liquid biopsy for lung cancer-a narrative review. *Translational Lung Cancer Research, 13*(11), 3241–3251. DOI: 10.21037/tlcr-24-828 PMID: 39669995

Shehata, D. G., Pan, J. M., Pan, Z., Vigneswaran, J., Contreras, N., Rodriguez, E., Sakowitz, S., Magarinos, J., Pereira, S., Wilder, F. G., & Watkins, A. A. (2025). Equity and Opportunities in Lung Cancer Care-Addressing Disparities, Challenges, and Pathways Forward. *Cancers (Basel), 17*(8), 1347. Advance online publication. DOI: 10.3390/cancers17081347 PMID: 40282525

Shen, Y., Chen, J.-Q., & Li, X.-P. (2025). Differences between lung adenocarcinoma and lung squamous cell carcinoma: Driver genes, therapeutic targets, and clinical efficacy. *Genes & Diseases, 12*(3), 101374. https://pubmed.ncbi.nlm.nih.gov/40083325/. DOI: 10.1016/j.gendis.2024.101374 PMID: 40083325

Shen, Z., & Wan, Y. (2018). Emerging strategies of cancer therapy based on ferroptosis. *Advanced Materials, 30*(12), 1707342. DOI: 10.1002/adma.201707342

Sibuyi, N. R. S., & Moabelo, K. (2021). Multifunctional gold nanoparticles for improved diagnostic and therapeutic applications: A review. *Critical Reviews in Oncology/Hematology, 167*, 103529. DOI: 10.1016/j.critrevonc.2021.103529

Siddique, S., & Chow, J. C. L. (2022). Recent advances in functionalized nanoparticles in cancer theranostics. *Nanomaterials (Basel, Switzerland), 12*(16), 2826. DOI: 10.3390/nano12162826

Sivan, A., Corrales, L., Hubert, N., Williams, J. B., Aquino-Michaels, K., Earley, Z. M., Benyamin, F. W., Lei, Y. M., Jabri, B., Alegre, M.-L., Chang, E. B., & Gajewski, T. F. (2015). Commensal Bifidobacterium promotes antitumor immunity and facilitates anti-PD-L1 efficacy. *Science, 350*(6264), 1084–1089. DOI: 10.1126/science.aac4255 PMID: 26541606

Souza, V. G. P., Forder, A., Pewarchuk, M. E., Telkar, N., de Araujo, R. P., Stewart, G. L., Vieira, J., Reis, P. P., & Lam, W. L. (2023). The complex role of the microbiome in non-small cell lung cancer development and progression. *Cells*, *12*(24), 2801. https://pubmed.ncbi.nlm.nih.gov/38132121/. DOI: 10.3390/cells12242801 PMID: 38132121

Sozzi, G., Boeri, M., Rossi, M., Verri, C., Suatoni, P., Bravi, F., Roz, L., Conte, D., Grassi, M., Sverzellati, N., Marchiano, A., Negri, E., La Vecchia, C., & Pastorino, U. (2014). Clinical utility of a plasma-based miRNA signature classifier within computed tomography lung cancer screening: A correlative MILD trial study. *Journal of Clinical Oncology*, *32*(8), 768–773. DOI: 10.1200/JCO.2013.50.4357 PMID: 24419137

Su, S., Chen, F., Xu, M., Liu, B., & Wang, L. (2023). Recent advances in neoantigen vaccines for treating non-small cell lung cancer. *Thoracic Cancer*, *14*(34), 3361–3368. DOI: 10.1111/1759-7714.15126 PMID: 37905603

Sui, C., Wu, H., Li, X., Wang, Y., Wei, J., Yu, J., & Wu, X. (2024). Cancer immunotherapy and its facilitation by nanomedicine. *Biomarker Research*, *12*(1), 77. DOI: 10.1186/s40364-024-00625-6 PMID: 39097732

Sun, X., Ou, Z., Chen, R., Niu, X., Chen, D., Kang, R., & Tang, D. (2016). Activation of the p62-Keap1-NRF2 pathway protects against ferroptosis in hepatocellular carcinoma cells. *Hepatology (Baltimore, Md.)*, *63*(1), 173–184. DOI: 10.1002/hep.28251

Sun, X., Ou, Z., Xie, M., Kang, R., Fan, Y., Niu, X., Wang, H., Cao, L., & Tang, D. (2015). HSPB1 as a novel regulator of ferroptotic cancer cell death. *Oncogene*, *34*(45), 5617–5625. DOI: 10.1038/onc.2015.32

Sun, Y., Yang, J., Li, Y., Luo, J., Sun, J., Li, D., Wang, Y., Wang, K., Yang, L., Wu, L., & Sun, X. (2022). Single low-dose INC280-loaded theranostic nanoparticles achieve multirooted delivery for MET-targeted primary and liver metastatic non-small cell lung cancer. *Molecular Cancer*, *21*, 212. Advance online publication. DOI: 10.1186/s12943-022-01681-y

Šutić, M., Vukić, A., Baranašić, J., Försti, A., Džubur, F., Samaržija, M., Jakopović, M., Brčić, L., & Knežević, J. (2021). Diagnostic, Predictive, and Prognostic Biomarkers in Non-Small Cell Lung Cancer (NSCLC) Management. *Journal of Personalized Medicine*, *11*(11), 1102. Advance online publication. DOI: 10.3390/jpm11111102 PMID: 34834454

Tai, Y., Chen, K., Hsieh, J., & Shen, T. (2018). Exosomes in cancer development and clinical applications. *Cancer Science*, *109*(8), 2364–2374. https://pubmed.ncbi.nlm.nih.gov/29908100/. DOI: 10.1111/cas.13697 PMID: 29908100

Tanaka, F., Yoneda, K., Kondo, N., Hashimoto, M., Takuwa, T., Matsumoto, S., Okumura, Y., Rahman, S., Tsubota, N., Tsujimura, T., Kuribayashi, K., Fukuoka, K., Nakano, T., & Hasegawa, S. (2009). Circulating tumor cell as a diagnostic marker in primary lung cancer. *Clinical Cancer Research, 15*(22), 6980–6986. https://pubmed.ncbi.nlm.nih.gov/19887487/. DOI: 10.1158/1078-0432.CCR-09-1095 PMID: 19887487

Tang, S., Qin, C., Hu, H., Liu, T., He, Y., Guo, H., Yan, H., Zhang, J., Tang, S., & Zhou, H. (2022). Immune Checkpoint Inhibitors in Non-Small Cell Lung Cancer: Progress, Challenges, and Prospects. *Cells, 11*(3), 320. Advance online publication. DOI: 10.3390/cells11030320 PMID: 35159131

Teo, S. P. (2022). Review of COVID-19 mRNA Vaccines: BNT162b2 and mRNA-1273. *Journal of Pharmacy Practice, 35*(6), 947–951. DOI: 10.1177/08971900211009650 PMID: 33840294

Tetzlaff, M. T., Teh, B. S., Timme, T. L., Fujita, T., Satoh, T., Tabata, K.-I., Mai, W.-Y., Vlachaki, M. T., Amato, R. J., Kadmon, D., Miles, B. J., Ayala, G., Wheeler, T. M., Aguilar-Cordova, E., Thompson, T. C., & Butler, E. B. (2006). Expanding the therapeutic index of radiation therapy by combining in situ gene therapy in the treatment of prostate cancer. *Technology in Cancer Research & Treatment, 5*(1), 23–36. DOI: 10.1177/153303460600500104 PMID: 16417399

Tomasik, B., Skrzypski, M., Bieńkowski, M., Dziadziuszko, R., & Jassem, J. (2023). Current and future applications of liquid biopsy in non-small-cell lung cancer—A narrative review. *Translational Lung Cancer Research, 12*(3), 594–614. https://pubmed.ncbi.nlm.nih.gov/37057121/. DOI: 10.21037/tlcr-22-742 PMID: 37057121

Travis, W. D., Brambilla, E., Nicholson, A. G., Yatabe, Y., Austin, J. H. M., Beasley, M. B., Chirieac, L. R., Dacic, S., Duhig, E., Flieder, D. B., Geisinger, K., Hirsch, F. R., Ishikawa, Y., Kerr, K. M., Noguchi, M., Pelosi, G., Powell, C. A., Tsao, M. S., & Wistuba, I. (2015). The 2015 World Health Organization Classification of Lung Tumors: Impact of Genetic, Clinical and Radiologic Advances Since the 2004 Classification. In *Journal of thoracic oncology : official publication of the International Association for the Study of Lung Cancer* (Vol. 10, Issue 9, pp. 1243–1260). DOI: 10.1097/JTO.0000000000000630

Tsay, J.-C. J., Wu, B. G., Badri, M. H., Clemente, J. C., Shen, N., Meyn, P., Li, Y., Yie, T.-A., Lhakhang, T., Olsen, E., Murthy, V., Michaud, G., Sulaiman, I., Tsirigos, A., Heguy, A., Pass, H., Weiden, M. D., Rom, W. N., Sterman, D. H., & Segal, L. N. (2018). Airway Microbiota Is Associated with Upregulation of the PI3K Pathway in Lung Cancer. *American Journal of Respiratory and Critical Care Medicine, 198*(9), 1188–1198. DOI: 10.1164/rccm.201710-2118OC PMID: 29864375

Tsoulos, N., Papadopoulou, E., Metaxa-Mariatou, V., Tsaousis, G., Efstathiadou, C., Tounta, G., Scapeti, A., Bourkoula, E., Zarogoulidis, P., Pentheroudakis, G., Kakolyris, S., Boukovinas, I., Papakotoulas, P., Athanasiadis, E., Floros, T., Koumarianou, A., Barbounis, V., Dinischiotu, A., & Nasioulas, G. (2017). Tumor molecular profiling of NSCLC patients using next generation sequencing. *Oncology Reports*, *38*(6), 3419–3429. DOI: 10.3892/or.2017.6051 PMID: 29130105

Vadakara, J., & Borghaei, H. (2012). Personalized medicine and treatment approaches in non-small-cell lung carcinoma. *Pharmacogenomics and Personalized Medicine*, ●●●, 113–123. https://pubmed.ncbi.nlm.nih.gov/23226067/ PMID: 23226067

Van Den Broeck, A., Brambilla, E., Moro-Sibilot, D., Lantuejoul, S., Brambilla, C., Eymin, B., & Gazzeri, S. (2008). Loss of histone H4K20 trimethylation occurs in preneoplasia and influences prognosis of non-small cell lung cancer. *Clinical Cancer Research*, *14*(22), 7237–7245. DOI: 10.1158/1078-0432.CCR-08-0869

Van der Meij, B. S., Langius, J. A. E., Spreeuwenberg, M. D., Slootmaker, S. M., Paul, M. A., Smit, E. F., & van Leeuwen, P. A. M. (2012). Oral nutritional supplements containing n-3 polyunsaturated fatty acids affect quality of life and functional status in lung cancer patients during multimodality treatment: A randomized controlled trial. *European Journal of Clinical Nutrition*, *66*(3), 399–404. DOI: 10.1038/ejcn.2011.214

Vanni, I., Coco, S., Truini, A., Rusmini, M., Dal Bello, M. G., Alama, A., Banelli, B., Mora, M., Rijavec, E., Barletta, G., Genova, C., Biello, F., Maggioni, C., & Grossi, F. (2015). Next-Generation Sequencing Workflow for NSCLC Critical Samples Using a Targeted Sequencing Approach by Ion Torrent PGM™ Platform. *International Journal of Molecular Sciences*, *16*(12), 28765–28782. DOI: 10.3390/ijms161226129 PMID: 26633390

Vétizou, M., Pitt, J. M., Daillère, R., Lepage, P., Waldschmitt, N., Flament, C., Rusakiewicz, S., Routy, B., Roberti, M. P., Duong, C. P. M., Poirier-Colame, V., Roux, A., Becharef, S., Formenti, S., Golden, E., Cording, S., Eberl, G., Schlitzer, A., Ginhoux, F., & Zitvogel, L. (2015). Anticancer immunotherapy by CTLA-4 blockade relies on the gut microbiota. *Science*, *350*(6264), 1079–1084. DOI: 10.1126/science.aad1329 PMID: 26541610

Vetsika, E.-K., Sharma, P., Samaras, I., Markou, A., Georgoulias, V., Whiteside, T. L., & Kotsakis, A. (2021). Small Extracellular Vesicles in Pre-Therapy Plasma Predict Clinical Outcome in Non-Small-Cell Lung Cancer Patients. *Cancers (Basel)*, *13*(9), 2041. Advance online publication. DOI: 10.3390/cancers13092041 PMID: 33922569

Vijayvergia, N., Shah, P. C., & Denlinger, C. S. (2015). Survivorship in Non-Small Cell Lung Cancer: Challenges Faced and Steps Forward. *Journal of the National Comprehensive Cancer Network : JNCCN, 13*(9), 1151–1161. DOI: 10.6004/jnccn.2015.0140 PMID: 26358799

von Plessen, C., Bergman, B., Andresen, O., Bremnes, R. M., Sundstrøm, S., Gilleryd, M., Stephens, R., Vilsvik, J., Aasebø, U., & Sörenson, S. (2006). Palliative chemotherapy beyond three courses conveys no survival or consistent quality-of-life benefits in advanced non-small-cell lung cancer. *British Journal of Cancer, 95*(8), 966–973. DOI: 10.1038/sj.bjc.6603383

Waldeck, S., Mitschke, J., Wiesemann, S., Rassner, M., Andrieux, G., Deuter, M., Mutter, J., Lüchtenborg, A.-M., Kottmann, D., Titze, L., Zeisel, C., Jolic, M., Philipp, U., Lassmann, S., Bronsert, P., Greil, C., Rawluk, J., Becker, H., Isbell, L., & von Bubnoff, N. (2022). Early assessment of circulating tumor DNA after curative-intent resection predicts tumor recurrence in early-stage and locally advanced non-small-cell lung cancer. *Molecular Oncology, 16*(2), 527–537. DOI: 10.1002/1878-0261.13116 PMID: 34653314

Wang, J., Zhou, T., Liu, Y., Chen, S., & Yu, Z. (2021). Application of Nanoparticles in the Treatment of Lung Cancer With Emphasis on Receptors. *Frontiers in Pharmacology, 12*, 781425. DOI: 10.3389/fphar.2021.781425 PMID: 35082668

Wang, L., Jia, Q., Chu, Q., & Zhu, B. (2023). Targeting tumor microenvironment for non-small cell lung cancer immunotherapy. *Chinese Medical Journal Pulmonary and Critical Care Medicine, 1*(1), 18–29. DOI: 10.1016/j.pccm.2022.11.001 PMID: 39170874

Wang, M., Yu, F., & Li, P. (2023). Intratumor microbiota in cancer pathogenesis and immunity: From mechanisms of action to therapeutic opportunities. *Frontiers in Immunology, 14*, 1269054. DOI: 10.3389/fimmu.2023.1269054 PMID: 37868956

Wang, S.-J., Li, D., Ou, Y., Jiang, L., Chen, Y., Zhao, Y., & Gu, W. (2016). Acetylation is crucial for p53-mediated ferroptosis and tumor suppression. *Cell Reports, 17*(2), 366–373. DOI: 10.1016/j.celrep.2016.09.022

Wang, S.-Q., Shuai, Z.-F., Zhang, X.-J., Wu, T., Dong, H.-Y., Liu, T., Wen, Q.-T., & Yu, X.-W. (2020). Detection of CTCs and CSCs in the staging and metastasis of non-small cell lung cancer based on microfluidic chip and the diagnostic significance. *European Review for Medical and Pharmacological Sciences, 24*(18), 9487–9496. DOI: 10.26355/eurrev_202009_23034

Watanabe, M., Kenmotsu, H., Ko, R., Wakuda, K., Ono, A., Imai, H., Taira, T., Naito, T., Murakami, H., Abe, M., Endo, M., Nakajima, T., Koh, Y., & Takahashi, T. (2018). Isolation and molecular analysis of circulating tumor cells from lung cancer patients using a microfluidic chip type cell sorter. *Cancer Science*, *109*(8), 2539–2548. DOI: 10.1111/cas.13692

Whiteside, S. A., McGinniss, J. E., & Collman, R. G. (2021). The lung microbiome: Progress and promise. *The Journal of Clinical Investigation*, *131*(15), e150473. Advance online publication. DOI: 10.1172/JCI150473 PMID: 34338230

Wilson, B. C. (2002). Photodynamic therapy for cancer: principles. *Canadian Journal of Gastroenterology = Journal Canadien de Gastroenterologie, 16*(6), 393–396. DOI: 10.1155/2002/743109

Wirtz, D., Konstantopoulos, K., & Searson, P. C. (2011). The physics of cancer: The role of physical interactions and mechanical forces in metastasis. *Nature Reviews. Cancer*, *11*(7), 512–522. https://pubmed.ncbi.nlm.nih.gov/21701513/. DOI: 10.1038/nrc3080 PMID: 21701513

Wistuba, I. I., Behrens, C., Lombardi, F., Wagner, S., Fujimoto, J., Raso, M. G., Spaggiari, L., Galetta, D., Riley, R., Hughes, E., Reid, J., Sangale, Z., Swisher, S. G., Kalhor, N., Moran, C. A., Gutin, A., Lanchbury, J. S., Barberis, M., & Kim, E. S. (2013). Validation of a proliferation-based expression signature as prognostic marker in early stage lung adenocarcinoma. *Clinical Cancer Research*, *19*(22), 6261–6271. DOI: 10.1158/1078-0432.CCR-13-0596 PMID: 24048333

Wong-Rolle, A., Wei, H. K., Zhao, C., & Jin, C. (2021). Unexpected guests in the tumor microenvironment: Microbiome in cancer. *Protein & Cell*, *12*(5), 426–435. DOI: 10.1007/s13238-020-00813-8 PMID: 33296049

World Health Organization. (1996). *Cancer pain relief: With a guide to opioid availability* (2nd ed.). World Health Organization.

Wu, J., & Chen, Y. (2024). Unraveling the Connection: Extracellular Vesicles and Non-Small Cell Lung Cancer. *International Journal of Nanomedicine*, *19*, 8139–8157. DOI: 10.2147/IJN.S477851 PMID: 39139506

Wu, P., Han, J., Gong, Y., Liu, C., Yu, H., & Xie, N. (2022). Nanoparticle-Based Drug Delivery Systems Targeting Tumor Microenvironment for Cancer Immunotherapy Resistance: Current Advances and Applications. *Pharmaceutics*, *14*(10), 1990. Advance online publication. DOI: 10.3390/pharmaceutics14101990 PMID: 36297426

Wu, Y.-L., Park, K., Soo, R. A., Sun, Y., Tyroller, K., Wages, D., Ely, G., Yang, J. C.-H., & Mok, T. (2011). INSPIRE: A phase III study of the BLP25 liposome vaccine (L-BLP25) in Asian patients with unresectable stage III non-small cell lung cancer. *BMC Cancer*, *11*(1), 430. DOI: 10.1186/1471-2407-11-430 PMID: 21982342

Xi, S., Xu, H., Shan, J., Tao, Y., Hong, J. A., Inchauste, S., Zhang, M., Kunst, T. F., Mercedes, L., & Schrump, D. S. (2013). Cigarette smoke mediates epigenetic repression of miR-487b during pulmonary carcinogenesis. *The Journal of Clinical Investigation*, *123*(3), 1241–1261. DOI: 10.1172/JCI61271

Xia, T., Du, W.-L., Chen, X.-Y., & Zhang, Y.-N. (2021). Organoid models of the tumor microenvironment and their applications. *Journal of Cellular and Molecular Medicine*, *25*(13), 5829–5841. DOI: 10.1111/jcmm.16578 PMID: 34033245

Xue, C., Chu, Q., Zheng, Q., Yuan, X., Su, Y., Bao, Z., Lu, J., & Li, L. (2023). Current understanding of the intratumoral microbiome in various tumors. *Cell Reports Medicine*, *4*(1), 100884. DOI: 10.1016/j.xcrm.2022.100884 PMID: 36652905

Yan, X., Yang, M., Liu, J., Gao, R., Hu, J., Li, J., Zhang, L., Shi, Y., Guo, H., Cheng, J., Razi, M., Pang, S., Yu, X., & Hu, S. (2015). Discovery and validation of potential bacterial biomarkers for lung cancer. *American Journal of Cancer Research*, *5*(10), 3111–3122. https://pubmed.ncbi.nlm.nih.gov/26693063/ PMID: 26693063

Yang, Y., Liu, H., Chen, Y., Xiao, N., Zheng, Z., Liu, H., & Wan, J. (2023). Liquid biopsy on the horizon in immunotherapy of non-small cell lung cancer: Current status, challenges, and perspectives. *Cell Death & Disease*, *14*(3), 230. DOI: 10.1038/s41419-023-05757-5 PMID: 37002211

Yuan, C.-S. (2007). Methylnaltrexone: Mechanisms of action and effects on opioid bowel dysfunction and other opioid adverse effects. *The Annals of Pharmacotherapy*, *41*(6), 984–993. DOI: 10.1345/aph.1K009

Yuan, H., Li, X., Zhang, X., Kang, R., & Tang, D. (2016). Identification of ACSL4 as a biomarker and contributor of ferroptosis. *Biochemical and Biophysical Research Communications*, *478*(3), 1338–1343. DOI: 10.1016/j.bbrc.2016.08.124

Zaman, F. Y., Subramaniam, A., Afroz, A., Samoon, Z., Gough, D., Arulananda, S., & Alamgeer, M. (2023). Circulating Tumour DNA (ctDNA) as a Predictor of Clinical Outcome in Non-Small Cell Lung Cancer Undergoing Targeted Therapies: A Systematic Review and Meta-Analysis. *Cancers (Basel)*, *15*(9), 2425. Advance online publication. DOI: 10.3390/cancers15092425 PMID: 37173891

Zhang, C., Bu, W., Ni, D., Zhang, S., Li, Q., Yao, Z., Zhang, J., Yao, H., Wang, Z., & Shi, J. (2016). Synthesis of iron nanometallic glasses and their application in cancer therapy by a localized Fenton reaction. *Angewandte Chemie International Edition, 55*(6), 2101–2106. DOI: 10.1002/anie.201510031

Zhang, D., Bian, G., Zhang, Y., Xie, J., & Hu, C. (2025). MOLUNGN: A multi-omics graph neural network for biomarker discovery and accurate lung cancer classification. *Frontiers in Genetics, 16*, 1610284. DOI: 10.3389/fgene.2025.1610284 PMID: 40534839

Zhang, J.-T., Liu, S.-Y., Gao, W., Liu, S.-Y. M., Yan, H.-H., Ji, L., Chen, Y., Gong, Y., Lu, H.-L., Lin, J.-T., Yin, K., Jiang, B.-Y., Nie, Q., Liao, R.-Q., Dong, S., Guan, Y., Dai, P., Zhang, X.-C., Yang, J.-J., & Wu, Y.-L. (2022). Longitudinal Undetectable Molecular Residual Disease Defines Potentially Cured Population in Localized Non-Small Cell Lung Cancer. *Cancer Discovery, 12*(7), 1690–1701. DOI: 10.1158/2159-8290.CD-21-1486 PMID: 35543554

Zhang, M., Deng, C., Fu, F., Li, Y., Zhang, Y., & Chen, H. (2025). Site-specific follow-up strategy for surgically resected patients with NSCLC based on ten-year follow-up data. *Lung Cancer (Amsterdam, Netherlands), 201*, 108451. https://doi.org/DOI. DOI: 10.1016/j.lungcan.2025.108451 PMID: 39983445

Zheng, H., Zhan, Y., Liu, S., Lu, J., Luo, J., Feng, J., & Fan, S. (2018). The roles of tumor-derived exosomes in non-small cell lung cancer and their clinical implications. *Journal of Experimental & Clinical Cancer Research : CR, 37*(1), 226. DOI: 10.1186/s13046-018-0901-5 PMID: 30217217

Zhou, J., Xu, Y., Liu, J., Feng, L., Yu, J., & Chen, D. (2024). Global burden of lung cancer in 2022 and projections to 2050: Incidence and mortality estimates from GLOBOCAN. *Cancer Epidemiology, 93*, 102693. https://pubmed.ncbi.nlm.nih.gov/39536404/. DOI: 10.1016/j.canep.2024.102693 PMID: 39536404

Zhou, Z., Song, J., Tian, R., Yang, Z., Yu, G., Lin, L., Zhang, G., Fan, W., Zhang, F., Niu, G., Nie, L., & Chen, X. (2017). Activatable singlet oxygen generation from lipid hydroperoxide nanoparticles for cancer therapy. *Angewandte Chemie International Edition, 56*(23), 6492–6496. DOI: 10.1002/anie.201701181

Zhu, X. R., Li, Y., Yang, M., Whitaker, T. J., Taylor, P. A., Zhang, X., Poenisch, F., Sahoo, N., Liao, Z., & Chang, J. Y. (2023). Stereotactic body proton therapy for early stage non-small cell lung cancer - Technical challenges and solutions: The MD Anderson experience. *Journal of Radiosurgery and SBRT, 9*(1), 75–82. https://pubmed.ncbi.nlm.nih.gov/38029015/ PMID: 38029015

Zografos, E., Dimitrakopoulos, F.-I., & Koutras, A. (2022). Prognostic Value of Circulating Tumor DNA (ctDNA) in Oncogene-Driven NSCLC: Current Knowledge and Future Perspectives. *Cancers (Basel)*, *14*(19), 4954. Advance online publication. DOI: 10.3390/cancers14194954 PMID: 36230877

Zou, J., Chen, W., & Wang, Z. (2022). Ferroptosis in non-small cell lung cancer: Progression and therapeutic potential. *International Journal of Molecular Sciences*, *22*(24), 13335. DOI: 10.3390/ijms222413335

About the Contributors

Pallavi Singh has been a Seasoned academician and versatile Researcher with more than 17 years of experience in teaching, research, Innovation, and leadership experience in the domain of Biotechnology. She holds B.Tech, M.Tech and Ph.D degree in Biotechnology. She is currently serving as Professor and Program Coordinator (B.Tech. Biotechnology) in Department of Biotechnology at Graphic Era Deemed to be University, Uttarakhand, India. She has published over 57 research papers in reputed National and International journals which includes journals like International Journal of Surgery, Frontiers in Microbiology, Current Issues in Molecular Biology, Computational Toxicology, Scientific reports, Journal of Nanomaterials etc. She has further published 2 Books, 5 Book chapters along with many International and National conference presentations. Further, She has published 17 patents in the domain of computational biology, Cancer and Bioprocess Engineering. 6 of her patents have been granted in years 2023 and 2024. She has h index of 11 and i10 index of 11 and is in Editorial Board of many Scopus and SCI journals. She has guided 35 projects at B.Tech and M.Tech level and 5 students are currently pursuing their Ph.D under her guidance.

Shiva Prasad Kollur is working as Associate Professor in Chemistry at Amrita Vishwa Vidyapeetham, Mysuru Campus, India. His research interests included Anticancer therapeutics, Bioinorganic and Materials Chemistry. He has published over 250 scientific research articles in international peer-reviewed journals and several of his research findings are patented. He has mentored more than 40 scholars (Grads/Postgrads) for their degree fulfilment and 8 PhD scholars are presently working under his supervision.

Raghavendra G. Amachawadi is currently working as an Associate Professor in Department of Clinical Sciences, Kansas State University, Manhattan. He has published 116 research articles and has h index of 28 and i10 index of 65. He has handled National level projects in United states and has obtained total funding of dollars14,244,503 from prominent agencies in United states like USDA-NIFA, USAID-Global Food Systems, FDA, National Pork Board, Elanco Animal Health, National Cattlemen's Beef Association (Beef check-off), ICASA-FFAR, and Animal Health Commodity groups.He has expertise in microbiome, metagenomics, and metabolomics research, and investigates the complex interactions between host, microbial communities, and pathogens, aiming to develop innovative, antibiotic-free intervention strategies to control critical issues such as liver abscesses in feedlot cattle, bovine respiratory disease, and swine colibacillosis. He has thorough expertise in animal research and translational medicine.

***

Reyhaneh Alidoosti Shahraki received her master's degree in molecular genetics from Tarbiat Modares University in Iran, one of the leading universities in the field of life sciences in Iran. She began her studies in the field of cancer genetics at this university, and after completing her postgraduate studies, she continued her work in the field of cancer genetics. She is currently working as a researcher in this field and has published articles and works in this field.

Sonalika Bhalla is a Junior Research Fellow at Chitkara School of Pharmacy, Chitkara University, Himachal Pradesh with specialization in neuropharmacology. She has 1 year of experience in medical underwriting and pharmacovigilance operations and 1 year of teaching experience. With expertise in pharmacology and analytical techniques, she has contributed to 4 research articles and 5 review articles.

Sumitha Elayaperumal is an Assistant Professor at JSS Academy of Higher Education and Research (JSS AHER) in Mysuru, Karnataka. She has a robust background in molecular biology and biotechnology, with research interests spanning haemostasis, genotype-phenotype correlations, and molecular mutations. Dr. Elayaperumal earned her Ph.D. in molecular genetics from Christian Medical College, Vellore, focusing on von Willebrand disease. Her postdoctoral research at Vellore Institute of Technology involved developing novel purification strategies for recombinant Factor VIII biosimilars. Previously, she served in the Department of Medical Oncology at Meenakshi Mission Hospital & Research Centre, Madurai, where she conducted molecular analyses for myeloproliferative disorders, chronic myeloid leukemia, and acute promyelocytic leukemia. Dr. Elayaperumal has authored over 35 publications, including articles on plant-based nanotherapeutics, biofilms in cancer development, and eco-friendly biosurfactant solutions for petroleum hydrocarbon cleanup. She has also contributed to book chapters on encapsulated omega-3 delivery systems in functional foods and genetic modification in vitamin-rich crop biofortification. Her interdisciplinary expertise and dedication to research have significantly advanced the fields of biotechnology and molecular medicine. Dr. Elayaperumal continues to inspire students and contribute to scientific knowledge through her teaching and research endeavors at JSS AHER.

Manideepa Govindarajan is a dedicated B.Tech Biotechnology student specializing in clinical pathology, molecular biology, and computer-aided drug discovery. She is passionate about unraveling the mysteries of the human body through cutting-edge laboratory techniques, with a strong interest in cancer biology, particularly in exploring the molecular basis of cancer development and progression. She has also contributed to the field through her co-authored book chapter titled 'Recent Advancements in CAR-T Cell Therapy,' highlighting her engagement with innovative cancer immunotherapies.

Mohammad-Salar Hosseini, MD, MPH, Fellowship in Palliative Care, is a physician-researcher, graduated from Tabriz University of Medical Sciences. As a Member of the European Society for Medical Oncology (ESMO), he looks forward to linking preclinical research and clinical practice in oncology throughout his career in order to obtain the highest standards of patient care and effective bench-to-bedside research.

Hossein Jabbari Beyrami, PhD in Healthcare Services Management and Fellowship in Palliative Care, is a professor of community medicine at Tabriz University of Medical Sciences. As a member of the Iranian Academy of Medical Sciences and a former head of department and director of university hospitals with over 35 years of educational and administrative experience, he is one of the pioneers in the provision of palliative care services in East Azerbaijan, Iran.

Prerna Mehta is a distinguished academic and accomplished author with a robust educational background. She completed her BSc in Biotechnology at Rungta College of Science and Technology in Bhilai, Chhattisgarh, where she was honored with a gold medal for her exceptional performance. She then pursued a Master of Science in Biotechnology from Government V.Y.P.T. College, Durg, and obtained a B.Ed. degree from Ghanshyam Singh Arya Kanya College in Durg. Prerna's expertise covers a range of fields, including genetics, nanoparticles, biochemistry, and genetic engineering.Additionally, she is a lifetime member of the International Organization of Academic and Scientific Development (IOASD) and serves as a reviewer for the East African Scholars Journal of Biotechnology and Genetics. Prerna is also a lifetime member of The Indian Science Congress Association in Kolkata. As an accomplished author, she has written three books and holds utility patents for innovative projects: “A chamber to detect radiation and a method to shower melanin to protect the user against radiation" and "AI-Powered Rural Enhancement System for Tackling Hunger & Ensuring Water Conservation through Smart Resource M

Vivek Pazhamalai working as Associate Professor at Vels Institute of Science, Technology and Advanced Studies, and has teaching experience of 15 years. He has published more than 60 research articles in international and national journals to his credit.

Mathumida Rajendran is a committed B.Tech Biotechnology student with a keen focus on clinical pathology, molecular biology, and computer-aided drug discovery. She is deeply fascinated by the complexity of the human body and enjoys exploring it through advanced laboratory techniques. Her primary interest lies in cancer biology, especially in understanding the molecular mechanisms behind cancer initiation and progression. Demonstrating her dedication to research and innovation, Mathumida has co-authored a book chapter titled "Recent Advancements in CAR-T Cell Therapy," reflecting her involvement in cutting-edge cancer immunotherapy approaches and her drive to contribute meaningfully to the scientific community.

Jayasri Rajkumar is a Biotechnology student at Vels University, specializing in microbiology, molecular biology, phytomedicine, and bioinformatics. With a strong interest in advanced molecular biology, Jayasri has also enhanced her understanding of computational tools in biotechnology through bioinformatics studies. Her academic journey is driven by a passion for bridging theoretical knowledge with hands-on experiences, aiming to contribute to the dynamic and growing biotechnology research and industry

Anjali Roy is currently a second year Ph.D research scholar at the Department of Life Science & Bioinformatics, Assam University, Silchar. Her field of research is associated with microbial biotechnology, dealing with yeasts. She received a bachelor's degree with honors in botany from Gurucharan University, Silchar and a master's degree in botany as well from the Department of Life Science and Bioinformatics, Assam University.

Meenambiga S S Assistant Professor completed 6 years of teaching experience and 4 years of research experience in the field of Biotechnology. Passionate about teaching and have trained many young students in the field of Mycology, Natural Product Research, Nanoparticle synthesis, Drug Discovery from Plants and fungal sources and in-silico analysis of drug targets using modern Bio-informatics tools. Skilled in scientific writing covering the following aspects: Proposal submission, research articles suitable for national and international publications,drafting, proof reading and editing research thesis and expertise in critically reviewing the research manuscript for indexed journals. Member of Board of Studies for B.Tech Biotechnology curriculum in VISTAS. Guided more than 20 undergraduate students projects and served as Principal Investigator in the student's project funded by Tamilnadu State Council for Science and Technology. Published more than 30 research and review articles in national and international indexed journal and has volunteered as reviewer for many reputed journals. Life member of Mycological Society of India, BRSI, IARA, IAENG and many other professional organizations. Completed

Sarvin Sanaie, MD, PhD in Nutrition, has been an academic staff member of Tabriz University of Medical Sciences for over 10 years. With over 150 peer-reviewed publications and a Scopus h-index of 26, her fields of interest include medical nutrition therapy for patients with neurodegenerative disease, critically ill patients, and cancer patients, as well as the use of functional foods in these groups.

Sharmistha Sharma is a Ph.D. research scholar at the Department of Life Science & Bioinformatics, Assam University, Silchar. Her interest lies in the research associated with microbial biotechnology, which deals primarily with fungi. She received a bachelor's degree with honors in botany from Gurucharan University, Silchar, and a master's degree in botany from the Department of Life Science & Bioinformatics, Assam University.

Vivek Sharma is a dedicated researcher and academician with a strong foundation in pharmacology and toxicokinetics. Currently pursuing his Ph.D. as a Research Scholar at UPES (since February 2025), he has previously served as a Junior Research Fellow at Chitkara University, where he focused on novel aspects of pharmacological and toxicokinetic studies. With prior academic experience as an Assistant Professor at Haridwar University Roorkee and Baddi University of Emerging Sciences and Technology (BUEST). His passion for scientific research and teaching has driven him to stay actively involved in academia. Mr. Sharma holds a Master of Pharmacy (Pharmacology) degree from BUEST, where he conducted dissertation work on the neuroprotective effect of a nitrate ester derivative of paracetamol in scopolamine-induced amnesia in zebrafish. His choice of zebrafish was driven by their high genomic similarity (70%) to humans, making them an ideal model for cognition-related studies.

Naveen Singh is a Junior Research Fellow at the Chitkara School of Pharmacy, Chitkara University, Himachal Pradesh. He is currently working on a DST-SERB-sponsored project focused on PFAS exposure in water sources. He holds an M. Pharm in Pharmacology and is pursuing a Ph.D. in Pharmaceutical Sciences at Chitkara

University. His research interests include Neuropharmacology, phytopharmacology, and diabetes-related complications. With expertise in pharmacology and analytical techniques, He has one year of academic experience as an Assistant Professor. He is also a lifetime member of APTI.

Rajnish Srivastava has 11 years of extensive experience in academics and research. He presently serves as an Associate professor in the Department of Pharmacology, Chitkara University School of Pharmacy, Chitkara University, Himachal Pradesh. He is involved in various consultancy pro-jects sponsored by national institutes and industries related to dermal and neurodegenerative diseases. His field of specialization consists of the formulation and development of nanostructured drug delivery systems by low-energy methods, and the identification of targets/biomarkers for neurological, metabolic, and dermal diseases. He has developed hybrid therapeutic interventions for diabetes and associated complications like neuropathy. He Proficiently worked with the ad-vanced video tracking system ANYMAZE for the assessment of neurobehavioral activity in ro-dents. He is skilled in protocol designing and carrying out in vivo pharmacological studies and is expert in the development and testing of preclinical pharmacological screening models. He is also proficient in regulatory and safety pharmacology and performing toxicological studies of chemi-cals and drugs using clinically relevant animal models. He has published more than 40 research papers in international and national journals of different reputes. He has 2 patents and 4 interna-tional book chapters. He has attended more than 50 national and international conferences. He is a potential reviewer for more than 20 internationally reputed journals like Phytomedicine, Journal of Biochemical and Molecular Toxicology etc. Dr. Srivastava has been serving as Committee for the Control and Supervision of Experiments on Animals (CCSEA) nominee from last 10 years. He was awarded the Best Faculty Facilitation award for the subject of human Anatomy Physiol-ogy, and Health Education in 2015 by the Madhya Pradesh Council for Science and Technology (MPCST).

Ankita Thakur is a Junior Research Fellow at the Chitkara School of Pharmacy, Chitkara University, Himachal Pradesh, India. She holds a Master's degree in Pharmaceutics and was awarded a gold medal for academic excellence. She also has experience in academia as an Assistant Professor. Her research focuses on the development of novel drug delivery systems, especially nano based formulations for challenging molecules.

Yosra Vaez-Gharamaleki, MD, is a postdoctoral researcher at the Hematology and Oncology Research Center, Tabriz University of Medical Science, Iran. She has a strong clinical and translational research background to explore innovative therapeutic strategies and improve patient-centered care.

Nitin Verma has more than 18 years of teaching, research and administrative experience. He has published more than 45 International and national research papers in peer reviewed journal, contributed more than 15 chapters in books and presented research work in 65 national and international conferences, seminars, and workshops. He is actively engaged in the field of research on toxicology, risk assessment of chemicals and their impact on environment and human health with special focus on PFAS and computational toxicity studies etc. He is a Member of Board of Studies, Academic Council, Academic and Research Committee, Coordinator- Academic Industry Partnership Programme with CIPLA, Mankind Pharma, Fresenius Kabi, Glenmark and Abbott Healthcare and handling projects of INR more than 40 million. He is a member of the various professional societies and in reviewer board of various Journals. He has recently visited countries viz USA, Greece, Rome, Slovakia, Australia, Japan, Switzerland, and Singapore.

Index

A

B

C

D

E

M

N

www.ingramcontent.com/pod-product-compliance
Lightning Source LLC
LaVergne TN
LVHW062339300926
849161LV00007B/1747